Nursing Case Management

From Essentials to Advanced Practice Applications

Third Edition

www.mosby.com

Nursing Case Management

FROM ESSENTIALS TO ADVANCED PRACTICE APPLICATIONS

Third Edition

ELAINE L. COHEN, EdD, RN, FAAN
Director of Case Management
Utilization Management, Department of Quality & Outcomes
Associate Professor, School of Nursing
University of Colorado Hospital
University of Colorado
Health Sciences Center
Denver, Colorado

TONI G. CESTA, PhD, RN, FAAN
Director of Case Management
St. Vincents Catholic Medical Centers of New York
New York, New York

A Harcourt Health Sciences Company

With 85 Illustrations

A Harcourt Health Sciences Company

Vice-President, Nursing Editorial Director: Sally Schrefer
Editors: Lisa M. Potts and Yvonne Alexopoulos
Developmental Editors: Aimee E. Loewe and Kimberly A. Netterville
Project Manager: John Rogers
Project Specialist: Kathleen L. Teal
Designer: Kathi Gosche

THIRD EDITION

Mosby, Inc.
A Harcourt Health Sciences Company
11830 Westline Industrial Drive
St. Louis, Missouri 63146

ISBN 0-323-01135-7

00 01 02 03 04/9 8 7 6 5 4 3 2 1

*To all the pioneers and their efforts
in the development, research, and
evaluation of nursing case management*

Contributors

SHERRY L. ALIOTTA, BSN, RN, CCM
President/CEO
S.A. Squared, Inc.
Los Alamitos, California

AMY J. BARTON, PhD, RN
Associate Dean for Practice/Assistant Professor
School of Nursing
University of Colorado Health Sciences Center
Denver, Colorado

ARTHUR E. BLANK, PhD
Director, Research Support
Beth Israel Medical Center
New York, New York

JEANNE BOLING, MSN, CRRN, CDMS, CCM
Executive Director
Case Management Society of America
Little Rock, Arkansas

MICHAL BOYD, RN, MSN, ND, CANP
Assistant Professor
School of Nursing
University of Colorado Health Sciences Center
Denver, Colorado

MICHELLE M.O. BOYLAN, DM(c), RN
Manager
Quality and Outcomes Management
University of Colorado Hospital
Denver, Colorado

BILL BRODIE, BSN, MHSA, RN
Director of Medical Professional Services
Brookwood Medical Center
Birmingham, Alabama

NANCY J. BROWN, PhD, RN, FAAN
Associate Professor/Chair
Division of Community, Health Systems, and
  Policy
School of Nursing
University of Colorado Health Sciences Center
Denver, Colorado

REBECCA F. CADY, BSN, RNC, JD
Associate Attorney
Grace, Brandon, and Hollis, LLP
San Diego, California

MARY ALLEN CAREY, PhD, RN, CS
Associate Professor/Division Director
College of Nursing
University of Oklahoma Health Sciences Center
Oklahoma City, Oklahoma

TINA GERARDI, MS, RN, CPHQ
Deputy Executive Director
New York State Nurses Association
Latham, New York

MARY LU GERKE, MSN, BSN, CCRN
Administrative Director, ICU/Perioperative
Gundersen Lutheran Medical Center
LaCrosse, Wisconsin

COLLEEN J. GOODE, PhD, RN, FAAN
Vice-President/Chief Nursing Officer
Patient Services
University of Colorado Hospital
Denver, Colorado

SHAROL F. JACOBSON, PhD, RN, FAAN
Professor/Director of Nursing Research
College of Nursing
University of Oklahoma Health Sciences Center
Oklahoma City, Oklahoma

EVELYN KOENIG, MSW, ACSW
Director
Office of Case Management
Vanderbilt University Medical Center
Nashville, Tennessee

GERRI S. LAMB, PhD, RN, FAAN
Associate Dean for Clinical & Community
   Services
College of Nursing
University of Arizona
Tucson, Arizona

CARRIE B. LENBURG, EdD, RN, FAAN
President and Consultant
Creative Learning and Assessment Systems
Roan Mountain, Tennessee

PATRICIA HRYZAK LIND, MS, RN
Director
Health Management and Product Support
   Preferred Care
Rochester, New York

MARGO MacROBERT, MS, RN, CNAA
Case Management Program Director
College of Nursing
University of Oklahoma Health Sciences Center
Oklahoma City, Oklahoma

JOAN K. MAGILVY, PhD, RN, FAAN
Professor/Director, PhD Program in Nursing
School of Nursing
University of Colorado Health Sciences Center
Denver, Colorado

CATHY MICHAELS, PhD, RN, FAAN
Post-Doctoral Fellow in Community-Based
   Interventions
College of Nursing
The University of Arizona
Tucson, Arizona

PATRICIA MORITZ, PhD, RN, FAAN
Associate Dean for Research/Associate Professor
School of Nursing
University of Colorado Health Sciences Center
Denver, Colorado

JEAN A. NEWSOME, DSN
Operations Leader
Brookwood Medical Center
Birmingham, Alabama

KATHRYN NOLD, RN, MSHA
Administrator of Analysis
Strategic Development & Managed Care
University of Colorado Hospital
Denver, Colorado

THERESA J. ORTIZ, MSW, ACSW, LCSW
Manager of Social Services
University of Colorado Hospital
Denver, Colorado

BARI K. PLATTER, MS, RN
Clinical Nurse Specialist/Educator
University of Colorado Hospital
Colorado Psychiatric Health
Denver, Colorado

GAYLE PREHEIM, EdD, RN, CNAA
Associate Professor
School of Nursing
University of Colorado Health Sciences Center
Denver, Colorado

RICHARD W. REDMAN, PhD, RN
Associate Dean for Academic Affairs
Professor
School of Nursing
University of Colorado Health Sciences Center
Denver, Colorado

LYNN RIIPPI, BSN, RN
Health Plan Case Manager
University of Colorado Hospital
Denver, Colorado

JILL SCOTT, PhD, RN
Assistant Professor/Associate Director for
  Nursing, AHEC
School of Nursing
University of Colorado Health Sciences Center
Denver, Colorado

MARLYS SEVERSON, BSN, RN, CCM
President/CEO
SCM Associates
Bellflower, California

ROY L. SIMPSON, RN, C, CMAC, FNAP,
FAAN
Vice-President
Nursing Informatics
Cerner Corporation
Kansas City, Missouri

DIANE J. SKIBA, PhD
Associate Dean for Informatics/Director,
  Academic Innovations
University of Colorado Health Sciences Center
Denver, Colorado

KATHLEEN SMITH, MS, RN
Clinical Informatics Nurse Specialist
University of Colorado Hospital
Denver, Colorado

VIVIENNE SMITH, BSN, RN
Informatics Nurse Specialist
University of Colorado Hospital
Denver, Colorado

HUSSEIN A. TAHAN, MS, DNSc(C), RN,
CNA
Manager
Nursing Professional Practice Programs
Mount Sinai Hospital
New York, New York

SISTER CAROL TAYLOR, CSFN, PhD, MSN,
RN
Associate Director
Center for Clinical Bioethics
School of Nursing
Georgetown University
Washington, D.C.

MARY CRABTREE TONGES, PhD, MBA,
FAAN
Senior Vice-President
Nursing and Patient Services
Robert Wood Johnson University Hospital
New Brunswick, New Jersey

KAY VAUGHN MS, RN, CS
Senior Instructor/Faculty
School of Nursing
University of Colorado Health Sciences Center
Denver, Colorado

CAROLEE WHITEHILL, MS, RN
Case Manager
Emergency Services
University of Colorado Hospital
Denver, Colorado

JOANNE WOODALL, MSN, RN, CM
Director
Case Management
Tucson Medical Center
Tucson, Arizona

BONNIE COX YOUNG, MS, RN
Senior Director of Psychiatric Patient Services
University of Colorado Hospital
Colorado Psychiatric Health
Attendant Instructor/Adjoint Faculty
Department of Psychiatry
School of Medicine
Denver, Colorado

DONNA ZAZWORSKY, MS, RN, CCM
Program Director
St. Elizabeth of Hungary Clinic
Principal, CaseManagerSolutions.com
Tucson, Arizona

Reviewers

MANUSCRIPT REVIEWER

VIVIEN DE BACK, PhD, RN, FAAN
Editor
International Nursing Review
Franklin, Wisconsin

JACKIE BIRMINGHAM, MS, BSN, RN, A-CCC, CMAC
Executive Director
Continuum Care Services
Suffield, Connecticut

ELIZABETH FALTER, MS, RN, CNAA
President
Falter and Associates, Inc.
Croton-on-Hudson, New York

MARGARET MURPHY, PhD, RN
Nurse Consultant
Empowering Change
Milwaukee, Wisconsin

DONNA ZAZWORSKY, MS, RN, CCM
Program Director
St. Elizabeth of Hungary Clinic
Principal, CaseManagerSolutions.com
Tucson, Arizona

LISA ZERULL, MSN, RN
Program Director
Case Management
Winchester Medical Center
Winchester, Virginia

Foreword

What happens when new knowledge is presented to the health care community? Putting aside the resistance that occurs with change, new information tends to shift the perspective we have on a subject. Change the way you view an activity and the activity takes on a new form. Such changes in perception occur throughout the health care industry each time we are exposed to the results of research, are informed of improved health outcomes related to a new practice model, or affected by external challenges. This evolutionary process of infusing new knowledge into the system results in a better understanding of our former work and ultimately, transforms the way we practice. Even our history changes with new perceptions once we understand the effect of work done in the past.

In this third edition of *NURSING CASE MANAGEMENT: FROM ESSENTIALS TO ADVANCED PRACTICE APPLICATIONS,* Cohen and Cesta bring us lessons learned from the past and provide us with new perceptions on well known models. We are given the historic underpinnings and origination of nursing case management. The value of former editions is not lost but we find that past work is placed in a new time and a new place. What was known then is understood as an early expression of present work. In some instances we find former models of nursing case management no longer exist. However from that work we encounter a new generation of practice models. We discover within these pages nursing models with new applications or approaches implemented in a different geographical site. We learn that at one time nursing case management was synonymous with hospital nursing, but now these new generations of models are found wherever health care is delivered and in some instances the common strategy across a continuum of care.

There are lessons to be learned here. The history of practice, in particular nursing case management, offers a perspective of where we came from and how far we have advanced. The changes in practice we read about here offer us a view of the bigger picture of health care and how we as nurses influence those environments. These perspectives on the past and present help the reader know the system as a whole while offering expert opinion on what to expect in the future.

Cohen and Cesta have accomplished more than simply updating a text. They have led us through the years of nursing case management offering insights into the internal and external pressures that have resulted in model redesign. And they have given voice to the many nurses whose work and research result in the evolution of systems. Health care environments change, reimbursement systems are revised, technology advances and nurses who work under all these pressures respond.

Probably the most dramatic change seen in nursing case management and described in this text is the emergence and wide acceptance of interdisciplinary models of care. Little today can be accomplished in isolation resulting in more collaborative relationships. Studies are showing that outcomes of care are more positive when that care is directed and provided by a group or a team who are knowledgeable about the family and community.

A final lesson to be learned from this updated version is a reminder that what is written today will be our history in future years. The speed of change and the speed of technology assure us that nurses' present work as "history" is not very far away.

Vivien De Back, PhD, RN, FAAN
Editor
International Nursing Review
Franklin, Wisconsin

Preface

Our first edition was a comprehensive text to explore nursing case management and promote the development of a critical mass of information around this model of care delivery. It spoke to the diversity and challenges we faced in professional practice settings.

This book has since grown into a "classic" resource, establishing a foundation and springboard for other work in nursing case management to evolve. Building upon this heritage and looking at nursing case management through the filters of a new era, we rewrote, reformatted, and redesigned the content for the third edition.

Since our book is used as a basic text on the subject of nursing case management and managed care, it requires a framework that includes both a historical perspective and new concepts common to health care today. Therefore a true update does not just describe where we stand currently with these approaches but also returns to the original work and reflects on it through current perspectives. A new subtitle was added to reflect this change.

Now eight years later, we have attempted to present what occurred with nursing case management and how it changed professional practice. We were fascinated with discovering what elements caused case management to thrive in some settings and which issues spoke to its vulnerabilities. What we once thought would be successful as a pure nursing model has been shown to be more effective when implemented in an interdisciplinary fashion.

The health care environment forced us as professional nurses to rethink the direction we were going. Faced with the realities of a managed care market we recognized the value of other disciplines and collaboration in the process and management of care. This paradigm shift allowed us to refocus our professional objectives to include other players on the health care team. In the end the recipient of that care benefits from the collective wisdom and expertise of the team members.

New concepts and fresh ideas grow out of the tension that is created when a need is not met. In nursing case management we discovered that it was more effective when all the people involved in providing care were part of the case management approach. That is the beauty of an integrated and collaborative team—responsibility is shared.

Subsequent editions were written during a historic time that nursing case management was being developed. We were living it and projecting where case management would go hereafter. We were also being called to evaluate the effectiveness of what the nursing profession had created. Consequently, we have become the beneficiaries of outcomes of the initial approach to nursing case management. This provides the platform to project where we need to be in the future.

We have honored that past by holding on to the historic pieces—however, they are set in the context of the 21st century. We have moved beyond the critical mass and have taken a fresh look at case management approaches to the delivery of care. To get into the depth of full understanding of this model, one needs to be the vehicle for the expression of others views, perspectives, and ideas. Thus the many contributors to this book. Nursing case management has been played out in multiple ways and in different context and thus, its usefulness and effectiveness is validated in multiple arenas. This edition addresses the diverse facets of contemporary practice in nursing case management. It reflects a less dated and more system focused approach which makes this text a "lived" document.

With the globalization of every element of our lives, professionals and consumers benefit from the cooperation received from partnering. General concepts of partnerships are explored as we describe how case managers partner with other disciplines and groups. As we witness the emergence of collaborative models in health care we see how new generations of nursing case management exemplify care of individuals and communities, begin to address population based services and respond to increased consumerism in health care. In a health care environment where all social, political, economic, and cultural issues intersect we realize how an understanding of public policy enhances the practice of the case manager.

With numerous changes in health care taking center stage in practice settings, this edition affords the opportunity to view the impact of public policy on health care delivery. The implementation of new case management models addresses the importance of educational requirements, promotion of practice competencies, and role definition for the full development of future nurse case managers.

We now reside in a data-driven health care environment and methods for gathering, evaluating, and presenting relevant data about care systems is paramount. The evaluation component of case management that focuses on clinical, financial, utilization, and quality elements and its applicability to the day to day practice of the case manager is covered in this edition. This book expands on the importance of evaluating the outcomes of care and how collecting data can provide an infrastructure on which to base future decisions. Issues such as outcomes effectiveness data and the influence of evidenced-based practice are presented. Understanding the effects of health care reimbursement and its application at the patient level, compliance and regulatory issues, and principles needed to effect successful change, are covered extensively.

In looking back at our rich past, we realized that our books on nursing case management incorporate a broader scope of coverage and are written to compliment other texts on this subject. We have been able to set the underpinning and foundation of case management practice by offering practical application to the theory presented as well as how case management is changing to meet the dynamic challenges of our health care settings. Our book is for the leaders of nursing case management.

There is a purposeful ebb and flow in the 3rd edition as we attempt to capture the depth and breath of contemporary practice and strike a balance between former approaches to nursing case management and their newer examples. Some foundational models are no longer in their original form. They have transitioned and by doing so offer lessons in the evolution of practice. These nursing case management models embraced change and left a living heritage for us to mature. Most importantly, the innovators of these models gave us a wonderful future to behold. It is in this spirit that we offer our current edition.

ACKNOWLEDGMENTS

We have reached an unprecedented time in this book's history. Now in its third edition we wish to formally acknowledge our many readers for making this book a success. We are thankful and humbled by the many insights you impart. To our numerous contributors, sincere thanks for sharing your expertise and wisdom. Your diversity of opinion and powerful reflection speaks to the future of health care. To our reviewers, your perspectives helped frame the context of this edition. We are deeply grateful to Dr. Vivien De Back for her perceptive foreword and her invaluable contributions as our manuscript reviewer. Your generosity of time and sage advice is extremely appreciated. We are indebted to Lisa Potts, Yvonne Alexopoulos, Kathy Teal, and the entire staff of Nursing Editorial for their expert assistance. Their caring manner, commitment to quality publications, and professionalism is outstanding. Heartfelt thanks to our families and friends for your graciousness, indomitable spirits, and loving support.

Elaine L. Cohen and Toni G. Cesta

Contents

Unit V   ADDRESSING HEALTH CARE DELIVERY THROUGH CASE MANAGEMENT: PUBLIC POLICY IMPLICATIONS

Unit VI   THE PLANNING PROCESS: DEVELOPING COLLABORATIVE RELATIONSHIPS

Unit VII   IMPLEMENTATION: TAKING A SYSTEMS PROCESS APPROACH

EVOLUTION OF CASE MANAGEMENT

Health care delivery in the 21st century holds great promise and formidable challenges for nursing case management. The complex variations in the practice of nursing case management and its integration into the business of health care are the focus of Unit I. Understanding the development of case management is critical to evaluating how it is evolving to meet the needs of the future. Although many of its historical manifestations hold true to present-day practice, nursing case management remains challenged by the multitude of issues posed by a transforming health care system, our individual health care settings, and professional practice. Its strength, however, resides in the ability to mature in concert with the changing health care marketplace.

Evolution of Nursing Case Management in a Changing Health Care System

CHAPTER OVERVIEW

Many dramatic changes in the practice and delivery of health services have contributed to the new realities and complexities of the current health care system. This chapter presents how the changing health care system and emerging issues have shaped current nursing case management practices. The chapter also identifies opportunities for innovation and provides an overview of the trends that have led to the development of the nursing case management approach in the delivery of patient care.

This section also discusses the reasons for the success of the nursing case management model in increasing cost-effectiveness, quality of care, and job satisfaction. Included in this discussion are nurse-physician collaborative practice, management of the patient's environment by coordinating and monitoring the appropriate use of patient care resources, monitoring of the patient's length of stay and patient-outcome standards to produce measurements for evaluating cost-effectiveness, and enhanced autonomy and increased decision making by direct health care providers.

Nursing case management offers the nursing profession an opportunity to define its role in the health care industry and challenges the profession to identify the work that nurses do in terms of its autonomous value to the patient.

DYNAMICS OF THE CARE CLIMATE

The 1990s marked a decade of major transition in health care as the system shifted from traditional fragmented approaches of health service delivery to greater integration and control brought on by managed care. However, as the 1990s recede and give way to the 21st century, many of the same issues of access, cost containment, and quality persist. Why these challenges continue is evident by the following:

- Diminished access to health care services for the uninsured population
- Rationed and multitiered distribution of health services

- Mixing of government pricing regulation and market-based competition, resulting in fragmented and cumbersome cost-control initiatives
- Increased control mechanisms for continuous quality improvement and compliance
- Greater demand for concrete, documented information on measurable outcomes at the individual and community levels
- Rising ethical concerns and legal liability resulting in the practice of defensive medicine
- Shifting in the delivery of services from acute care settings to more inclusive services across the health/illness continuum
- Lack of consensus and definition of what constitutes health and the impact of socioeconomic, environment, and public health etiologies on the delivery of cost-effective, quality health care (Cohen & De Back, 1999; De Back & Cohen, 1996; Kindig, 1999; Shi & Singh, 1998).

Archetypal Changes

Major paradigm shifts that have unfolded in the decade of the 1990s underpin the current practice of health care professionals. These changes represent the focus and direction that the leadership in nursing case management will be taking for delivery of health care services well into the next century.

REVISITING PRIMARY HEALTH CARE

These new paradigms converge to offer health, wellness, and care rather than exclusively focusing on illness and cure. To reduce costs and assure access, the new environment for health care supports primary care–based health care interventions on the community level, the hallmark of which emphasizes an integrated approach to continuous and seamless health care delivery across an individual's lifetime (De Back & Cohen, 1996). Primary care is population based and wellness care focused and demands a shift in the commitment of health care professionals to safeguard the population's and society's health and well-being (Campbell, 1997; Issel & Anderson, 1996; Taylor & Barnet, 1999). As the emphasis of care shifts toward wellness and prevention, nonmedical determinants such as socioeconomic status, lack of housing, inadequate nutrition, family violence, and public health will play a greater role in contributing to population health outcomes (Issel & Anderson, 1996; Kindig, 1999).

Reimbursement in a primary care–based wellness-focused system will embrace new criteria for payment as health promotion strategies, surveillance, health maintenance, and care activities take the forefront. Present fee-for-service arrangements will be outpaced by population-based capitation, contractual arrangements for group services, and other innovative financial models (De Back & Cohen, 1996). Kindig (1999) proposes a realignment of financial incentives that is based on an aggregate measure of health for large populations or health plans that could be used for the maintenance and improvement of the health of populations. The measurement of health status proposed by Kindig (1997) must incorporate both quantity (i.e., mortality) and quality of life.

The technological challenges in providing population-based care are numerous; as outlined by Adkins and Morgan (1995) they include defining "community" within a statistical and epidemiological perspective, establishing data collection methods and aggregation of information, developing information in the most meaningful and accessible format, and determining the efficacy of treatment and care outcomes. These authors refer to the integration of communication, computing, and content processes as an "Infocosm" similar to what is commonly defined as the information superhighway. This technology medium will enhance the management of data for population-focused care by linking knowledge management (communication capability), ensuring public data access (transcending from individual care record to community plans), accessing virtual information to determine population-based care protocols, and processing a large volume of data to meet the needs of an expanded customer infrastructure (Adkins & Morgan, 1995).

One key to a well-developed, coordinated system of health care involves partnership. The importance and power of partnering are evident in the outcomes generated by these relationships. Affiliations that facilitate the improvement of health and plan wellness and illness care to meet the needs of individuals, communities, and populations are emerging through the efforts of health care professionals involved on numerous local, regional, national, and international levels. These endeavors are not limited by geographic or system boundaries and demand involvement and integration across educational, legislative, economic, and public arenas (Cohen & De Back, 1999). Case management will have a significant role in the development of population-based health management as exemplified by the case manager's ability to provide health services for individuals, communities, special populations, institutions, and health plans, while addressing health status, quality of life, and effectiveness of health care utilization issues (Chapman, 1999).

CONSUMER STRENGTH

Additional forces are moving the traditional models of fragmented and dehumanized care to those that are comprehensive, coordinated health care networks. Basic premises that relied on exclusionary provider-based decision making have shifted to principles that place emphasis on increased responsiveness to the health care needs of consumers and the development of collaborative partnerships with the recipients of health care.

As customers who purchase health care, consumers are much more sophisticated and savvy about their options for health care services and are demanding better communication with health care professionals (Campbell, 1998; Golodner, 1999). Several strategies, such as HCFAs Conditions of Participation (federal regulations that assure a hospital's compliance with certain practice criteria) and the House and Senate proposed patients' bill of rights, are aimed at ensuring that consumers are included in health care/treatment decision-making processes. A report titled "Eye on Patients," conducted by the American Hospital Association (1996) and the Picker Institute, demonstrated that regardless of the setting in which they received health care (ambulatory or acute care), patients claimed that they were not involved in decisions about their care to the extent that they wanted to be (21% of patients in clinics or physician offices and 36% of patients in hospitals).

Smith and Brooks (1999) advocate structure, process, and outcome targets to improve customer relations. Some of these elements include promoting the use of the Internet as a source of health care information; widespread customization of health services; minimizing cultural, environmental, and attitudinal barriers to care; cultivating ways to partner with the consumer in promoting cost-effective services; and improving consumer knowledge and personal health care abilities.

Changes in the geographical locations where health care can be and is provided have given rise to multiple service settings distinguished by the movement from acute to primary care; from inpatient to ambulatory settings; and from institution-based to integrated delivery systems. These changes have resulted in the prevailing mindset to realign and adjust itself to what Taylor and Barnet (1999) identify as the "nonnegotiables of moral health care" (Box 1-1), which one of these principles speaks to the collaborative efforts of accepting the consumer as a partner in care. These practice elements strike at the very core of our professional and moral obligations to society and demand fundamental changes in our approaches to health care delivery.

DIMENSIONS OF CARE SYSTEMS

Within this context, the infrastructure of nursing case management has evolved to provide care and manage services in the new care system. The intricacies of delivering health care have greatly influenced

Box 1-1 ▸ NONNEGOTIABLES OF MORAL HEALTH CARE

JUST SYSTEM OF HEALTH CARE
- Views health care as an obligation of a moral society rather than a mere business commodity
- Ensures a basic, decent minimum of care for all
- Responsive to the needs of the most vulnerable members of society
- Distributes the benefits and burdens of care giving justly

"PATIENT-FIRST" ORIENTATION
- Commits system resources and professional competencies and will to an orientation that consistently puts patients first
- Demands the subordination of self-interest to the promotion of patient well-being when patient interests are at stake

BROAD NOTION OF HEALTH THAT ENCOMPASSES MORE THAN PHYSIOLOGICAL FUNCTIONING
- Commitment to wholeness of being versus wholeness of body; to cure as *one* of the manifestations of care
- Commitment to quality of life that is multidimensional (i.e., physiological, emotional, social, and spiritual functioning) and subjective
- Range of therapeutic interventions to include more than the "technological fix," that is, com-

passionate presence, development of coping strategies that address problems related to life's meaning and purpose, and so on

TRUSTING PROFESSIONAL RELATIONSHIPS
Includes relationships among the health care system and the public at large; patients, families, and employees; and health care professionals and patients, families, and other health care professionals.
- Grounded in the system's and the health care professional's commitment to secure the patient's and/or society's health and well-being (i.e., fidelity to fiduciary responsibilities)
- Based on a respect for human dignity, which affirms the worth of everyone with whom one interacts
- Provide the individualized knowledge that guides collaborative efforts to achieve valued health outcomes

CLINICAL COMPETENCE
- Encompassing interpersonal, intellectual, technical, and ethical competencies
- Demonstrated ability to "work the system" to achieve valued health outcomes

From Cohen EL, De Back V: *The outcomes mandate: case management in health care today,* St Louis, 1999, Mosby.

the relationships between managed care and the case management model, thereby reconfiguring the approach from managing costs to managing care. An example of this trend is illustrated in the Institute of Medicine (1996) treatise "2020 Vision: Health in the 21st Century," whereby the influx of high-risk individuals (i.e., chronically ill elderly with complex medical problems and the indigent, whose risk factors are related to socioeconomic origins) will potentially shift managed care from an episode-driven system to a risk-driven one. To increase the quality of health care and reduce costs, identifying and intervening with individuals who are at risk for high service utilization will require providers to predict and manage health risk across a full continuum (Clough, 1996). The Healthy People 2010 Program takes national health initiatives even further by attempting to improve the quality of life for all Americans. Through implementation of national benchmarking standards, Healthy People 2010 will hopefully eliminate the health disparities that exist between racial, ethnic, and economic groups (Healthy People 2010, Department of Health and Human Services, January, 2000.) These possibilities reflect the complex variations in the practice of case management and its integration into the business of health care.

To establish accountability and guarantee value, nursing case management must embrace the panorama of health care processes and retain a broader, more global political, public, and social systems perspective. Rethinking the future processes and outcomes of nursing case management places this model in sync with evolving population-based care delivery systems. The concomitant effects of such an approach are not just in one system in which the case manager works, but the variety of systems that affect the work of providers and enhance the understanding, role, and practice of the nurse case manager. Subsequent chapters focus on the interdisciplinary integration and coordination elements so vital to the successful evolution of case management.

As we move into the new millennium, some of the primary system challenges that will continue to influence the provision of health care in general and nursing case management specifically are the growth and consequences of managed care; caring for the long-term and chronic illness population; attending to the uninsured; increased technology, practice, quality, and outcome issues; and consumer service and empowerment—subjects that are covered in later chapters.

PRESERVING THE PAST AND PROJECTING THE FUTURE

What is Nursing Case Management?

Understanding the development of nursing case management as a model is critical to evaluating how it is evolving to meet the needs of the future. Nursing case management, which was first introduced in 1985 and is considered an outgrowth of primary nursing, allows for quality, outcomes-focused care while containing costs. This approach to managing the delivery of health care has emerged as a professional practice model that increases nurse involvement in decisions regarding standards of practice and integrates the cost and quality components of nursing services (Zander, 1985). The historical manifestations of nursing case management hold true to present-day practice in that this model provides outcome-oriented patient care within an appropriate length of stay, uses appropriate resources based on specific case types, promotes the integration and coordination of clinical services, monitors the use of patient care resources, supports collaborative practice and continuity of care, and enhances patient and provider satisfaction (Ethridge & Lamb, 1989; Henderson & Wallack, 1987; Stetler, 1987; Zander, 1987, 1988a).

The practice of case management itself can vary from one practice setting to another, with its identifying characteristics dependent on the discipline that employs it, the personnel and staff mix used, and the setting in which the model is implemented. Nursing case management, however, is a collaborative approach that focuses on the coordination, integration, and direct delivery of patient services and places internal controls on the resources used for care. Such management emphasizes early assessment and intervention, comprehensive care planning, and inclusive service system referrals.

Several health care settings have adopted unique methods of monitoring patient care activity and resource distribution, such as critical paths (a description of patient care requirements in outline form), case management care plans (similar to the standard nursing care plan but adapted to nursing case management outcome standards), and multidisciplinary action plans (MAPs).

Nursing case management has been described as within the walls (WTW), which emphasizes case management activities in the acute care hospital setting, and as beyond the walls (BTW), which refers to case management in outpatient and community-based environments as well as health maintenance organization (HMO) arrangements (Ethridge, 1991; Ethridge & Lamb, 1989; Rogers, Riordan, & Swindle, 1991). In addition, collaborative models of case management that embrace the elements of joint decision-making responsibility and shared accountability have emerged to assure comprehensive patient care and overall system improvement. Mergers of organizations, which have become commonplace in health care, have led to the development of integrated case management models. Case management practices have been successfully incorporated into population-based disease management models as well.

However one views it, because nursing case management balances the cost and quality components of nursing service and patient care outcomes, it has successfully evolved into a professional model that is both sensitive and responsive to current practice demands. A more detailed and differential analysis of case management models is provided in following chapters of this book.

Why Nursing Case Management?

Although appropriate for their time, the efficacy of the traditional models of nursing care delivery is challenged by the multitude of issues posed by the evolving health care system, our individual health care settings, and professional practice. The cutbacks in Medicare reimbursements along with numerous shifts in the configurations of managed care, and demographic changes in work force composition, have compelled providers of health care services to engage in the restructuring and innovative rethinking of priorities related to the delivery and management of patient care. The focus on different approaches to care delivery has prompted health service settings to look at alternative delivery systems as a means of improving patient outcomes and controlling costs.

Restructured Reimbursement

In an era of managed care and government cutbacks, current health care financing and reimbursement methodologies present a dizzying array of options and alternatives. In its most simplistic form, the concept of managed care within the acute care setting has evolved as an approach by which the directives on patient care are determined by predicted patterns of resource use. The managed care system places emphasis on managing the patient's environment by coordinating and monitoring the appropriate use of resources and is an integral component of the nursing case management model (Cohen, 1991). This model seeks to increase accountability for nursing practice and to reduce costs and fragmentation associated with patient care by establishing a mechanism for the regulation and integration of services over the course of an individual's illness (Henderson & Wallack, 1987; Zander, 1988a). Through the coordination of such processes as utilization review/utilization management (the evaluation of medical necessity, appropriateness of level of care, efficiency, and quality of health care services) and discharge planning (evaluation of the patient's care needs early in the admission process that assures appropriate support services and/or placement along the continuum), optimum patient outcomes can be achieved.

Chapter 21, The Managed Care Market: Nurse Case Management as a Strategy for Success, examines case management in the context of the current health care market, expresses the nurse case manager's role within the managed care environment, and discusses new opportunities that managed care has generated for nurses.

Assessment criteria related to hospital-based nursing case management must be able to assess quality while monitoring and evaluating the outcomes of professional practice. The method used demands the following from the provider:

- Independent assessment and adjustment to variations in patients' needs as defined in terms of patient diagnosis, severity level, and spiritual, emotional, and family concerns
- Identification and utilization of appropriate health care resources
- Comprehensive monitoring of patient discharge programs to ensure continuous access to care (Ethridge & Lamb, 1989; Zander, 1988b).

The basic principles used in case management have universal application and are widely used by insurers to control escalating health care costs. These principles are also used by providers in acute care settings to contain inpatient expenditures and provide quality patient care (McIntosh, 1987; Ricklefs, 1987).

The findings of research studies indicate that the changes in inpatient nursing practice patterns associated with nursing case management have helped reduce costs related to the hospitalization of defined groups of patients within certain DRG categories (Cohen, 1991; Ethridge & Lamb, 1989; Zander, 1988b). These changes have promoted cost-effectiveness, allowed nurses to maintain professional autonomy, improved relationships between nurses and physicians, and improved care provider satisfaction (Cohen, 1991; Ethridge & Lamb, 1989; Olivas et al., 1989a; 1989b; Zander, 1988c).

CURRENT ISSUES IN NURSING CASE MANAGEMENT

Nursing case management continues to evolve in concert with the changing health care marketplace. Among the trends and issues shaping case management today are the continual need for concrete, documented information on the measurable outcomes of nursing case management interventions and the importance of future nursing case management research in shaping the structure and process of care. Other important influences are the expanding role and implications of information technology and data reporting processes, the increasing use of standardized language and documentation systems that allow for systematic tracking and management of patients across a health care continuum; outcomes effectiveness and evidence-based practice; education and competencies of future nurse case managers; understanding compliance, regulatory, and reimbursement issues; and emphasis on ethical competence in nursing case management. Later chapters address each of these issues in turn.

Traditional nursing care delivery systems are ill equipped to deal with the many constraints, economic limitations, and continual changes in today's health care settings. Cost containment and concerns about quality of care are pushing health care institutions to consider case management as a way to improve patient care and control costs. Assigning a case manager to oversee the provision of patients' care is an increasingly used and widely recognized strategy to help ensure that patients receive needed care and services and that those services are delivered in an efficient, cost-effective manner.

References

Adkins, K., & Morgan, G. (1995, Jan.). Focusing care: Away from the patient and toward the population. *Healthcare Informatics, 12*(1), 76-78.

American Hospital Association (1996). *The Picker Institute: Eye on patients: A report from the American Hospital Association and the Picker Institute.* Chicago: American Hospital Association.

Campbell, S. (1997). A population-based approach to managing risk, access and care in a managed care market. *Healthcare Strategic Management, 15*(7), 14-15.

Campbell, S. (1998). Healthcare organizations are listening to the newly found voice of the consumer. *Healthcare Strategic Management, 16*(3), 14-15.

Chapman, L. (1999, Nov./Dec.). Population health management and the role of the case manager. *The Case Manager, 10*(6), 60-63.

Clough, J. (1996). Risk identification: Management versus avoidance. In E. Cohen (Ed.), *Nurse case management in the 21st century* (pp. 168-180). St. Louis: Mosby, Inc.

Cohen, E. (1991). Nursing case management: Does it pay? *Journal of Nursing Administration, 21*(4), 20-25.

Cohen, E., & De Back, V. (1999). *The outcomes mandate: Case management in health care today.* St. Louis: Mosby, Inc.

De Back, V., & Cohen, E. (1996). The new practice environment. In E. Cohen (Ed.), *Nurse case management in the 21st century* (pp. 3-9). St. Louis: Mosby, Inc.

Department of Health and Human Services (2000, January). *Healthy People 2010.* (Author.)

Ethridge, P. (1991). A nursing HMO: Carondelet St. Mary's experience. *Nursing Management, 22*(7), 22-27.

Ethridge, P., & Lamb, G. (1989). Professional nursing case management improves quality, access, and costs. *Nursing Management, 20*(3), 30-35.

Golodner, L. (1999). Consumer voice: From whimper to roar. In E. Cohen & V. De Back (Eds.), *The outcomes mandate: Case management in health care today* (pp. 20-26). St. Louis: Mosby, Inc.

Henderson, M.G., & Wallack, S.S. (1987). Evaluating case management for catastrophic illness. *Business and Health, 4*(3), 7-11.

Institute of Medicine (1996). *2020 vision: Health in the 21st century.* Washington, DC: National Academy Press.

Issel, L.M., & Anderson, R. (1996). Take charge: Managing six transformations in health care delivery. *Nursing Economics, 14*(2), 78-85.

Kindig, D. (1997). *Purchasing population health: Paying for results.* Ann Arbor, MI: University of Michigan Press.

Kindig, D. (1999). Purchasing population health: Aligning financial incentives to improve health outcomes. *Nursing Outlook, 47*(1), 15-22.

McIntosh, L. (1987). Hospital based case management. *Nursing Economics, 5*(5), 232-236.

Olivas, G., Del Togno-Armanasco, V., Erickson, J.R., & Harter, S. (1989a). Case management: A bottom-line care delivery model: Part I: The concept. *Journal of Nursing Administration, 19*(11), 16-20.

Olivas, G., Del Togno-Armanasco, V., Erickson, J.R., & Harter, S. (1989b). Case management: A bottom-line care delivery model. II: Adaptation of the model. *Journal of Nursing Administration, 19*(12), 12-17.

Ricklefs, R. (1987, Dec. 30). Firms turn to case management to bring down health care costs. *Wall Street Journal.*

Rogers, M., Riordan, J., & Swindle, D. (1991). Community-based nursing case management pays off. *Nursing Management, 22*(3), 30-34.

Shi, L., & Singh, D. (1998). *Delivering health care in America: A systems approach.* Gaithersburg, Maryland: Aspen Publication.

Smith, T., & Brooks, A.M. (1999). Redefining quality: Designing new partnerships for consumer and provider. In E. Cohen & V. De Back (Eds.), *The outcomes mandate: Case management in health care today* (pp. 198-206). St. Louis: Mosby, Inc.

Stetler, C.B. (1987). The case manager's role: A preliminary evaluation. *Definition, 2*(3), 1-4.

Taylor, C., & Barnet, R. (1999). The ethics of case management: The quality/cost conundrum. In E. Cohen & V. De Back (Eds.), *The outcomes mandate: Case management in health care today* (pp. 30). St. Louis: Mosby, Inc.

Zander, K. (1985). Second generation primary nursing: A new agenda. *Journal of Nursing Administration, 15*(3), 18-24.

Zander, K. (1987). Nursing case management: A classic. *Definition, 2*(2), 1-3.

Zander, K. (1988a). Managed care within acute care settings: Design and implementation via nursing case management. *Health Care Supervisor, 6*(2), 24-43.

Zander, K. (1988b). Nursing case management: Strategic management of cost and quality outcomes. *Journal of Nursing Administration, 18*(5), 23-30.

Historical Perspective of Nursing Care Delivery Models Within the Hospital Setting

CHAPTER OVERVIEW

This chapter reviews the history and theory of various models of professional practice and institutional patient care systems. The restructuring of health care delivery systems has become a promising and successful solution in dealing with cost containment, patient care, and quality assurance issues. Benefits include managing the appropriate use of health care and personnel resources; providing effective and efficient patient care through comprehensive assessment, planning, and coordination efforts; promoting opportunities for professional development and growth across all health care disciplines through participatory and collaborative practice models; and meeting the needs of both the provider and the recipients of care through integrated networks of health services.

EVOLUTION OF NURSING CARE

A historical perspective will help readers see how professional practice and nursing care delivery models evolved and how some of the methods used by previous approaches have contributed to the development of nursing case management today.

Various configurations for the delivery of nursing care have matured within the rapidly changing health care industry. These changes have paralleled major economic, societal, and demographic trends. Most recently, changes in patient requirements have occurred as a result of imposed economic constraints brought on by managed care. Currently, patients are being discharged with increased severity of illness levels, and alternative access to care is not always available or affordable. The rise of consumerism, with its emphasis on patient involvement, the advances in scientific technology, and the change in societal values and expectations all contribute to the multifaceted nature of nursing care delivery systems. Several approaches have emerged to meet specific market demands.

Models of Nursing Care

The traditional modes of delivery were defined by patient selection and allocation and assignment systems of personnel (Arndt & Huckabay, 1980; Stevens, 1985).

The case method was one of the earliest staffing assignments developed. It involved assigning the nurse to either one patient or a caseload of patients to provide complete care. Sometimes referred to as private duty, the case method used a patient-centered approach by giving the professional nurse full responsibility for the care of the patients on an 8-hour basis (Poulin, 1985; Stevens, 1985). This method, considered the precursor of primary nursing (Poulin, 1985), was inefficient because only one nurse provided all direct care for the patient.

The functional method required a division of labor according to specific tasks and was a popular improvement of the case method (Stevens, 1985). The functional model, a task-oriented approach, involved the use of a variety of personnel. It was regarded as a highly efficient, regimented system and was designed to take advantage of different levels of caregiver skill (Stevens, 1985). In functional care the nurse was required to organize and manage a number of given tasks within a certain time.

The issue associated with the functional approach in nursing care delivery was the fragmentation that occurred in the effort to meet the needs of both patient and staff. Components of patient care that were not addressed raised the frustration levels of both the provider and the patient (Poulin, 1985; Stevens, 1985). The sole reliance on regimented tasks was one of the functional model's major drawbacks and resulted in dissatisfaction for both the patient and the nurse. The functional method also did not offer the opportunity to provide comprehensive, continuous care. Nursing's use of the functional method was the adaptation of an industrial mode of practice to a service system (Poulin, 1985; Stevens, 1985).

Team nursing changed the assignment orientation from tasks to patients and addressed the problems of the functional system (Shukla, 1982; Van Servellen & Joiner, 1984). For instance, patient care needs that might have been missed in a functional nursing model could be picked up by the team approach. The team method was developed in the early 1950s by Dr. Eleanor Lambertsen as a way to use all nursing personnel with various skill levels (professional nurses, practical nurses, and nurses' aides). This approach developed in response to the improved technology and shortage of professional nurses (Lambertsen, 1958). The system began to evolve, with greater efforts being made to improve the quality of patient care by focusing on patient outcomes. The professional nurse was responsible for the delivery of patient care services and the supervision, coordination, and evaluation of the outcomes of nursing care provided by the team members.

The advantage of team nursing over functional nursing included increased availability of professional nursing skill for a larger number of patients, greater continuity of care, increased interaction between nurses and patients, and less time spent by professional staff on nonprofessional tasks. The anticipated outcome of such a system was cost-effective nursing care (Chavigny & Lewis, 1984; Hinshaw, Chance, & Atwood, 1981; Lambertsen, 1958; Shukla & Turner, 1984).

The team approach was more than a system for the assignment of personnel. The approach relied heavily on the education, experience, clinical skill, and values of all staff involved in the care of patients. The specifics of nursing care were delineated in the nursing care plan, which included therapeutic, preventive, and rehabilitative steps. Because the care plan was initiated on admission and developed throughout the course of the patient's hospitalization, it was considered cumulative. The plan served as an evaluative measure of patient care and later was adapted as a standard for nursing practice by the Joint Commission on Accreditation of Healthcare Organizations (JCAHO). Although team nursing increased the professional nurse's responsibility for patient outcomes, the limitation in the team approach was related to a greater complexity of role functions and an inability to fit into existing practice systems.

Primary nursing is a configuration of care that promotes greater professional accountability and autonomy and improves continuity of care. This model picks up where team nursing leaves off by making the individual nurse responsible for the assessment, planning, coordination, and evaluation of the effectiveness of care for a certain number of patients. Primary nursing encourages collaborative practice and promotes patient advocacy (Dieman, Noble, & Russel, 1984; Halloran, 1983; Poulin, 1985; Zander, 1985).

Primary nursing is viewed as a care planning system rather than a caregiving one. The focus in this model is on the planning process for comprehensive and individualized delivery of care. The process uses the nursing care plan, which outlines preferred patient outcomes (Dieman et al., 1984; Stevens, 1985). Nurses are held responsible and accountable for the outcome of patient care during hospitalization. The nurse is also expected to use the nursing process as a framework for administering professional and direct care responsibilities (Halloran, 1983).

Studies have compared the economic and cost-effective variables of primary nursing (Daeffler, 1975; Felton, 1975; Hancock et al., 1984; Hinshaw et al., 1981). These studies report that primary nursing contributes to greater patient and staff satisfaction and is less expensive than team nursing (Daeffler, 1975; Felton, 1975). However, the validity of these studies has been questioned. It appears that the reported cost savings and improvement in the quality of care are a result of the competency levels of the professional staff rather than of the structure of primary nursing (Shukla, 1981).

For primary nursing to be effective, compatible support systems, such as unit secretaries, need to be in place to provide for the routine and nonprofessional activities of the care setting. However, because of current budget constraints, increased severity of patient conditions, and shortened length of stay, hospitals have difficulty maintaining this system of care. Initially, the concept of primary nursing required an all-professional nursing staff. However, a mix of nursing service staff skills and competencies is currently being used successfully in many hospitals (Poulin, 1985; Stevens, 1985). As a result, this patient care delivery system is assuming characteristics of other patient care models and is evolving into a prototype that can be adapted to alternative delivery models of nursing care.

PROFESSIONAL PRACTICE AND ALTERNATIVE PATIENT CARE DELIVERY MODELS

The unstable nature of health care economics and managed care has made it necessary to focus attention on developing and implementing alternative systems for the delivery of patient care. A decade ago, the need to deliver health care effectively and efficiently stimulated the promotion of national initiatives directed by the Department of Health and Human Services and supported by the National Commission on Nursing. The purpose of these efforts was to decrease length of stay, reduce costs, and improve the quality of patient care (National Commission on Nursing Implementation Project [NCNIP], 1986; Secretary's Commission on Nursing, 1988).

The same principles hold true today that to achieve these goals while maintaining viability, patient care delivery systems must be sensitive to limited fiscal and resource appropriation. The systems must also incorporate cost-effective standards, establish quality assurance outcomes of professional practice, and broaden accountability for the outcomes of care. Several professional practice and alternative care delivery models have been successfully developed and implemented. These models have prompted major adjustments in the practice environments of their settings.

Some of the fundamental characteristics of these professional practice and care delivery approaches are the adaptability and receptiveness of the approaches to differentiated and professional competency levels of practice, the reconfiguration of patient care and maximum use of nursing personnel resources, the use of collaborative practice arrangements among nurses, physicians, and other health care workers, the redesigning of the relationship between the providers and recipients of health care to improve patient care outcomes, and the enhancement of the relationship between the providers of patient care and the organizational culture supporting them. A description of some of the models used in practice follows.

Integrated Competencies of Nurses Model (ICON)

ICON models I and II are examples of the earliest alternate care delivery approaches blending the professional and educational competency levels of staff with the health care needs and requirements of patients (Rotkovich, 1986). The nursing care responsibilities in these models, which were set up as demonstration projects, are differentiated on the basis of the nurse's educational preparation. Head nurses are required to have a master's degree and are responsible for the management and distribution of personnel and resources and overall quality of care delivered on the unit. Nurses with baccalaureate degrees are accountable for the assessment, planning, and evaluation activities of the nursing process. Nurses with associate degrees complement the professional nurse in patient care and carry out nursing decisions. In ICON I model, licensed practical nurses (LPNs), nurses with diplomas, and nursing assistants are excluded from the staffing complement.

Although ICON I was considered the nursing care delivery system for the future, another model, ICON II, had been implemented and ran concurrently to help LPNs and nurses with diplomas or associate degrees make the transition into their respective practice roles (Rotkovich & Smith, 1987). The goal of this model was to assist through in-service programs, continual education, and clinical preceptors the grandfathering of the associate degree and diploma nurses into the professional nurse's role and the LPNs into the associate nurse's role. This objective is in line with the profession's broader goal of achieving two entry levels of nursing practice.

Cost-effectiveness, quality, and job satisfaction variables were measured and evaluated on an ongoing basis. No data have been published relating the effects of staff mix and competency levels of nursing staff on the productivity and quality of patient care using the ICON I and II models. Information on nursing personnel satisfaction and retention is also missing.

Partners in Practice

The partners-in-practice system, defined by Manthey (1989) as a progression from primary nursing, is a partnership established between an experienced senior registered nurse and an individual who supports the nurse as a technical assistant. The technical assistant is assigned to the nurse, not to a caseload of patients. Consequently, by delegating tasks to the technical assistant, the registered nurse can concentrate on providing professional patient care.

The registered nurse is responsible for defining the role, standards, and nursing care activities. By providing direction and supervision, the registered nurse is also accountable for the overall care delivered in the partnership. An official contract is used to confirm the relationship, and both members are paired on the same time schedule.

This system of care delivery is highly sensitive to unit-based human resource distribution requirements, skill mix, competency levels, and patient care needs. Because of the emphasis placed on the delivery of productive and efficient health care services, the partners-in-practice system can yield substantial benefits. These benefits include savings in overall budget and personnel salary expenditures as a result of reduced turnover rates, decreased use of staffing agencies, and improved management of supplemental nursing resources. The system enhances nursing staff retention by offering opportunities for advanced clinical training and education.

Contract and Group Practice Models

Contract and group practice models have been implemented at Johns Hopkins Hospital. They focus on building up the relationship among nursing care providers, the organization, and the environments in which they work. The contract model concentrates on promoting job satisfaction and retention by engaging nursing staff in autonomous decision making related to unit-based staffing levels and coverage, scheduling activities, standards of practice, quality assurance, and peer review (York & Fecteau, 1987). Another characteristic of this model is that it uses primary nursing. The staff benefits from the associated practice arrangements, which include salaried (versus hourly wage) compensation programs.

The group practice model is another innovative system developed for nurse practitioners who work in the emergency department and provide services to a group of patients needing primary health care (York & Fecteau, 1987). This model, which is built on the same objectives and goals as the contract model, initiates a productivity incentive that compensates nurse practitioners for the amount of care they provide per patient visit. This model calls for creation of an incentive fund that is allocated as patient target volumes are met.

Both these models prove their economic viability and organizational effectiveness by decreasing costs related to staff turnover and sick time, increasing patient visits and admissions, and decreasing length of stay. Reallocation of staff mix, skill, and competence levels leads to greater productivity and better use of the professional nursing staff. Additional gains include increased job satisfaction because of greater continuity of patient care, increased professional responsibility and autonomy, and reciprocal compensation packages.

NURSING CASE MANAGEMENT

A review of the literature indicates that aspects of some of the past and current nursing practice approaches and delivery models of care were incorporated into the development of nursing case management. The strength of nursing case management comes from the philosophy and collaborative practice strategies of both primary and team nursing. In fact, some of the care planning and coordination processes used in these models are reflected in the critical paths and care plans of nursing case management. These plans are used to monitor patient care requirements and activity as well as the resources for meeting those needs.

With former models, nursing care revolved around the nursing care plan, which provided a broad-based outline for the delivery of nursing services for the patient. These plans gave little direction in establishing a structure for achieving expected outcomes of nursing care for each day of hospitalization. The nursing case management model, however, provides a framework for nurses to manage the patient's hospital stay. Directing the delivery of patient care services allows the nurse to anticipate needs, thereby providing the opportunity for overall coordination and integration of outcomes and cost (Cohen & Cesta, 1994; Zander, 1990).

Nursing case management also integrates many of the professional practice demands and initiatives characteristic of alternative patient care delivery models. By emphasizing care that is patient-centered, the nursing case management approach embraces techniques of business in which the patient is seen as a valuable consumer who has the right to demand the best in health care. Placing the patient at the core of nursing's power base authorizes the profession to reconfirm its commitment to society. Nursing case management incorporates a new way of looking at the relationships among cost, quality, and nursing care. It places an emphasis on the autonomy, authority, and accountability of professional nursing practice by promoting an open system of care in which information is shared among all disciplines. A team whose members work collaboratively replaces the individual method of providing patient care. Because of its universal applicability, an in-depth discussion and treatment of the nursing case management model will be provided in Unit II.

References

Arndt, C., & Huckabay, L. (1980). *Nursing administration theory for practice with a system approach.* Chicago: American Hospital Association, pp 65-111.

Chavigny, K., & Lewis, A. (1984). Team or primary nursing care? *Nursing Outlook, 32*(6), 322-327.

Cohen, E., & Cesta, T. (1994, Fall). The economics of health care and the realities of nursing in the 1990s. Case management in the acute care setting: a model for health care reform. *Journal of Case Management, vol. 3*(3), 110-116, 128.

Daeffler, R.J. (1975). Patient's perception of care under team or primary nursing. *Journal of Nursing Administration, 6*(3), 20-26.

Dieman, P.A., Noble, E., & Russel, M.E. (1984). Achieving a professional practice model: How primary nursing can help. *Journal of Nursing Administration, 14*(7), 16-21.

Felton, G. (1975). Increasing the quality of nursing care by introducing the concept of primary nursing: A model project. *Nursing Research, 24*(1), 27-32.

Halloran, E. (1983). Staffing assignment: By task or by patient. *Nursing Management, 14*(8),16-18.

Hancock, W.N., et al. (1984). A cost and staffing comparison of an all-RN staff and team nursing. *Nursing Administration Quarterly, 8*(2),45-55.

Hinshaw, A.S., Chance, H.C., & Atwood, J. (1981). Staff, patient and cost outcomes of all-RN registered nurse staffing. *Journal of Nursing Administration, 11*(11), 30-36.

Lambertsen, E. (1958). *Education for nursing leadership.* Philadelphia: J.B. Lippincott Co.

Manthey, M. (1989). Practice partnerships: The newest concept in care delivery. *Journal of Nursing Administration, 19*(2), 33-35.

National Commission on Nursing Implementation Project (1986, Nov. 7). *Invitational Conference.* Milwaukee: W.K. Kellogg Foundation.

Poulin, M. (1985). Configuration of nursing practice. In American Nurse's Association (Ed.), *Issues in professional nursing practice* (pp. 1-14). Kansas City, Mo.: The Association.

Rotkovich, R. (1986). ICON: A model of nursing practice for the future. *Nursing Management, 17*(6), 54-56.

Rotkovich, R., & Smith, C. (1987). ICON I—The future model, ICON II—The transition model. *Nursing Management, 18*(11), 91-96.

Secretary's Commission on Nursing (1988, Dec.). *Final report (Volume I).* Washington, D.C.: Department of Health and Human Services.

Shukla, R.K. (1981). Structure vs. people in primary nursing: An inquiry. *Nursing Research, 30*(7), 236-241.

Shukla, R.K. (1982). Primary or team nursing? Two conditions determine the choice. *Journal of Nursing Administration, 12*(11), 12-15.

Shukla, R.K., & Turner, W.E. (1984). Patient's perception of care under primary and team nursing. *Research in Nursing and Health, 7*(2), 93-99.

Sovie, M.D. (1987). Exceptional executive leadership shapes nursing's future. *Nursing Economics, 5*(1), 13-20.

Stevens, B.J. (1985). *The nurse as executive* (pp. 105-137). Rockville, Md.: Aspen Publication.

Van Servellen, G.M., & Joiner, C. (1984). Convergence among primary nurses in their perception of their nursing functions. *Nursing and Health Care, 5*(4), 213-217.

York, C., & Fecteau, D. (1987). Innovative models of professional nursing practice. *Nursing Economics, 5*(4), 162-166.

Zander, K. (1985). Second generation primary nursing: A new agenda. *Journal of Nursing Administration, 15*(3), 18-24.

Zander, K. (1990). Managed care and nursing case management. In G.G. Mayer, M.J. Madden, & E. Lawrenz (Eds.), *Patient care delivery model* (pp. 37-61). Rockville, MD: Aspen Publishers, Inc.

Historical Development of Case Management

CHAPTER OVERVIEW

The case management approach represents an innovative response to the demands of providing care in the least expensive setting and coordinating and planning for needed community resources. For the past 30 years there has been a growth in the variety of case management delivery systems of care.

This chapter reviews the historical development of the case management concept. Descriptions of different nonnursing case management models are given to make the reader aware of the vastness and complexity of this approach. This is not intended to suggest limited use of the case management model. On the contrary, its great potential and applicability should be promoted. Studies show that this model can be an effective and efficient system by focusing on and caring for the health and social needs of the individual.

INTRODUCTION OF CASE MANAGEMENT

Most of the literature on nursing case management practiced in the acute care setting is evolving. However, case management has been used by mental health and social services for years. For more than two decades the case management approach has been used as an alternate design for the delivery of health care. The first federally funded demonstration project began in 1971 and has been associated with a number of methods to coordinate and provide comprehensive services of care for the individual (Merrill, 1985). Regardless of the different approaches, the main principle underlying case management is ensuring the quality as well as the efficiency and cost-effectiveness of services provided (Weil & Karls, 1985). Emphasis is placed on the recipient of case managed care and the coordination and networking of services (Weil & Karls, 1985; White, 1986).

Research related to the outpatient and community-based population has studied the effects of health care case management in areas other than nursing. The specific target groups included the frail elderly, the chronically ill who are functionally or emotionally challenged, and clients who require long-term care services. These case management projects were designed to use less expensive, community-based services to prevent unnecessary institutionalization (Steinberg & Carter, 1983; Zawadski, 1983). Various services, from companionship to homemaking, were provided to assist individuals in their daily activities.

Findings of these studies show that case-managed, in-home support services, such as mental health, respite care, and homemaker or personal care services, have been effective in improving access (evidenced by shorter service waiting lists), assessment, and care planning needs of elderly clients (EISEP, 1988; Raschko, 1985). Additional studies illustrate the efficacy of case management in coordinating and integrating health and social services for long-term care, assessing quality-of-life outcomes (quality-of-living conditions), and reducing time spent in long-term care facilities (Carcagno & Kemper, 1988; Eggert, Bowlyow, & Nichols, 1980; Sherwood & Morris, 1983).

Because the nursing profession recognizes the need for changes in the system of health care delivery, more and more nurses are being designated as case managers. This change results from nurses' expertise and knowledge in managing patient care. Case managers are involved in the assessment, coordination, referral, and individualized planning, monitoring, and follow-up activities associated with case management (Grau, 1984; Johnson & Grant, 1985; Mudinger, 1984).

Primarily used with long-term care populations, case management arrangements have been developed by private insurance carriers as cost-containment strategies and have been integrated into the acute care setting (Henderson & Collard, 1988; McIntosh, 1987). Consequently, different models of case management have evolved. Merrill (1985) identified three categories of case management: social, primary care, and medical-social.

SOCIAL CASE MANAGEMENT

Social case management models emphasize comprehensive long-term community care services used to delay hospitalization. Both health and social needs are addressed in this setting. Primarily successful with the elderly population, this model focuses on ensuring the independence of the individual through family and community involvement. It is based on a multidisciplinary approach to coordinate the care of the patient.

Various services, from companionship to homemaking, are offered to assist individuals in their daily activities. One example of the social case management approach is the U.S. Department of Housing and Urban Development's Congregate Housing Services Program, in which non-health services are provided to the elderly living in a housing project.

PRIMARY CARE CASE MANAGEMENT

Primary care case management takes on the role of gatekeeper based on the medical model of care. This approach focuses on the treatment of a particular health problem and tries to prevent institutionalization. In this model the physician functions as the case manager and is responsible for coordinating services and managing the patient (Johnson & Grant, 1985).

Primary care case management emphasizes the need to regulate resource use to assure cost-effectiveness. Examples mentioned include health management organizations (HMOs), which originally served Medicaid beneficiaries and have become increasingly popular among insurance companies as a means of controlling the disproportionate use of medical care.

Since the patient population accommodated by primary care case management is defined by health status, the type of case management services required varies according to the health needs of the patient. The financial imperatives to curtail high-cost medical technology are strong under the primary care case management system. However, a major liability of this approach is the exclusion of necessary medical services and hospitalization. Johnson and Grant (1985) recommend that quality assurance standards be incorporated into this mode of health care delivery.

MEDICAL-SOCIAL CASE MANAGEMENT

The medical-social case management model focuses on the long-term-care patient population at risk for hospitalization. This model combines available resource utilization with additional services, which are not traditionally covered by health insurance, to maintain the individual in the home or community. The case manager(s) in this system may be drawn from nurses, physicians, social workers, and family members who have input into the assessment, coordination, care planning, and care monitoring.

An example of the medical-social case management model is the social-HMO demonstration project, which integrates both medical and social services on a prepaid capitated basis to meet the multiple needs of the chronically ill patient. This model emphasizes providing the least restrictive and least costly long-term care by identifying the appropriate services and coordinating its delivery.

Additional definitions of the case management model are offered by White (1986), who bases the case management approach on a continual process of responsibility and authority for the provision of care and resource appropriation and use. Along this spectrum, situations arise that either preclude the use of case management or facilitate case management arrangements with direct health service delivery.

Five case management models were also characterized. These models are differentiated on the basis of authority level of the client, support and financial systems, and payment allocation (White, 1986).

1. Restricted market: In this arrangement the clients become their own case managers and negotiate for services among independent providers.
2. Multiservice agency: This system allows an agency to provide its own health care.
3. Advocacy agency: With this model, some case management is provided along with direct patient care services.
4. Brokerage agency: The agency in this system acts as a broker in coordinating, controlling, and monitoring services and resources.
5. Prepaid long-term-care organization: With this arrangement a company contracts for case management services and coordinates resources on a prepaid, capitated basis.

Weil and Karls (1985) further characterized case management into three practice models: the generalist case manager or broker model, the primary-therapist-as-case-manager model, and the interdisciplinary team model.

The generalist case manager model is structured to provide direct service, access, planning, and monitoring activities to clients. The case manager in this system acts as a broker and is involved in the intake, coordination, and evaluation processes.

A broad range of professional disciplines may be represented; therefore the case managers in this model may include social workers, nurses, and mental health or rehabilitation specialists. Continuous and efficient service is assured because of the close working relationship between the case manager and client. The case manager also benefits from autonomous decision making and other independent management responsibilities.

The primary therapist model emphasizes a therapeutic relationship between the case manager and client. The case manager in this system is required to have a master's degree and training in psychology, social work, psychiatry, or psychiatric clinical nursing specialties.

As in the generalist model the case manager-patient relationship is a close one with the case manager responsible for coordination and evaluation services. Because of this one-on-one relationship, the primary therapist model works well with small, community-based programs and has been successful in coordinating and planning efforts and resources with larger networking systems.

Initiatives to ensure the delivery of case management are strong under the primary therapist model. However, therapeutic services have been known to take precedence at the expense of case management functions. Weil and Karls (1985) recommend the supplementation of case management responsibilities with therapeutic care.

The interdisciplinary team model focuses on providing case management services through a collaborative team approach. The responsibilities and designated case management functions are divided among the team members according to their area of specialization and expertise.

In this system the case managers may include nurses, social workers, or therapists who have accountability and provide services within their own area of concentration. One team member, however, is appointed to maintain overall service coordination and evaluation.

The benefits of the interdisciplinary team approach include improved continuity of care and enhanced coordination of services and staff support systems to promote mutual program planning, problem solving, and client advocacy.

PRIVATE CASE MANAGEMENT

Private case management systems have evolved to meet the needs of clients outside publicly funded programs or those who prefer more personalized services (Parker & Secord 1988). Parker and Secord cite the findings of a major survey conducted by Inter-Study's Center for Aging and Long-Term Care and funded by the Retirement Research Foundation.

This study investigated the characteristics, services, referral, and funding sources of private geriatric case management firms across the United States. According to Parker and Secord (1988), this model evolved as a result of an increase in the elderly population, escalating health care costs, growing need for integrated social and health services for the elderly, and increasing emphasis placed on long-term care issues. Survey findings are discussed in the following five paragraphs.

Private case management firms were in business an average of 3 years, and most (98.9%) were independently owned, run for profit, and self-managed. Some affiliations existed with hospitals, public and private social service agencies, and nursing homes. Clientele consisted of elderly individuals with mean annual incomes ranging from $5,000 to $15,000. Case managers in this system were college graduates who were prepared in social work or nursing and who carried a small caseload of clients.

In most instances, private case management functions included coordination of services, social, functional, and financial; mental health assessment and counseling; and referral, monitoring, and evaluation services. Medical assessments were done by physicians in 44% of the private case management businesses. Some of the other services consisted of nursing home and housing placement, retirement planning, companion and homemaker services, and transportation and respite care. These direct services were provided more frequently by for-profit and unaffiliated private case management businesses than by the nonprofit and affiliated companies. Those firms that employed registered nurses as case managers tended to provide more direct care services as well.

Services most often referred by private case managers included home health care, homemaker, and personal care services, family and legal counseling, and physical therapy. Referral sources were composed of physicians, social workers, family members, and self-referrals.

Private case managers were able to provide more individualized services and were also accessible on off hours, weekends, and holidays.

Reimbursement for services provided by private case managers ranged from hourly and set rates per session to service and package rates. Unaffiliated and for-profit businesses used more hourly and set rate methods and also segregated their services to charge for case management functions involving more time and attention. Sliding fee scales were more common in affiliated and nonprofit organizations. Funding sources to private case management businesses included out-of-pocket payments by client or family members, private insurance, Medicare, Medicaid, and other sources that consisted of public funds, trusts, and grants.

Benefits of private case management approaches for staff members include increased flexibility and autonomy in decision making, independent planning and coordinating of services, greater income, and professional satisfaction. Clients and their families also reported improved accessibility to case managers, less duplication and redundancy of services, individualized care, and long-term association with one case manager. However, further evaluation is needed regarding access to other health care services, overall quality of private case management care, cost, and reimbursement issues.

COMPONENTS OF CASE MANAGEMENT

Weil and Karls (1985) extensively outlined the main service components common in all case management models.

CLIENT IDENTIFICATION AND OUTREACH

Individuals who are eligible or need case management services are identified. Admission to a case management program is determined by interview process, referral, and networking systems or by the case manager actively promoting eligibility for individuals who might not inquire about case management services for themselves (for example, individuals who are indigent or have mental illness).

INDIVIDUAL ASSESSMENT AND DIAGNOSIS

Case managers use their comprehensive knowledge and skill to assess the physical, emotional, and psychological needs as well as the social and support requirements of their clients. This process aids in the coordination, facilitation, monitoring, and access of case management services.

SERVICE PLANNING AND RESOURCE IDENTIFICATION

With the collaboration of the client the case manager assumes the responsibility for coordinating and planning care services. This includes the development of care plans and determining resource and networking systems.

LINKING CLIENTS TO NEEDED SERVICES

Case managers act as brokers to expedite and follow through with the coordination and planning needs of the client. Both community and agency resources may be used. In some systems this responsibility involves actually transporting the client to a recommended service.

SERVICE IMPLEMENTATION AND COORDINATION

The case manager ensures that the identified needs are satisfied and follows the formal agreements made with the networking agencies. This is done by extensive documentation and record keeping of the efficiency, effectiveness, and quality of case management care services. A participative relationship of client and case manager and autonomous decision making on the part of the case manager are crucial to both groups' engagement in the system.

MONITORING SERVICE DELIVERY

The case manager is responsible for directing and overseeing the distribution of services to the client. A multidisciplinary and multiservice relationship is promoted to assure appropriate and effective delivery of case-managed services.

ADVOCACY

Case managers act on behalf of the client in assuring that needed interventions are obtained and that the client is making progress in the program. As explained by Weil, the advocacy strategy is used not only for the individual client but also for the benefit of all individuals in common predicaments.

EVALUATION

The case manager is responsible and accountable for appraising the specific as well as the overall usefulness and effectiveness of case managed services. The evaluation process involves continuous monitoring and analysis of the needs of the individuals and services provided to the clients. Early identification of changes or problems with the client or the provider of services is made, ensuring timely intervention and re-planning by the case manager.

References

Carcagno, G.J., & Kemper, P. (1988). The evolution of the National Long Term Care Demonstration: An overview of the Channeling Demonstration and its evaluation. *Health Services Research, 23,* 1-22.

Eggert, G.M., Bowlyow, J.E., & Nichols, C.W. (1980). Gaining control of the long term care system: First returns from Access Experiment. *The Gerontologist, 20,* 356-363.

EISEP (1988, November 30). *An evaluation of New York City's home care services supported under the expanded in-home service for the elderly program.* Health Research: New York University. Funded by New York City's Department for the Aging (contract #11000100).

Grau, L. (1984). Case management and the nurse. *Geriatric Nurse, 5,* 372-375.

Henderson, M.G., & Collard, A. (1988). Measuring quality in medical case management programs. *Quality Review Bulletin,* 14(2), 33-39.

Johnson, C., & Grant, L. (1985). *The nursing home in American society.* Baltimore: Johns Hopkins University Press, pp 140-200.

McIntosh, L. (1987). Hospital based case management. *Nursing Economics,* 5(5), 232-236.

Merrill, J.C. (1985). Defining case management. *Business and Health,* 3(5-9), 5-9.

Mudinger, M.O. (1984). Community based case: Who will be the case managers? *Nursing Outlook,* 32(6), 294-295.

Parker, M., & Secord, L. (1988). Private geriatric case management: Providers, services and fees. *Nursing Economics,* 6(4), 165-172, 195.

Raschko, R. (1985). Systems integration at the program level: aging and mental health. *The Gerontologist, 25,* 460-463.

Sherwood, S., & Morris, J.N. (1983). The Pennsylvania Domiciliary Care Experiment: Impact on quality of life. *American Journal of Public Health, 73,* 646-653.

Steinberg, R.M. & Carter, G.W. (1983). *Case management and the elderly: A handbook for planning and administering programs.* Lexington, Mass.: Lexington Books.

Weil, M., & Karls, J. (1985). Historical origins and recent developments. In M. Weil & J. Karls (Eds.), *Case management in human service practice* (pp. 1-28). San Francisco: Jossey-Bass Publishers.

White, M. (1986). Case management. In G.L. Maddox (Ed.), *The encyclopedia of aging* (pp. 92-96). New York: Springer Publishing.

Zawadski, R.T. (1983). The long-term care demonstration projects: What are they and why they came into being? *Home Health Care Services Quarterly,* 4(3-4), 5-26.

II

CONTEMPORARY MODELS OF CASE MANAGEMENT

Unit II highlights the emergence of collaborative models of nursing case management that embrace elements of joint decision making and shared accountability. This approach assures comprehensive patient care delivery and overall system improvement. In the 21st century, case management models will include the integration of care across the continuum. Both care management and disease management approaches build on interdisciplinary systems of care and are evolving as complimentary strategies to nursing case management.

Dimensions of Nursing
Case Management

CHAPTER OVERVIEW

As the demand for cost-effective high-quality health care continues to grow, innovative approaches to improving patient care delivery must be explored. The goals of cost-effectiveness combined with high quality care can only be achieved within a framework of total organizational commitment to restructuring care to meet the needs of today's health care provider and the present patient population.

Case management is an effective approach that can be used in the reorganization process. As discussed, this model helps define the role and scope of the nurse's responsibilities in the delivery setting. Case management models can enhance the productivity and competency levels of staff by organizing personnel to use their varying skills and expertise in better ways. This could increase professionalism and the satisfaction of all providers.

By ensuring that appropriate outcomes are achieved, case management provides a framework for continuous and refined planning of nursing and interdisciplinary care and ensures appropriate and cost-effective use of patient resources. Finally, case management models can contribute to the foundation of total quality improvement and ensure continued delivery of high-quality patient care.

PRECURSER OF CONTEMPORARY APPROACHES TO NURSING CASE MANAGEMENT

Cost management issues and quality care, which at one point were on opposite sides of the health care delivery spectrum, are now being integrated into one system. The economic power once reserved for physicians and hospitals has been transferred to the purchasers of health services, which include business corporations, insurance companies, and individuals. The buyers' objectives are coordinating and managing the use of health services and allocating resources for future distribution.

Managed care emerged as control shifted from the provider to the purchaser of health services. The managed care system links the provider with the patient to manage cost, access, and quality components of health care delivery. Major health policies like the federal Health Maintenance Organization Act, adopted in the early 1970s, established a trend for the growth of managed care programs. The health maintenance organizations (HMOs) and preferred provider organizations (PPOs), two popular examples, offered an alternative to costly inpatient care through the provision of cost-effective treatments and multiple preventive and outpatient services.

Case management is used in these managed care plans as a cost-containment initiative. It further grounds the managed care approach by focusing on the individual health care needs of the patient. Case management is effective because it targets the coordination, integration, and outcome evaluation processes of care. The inherent strengths in case management systems have led to a renewed interest in the utility and effectiveness of such systems.

TRENDSETTING IN NURSING CASE MANAGEMENT

Managed care is a system that provides the generalized structure and focus for managing the use, cost, quality, and effectiveness of health care services. Managed care then becomes an umbrella for several cost containment initiatives that may involve case management. On the other hand, nursing case management can be conceptualized as a process model, the underpinnings of which are essential in attending to the many components and services used in the delivery aspects of patient care.

With case management the accountability and responsibility for the delivery of care are based on an entire occurrence of hospitalization for a targeted DRG group of patients and is not geographically confined to that patient's unit (Etheredge, 1989; Zander, 1990). This widens the circumscribed area of patient services to include patient care planning and coordination across health care settings. Case management, then, implies consistency of provider: even though different, formal, informal, and even very esoteric resources are used, the coordinator or provider (usually an individual) remains the same (Zander, 1991).

Collaborative practice arrangements in the form of group practice are supported, and interdisciplinary decision making is facilitated to ensure appropriate use of patient resources and achievement of expected clinical outcomes. Collaboration usually includes members of the health care team and the patient or family to help accomplish anticipated care outcomes. Participants of the health care team use critical paths, clinical pathways, and case management plans. Variance analysis and evaluation of patient care are expanded beyond the confines of the patient unit and encompass all patients in the specific caseload (Etheredge, 1989; Zander, 1990).

An example of a case management model—the Beth Israel Multidisciplinary Patient Care Model (Cesta, 1991)—was developed for use within an acute care setting. Using the practice concepts of both primary and team nursing, this model supported the coordination and management of patient care from admission to discharge. The objectives of the model were as follows:

Improve quality of care
Control resource utilization
Decrease length of stay
Increase patient satisfaction
Increase staff satisfaction

This case management model, which was implemented through a reorganization of the nursing department structure, provided the opportunity for advancement of selected registered nurses working at the bedside. When a case management career ladder is used, nurses who have a baccalaureate degree and who have demonstrated advanced clinical and leadership skills can remain in the direct patient care environment and expand their professional careers by working as case managers.

The case manager was removed from direct care delivery to coordinate overall patient services. This individual is also part of a multidisciplinary team that continually assesses, evaluates, and plans patient care. The assessment is based on expectations regarding outcomes of care of the physician, nurse, and all other individuals involved in the patient's care.

Case managers assumed responsibility for a caseload of patients who met high-risk criteria developed for each clinical area. Patients were referred to utilization management or social work as needed. Care was managed through prospective protocols called multidisciplinary action plans (MAPs). Outcome data, including variances, were collected and used to improve clinical and system processes.

A MAP projected patient care outcomes for each day of hospitalization. Because care plans were a group effort, they promoted greater satisfaction for the patient, family, and health team members. These plans involved all patient care areas and specialties and covered a wide range of diagnoses or surgical procedures, such as neurosurgery, orthopedics, acquired immunodeficiency disease (AIDS), general medicine, pediatrics, maternal and child health, oncology, detoxification, and rehabilitation. Ultimately the model increased professional development and improved recruitment, motivation, and retention of staff (Ake et al, 1991).

Case managers, who were unit based, coordinated the care being delivered by the registered nurses and nursing assistants working on the team. The manager also served as a role model to the novice nurse or orientee. By consulting with less-experienced registered nurses, the manager helped to improve the professionalism and clinical skills of the unit's personnel and promoted collegial relationships with all health care providers. Other responsibilities of the case manager included patient and family teaching and support and discharge planning with the social worker.

This model enhanced the use of personnel by expanding support or ancillary staff role responsibilities. Because the nursing attendants were included as part of the care team, they better understood the medical and nursing needs of their patients.

The multidisciplinary patient care model was an integral component of the organizational restructuring of patient care delivery. Because it was research based and part of the planned change process, several clinical and quality care indicators were evaluated to determine the model's effectiveness. This model required ongoing assessment of quality improvement data, job and patient satisfaction ratings, and length-of-stay data.

Another example of a comprehensive case management model was developed at The Long Island College Hospital, Brooklyn, New York. This model incorporated the same goals as the Beth Israel model, with emphasis on the use of product and personnel resources. Process and structure redesign for this model began with a review of the role functions of nurses, social workers, utilization managers, and discharge planners. The existing care process for each discipline was entered in a flow chart, and process barriers were identified. Each discipline identified ways in which personnel might be redeployed to assure the best use of available personnel as well as to reduce duplication. Interventions were moved to preadmission whenever possible. For example, discharge planning and home care referrals were moved to the preadmission arena. Social workers began to divide their time between the inpatient and outpatient care settings.

Another significant component of this model was the redeployment of the existing clinical nurse specialists as case managers. Long Island College Hospital identified the case manager as an advanced practice role, and the clinical nurse specialists were best prepared to assume the additional responsibilities associated with case management. Generic staff development functions that they were performing were returned to the Department of Nursing Education and Research.

The Professionally Advanced Care Team (ProACT) Model

The ProACT model was developed at the Robert Wood Johnson University Hospital (RWJUH) to meet the demand-induced nursing shortage, differentiated practice, and prospective payment initiatives (Tonges 1989a, 1989b). This model expanded the role and professional practice of the registered nurse by establishing two roles for the nurse. The first role is that of the clinical care manager (CCM), and the second is that of primary nurse.

The CCM role required a nurse with a baccalaureate degree who managed the care for a caseload of patients throughout their hospitalization. This position involved managerial, personnel, clinical, and fiscal accountability. Primary nurses, who had graduated from accredited registered-nurse programs, were give responsibility for 24-hour management of patients on the unit and all direct and indirect caregiving activities. They were also accountable for the assessment, planning, and evaluation components of patient care as well as the delegation of tasks to licensed practical nurses (LPNs) and nursing assistants providing direct patient care.

This system maximized primary nursing through the redistribution of support staff and a restructuring of ancillary services at the unit level. Patient care services that could be supported by nonnursing departments, such as housekeeping, dietary, supplies, and pharmacy, were assigned to the appropriate unit personnel. For example, support-service hosts were responsible for hotel-type functions such as bed making, and pharmacy technicians were responsible for ordering, obtaining, and preparing medications, among other duties. By placing accountability for nonclinical services on personnel from respective support departments, nurses were free to provide comprehensive and coordinated patient care.

The traditional reporting structures and organizational processes were altered to adapt to the ProACT model's premise of restructuring care with the patient as the central focus. Luckenbill and Tonges (1990) reported in a preliminary evaluation that job satisfaction increased through collaborative care efforts among nurses, physicians, and other health care workers and through a well-coordinated support-service system for staff and patients. Additional findings included a 10% decrease in length of stay with specific DRG patients and a concomitant increase in patient revenues that were attributable to nursing interventions.

As part of an iterative process of work redesign at RWJUH, the clinical care manager role was re-examined and substantially changed in the mid-1990s. The first change broadened the CCM's scope from a unit-based to a service-based approach. This review subsequently identified an opportunity to decrease duplication of effort and redundancy in the nursing case management, utilization management, and discharge planning functions (Brett, Bueno, Royal, & Sengin, 1997). It was felt that all three roles centered on expediting patient throughput, primarily by reviewing and using data from the medical record, resulting in overlap among responsibilities. To streamline processes and improve efficiency, the case management, utilization management, and discharge planning functions were integrated into a new outcomes manager role. Several key processes were automated to support this transition, including home care referrals. A number of variables were evaluated to assess the outcomes of this change, and the most striking results appear to be a 41.5% increase in home care referrals and a reduction of 17 full-time equivalents (Brett et al., 1997).

South Dakota Demonstration Project—Differentiating Outside the Walls

A nursing delivery model expanding on the theme of differentiated practice has been developed and implemented at Sioux Valley Hospital in South Dakota. This hospital was one of several institutions participating in a statewide demonstration project. The project demonstration sites consisted of a consortium of institutions, with representation from the acute care setting, long-term care (nursing home), and home health agencies (Koerner, Bunkers, Nelson, & Santenna, 1989).

Differentiating Outside the Walls*

Nursing case management has been in existence in this 400-bed hospital since the practice differentiated in 1989 (Koerner & Karpiuk, 1994). That model was founded on principles of the original primary nursing concepts of the 1970s and 1980s: consistent caregivers; holistic, patient-centered planning; and coordinated acre and services within a hospital setting. The primary nurse, or case manager, had the authority and autonomy for care decisions and was accountable to guide care delivery toward financially sound goals. Early outcomes of primary nursing models included reduced hospital length of stay and cost of care, reduced recidivism, and increased patient satisfaction. However, this early single-case or unit-based approach to care delivery in the hospital setting lacked aggregate analysis of populations and did not extend across the continuum. It also lacked measures related to physiological outcomes, quality of life, functional status, and identification of high-risk subgroups within populations.

In the first generation of an Advanced Practice RN (APRN) case management model, focus was on the one-to-one relationship of an APRN and single high-resource-user cases, or HULAS (heavy users, losers, and abusers). This model was usually initiated after an inpatient acute care stay and extended into the patient's home setting after discharge. Case finding was based on case complexity, recidivism, or other pattern of unusual utilization or high cost. This method of case finding during or after crisis and in the midst of intensive resource use is a high-cost method for subscriber systems. As the concept of outcomes management developed in the literature, the one-to-one nursing case management model within its differentiated practice context began to shift. Episodic care gave way to longitudinal management of whole populations of patients. Risk assessment of managed subscribers increased. Evidence-based care practices and evolving national guidelines mandated continuous scrutiny of local practice patterns, care methodologies, and outcomes of care. Interdisciplinary collaborative management of increasingly complex patients replaced the old paradigm of care planning and task completion, while broadening the accountability of outcomes of care. The advent of integrated clinical pathways (ICPs), reflective of "re-modeling" in the next generation, provided a collaborative, multidisciplinary foundation for care delivery coordination, and , later, for outcomes management. Clinical pathways are evolving to facilitate coordination of complex, longitudinal care driven by evidence-based care methodologies. They assist in targeting, documenting, and tracking abstractable outcomes reflecting physiological, functional, utilization, and cost outcomes. As hospital-based care moves into the community, longitudinal clinical pathways, with greater emphasis on health maintenance and self-care of chronic disease, help to focus attention on longitudinal outcomes. In the future, visual trajectories from these outcomes may be consumer-friendly tools to help client-provider partnerships to understand and manage self-care and health maintenance (Jensen & Koerner, 1999).

References

Ake, J.M., Bower-Ferris, S., Cesta, T., Gould, D., Greenfield, J., Hayes, P., Maislin, G., & Mezey, M. (1991). The nursing initiatives program: Practice based models for care in hospitals. In *Differentiating nursing practice: Into the twenty-first century.* Kansas City, MO: American Academy of Nursing.

Brett, J.L., Bueno, M., Royal, N., & Sengin, K. (1997). PRO-ACT II™, Integrating utilization management, discharge planning, and nursing case management into the outcomes manager role. *JONA* 27(2), 37-45, 1997.

Cesta, T. (1991, Nov.). *Managed care,* personal correspondence and paper presented at the Annual Symposium on Health Services Research, New York.

Etheredge, M.L. (1989). *Collaborative care nursing case management.* Chicago: American Hospital Publishing, Inc. (American Hospital Association).

---

*Reprinted from Cohen and De Back (1999). *The outcomes mandate: Case management in health care today.* St Louis: Mosby.

Jensen, G.C., Koerner, J. (1999). Longitudinal profiling: A differential community nursing model. In E. Cohen & V. De Back (Eds.), *The outcomes mandate: Case management in health care today* (pp. 153-155). St. Louis, Mosby.

Koerner, J.G. & Karpiuk, K.L. (1994). *Implementing differentiated nursing practice: Transformation by design.* Gaithersburg, Md: Aspen Publishers, Inc.

Koerner, J.E., Bunkers, L., Nelson, B., & Santenna, K. (1989). Implementing differentiated practice: The Sioux Valley Hospital experience. *Journal of Nursing Administration, 19*(2), 13-20.

Luckenbill, J., & Tonges, M. (1990). Restructured patient care delivery: Evaluation of the ProACT TM model. *Nursing Economics, 8*(1), 36-44.

Tonges, M. (1989a). Redesigning hospital nursing practice: The professionally advanced care team (ProACT™) model, part I. *Journal of Nursing Administration, 19*(7), 31-38.

Tonges, M. (1989b). Redesigning hospital nursing practice: The professionally advanced care team (ProACT™) model, part II. *Journal of Nursing Administration, 19*(9), 19-22.

Zander, K. (1990). Managed care and nursing case management. In G.G. Mayer, M.J. Madden, & E. Lawrenz (Eds.), *Patient care delivery models* (pp. 37-61). Rockville, MD: Aspen Publishers.

Zander, K. (1991, April). Presentation at *Nursing care management: Transcending walls opening gates,* Saint Joseph Medical Center, Wichita, Kan.

Two Strategies for Managing Care

Care Management and Case Management*

Cathy Michaels, Elaine Cohen

CHAPTER OVERVIEW

In the 21st century case management models will include the management of care across the continuum. Various complementary strategies have evolved that build on an interdisciplinary system of care. Care management is one such approach that is designed to provide health planning for groups of individuals with like situations across the continuum of care.

CARE MANAGEMENT—A COMPLEMENT TO CASE MANAGEMENT

Case Management is a way of managing unique and high-risk situations often associated with costly hospital use. Typically situations requiring case management involve patients whose self-care capacity and/or care giving is diminished when their disease process and its treatment is the most intense, even life-threatening. The outcome of these situations is frequent hospital and physician visits. Patients at high risk, however, represent a small percentage of the patient population.

Most patients do not face high-risk situations. The majority of health care experiences encompass situations that are usual, that is, there are resources to manage the situation or there is resolution of illness. In these instances, patients have the capacity for self-care, the support of caregivers, or an illness that can be successfully treated, like pneumonia, hip surgery, or wound care. Patients in less than high-risk situations like this do not require the one-to-one relationship of case management, but do need continuity of care. Well-known examples of care management are the multidisciplinary teams for organ transplant and rehabilitation.

Care management can provide needed continuity, establishing a system of care for a particular condition, across the continuum of care to ensure seamless transition to the right services and right providers at the right time. Patients and their caregivers who can be supported by care management can manage their own health concerns. From the risk of self-care capacity, patients at moderate or low risk merit care management, while case management is for patients at high risk. Who matches what risk status is a care management decision, as is who requires case management.

Care management is embedded in the work of all clinicians. Health care professionals who develop therapeutic relationships with patients know what works for people and what does not, within their own disciplinary context. Nurses have much to contribute given their emphasis on body, mind, and spirit, as well as the ability to serve people across the continuum of care.

Individuals from many disciplines serve as case managers for patients in unique and high-risk situations. Social workers, for instance, provide case management for frail elders and the behaviorally challenged. Nurses may best be the case managers for people with life-threatening chronic illnesses, since physical evaluation along with psychosocial assessment is critical for avoiding and minimizing the need for hospitalization. In general, our most recent experience with managing care has overrelied on approaches used in case management. Issues that relate to the clinical population are the domain of care management. Care management practices, however, are not as prevalent, since clinicians often have not knit together their collective expertise across the continuum of care and across time for groups of people in similar moderate- and low-risk situations.

Care management is a matter of clinical judgment, but decisions cannot be made in isolation of the other disciplines. Clinicians must connect and coordinate their efforts. What drives the system that is created and which discipline does what mainly depends on the available clinical resources. Boxes 5-1 and 5-2 present examples of care management teams.

Box 5-1 ▸ A CARE MANAGEMENT EXEMPLAR FOR A HOSPITAL IN A REMOTE AREA

An interdisciplinary team established a care management system for people with chronic obstructive pulmonary disease (COPD). The hospital nursing staff assumed assessment of the patient's self-care capacity, and the respiratory therapists, the knowledge, skill, and ability related to the use of inhalers and nebulizers. If the patient is at high risk, the respiratory therapist will continue to follow the patient through home care. If, however, the person with COPD is in the end stage, the nurse case manager will follow because of the disease's complexity and end-of-life issues. This care management strategy was developed by an interdisciplinary team in a small community hospital. Clinically and financially, it was important to create a system of care for people with COPD, a fairly large population in this area without many clinical resources. Outside unit staff nurses and respiratory therapists, it was important to focus the work of the nurse case manager on COPD at the end of life, the highest of high risk. But this care management strategy can be revisited and redesigned every year by evaluating annual outcomes for this population.

Box 5-2 ▸ A SECOND EXEMPLAR FROM A HOSPITAL IN AN URBAN AREA

The multidisciplinary team comes together to strengthen a hospital program for congestive heart failure (CHF) and ends up considering a post-hospital follow-up by phone and, if needed, home visit, and pre-hospital emergency room CHF clinic. This bolsters the work of nurse case managers who are already in place for patients whose hospital experience exceeds more than 2 hospital visits in 6 months. The team reached the consensus that a system of care was needed to bolster the work of the nurse case managers.

LAUNCHING CARE MANAGEMENT

Launching a care management effort needs to build on an interdisciplinary system of care that complements case management. This can be achieved by maximizing success in improving health and well-being for people in both high-risk and less than high-risk situations at the same time, decreasing cost to the health system. Care management is defined as a way for clinicians to link their disciplinary efforts, programs, and services across the continuum of care for the clinical benefit of patients in like situations who are at moderate- or low-risk status with a similar health care situation and to identify when case management is called for and which discipline is in the best position to provide it. To be effective, care management must be cycled across the continuum—at a minimum from the hospital to home, and across primary or specialty care settings.

The necessary clinical mindset for care management is to consider one's patient care unit at the entire continuum of care, not just a single point on that continuum, like a medical-surgical unit or home health. As such, no patient is ever discharged, but moves along the continuum of care matched to self-care or whatever services are needed to support health and well-being. Then by developing clinical guidelines and linkages to weave together disciplinary efforts between the multiple points across the continuum of care, the therapeutic relationship between interdisciplinary providers and patients is supported rather than "taken over," as is the case with many clinical protocols and mandates (Box 5-3).

Organizing care management with a seamless and effective interdisciplinary, not just multidisciplinary, effort that best serves patients and their caregivers reflects three principles:

Principle 1: Care management is a community effort.
Principle 2: Patients are grouped by similar health and functional efforts.
Principle 3: A system of care is built to support the therapeutic relationship between providers and patients.

PRINCIPLE 1: CARE MANAGEMENT IS A COMMUNITY EFFORT

In many health settings today, we are learning how to streamline clinical connections. For example, to avoid hospitalizations, we need to be able to simplify initiating home health care in the community for patients with life-threatening chronic illnesses. Initiating home health care usually requires a physician to receive clinical information about the patient and respond by ordering home health services. Often this occurs when the physician is doing other things, like seeing patients in the office or making rounds

---

Box 5-3	**EXEMPLAR OF CARE MANAGEMENT OVER THE CONTINUUM OF CARE**

Clinical diabetes educators could be the case managers for high-risk diabetic groups who experience uncontrolled blood sugar levels and make frequent visits to the emergency department. Support groups at physician offices and/or at neighborhood centers could be developed for people with diabetes who are at moderate risk for managing their health concerns (these groups are diagnosed with diabetes, but their blood sugar level is controlled most of the time with diet, exercise, and medication). Quarterly education programs could be developed for people who are at low risk or predisposed to developing diabetes and those with diabetes who are at moderate risk.

in the hospital. Delays can only increase the likelihood that hospitalization will be extended—an unwelcome disruption of life for most patients and a cost to the health system.

Clinical connections comprise programs and services across the continuum of care and the disciplines that provide care. Streamlined, these connections represent a stage of integration where we have the disciplinary interdependence to provide accessible, quality, and cost-effective care across the continuum and across time.

Interdependence is the key to building a system of clinical connections, or a system of care. We can start shifting to interdependence by inviting all the appropriate clinicians to knit together their collective efforts to assist a group of patients, or a clinical population, presenting a challenge to the health system. This interdependence is similar to a community approach that is inclusive, not exclusive. We look to who will be the right provider to do what for whom, when, where, and why. The interdisciplinary community then becomes a vehicle for mutual exchange, dialogue, and active listening. The clinicians can then organize their efforts across the continuum of care and across time, honing in on the best approach for patients given the resources of the health system.

PRINCIPLE 2: GROUPING PATIENTS

One of the first tasks in care management is to identify groups of people in like situations who feel vulnerable and present a clinical and financial challenge to the health system. These clinically relevant groups or populations are then risk stratified into high-, moderate-, and low-risk situations. Individuals in the high-risk (unique) group may require case management interventions. The interdisciplinary team can then decide which discipline is best suited to become the case manager and develop a system of consultation with the other disciplines to support the designated primary case manager in their care responsibilities. The key in this situation is not to duplicate effort, since it can be confusing to the patient and expensive to the system, not just in dollars but in needless resource use. The interdisciplinary team can also develop care management approaches for improving the health and well-being of moderate- and low-risk groups of patients within that population.

PRINCIPLE 3: HONORING THE THERAPEUTIC RELATIONSHIP

A key to care management is building a system of care that supports the therapeutic relationship. Care management is not intended to provide a recipe or protocol for treating everyone the same. Rather, the intent is to build a system of care that streamlines the mechanics of health services so providers have more therapeutic time to spend with their patients.

In a letter to the editor, published in the *Arizona Daily Star* (1998), Isla Jacobs, a southern Arizona resident writes about the importance of relationship: "I lament the direction the medical profession has taken. It's a big business now and seems to be preoccupied with cold efficiency. Listening to a patient's problems, whether real or imagined, has gone by the wayside. Two of the most important areas of medicine are trust and patience. In days past the doctor was truly a member of the family." Although her remarks are addressed to physicians, Isla's words have meaning for every health care provider. Essential to a therapeutic relationship is the capacity to be heard by and be known to the professionals to whom you entrust your health. With meaningful relationships between patients and providers, successful outcomes can be maximized for patients, providers, and the entire health care system.

SUMMARY

Care management is important for every health system, whether or not the system is contracted to provide health care. An example of the Medicare reimbursement process will help illustrate this point. If a patient's hospitalization costs more than what Medicare pays (either by an extended length of stay or costly care within that stay), then the health system pays the difference. Managing care within the hospitalization period can increase efficiency and lower expenses. But managing care across the continuum can avoid and minimize the need for hospitalization in the first place and/or increase the likelihood that the patient's length of stay will be within predetermined limits. Care management is simply indispensable to a health system in that it serves as insurance for decreasing the need for costly hospital stays. The future bodes well for care management as a springboard for successful contracting.

Our current care challenges revolve around chronic conditions and aging and therefore require multiple strategies to manage care across the continuum. Case management and care management are two strategies for helping people with chronic conditions and aging issues to learn to optimize health, well-being, and self-care capacity. Case management is designed for unique and high-risk situations. Care management is the approach associated with a common diagnosis or life situation—that is for people in moderate and lower risk situations. By honoring the therapeutic relationship, both case and care management can improve health and well-being while generating cost savings.

Case management is better known. Care management is yet to unfold. But not unlike care planning for hospital patients, care management is simply health planning for groups of people with like situations across the continuum of care. Based on a foundation of clinical judgment and interdisciplinary effort, care management can be a winning proposition.

Reference

Jacobs, I. (1998, June 2). Lost family member (Letter to the editor). *Arizona Daily Star,* p. 8.

BIBLIOGRAPHY

Bower, K., & Falk, C. (1996). Case management as a response to quality, cost and access imperatives. In E. Cohen (Ed.), *Nurse case management in the 21st century.* St. Louis: Mosby-Year Book, Inc.

Cohen, E., & Cesta, T. (1997). *Nursing case management: From concept to evaluation.* St. Louis: Mosby-Year Book, Inc.

National Chronic Care Consortium (1995). *Risk identification.* Bloomington, MN: Author.

Newman, M., Lamb, G., & Michaels, C. (1992). Nurse case management—The coming together of theory and practice. *Nursing & Health Care, 12*(8), 404-408.

Stempel, J., Carlson, A., & Michaels, C. Walking in partnership. In E. Cohen (Ed.), *Nurse case management in the 21st century.* St. Louis: Mosby-Year Book, Inc.

Disease Management

Applying Systems Thinking to Quality Patient Care Delivery

Patricia Hryzak Lind

CHAPTER OVERVIEW

The concept of disease management is not new. It has taken on heightened interest and awareness with the evolution of managed care, cost containment, and consumerism. "Disease management is the comprehensive, integrated approach to care and reimbursement based on the natural course of the disease with treatment designed to address an illness with maximum effectiveness and efficiency" (Zitter, 1994, p. 1). To implement a successful disease management program, one must understand the natural course of the condition and treatment alternatives with attention to cost and quality of these options, understand how one educates an individual and a population about their condition and clinical and nonclinical treatment options, have knowledge and data about health care utilization and costs across all care settings, and include elements of prevention and health promotion to maintain clients at their optimal level of wellness for as long as possible.

EVOLUTION OF DISEASE MANAGEMENT

Population-based disease management has been used by individual clinical practices in examples such as identifying and inviting all patients with diabetes for diabetic education classes, or when mailing educational materials to all women of childbearing age in need of Pap screening tests. While these interventions target groups at risk, a more comprehensive approach to disease management should include the assessment of patient needs, identification of the problem, planning of a comprehensive group of interventions, evaluating the effectiveness of the approaches, and measurement of the clinical, cost, satisfaction, and functional outcomes.

Disease management is progressing from simply targeting those members most at risk for the disease to encompass educating populations at large about prevention and health promotion. Disease management continues to evolve from that of a chronic disease focus to a program designed to improve the health of populations served by organizations, provider groups, or the community at large. This evolution cannot occur without the integration of nursing knowledge and practice into all aspects of the program beginning with planning and throughout evaluation.

EVALUATING DISEASE MANAGEMENT PROGRAM

Success factors for a disease management program include several key components (Box 6-1) (Todd and Nash, 1997). The integration of information and data to include the continuum of the disease management program from the selection of patients for targeting to program implementation and outcome evaluation is essential to ensure program success. Linking program participation to cost and utilization data has become increasingly more critical as managed care organizations and employers evaluate the effectiveness of either targeted or prevention programs on their bottom lines. Targeted programs are aimed at specific patients with chronic conditions such as diabetes. Further specificity occurs in these programs by choosing patients at increased risk such as nonadherence to treatment plans or a lack of preventive care such as annual eye examinations. This aspect of disease management has become easier with the development of health care information systems that track and trend these data. However, the future holds additional opportunities with the integration of encounter-level data, increased accuracy at targeting at-risk patients, linkages to utilization data that can be trended for longitudinal studies, and additional research in guideline implementation and the refinement of valid and reliable instruments to assess progress toward outcome measures.

A sound method for calculating return on investment is also critical to program implementation and evaluation. Disease management programs must prove their worth in today's cost-conscious and competitive health care environment. Purchasers and developers of disease management programs are becoming more sophisticated in understanding how programs impact their health care costs, participant quality of life, functional status, and productivity of their employees. Statements about "return on investment" must be substantiated with actual health care costs and accurate calculations of cost avoidance. Estimates and approximations are increasingly being replaced with calculations based on actual health care expenditures. Innovative programs will continue to develop and flourish if these programs use data to demonstrate actual health care savings, increased worker productivity, and improved quality of life.

Determining the "teachable moment" for patients or providers or the point in a treatment algorithm when the greatest health impact can be achieved will continue to provide opportunities for research. A "teachable moment" is that point when the patient is ready and able to change behavior to achieve a healthier state. For providers of health care, it means recognizing where the patient is along the change continuum and providing information and support in concert with the patient's current status.

Using a quality improvement framework, determining what interventions have the most impact, is necessary to continuously advance patient care. The timing and type of intervention and how it is de-

Box 6-1 ▶ **KEY SUCCESS FACTORS**

KEY SUCCESS FACTORS FOR DISEASE MANAGEMENT
Understanding the course of the disease
Targeting patients likely to benefit from the intervention
Focusing on prevention and resolution
Increasing patient compliance through education
Providing full care continuity across health care settings
Establishing integrated data management systems
Aligning incentives

livered via media or technology will continue to change as new health and patient education innovations enter the market. Research as to the most appropriate and cost-effective type of provider will refine approaches to patient care as well as contain costs. The optimal timing and method of reinforcement of education to sustain a behavior change is critical to learning more about patient education and motivation. All of these areas are fruitful opportunities for research and program evaluation studies.

Disease management continues to change as new and different partnerships emerge. Partnerships between managed care organizations, employers, and disease management programs continue to develop. Employers are using data such as the Health Plan Employer Data Information Set (HEDIS) or the National Committee for Quality Assurance Quality Compass to identify health plans that improve the health and satisfaction of the work force. Contractual relationships between employers and disease management companies have emerged as employers search for ways to have healthy employees productively at work. Employers may evaluate each health plan's preventive and disease management interventions to select the insurer who offers well developed programs to assist employees maintain and improve their health and ultimately their work productivity.

Consumers are being charged by their employers, as well as their care providers, with taking responsibility for their own health status. Lifestyle concerns such as obesity, nutrition, and substance use contribute to overall health state. Although a health care provider can counsel and educate patients about these issues, the ultimate change rests with each patient. Employers in turn are shifting health care costs to their employees through higher premiums and co-payments. Some employers have charged a higher premium contribution for those employees who smoke, thus adjusting for increased health costs.

Consumers are actively seeking health information. Deering (1996) found that 80% of consumers with mental and physical health problems sought information about their condition, and 67% to 79% read advertisements or watched television, respectively, about health or medicine concerns. Clearly, consumers are seeking knowledge and are looking to partner with their practitioner, employer, or managed care company to support their health behaviors.

The alignment of incentives continues to support the success of any disease management program. Risk contracting within managed care organizations or capitation as a reimbursement mechanism encourages the determination of the most cost-effective treatment in the most cost-effective setting. The use of incentives or rewards with education of patients to seek optimal levels of health, as well as attain necessary preventive care, must be in concert with the financial aspects of physician reimbursement. If physicians are penalized for preventive service utilization or are not at risk for costly hospital services, the incentives for prevention are incorrectly aligned with disease management programs.

Employers have instituted wellness incentives through self-insured products. These programs consist of monetary incentives or rebates when specified health behaviors are achieved. Targeted changes may include smoking cessation, weight loss, or sustained exercise program attendance. Programs have been well accepted by employees with increased employee health and satisfaction.

Managed care plans provide physician profiling reports that include data on individual patients within selected populations. A sample annual profile might contain a list of all patients with asthma, the number of office and emergency room visits within the last year, the number of filled prescriptions for inhaled corticosteroids, and whether the patient had a flu shot the previous fall. These reports may be given to assist the physician in care provision or quality improvement opportunities identified by the managed care plans. Monetary incentives may be linked to the data if the managed care plan was trying to increase prescribed inhaled corticosteroids after an acute asthma exacerbation or if they were attempting to raise the percentage of at-risk members who receive a flu vaccination.

For disease management programs to be successful, the alignment of the incentive to the sought-after behavior is critical. To achieve this goal, data must be accurate and contain an actionable plan for the patient or provider. Barriers to care must be assessed and understood. Modes of receiving information may be varied and based on patient preference. Reinforcement of the desired behavior should be rewarded and sustained. Patient behavior includes adherence to treatment regimens, including drug therapy, diet, exercise, and lifestyle changes. Therefore understanding aspects of self-care, including how and when to self-medicate, is important in managing a chronic condition.

Evaluation of the program should be multidimensional and include patient satisfaction, health care utilization and cost, functional status and quality of life, and clinical outcomes. Additional information about evaluation will be included later in this chapter.

Disease management programs will continue to grow and evolve, as will the role of the nurse in the development, implementation, and evaluation of these programs. Consumerism and the patient's quest for health care information, the proliferation of the information through technology such as the Internet, and changing provider-patient relationships into partnerships also provide opportunities for nurses to influence the health and knowledge of populations. Nursing can do much to promote the concept of health management through the development and implementation of programs that support primary prevention while implementing disease management programs that target individuals who are in need of interventions at the secondary or tertiary levels of prevention.

DISEASE MANAGEMENT PROGRAM DEVELOPMENT

Defining the Population

In a great mystery, knowing "who done it" ahead of time will ruin the book. For disease management, knowing "who needs it" ahead of time will ensure program success and potentially guarantee customer satisfaction. Defining the population and knowing that you have selected the patients who truly have the condition and could benefit the most from your intervention would be disease management "utopia." "Targeted populations might include high-volume clinical services, high-cost health care expenditures, services that have great variation in clinical practice, services that may pose a significant risk to patients, clinical opportunities for improvement, or patient care situations where long-term complications are linked to provider risk" (Doxtator & Rodriguez, 1998, p. 186).

Disease management programs must be in concert with the needs of the organization. Using a framework for planning is helpful (see Figure 6-1). Understanding the program goals is essential. If the vision of the program is to decrease inpatient re-admissions after hospitalization for depression, the design of the program will be different than a program designed to increase worker productivity related to unscheduled absences for migraines. Knowing what the organization wants to achieve with the disease management program and why this change is needed is the first step in program design. Some conditions are more suitable for disease state management than others. Chronic conditions account for 75% to 80% of health care costs and treatment. Specific elements are necessary before a condition can be selected for disease management. These would include patient education for self-care, sharing of real-time patient care data and best practices with clinicians, and the ability to influence the continuum of care to improve outcomes and lower costs.

The next step is abstracting data to substantiate the need for the program. Employers might obtain the data from their worker's compensation files or from absentee records. Managed care organizations may analyze annual health care utilization data to determine those clinical conditions that are the drivers for inpatient, emergency, outpatient, primary care, or pharmaceutical health care costs. Physicians, through their office data base, may determine those clinical conditions seen frequently in their office. Each of these examples may identify one or more clinical conditions that, through a disease manage-

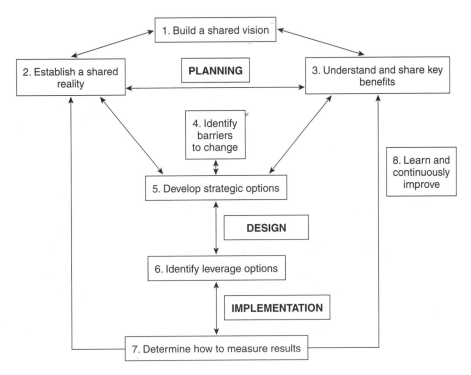

FIGURE **6-1**   Systems-thinking model: The disease management process.
Redrawn from *Todd, W.E. and Nash, D. (1996). Disease management—A systems approach to improving patient outcomes. Chicago: American Hospitals Publishing Co.*

ment program, could improve patient care, decrease health care costs, or shift utilization to a more appropriate level of care. Analyzing data over several years allows for a clear identification of the program rather than aberrant data due to patient outliers or unusual clinical conditions. Trending data and comparing the findings to regional or national benchmarks will validate incidence and prevalence to further ensure the methodology for correct patient identification.

A number of companies have entered the market with a variety of data abstraction systems to identify patients for interventions. Based on organizational needs and goals, a careful analysis of the data extraction systems, company and provider community acceptance of these types of systems and robustness of the educational interventions will assist in decision making. There are information systems that identify patients with the health condition as well as systems that attempt to detect patients at risk or those who are undiagnosed. Selection of a system based on goals with attention to confidentiality and state and federal legal considerations will vary based on practice location. For practices that span state lines, knowledge of legislation is essential.

Another organizational data need is a system to manage and evaluate individual case management clients. It is unlikely that a patient identification system and data tracking system for case management exist in one software package. The case management system should contain demographic information such as patient identification, data input capabilities for health outcome, satisfaction and functional status surveys, and a link to cost and utilization data. The ability to analyze this progress of individuals and populations is essential. The interface with current information systems and analysis software is part of the evaluation process in selecting software. In addition, patient confidentiality and security safeguards require careful scrutiny. Short-term tactical solutions such as database development projects, stand-alone PC-based software, or stand-alone reporting initiatives can provide helpful lessons for the selection of long-term strategic initiatives such as data warehouse systems (Matthews, 1999).

Disease management programs are built from a quality improvement perspective. The identification of strategic opportunities that achieve program planners' goals as well as participants' purpose is paramount to success. Early generations of disease management targeted "low hanging fruit" or those patient care opportunities that, with simple interventions, could realize cost savings and changes in health behavior. Examples of such first-generation programs included mailed flu shot reminders to at-risk patients or outbound calls to remind chronically ill patients about medication refills. Following these types of interventions, targeted case management programs emerged for high-risk patients.

Disease management programs attempt to educate everyone within a selected population. Individual case management interventions are aimed at high-risk patients and provide customized interventions to address their specific patient care needs. An example of this approach would be mailing educational interventions to all managed health care plan members with diabetes to remind them of preventive care and to provide information on diabetic education. Individualized case management would occur with newly diagnosed members, those recently prescribed insulin pumps, or those recently hospitalized for complications related to their diabetes. Individual case management reinforces the continuing relationship between the patient and the primary care provider, through the use of an individual plan of care.

Understanding who bears the financial risk for health care costs is also an important part of the planning process. Providers may share financial risk with managed care organizations. As the managed care organization communicates data related to quality improvement activities, the practitioner may be rewarded or penalized for compliance with these initiatives. Examples of data sharing would include profiles of patients with diabetes in need of retinal eye examination or lists of patients with congestive heart failure without evidence of prescribed ACE inhibitor medications. Monetary rewards or penalties may be tied to the level of patient compliance and/or physician education about preventive care and chronic conditions.

Todd and Nash (1997) predict that the next generations of disease management will include "truly integrated care" leading to "health management." They define integrated care as a program that aligns care and reimbursement, and they include risk stratification for patients with interventions that are matched to patient risk. Health management encompasses prevention as well as disease management through the "collection of health status, health risk and severity data, and the linkage of this information to clinical and economic outcomes data for the purpose of determining the predictors of health, disability, illness, disease, complications and probability of eventual outcome" (Peterson & Kane, 1997, p. 307).

PLANNING THE INTERVENTION

Planning the intervention includes researching the literature and interviewing colleagues who have implemented similar programs. Published research may contain the outcomes, instruments, and tools suggested to achieve goals. Actual implementation strategies may not be included. Unpublished program information may be presented at professional seminars that will assist with other avenues for planning interventions.

Understanding available human, information, communication, educational, and financial resources is essential. Determining who the organizational champions are to assist in gaining more of these resources is also paramount to program success. A clinical team approach to disease management would involve primary care and specialist practitioners including physicians, nurses and social workers as well as pharmacists. Additional assistance from data and financial analysts, quality improvement specialists, and outcome measurement experts would augment the team process and product. Integration of these champions in the planning process will assist greatly in achieving program goals.

The proliferation of pharmaceutical companies within this aspect of health care is remarkable. Often in partnership with data management companies or universities, pharmaceutical companies are attempting to strengthen their programs with the data to support their interventions and costs. The organization must decide if the disease management program will be purchased from a vendor or developed within the company or clinical practice. Each approach has its benefits and drawbacks. A careful analysis of resources also assists the planner and the decision makers in selecting the "buy or build" route.

Development of a business plan to determine whether to partner with a vendor or develop one's own program is required. A careful analysis of the partner's history, scope of services, implementation work plan, measurable outcome results, program costs, and data integrity is conducted. A review of the company's business alliances may also prove enlightening. If the vendor is linked to a pharmaceutical company, one might explore expectations about drug promotion or formulary placement. Review of sample data extractions against one's own data warehouse will validate if the correct patients have been selected for the intervention. A thoughtful review of each partner's objectives, skills, and patient care contributions will assist with the decision as to whether a disease management vendor will add value to the clinical initiative.

Contractual arrangements between the physician or managed care organization and the disease management vendor are necessary. Key elements in the contract should include "the type of agreement, identification of the intervention group, establishment of analysis for cost baselines, profiling of disease data elements, requirement for resource costing, seasonal adjustment procedures and definition of terms, contract dynamics and management" (Langley, Langley-Hawthorne, Martin & Armstrong, 1996, p. 1099). Legal review of the contract in concert with a clinician's scrutiny will determine how patients, providers, and employers will accept and embrace the program interventions.

New patient educational media and technology continue to enter the health management market. Patient reminders through interactive voice response systems, list serves and interactive websites on the Internet, and patient registration for educational program through cable television networks are just the start of new modes of providing patient education. Several of these approaches also include pre- and post-learning assessments and integration of standardized instruments to assess functional status or quality of life to measure the effect of the intervention on an individual. Individual and population data are then available for analysis about the effectiveness of the education and/or the technology. These types of program also allow consumers to access education when they desire and often in their home rather than through structured classroom sessions.

Determining the data source for identification of at-risk patients and measurement of intended outcomes early in the planning process is critical. When one understands the source of the data and data limitations, one can address these issues proactively or account for them in the intervention or analysis. Many managed care organizations use administrative claims data coupled with their own demographic database. These data are derived from paid health care claims and may vary based on provider coding or be delayed by billing procedures. Patients who should obtain care but do not are not identified for intervention because they have no paid health care claims. Patients without prescription coverage cannot be targeted for pharmaceutical interventions. Supporting administrative claims data with survey data or chart audits enriches patient identification and will add cost to the program.

Conduction of a barrier analysis also assists in program development. A barrier analysis involves the identification of obstructions to program development or resources. This information allows the planner to understand these obstacles and develop a proactive plan to address them. Comprehending the barriers to program implementation at this point is also crucial. Disease management programs with misaligned incentives or those that lack physician, patient, or employer cooperation are difficult to implement successfully. Identification of alternatives within the program for discussion with key constituents may assist greatly with overcoming these barriers.

Once the population is defined, a pilot approach will allow a "test run" of the intervention, including perceptions of the program participants and health care providers. For example, during the planning of a program to encourage pregnant women on Medicaid to obtain early and consistent prenatal care, focus groups might be held with women in their second pregnancies to determine the educational materials, appointment adherence rewards, and program barriers to patient implementation. Their helpful and constructive feedback would allow for changes in proposed printed materials and program processes before community implementation. A similar approach might be used with the high-volume obstetrical offices that assess operational processes in the physician's or midwife's practice.

Determining what type and format of patient education materials to be used is also essential. Most purchased or self-developed disease management programs offer mailed educational materials to assist consumers in learning more about a particular aspect of their condition. Some programs have developed web sites with educational materials, self-assessments, or hyperlinks to national organizations to assist patients. Telemedicine, interactive voice response programs, software programs, interactive laser disks, CD ROM materials, and other types of media continue to enter this market. Demand management companies offer outbound phone calls to at-risk members providing reminders, education, and support. Whatever the method chosen, the material must be understandable to the patient, be in concert with published national standards or guidelines, offer resources for additional information, and, if necessary, be approved by governmental agencies if provided to Medicare or Medicaid patients.

Some programs offer educational group sessions. Group educational sessions should use tested curricula that have been reviewed by health care providers and patients. Many national organizations such as the American Diabetes Association or the American Lung Association offer educational programs for patients and their families. Information about program availability, cost, location, and frequency of program offerings should be validated before distribution. A discussion with the agency is also helpful to review common goals, operational issues such as program promotion and attendance increases, the possibility of discounts, and a plan for data collection to assist with outcome evaluation. Some managed care plans have negotiated discounts or reduced rates for their members. Others offer rebates when a patient has completed a self-help course.

Consumer testing and validation of program incentives are helpful. Individuals and groups differ as to what is valued. What is acceptable to a pregnant woman on Medicaid may be different from what is appreciated by a Medicare patient with a chronic condition. In addition, the acceptability of incentives or prizes to the population, the providers, and any governmental regulations will affect the use of rewards.

If the planned disease management intervention also includes individual case management of high-risk members, planning for these resources in advance is also required. As more patients and health care providers become aware of the program, referrals for individual case management will increase. Some of these referrals will be for patients who are truly at-risk for complications or increased health care utilization. Other referrals will be for patients who desire additional information or resources to better self-manage their condition. Knowing the program goals and available resources and developing a plan to assist consumers who want to enhance their self-management will allow the case manager to blend the roles of disease management implementation with individual case management.

IMPLEMENTATION OF THE PROGRAM

If planning is everything, implementation is the icing on the cake. Well-planned programs with pilots allow developers to test interventions and their acceptability to the consumer and health care provider before full population implementation. Pre-testing instruments, determining readability of the consumer materials, developing processes for distributing materials or gathering data, and assessing practitioner acceptability of the program should all be completed. Implementation serves as a time of continuous quality improvement, making program adjustments as needed with a clear vision of the outcomes expected and desired.

One practitioner intervention may be the distribution of clinical practice guidelines. As has been widely published, national guidelines often need modifications for acceptability to local practitioners. At the implementation stage, these guidelines will be distributed to care providers beyond the program champions, developers, or provider test groups.

There are many benefits to using clinical practice guidelines, including the distillation of relevant scientific literature and national standards into a document that supports evidence-based practice, and identification of specific patients for interventions and practical recommendations for care management. Practice guidelines also allow the establishment of key intervention points and outcome measures to reduce variability in care.

Guidelines include challenges and controversy. Practitioners may be unreceptive to "cookbook" medicine, be concerned about the legal implications, or debate the content or literature used to substantiate their development. Practical aids such as profiling systems, reminder letters, or patient education materials that support guideline parameters, removal of barriers to care access, and office supports such as reminder stickers or check sheets are valuable supports to the disease management program goals.

Guidelines like those used in disease management programs are never stagnant. A scheduled annual or semi-annual review of their recommendations and usefulness is essential to their implementation and ongoing credibility with practitioners. Guideline success is built on access to ongoing evidence-based practice information, patient management tools, reliable data and evaluation parameters, continuing reminders about the guidelines, and their intended patient care outcomes and clinician involvement in the development, dissemination, and evolution of this practice tool.

EVALUATION OF THE DISEASE MANAGEMENT PROGRAM

Process and outcome measures for the disease management program should be determined at the development and planning phase and be based on program goals. A multi-dimensional approach to evaluating the disease management program is integral to assessing program efficacy and effectiveness.

In 1997 the National Committee on Quality Assurance (NCQA) released its first data using the Quality Compass 1997, a database containing performance, accreditation, and patient satisfaction information from more than 300 managed health plans throughout the United States. The concept of the Quality Compass 1997 is based on the use of standard measures and tools to assess specific aspects of care and service throughout managed care plans. This model provides the opportunity to assess care globally across many managed care plans and has relevance to other care delivery sites.

The Clinical Value Compass (Figure 6-2) was developed to assess quality evaluation in clinical settings. Using Donabedian's constructs of structure, process, and outcome, "the logic underpinning the compass is that providers will measure the value of care for similar patient populations, analyze the internal delivery processes that contribute significantly to the current levels of measured outcomes and costs, run tests of changed delivery processes and determine if these changes lead to better outcomes" (Nelson, Mohr, Batalden, & Plume, 1996, p. 246). The four poles of the compass represent member satisfaction, functional status, cost associated with care, and clinical status.

The applicability of the compass directions to measure program outcomes can be used within managed care plans, physician offices, integrated delivery systems, or employer-developed disease management programs. The Clinical Value Compass approach has four cardinal points: functional status, costs, satisfaction with care, and clinical outcomes. Based on outcomes management, this framework allows

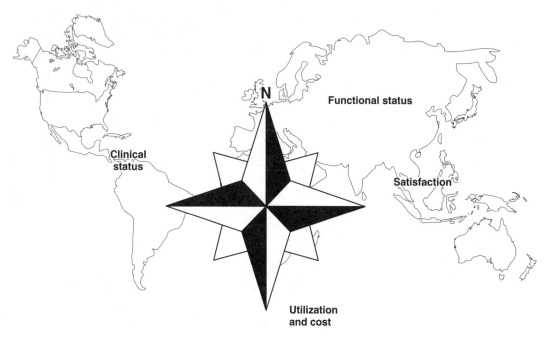

FIGURE **6-2**   Clinical value compass.

determination of specific results in each quadrant. These quadrants are representative of not only outcomes management but also the focus of health maintenance organizations, disease, or case management systems.

The directional points of the compass were developed through various research studies (Batalden & Stoltz, 1993; Batalden, Nelson, & Roberts, 1994; Nelson & Batalden, 1993; Nelson & Wasson, 1994). Functional status measures may include standardized instruments such as the Medical Outcomes Study Short Form 12 or 36 (Ware, Snow, Kosinski, & Gandek, 1993) or a quality of life measure specific to the program condition or disease process such as arthritis. Use of these types of tools allows comparison to other populations or published research. Instruments should be valid and reliable rather than homegrown to assure accurate measurement of the outcome. Permission to use the instrument must be obtained before use in order to comply with copyright regulations.

Patient satisfaction with the intervention is another measure that is part of the compass framework. Satisfaction surveys may measure participant satisfaction with the type of intervention they perceived they received, the amount of assistance offered by the intervention, and their satisfaction with their personal health outcome following the disease management intervention. Again, a standardized satisfaction survey that is found to be valid and reliable will serve as a measure of participant satisfaction.

Health care utilization can be measured through a pre- and post-test measure of service delivery. The number and cost of emergency room visits for a defined population of patients with asthma would be a utilization measure. Because of the seasonal or episodic variation of this illness as well as enrollment patterns within a managed care plan, continuous enrollment logic may be applied. To ensure accuracy and program evaluation over time, the selection of patients who have been constantly enrolled within the agency or health plan for 2 years will provide longitudinal data. The measurement would then include use of the emergency room for this population for 2 years before the intervention and for 2 years after the intervention. If a more timely measure is needed, the comparison of emergency room use within one spring allergy season to the following season may be used. When designing health care utilization measures, factor in any issues related to access that might affect this measure such as changes in co-payments, increased number of urgent care centers, or expanded primary care office hours.

Clinical outcome measures should also be thoughtfully chosen before intervention. For example, increased retinal eye examinations may be a process measure to the outcome measures of diabetic retinopathy as a complication of blindness. The timelines of the measure, as well as the access to data that may not be available for several years, must be considered as clinical outcome measures are chosen.

Another clinical measure may include a standardized HEDIS measure. HEDIS allows consumers and employers to compare performance across the managed care industry; to publish national, regional and state averages; and to establish benchmarks for care and service measures. The incorporation of an HEDIS measure would allow evaluators to compare findings across their own data and to benchmarks.

Two aspects of financial measures must be considered for the final pole of the compass framework. One measure is the health care costs affected through the disease management program intervention. For example, one might measure the costs associated with the emergency room visits in the previous example about the asthma disease management program. To determine this, elements such as copayments, negotiated rates for emergency room care, cost of medications, and treatments or professional services given in the emergency room would all be calculated into the pre- and post-intervention calculations.

When calculating the total program return on investment include all aspects of expenditures to support the program. A basic return on investment model will assist with the program analysis. Understanding the definitions of various types of costs and benefits such as direct versus indirect, fixed versus variable, and hard versus soft will assist with program calculations. "The use of an actual cost model is the most accurate and sophisticated accounting method; many health systems lack this advanced accounting capabilities" (Doxtator & Rodriguez, 1998, p. 189).

From the cost of the initial data extraction to target the population to the final measures based on the compass framework, accounting for costs is essential to a true analysis of return on investment. The collection of data to capture decreases and increases in utilization and revenue, ongoing program support costs, "soft" estimates, and initial program investment over periods of time, including the baseline and annually throughout the life of the program, are necessary. Determining the payback period is recommended. Because of the seasonal nature of some conditions, garnering physician buy-in to the program as well as patient enrollment, a 3-year payback period is often recommended. Assistance from the financial and quality analysts will be important to extract the financial costs and contrast them to the savings related to health care utilization and costs.

HEALTH MANAGEMENT FOR THE FUTURE

Disease management programs tend to be developed and proliferate where an over-supply of physicians or hospitals exist. Because of increased competition and demand from employers, the health care systems that focus on outcomes and can deliver these quality improvement changes initiate programs to meet these requirements. Often when the reimbursement structure changes to capitation or a set fee per patient, disease management programs will be instituted to promote education, self-help, and shift costly care to the most appropriate, cost-effective site of care. Some or all of these elements exist wherever health care is administered. Disease management program development is based on knowledge of the condition, finding the right population for information and self-management, aligning provider and patient incentives for care, developing information systems to allow sharing data and care across the continuum, and focusing on prevention.

While disease management will continue to be present as long as there are chronic conditions, health management will focus on chronically ill populations as well as healthy groups. Health promotion programs have long been the cornerstone of nursing. Optimal care for populations can be achieved through nursing leadership in the development, implementation, evaluation, and reimbursement for population-based health management.

References

Batalden, P.B., Nelson, E.C., & Roberts, J.S. (1994). Linking outcome measurement to continual improvement: The serial "V" way of thinking about improving clinical care. *The Joint Commission Journal of Quality Improvement, 20*(4), 167-180.

Batalden, P.B., & Stoltz, P.K. (1993). A framework for the continual improvement of health care: Building and applying professional and improvement knowledge to test changes in daily work. *The Joint Commission Journal of Quality Improvement, 19*(10), 424-447.

Deering, M.J. (1996). Consumer health information demand and delivery: Implications for libraries. *Bulletin of the Medical Library Association, 84*(2), 209-216.

Doxtator, R.F., & Rodriguez, D.J. (1998). Evaluating costs, benefits, and return on investment for disease management programs. *Disease Management, 1*(4), 185-192.

Eichert, J.H., & Patterson, R.B. (1998). Factors affecting the success of disease management. *The Journal of Oncology Management, 9*(1), 15-18.

Ichter, J.T. (1998). The link between disease management and capitation contracting: Financing population health. *Disease Management, 1*(1), 27-30.

Langley, P.C., Langley-Hawthorne, C.E., Martin, R.E., & Armstrong, E.P. (1996). Establishing the basis for successful disease management. *The American Journal of Managed Care, 2*(8), 1099-1108.

Lumsdon, K. (1995). Hard labor. *Hospitals & Health Networks, 69*(13), 34-42.

Matthews, P. (1999). Case management information systems: How to piece together now and beyond year 2000. *Nursing Case Management, 4*(2), 80-89.

National Committee for Quality Assurance. (January, 1997). *HEDIS 3.0—Health Plan Employer Data Information Set.* Washington, D.C.: National Committee for Quality Assurance.

National Committee for Quality Assurance. (October, 1997). *The state of managed care quality,* Press release: Washington, D.C.: American Association of Health Plans.

Nelson, E.C., & Batalden, P.B. (1993). Patient based quality improvement measurement systems. *Quality Management in Health Care, 21*(1), 18-30.

Nelson, E.C., Mohr, J.J., Batalden, P.B., & Plume, S.K. (1996). Improving health care, Part 1: The clinical value compass. *The Joint Commission Journal on Quality Improvement, 99*(4), 243-256.

Nelson, E.C., & Wasson, J.H. (1994). Using patient-based information to rapidly redesign care. *Healthcare Forum, 37*(4):25-29.

Peterson, K.W., & Kane, D.P. (1997). Beyond disease management: Population based health management. In W.E. Todd & D. Nash (Eds.), *Disease management—A systems approach to improving patient care* (pp. 305-346). Chicago: American Hospital Publishing Co.

Todd, W.E., & Nash, D. (1997). *Disease management—A systems approach to improving patient outcomes.* Chicago: American Hospital Publishing Co.

Toscani, M.R., & Patterson, R. (1995). Evaluating and creating effective patient education programs. *Drug Benefit Trends, 7*(9):36-39.

Ware, J.E., Snow, K.K., Kosinski, M., & Gandek, B. (1993). *SF-36 Health survey manual and interpretation guide.* Boston: The Health Institute, New England Medical Center.

Zitter, M. (1994). *The Zitter Group special report: Disease management.* San Francisco: The Zitter Group.

III

CONTEMPORARY MODELS OF CASE MANAGEMENT— WITHIN-THE-WALLS CASE MANAGEMENT

To become more responsive to the mandates of managed care environments and a rapidly changing health care system, new generations of acute care–based case management models have unfolded. Unit III offers a portrait of the many rich and varied models that have evolved across the country. These models have at their core the principles of interdisciplinary cooperation, relationship building, active communication, comprehensive support for continued health care needs, and client and family advocacy. These approaches speak to the contributions of all providers to maintaining the health of the public.

Within-the-Walls Case Management

An Acute Care-Based Nursing Case Management Model

CHAPTER OVERVIEW

This chapter reviews various models of within-the-walls case management. This approach became popular when hospitals began restructuring to improve productivity, manage effective use of resources, lower costs, and maintain quality.

Preliminary findings show that this patient care delivery model can have a great effect on resource use and quality patient care. Daily assessment and evaluation of the patient's clinical care, reduced length of stay and other financial benefits, general applicability of this model, and improved nurse, physician, and patient satisfaction demonstrate the merit and relevancy of this approach to patient care delivery and professional practice.

COST-EFFECTIVE CARE

The changing nature of health care economics has forced hospitals to view case management as an alternative to the delivery of direct care services. Hospital-based case management is founded on traditional approaches. It ensures the most appropriate use of services by patients. A case management system in the hospital setting avoids duplication and misuse of medical services, controls costs by reducing inefficient services, and improves the effectiveness of care delivery (Lavizzo-Mourey, 1987). Lavizzo-Mourey (1987), McIntosh (1987), and Henderson and Collard (1988) reported several advantages of hospital-based case management. First, the hospital setting offers a wide range of specialized skills that can be made available to both the provider and recipient of case management services. Second, because most of the resources needed for patient care are centralized within the acute care setting, early assessment of patient needs, planning and coordination of care delivery, and evaluation of alternative systems are enhanced. Third, because space and overhead costs are factored into hospital-based care, the management of expenditures associated with high-cost patients is minimized. Fourth, systems for monitoring and measuring the cost-effectiveness of case management arrangements are present within the hospital setting.

Many hospital-based case management systems have engaged registered nurses (RNs) as case managers (Henderson & Collard, 1988; Henderson & Wallack, 1987; McIntosh, 1987). Nurse involvement in case management allows nurses to influence and direct the delivery and quality of patient care. Such involvement allows for more control, visibility, and recognition for nursing services delivered. The involvement also offers more consistent outcome attainment and demonstrates nursing personnel contributions to patient care (Zander, 1988a).

Because it would be virtually impossible to cover all patient models of nursing case management that may currently exist, this chapter will focus on some of the systems that have served as the foundation for the development of within-the-walls case management. The chapter also highlights those approaches to patient care delivery and professional practice that have received national attention.

PRIMARY NURSE CASE MANAGEMENT MODEL

Nursing case management has emerged in the acute care setting as a professional model of practice. One model, characterized as a primary nurse case management model, has been used at the New England Medical Center in Boston, Massachusetts. Stetler (1987), Woldum (1987), and Zander (1988a, 1988b, 1990) have identified the following factors that distinguish this case management system of care.

Primary nurse case management is based on the concept of managed care. Managed care is defined as care that is unit based, outcome oriented, dependent on a designated time frame, and focused on the appropriate use of resources for both the inpatient and outpatient populations.

Primary nurse case management services and caseloads are designated for specific patient case types or case mixes. Some examples of case types coordinated by primary nurse case management are cardiac, leukemia, pediatric, gastrointestinal, stroke, craniotomy, and some gynecological.

Nursing case managers are the primary caregivers for patients. The managers provide direct care to patients in their caseloads while the patients are housed in their units, and they continue to coordinate the care of these patients throughout hospitalization, regardless of the patient's physical location.

The process of care is monitored by the use of case management plans, which include DRG length of stay; critical path reports, which outline the components of appropriate care; and variance analysis, which ensures the continuous evaluation of patient care activities.

Care is coordinated through collaborative group practice arrangements across geographic units, case consultation, and health care team meetings. Patient discharge planning is outlined before admission and updated throughout hospitalization until the time of discharge.

The New England Medical Center's nursing case management model presents an innovative alternative to the delivery of nursing care within the acute care setting. The model has evolved since its introduction and has been widely adapted.* The development of care multidisciplinary action plans (MAPs) increases the potential for evaluating the cost-effectiveness and quality of care standards proposed by this model. Care MAPS have expanded on case management plans and critical paths by focusing on standards of care and practice for a specific case type, responding to variances in the delivery of care, linking continuous quality improvement (CQI) to practices, and integrating resource allocation, patient care outcomes, and cost reimbursement systems (Zander, 1991, 1992a, 1992b).

The competence and experience of the case manager are critical to the effective delivery of patient care services (Henderson & Wallack, 1987). The case management model at the New England Medical Center, along with most nurse case management programs, primarily uses RNs as case managers. A case manager must have at least 1 year of nursing experience and charge responsibilities and must demon-

---

*Conceptually, case management is now considered a strategy for the coordination of care and is evolving into a sophisticated resource for managing access, quality, and cost (Bower & Falk, 1996).

strate leadership ability. Henderson and Wallack (1987) and Henderson and Collard (1988) recommend that to ensure cost-effective care and quality assurance standards, the nurse case manager should have expertise related to the care of designated types of patients and specific diagnostic categories. Because of the model's reliance on a primary nursing care delivery system, staffing mix allocation was not differentiated in the New England Medical Center's model. Some case management programs have successfully employed a variety of personnel other than professional nursing staff. Studies are needed to determine the best staffing mix for nursing case management programs.

Contrary to what Zander (1990) reported about the nursing case management model at the New England Medical Center, a study in another institution has shown a preliminary increase in direct nursing care hours and greater use of resources during the initial phase of hospitalization. These changes resulted in an overall decrease in length of stay, an increase in patient turnover, and a potential increase in patient revenues generated for the hospital (Cohen, 1991).

LEVELED PRACTICE MODEL

Another nursing case management model, identified as the leveled practice model, has focused on the management and coordination of patient care needs. This system differs from the primary nurse case management model in that the case manager's functions are focused on the management activities of patient care and not on the responsibility for patient care delivery (Loveridge, Cummings, & O'Malley, 1988; O'Malley & Cummings, 1988). A work group consisting of RNs, licensed practical nurses, and nurses' aides provides direct care on a specific patient unit. The professional nurse is designated as the case manager and is responsible for coordinating and monitoring patient care of an assigned caseload through collaboration with the work group, patient, family, and interdisciplinary health team members. In addition, the case manager relies on information related to case mix, hospital costs, patient resource use, insurance, and reimbursement data (O'Malley & Cummings, 1988).

The leveled case management model has promoted differentiated practice arrangements by delineating functional role responsibility and accountability between those nurses with baccalaureate degrees and those with associate degrees (Loveridge et al., 1988). Differentiated competence levels in nursing practice were classified extensively by Primm (1986). Because of the principles inherent in leveled practice case management, the role of the professional staff nurse becomes an autonomous one. Consequently, this change in practice places different obligations on the nurse manager. The nurse manager's role becomes what MacGregor-Burns (1978) described as transformational leadership, which focuses on teaching, mentoring, and coaching activities. In the leveled practice nursing case management model, management responsibility emphasized overall administrative and fiscal support, as well as patient outcome assessment and quality care improvement (Loveridge et al., 1988; O'Malley & Cummings, 1988).

PRIMARY CASE MANAGEMENT

The primary case management model, which was developed and implemented at Hermann Hospital in Houston, embraced the primary nursing philosophy of care and used a clinical career ladder for RNs (Cavouras et al., 1990). The clinical ladder consisted of six levels of clinical expertise, which progressed from a patient-focused orientation at the beginning levels to interdisciplinary and general service practice responsibility and accountability as nurse case managers at the top level.

The primary case management model used unit-based case managers who were responsible for coordinating, developing, and evaluating the delivery and the quality of patient care. Staff nurses and nurse extenders provided the care, which was based on standard protocols. The care plans outlined the daily care requirements and activities and served as a mechanism for monitoring and evaluating issues related to quality and as a patient care resource for nursing and hospital-wide support services such as laboratory, pharmacy, and respiratory therapy. Quality improvement was also monitored through unit-based quality assurance programs.

Cost-effectiveness, quality of care, and nurses' job satisfaction were also evaluated through retrospective variance analysis of patient charges and length of hospital stay, quality-assurance monitoring, and nurse satisfaction surveys. To date, no data have been published.

SAINT VINCENTS HOSPITAL AND MEDICAL CENTER INTEGRATED CASE MANAGEMENT MODEL

Case management models in the late 1990s are beginning to reflect the need to integrate previously disconnected services. Saint Vincents Hospital and Medical Center in New York City designed and implemented an integrated design model in 1997. The model integrates three functions of the case manager under one umbrella. These include the clinical coordination/facilitation role of the case manager, utilization management, and discharge planning. Each acute care case manager is unit based and performs these interrelated functions for all patients on the unit to which they are assigned. In the past, each of these functions was performed by a separate care provider. This fragmentation resulted in higher cost, longer length of stay, and an inefficient system.

To make the system more efficient and more responsive to a managed care environment, a number of structural changes were made. These included a redefinition of the functions listed above with a re-alignment of the functions under the role of the case manager. This more streamlined approach to care delivery resulted in a more efficient, integrated care delivery process and reduced the need to "pass the baton" from one team member to the next.

Case managers use guidelines and multidisciplinary action plans as tools in the clinical coordination/ facilitation aspect of their role (see Appendix 7-1). The guidelines delineate the appropriate resources and length of stay for various case types. The case managers are responsible for collecting variations from the guidelines as part of their daily variance collection process. Other variances collected identify system delays and clinical issues, quality issues, and unmet clinical outcomes.

The data are reviewed daily, and individual issues are addressed. The data are also aggregated and reviewed for potential quality improvement efforts. For example, magnetic resonance imaging (MRI) delays are collected in four categories that identify the cause of the delay:

Delays related to scheduling
Delays related to lack of weekend availability
Delays related to unavailable reports
Delays related to equipment failure

Repetitive, substantive delays are addressed in terms of the cause of the problem and potential solutions. An interdisciplinary team is often assembled to address the problem and develop an action plan for correcting the problem.

In the role of clinical coordinator and facilitator, a number of functions may be performed. Among these are development of the interdisciplinary plan of care and expediting diagnostic testing and treatments as identified by the plan of care. This clinical focus fosters a partnership with the physicians and other members of the health care team. It allows the case manager to identify and suggest opportunities to deliver care more efficiently and/or at lower cost.

The case managers are also responsible for performing utilization management functions. This includes using established review criteria such as the Milliman and Robertson Guidelines (1997) to perform insurance reviews. They are in daily communication with the third party payer and work to assure that the hospital gets reimbursed for every day that the patient is in the acute care setting. Services are reviewed to ensure that they are medically necessary and reasonable, provided in the most appropriate setting, and at or above quality standards.

Discharge planning functions were moved from under the responsibility of social work to the responsibility of the registered nurse case manager. This required a redefinition of the role of the social worker from one of discharge planning *coordinator* to discharge planning *collaborator*. Social workers were redeployed to perform other, more comprehensive social work functions such as those listed below:

Counseling and psychosocial support
Coping with end-stage-of-life issues
Substance abuse
Financial issues
Family support issues

Case managers perform the initial assessment and refer patients to the social worker based on high-risk screening criteria developed for specific clinical areas. For example, medical/surgical has their specific list of criteria, while the emergency department has a different list of criteria (see Table 7-1). The coordination function of discharge planning is performed by the RN case manager.

In an effort to better manage the routes of entry to the hospital, case managers are also assigned to the emergency and admitting departments. The case managers in the emergency department review all potential admissions for appropriateness and make referrals to outside agencies when needed. Their initial case management assessment is made and included as part of the in-hospital patient documentation on all admitted patients. The care processes of treat and release patients are expedited by the case manager and through the use of emergency department clinical practice guidelines that differentiate the appropriate interventions and time frames for treating various emergency conditions.

The case manager in the admitting department performs parallel functions. She reviews all planned admissions and transfers for appropriateness. She also performs a case management assessment on surgical patients in pre-admission testing. This documentation and a preliminary discharge plan is transferred electronically to the unit-based case manager. The collaborative effort performed by the admitting and emergency department case managers helps prevent inappropriate or unnecessary admissions and assures that the patient is receiving the care needed in the most appropriate setting.

The design of the case management model at Saint Vincents connects three role functions that had been disconnected in the previous care delivery system. This integrated approach reduces redundancy, duplication, and delays. Within the first year of implementation, the hospital achieved its target goal length of stay reduction of 1.1 days. Insurance denials were reduced by 30% in medical/surgical and 80% in psychiatry. Patient complaints regarding discharge planning and communication of the plan of care were reduced by 20%.

┃ TUCSON MEDICAL CENTER CASE MANAGEMENT MODEL

JoAnne Woodall

Past

A case management model developed at Tucson Medical Center (TMC) addressed the cost and quality aspects of patient care delivery (Del Togno-Armanasco, Olivas, & Harter 1989). This approach incorporated elements of the New England Medical Center's case management model and differentiated

Table 7-1	**GUIDELINES FOR REFERRALS** **RN Case Managers/Social Workers Medical/Surgical** **In-Patient Adult Services**

RN CASE MANAGER	**SOCIAL WORKER**
• Performs admission and concurrent utilization management, including insurance calls • Coordinates/facilitates plans of care • Facilitates daily rounds and team meetings • Assessments of all patients for psychosocial needs • Discharge planning, including equipment, home care, rehabilitation, and long-term care facilities • Orders transportation • Completes PRIs • Oversight of clinical guidelines • Tracks data (e.g., variances in patient care and systems standards) • Provides ALC notification • Issues HINN Letters	• Patient/family difficulty coping with new diagnosis (e.g., cancer, ventilator dependency, difficulty understanding/accepting decision making the long-term discharge planning options) • Psychiatric, cognitive, or behavioral factors that may impede delivery of care and discharge planning process • Inadequate supports that may impact on compliance with continuing care needs (NOTE: Social workers can provide case managers with information to give to patients and families, concerning entitlements) • Ethical or legal concerns (e.g., patient, family, team conflicts related to medical plan of care, guardianship cases or end-of-life issues around advance directives, DNR) • Suspicion or evidence of domestic violence, elder abuse or neglect, child abuse or neglect, rape, or sexual assault; known to protective services for adults (PSA) • Substance abuse counseling referrals where patient requests or is viewed as amenable to intervention • The unidentified patient or patients are seriously ill and there is difficulty locating significant others • Patients signing out against medical advice (AMA) (the hospital's AMA policy is currently under review) • Homelessness (e.g., new onset, patient is unable to return to prior living situation) • Long-term nursing facility placements for patients with complex family or financial situations

Courtesy *St. Vincents Hospital and Medical Center,* New York, New York, Revised 5/99.

practice models in addition to basic philosophic practice components of primary nursing and shared governance.

Called collaborative nursing case management, this model primarily focused on standardizing the use of patient care resources and the delivery of services during the patient's hospitalization for selected DRG case types. Both patient mix and service volume management strategies were used to attain cost-effective, quality patient care (Olivas et al., 1989a).

A collaborative case management plan (CCMP) and a care plan MAP were used to identify the contributions of all health care providers and support a unit-specific standard of patient care. Variations

	SHARED RESPONSIBILITIES: RN CASE MANAGER/SOCIAL WORKER	
RN CASE MANAGER		**SOCIAL WORKER**
• Admission utilization review: intake assessment of admitted patients • Utilization/insurance calls • Coordinate/facilitate plans of care for admitted patients • Screening/assessments of patients for psychosocial needs in conjunction with plan of care • Discharge planning, including equipment, home care, infusion treatment • Initiate in-patient discharge planning • Participates in the development of emergency department guidelines for care • Track data (e.g., variances in patient care standards, systems standards) • Clinical resource for staff • Facilitates patients' progress through the emergency department to disposition • Oversees/facilitates transfers from institution to institution	• Coordinate/facilitate plans of care for discharged patients • Transportation • Patient education (e.g., reinforcement regarding follow-up with medical appointments, medical regimen) • Crisis intervention needed for patient/family having difficulty coping with illness, family dysfunction, trauma, death, accidents, injuries, substance abuse • Referrals for nursing homes, adult homes, shelters	• Patient/family having difficulty understanding/accepting and/or following through on medical plans of care and continuing care options • Interventions regarding issues impacting access to continuum of care (e.g., immigration problem, primary caregiver or disabled person) • Advocacy and counseling around entitlements or other essential services (e.g., Medicaid, Food Stamps, housing, medications) • Suspicion or evidence of domestic violence, elder abuse or neglect, child abuse or neglect, sexual assault • Ethical or legal concerns (e.g., patient, family, team conflicts related to medical plan of care, guardianship or PSA cases, end of life issues around advance directives) • Referrals for home supports for psychosocially complex patients • Referrals needed for marital, individual, or family treatment • Assistance needed in locating families of unidentified, seriously ill patients • Tracking of difficult-to-locate patients for follow-up medical care

Table 7-1 ▶ **GUIDELINES FOR REFERRALS**
RN Case Managers/Social Workers Medical/Surgical In-Patient Adult Services—cont'd

from practice standards are also monitored and evaluated. The care plan MAP was revised in 1991 to meet requirements of the Joint Commission on Accreditation of Healthcare Organizations (Gwozdz & Del Togno-Armanasco, 1992). It was also used as a basic documentation form.

Hospital-wide and unit-specific multidisciplinary practice committees were established to assist in clinical decision making and overall evaluation processes of the patient care model. These groups consisted of physical therapists, dietitians, social workers, physicians, and home care professionals (Olivas et al., 1989b). Patients were encouraged to participate and were included in the planning of their care regimens, which are carried out on a continuous basis from the time of admission to after discharge.

Various evaluation mechanisms were developed to measure the potential impact of this case management model on outcomes of care. A patient satisfaction questionnaire and a retrospective chart review were implemented along with a physician-satisfaction-with-care questionnaire to ascertain variables related to patient care and job satisfaction. Information on cost of care, rate of absenteeism, and staff turnover also were collected. Findings showed increased satisfaction with both nursing and medical care (at the .05 alpha level) for case-managed, total hip replacement, coronary bypass, and valvular surgery patients. There was no turnover of nurse case managers, and a marked decrease in turnover rates was demonstrated for nursing staff on the oncology and orthopedic units.

Outcome data also showed a decreased length of stay among patients who underwent total hip and knee replacements. The decrease was 3.48 and 2.82 days, respectively, over a 3 1/2 -year period. Length of stay for valvular replacement and coronary bypass patients also decreased. In addition, a positive cost variance of $9,273 was realized for the valvular replacement and coronary bypass patient populations (Del Togno-Armanasco, 1992).

As noted, case management of TMC started as a unit-based nursing clinical model. Within a short time, notable success was demonstrated in the areas of satisfaction and cost savings. Lengths of stay decreased, costs diminished, and patient and physician satisfaction increased. When case management was initiated, TMC had a department of Patient and Family Services made up of social workers who did discharge planning, crisis counseling, and medical-legal intervention on a consulting basis. Additionally, the Department of Utilization Management (UM), made up of nurses, performed the required utilization review and utilization management functions. These departments co-existed and interfaced with case management. It became apparent that these departments were frequently involved with the same patients, the same charts, and the same issue. The resulting redundancy offered an opportunity for improvement.

Present

In 1996, in response to efforts to maximize efficiency and reduce redundancy, a number of significant changes were made. The unit-based case managers were centralized into a case management team (CMT) led by a steering committee of administrative leaders, director of budget and finance, and vice president for patient care. The Department of Patient and Family Services soon became part of this team, combining the social workers and nurse case managers into the same centralized department. UM was downsized to two nurses, and these nurses were also moved into the CMT. UM functions became part of the nurse case manager's role, with the designated UM nurses doing education and oversight for this function. The net result of these moves was to create one department with a net savings of FTE's.

The decision to combine these specialties into one department was grounded in solid rationale. Both social workers and nurse case managers use the tools of expert assessment, planning, coordination, and communication to do effective and timely discharge planning. This facilitates early discharge by eliminating delays for nonmedical reasons and ensuring a safe discharge with a plan in place to meet the patient's continuum health care needs. Recognizing that both medical and social complexity can contribute to extended lengths of stay and recidivism, the expertise of the nurse case manager and the social worker can each be used to greatest advantage, depending on the predominant risk factors presented by individual patients.

Similarly, both UM nurses and nurse case managers are involved in ensuring appropriate level of care, expediting the medical plan of care by eliminating system barriers, and ensuring accountability for utilization of expensive and finite resources. Both of these roles require review of the chart, communication with the physician, and coordination with payers to ensure reimbursement for services. Clearly, the roles of nurse case manager, social worker, and utilization management (UM) have significant areas of overlap (Del Togno-Armanesco et al, 1995). It is also apparent that the goals of each specialty are the same—to meet the health needs of the patient in the most effective and resource-efficient way.

Combining departments that share the same goals and many of the same functions seems like an obvious path to increased efficiency. However, bringing people together into the same department does not ensure the successful creation of a functional team. The literature is full of examples of territory conflict between nurse and social worker case managers. The difficulty in combining the roles of UM nurse and nurse case manager is also well documented (McKenzie, 1989; Hospital Case Management, 1996). The merging of these groups requires a change in identity, clarity of purpose, flexibility, and a high level of trust and willingness to learn. As TMC moved forward to make these changes, the following barriers were identified:

1. No unified model for case management was in place throughout the system.
2. The case managers frequently operated in isolation from each other and developed many procedures and processes that differed from one area to another. This was frequently confusing for physicians and other staff and impaired the smooth transition of patients from one unit to the next and from one case manager to the next. Case managers receiving patients from another area frequently felt as though they were "re-inventing the wheel" because elements of the case management plan were lost and patients were subjected to redundant assessments and intakes.
3. Social workers were redefined as case managers when they joined the case management team, but for the most part continued to function as social work consultants, much as they had in the past. Nurse case managers and social workers triaged tasks rather than designating patients to their respective case loads based on either medical or social risk criteria.
4. Nurse case managers verbalized that they viewed UM as another task to be added to that which they already did. They were resistant to letting go of clinical functions, which they knew, liked, and valued, to make room for the utilization review/utilization management function. The UM nurses, on the other hand were uncomfortable letting go of their UM/UR responsibilities to the case managers, who did not value them in the same way, and verbalized their concern that the quality of UM was diminishing.
5. The members of the new CMT did not feel or function like a team. They were various pieces put together for organizational purposes. Their comfort level with their jobs as they knew them was threatened. They were expected to do new things in a different way, but were unsure how to go about it or even if they wanted to.

The challenge at TMC was to overcome the barriers and emerge with a unified and highly functional CMT, fully utilizing the tremendous resources of knowledge, expertise, and experience brought to the group by each of the specialties. The expected outcomes were to enhance the effectiveness of all of the group members by sharing and expanding skill sets and to more successfully and efficiently promote the goals of case management and the organization.

The following strategies were employed to overcome barriers and accomplish the outcomes:

1. Clearly define a mission and purpose statement for the CMT that directly supports the overall vision and goals of the organization (Appendix 7-2).
2. Develop a model for case management that incorporates nursing, social work, and UM into one cohesive team.
3. Define and differentiate core case management functions common to all of the team members and specialty case management functions that belong to the expertise of each specialty area (Appendix 7-3).
4. Write job descriptions for nurse case manager, social worker case manager, and UM case manager that clearly reflect the above functions and competencies.
5. Develop a model by which patients are triaged either to the nurse or social worker case manager, depending on medical or social high-risk criteria (*Appendix 7-4*). This model was developed through a process of defining medical and social high-risk criteria for case management of inpatients. It is acknowledged that patients are at risk for high-cost/high-utilization care for reasons that relate to medical complexity as well as social complexity. High-risk patients are designated to the caseload of the nurse or social work case manager, whichever is most qualified to deal with the identified issues.

For patients with both medical and social complexities, the social worker and nurse collaborate and consult.

6. Offer continuing education opportunities on case management topics. The case management team compiled a list of educational requests and needs. This list was used as a springboard to develop a staff development calendar, using internal and external experts to present information on designated topics at biweekly meetings. The TMC case management team also cooperated with the Southern Arizona Chapter of Case Management Society of America (CMSA) to offer a preparatory course for the CCM exam. An on-site case management seminar was brought to TMC and attended by all of the CMT.

7. Have biweekly team meetings to discuss issues, celebrate successes, process decisions, and share information. CMT staff meetings are held on weeks alternating with the staff development presentations. These meetings give opportunities for disseminating organizational information, discussing case management issues, communicating projects and successes of individuals and clinical clusters within the CMT, problem solving, and giving sub-team reports.

8. Develop case management processes that move with the patients across the lines of specialty units to create seamless flow and continuity and reduce redundancy. One of the identified goals of case management is to facilitate seamless patient movement through the system. Since the case manager is a critical communication link, the case management processes must reduce redundancy and ensure continuity. The key touch points identified are admission, transfer, and discharge. Case management assessment and communication forms and processes have been developed and standardized by the team to see that these touch points do not become gaps and that continuity and quality are protected.

9. Implement individualized learning plans for case managers having difficulty in role definition. Because of the inconsistencies in how case management originated in various clinical units at TMC, role definition was an obstacle for some of the case managers. In several instances, individualized re-orientation plans were created and implemented to assist case managers to more clearly define their role and function. These learning plans included mentoring, rotations with other case management specialists, and observational experiences with community case managers. This approach was very successful, and, in some cases, the recipients of this re-orientation opportunity are now functioning as mentors and role models for others.

10. Promote a case management identity, both for individual team members and for the team as a whole. On occasion, the case management team meeting is replaced by a potluck, where food and fun are the agenda. Team-building programs and human dynamics seminars have been developed and offered as a means of improving communication, appreciating differences, and working effectively as a group.

These strategies, employed in the past 6 months, have had measurable success. Some examples of this are 10 out of 15 of the top DRGs admitted to TMC have shown decreased lengths of stay since the nurse case managers have taken over the utilization function; social workers are called less frequently to the emergency room since nurse case managers have been staffed there; medical and social high-risk criteria are used to screen every patient and assign the appropriate nurse or social work case manager; one-third of the nurse case managers have national certification in case management; case management team members are taking responsibility for planning and presenting staff development programs for the rest of the team; and numerous process improvement projects are underway, including critical pathways and a readmissions project. These indicators of team success enhance the goals of cost and quality improvement, which are the ongoing objectives of case management.

References

Bower, K.A., & Falk, C.D. (1996). Case management as a response to quality, cost, and access imperatives In E. Cohen (Ed.), *Nurse case management in the 21st century* (pp. 161-167). St Louis: Mosby-Year Book, Inc.

Cavouras, C.A., Walts, L., Taylor, S., Garner, A., & Bordelon, P. (1990). Alternative delivery system: Primary case management. In G. Mayer, M. Madden, & E. Lawrenz (Eds.), *Patient care delivery models* (pp. 275-282), Rockville, Md.: Aspen Publishers, Inc.

Cohen, E. (1991). Nursing case management: Does it pay? *Journal of Nursing Administration, 21*(4), 20-25.

Del Togno-Armanasco, V. (1992). [Collaborative Case Management: Outcome data]. Unpublished raw data.

Del Togno-Armanasco, V., Olivas, G., & Harter, S. (1989). Developing an integrated nursing case management model. *Nursing Management, 20*(5), 26-29.

Del Togno-Armanasco, V., Hopkin, L., & Harter, S., (1995). How case management really works. *American Journal of Nursing* 24I-24L.

Doyle, R.L., & Schibanoff, J.M. (1997). Healthcare management guidelines, Vol. 1, Milliman & Robertson, Inc.

Gwozdz, D.T., & Del Togno-Armanasco, V. (1992). Developing an integrated nursing case management model. *Nursing Management, 20*(5), 26-29.

Henderson, M.G., & Collard, A. (1988). Measuring quality in medical case management programs. *Quality Review Bulletin, 14*(2), 33-39.

Henderson, M.G., & Wallack, S.S. (1987). Evaluating case management for catastrophic illness. *Business and Health, 4*(3), 741.

Lavizzo-Mourey, R. (1987). Hospital based case management. *DRG Monitor, 5*(1), 1-8.

Loveridge, C., Cummings, S., & O'Malley, J. (1988). Developing case management in a primary nursing system. *Journal of Nursing Administration, 18*(10), 36-39.

MacGregor-Burns, J. (1978). *Leadership.* New York: Harper & Row.

McClelland, M., & Foster, D. (1991). The Mercy Hospital, Port Huron Project. *Nursing Administration Quarterly, 15*(4), 58-60.

McIntosh, L. (1987). Hospital based case management. *Nursing Economics, 5*(5), 232-236.

McKenzie, C.B., Torkelson, N.G., & Holt, M.A. (1989) Care and cost: Nursing case management improves both. *Nursing Management* 90(1), 30-34.

Olivas, G., Del Togno-Armanasco, V., Erickson, J.R., & Harter, S. (1989a). Case management: A bottom-line care delivery model. Part 1: The concept. *Journal of Nursing Administration, 19*(11), 16-20.

Olivas, G., Del Togno-Armanasco, V., Erickson, J.R., & Harter, S. (1989b). Case management: A bottom-line care delivery model. Part 2: Adaptation of the model. *Journal of Nursing Administration, 19*(12), 12-17.

O'Malley, J., & Cummings, S. (1988). Nursing case management. 3: Implementing case management. *Aspen's Advisor for Nurse Executives, 3*(7), 8-9.

Primm, P.L. (1986). Entry into practice: Competency statements for BSNs and ADNs. *Nursing Outlook, 34*(3), 135-137.

Schifalacqua, M. (1992). Personal communication.

Should case managers absorb UR, discharge planning? (1996, October), *Hospital Case Management,* 145-148.

Sinnen, M.T., & Schifalacqua, M. (1991). Coordinated care in a community hospital. *Nursing Management, 22*(3), 38-42.

Stetler, C.B. (1987). The case manager's role: A preliminary evaluation. *Definition, 2*(3), 1-4.

Wesley, M.L., & Easterling, A. (1991). The St. Joseph Mercy Hospital, Pontiac Project. *Nursing Administration Quarterly, 15*(4), 50-54.

Woldum, K. (1987). Critical paths: Marking the course. *Definition, 2*(3), 1-4.

Zander, K. (1988a). Managed care within acute care settings: Design and implementation via nursing case management. *Health Care Supervisor, 6*(2), 24-43.

Zander, K. (1988b). Nursing care management: Strategic management of cost and quality outcomes. *Journal of Nursing Administration, 18*(5), 23-30.

Zander, K. (1990). Managed care and nursing case management (pp. 37-61). In G.G. Mayer, M.J. Madden, & E. Lawrenz (Eds.), *Patient care delivery models.* Rockville, Md. Aspen Publishers, Inc.

Zander, K. (1991, Fall). Care Maps TM: The core of cost/quality care. *The New Definition, 6*(3), 1-3.

Zander, K. (1992a, Winter). Physicians, Care Maps and collaboration. *The New Definition, 7*(1), 1-4.

Zander, K. (1992b, Spring). Quantifying, managing, and improving quality. 1: How Care Maps link CQI to the patient. *The New Definition, 1*(2), 1-3.

APPENDIX 7-1

Saint Vincents Hospital and Medical Center

MULTIDISCIPLINARY ACTION PLAN

Diagnosis: Carotid Stenosis

Procedure: Carotid Endarterectomy
- ☐ Left
- ☐ Right
- ☐ Bilateral

Date/Time of arrival on unit: _____

Anticipated length of stay (including day of surgery): 1 day

Case Manager: _____

Social Worker (if applicable): _____

Goals mutually set with patient and/or family:
Yes ☐
No ☐ Explain: _____

INITIALS	SIGNATURE/TITLE	INITIALS	SIGNATURE/TITLE

MAP009 7/98

SAINT VINCENTS HOSPITAL AND MEDICAL CENTER
MULTIDISCIPLINARY ACTION PLAN
DAY OF SURGERY
Procedure: Carotid Endarterectomy

MD: _____

RN: _____

Date: _____

MAP DOES NOT REPLACE MD ORDERS		NOTES
Tests/Procedures/ Treatments	Nursing assessment and A-line monitoring q1hr × 4-6 hr Maintain systolic BP > 100 & < 180. Discontinue A-line after 4-6 hrs if systolic BP stable. If stable and A-line D/C'd, nursing assessment q2hr × 6 & if stable then q4hr Complete nursing admission assessment. Notify MD if T≥101° Measure intake and output × 8 hr; D/C if urinary output sufficient. HOB ↑ 30° Incentive spirometer 10 × q1hr while awake.	
Medication:	IV - 1 liter _____ @ _____ cc/hr. D/C when stable & tolerating PO fluids. Demerol _____ mg. & Vistaril _____ mg. IM q3-4 hr PRN pain. When tolerating PO, Percocet 1-2 tab PO q3-4 hr PRN pain. ASA 325 mg. PO qd.	
Activity:	OOB to chair within 4 hr, then progressive ambulation as tolerated.	
Nutrition:	NPO until alert, then clear fluids. Advance to cardiac prudent diet as tolerated.	
Consults:		
Patient Education:	Assess, instruct, and evaluate re: • Unit orientation • Pain modalities • Post-operative preventive care Give and review carotid endarterectomy patient MAP, if not previously received.	
Social Work:	Psychosocial assessment and intervention, and D/C plan, as indicated	
Case Management:	Evaluate individual patient/family needs. Initiate referrals and consults, as indicated.	

SAINT VINCENTS HOSPITAL AND MEDICAL CENTER
MULTIDISCIPLINARY ACTION PLAN
DAY OF SURGERY
Procedure: Carotid Endarterectomy

MD: _____

RN: _____

Date: _____

PATIENT PROBLEM AND NURSING INTERVENTIONS	EXPECTED PATIENT OUTCOME AND/OR DISCHARGE OUTCOME	ASSESSMENT/EVALUATION		
Alteration in Body Systems	Complications will be Prevented/Minimized			
1. Nursing Assessment A. *Vital signs & neurovascular check* B. *A-line* C. *Assess orientation to person, place & time.* D. *Assess lung sounds & RR.* E. *Assess if neck dressing is intact, and/or for the presence of drainage/bleeding. HOB ↑ 30°.* F. *Palpate abdomen, noting distention or discomfort. Auscultate for bowel sounds. Assess presence or absence of nausea, vomiting and flatus. Advance diet.* G. *Assess bladder for distention.* H. *Assess circulation and mobility of extremities.* I. *Assess IV site for redness, edema, & Pain. Ascertain IV is patent & infusing.*	A. VS & neurovascular status WNL. B. Hemodynamically Stable. C. Oriented to person, place, & time D. Respirations unlabored & even; lungs clear. Using incentive spirometer, coughing and deep breathing. E. Neck dressing dry and intact. F. Abdomen soft, not distended. Minimal/No nausea/vomiting. Tolerating diet. G. No signs/symptom of complications. Voiding without difficulty. H. No signs/symptoms of complications. I. No signs/symptoms of complications. IV D/C'd when stable & tolerating fluids.	1. A. (Flow sheet) B. (Flow sheet) C. (Flow sheet) D. (Flow sheet) E. (Flow sheet) F. (Flow sheet) G. (Flow sheet) H. (Flow sheet) I. (Flow sheet)	1. A. (Flow sheet) B. (Flow sheet) C. (Flow sheet) D. (Flow sheet) E. (Flow sheet) F. (Flow sheet) G. (Flow sheet) H. (Flow sheet) I. (Flow sheet)	1. A. (Flow sheet) B. (Flow sheet) C. (Flow sheet) D. (Flow sheet) E. (Flow sheet) F. (Flow sheet) G. (Flow sheet) H. (Flow sheet) I. (Flow sheet)
Alteration in Comfort	Pain R/T Postoperative Period will be Prevented/Minimized			
1. Incisional pain: A. *Assess level of pain (use 1-10 pain scale).* B. *Administer pain medications.* C. *Assess effect of pain medication.* D. *Use comfort measures and diversional measures.*	1. Verbalize minimal discomfort after Intervention implemented. 2. Attain identified goal of pain relief.	1. (Flow sheet)/ (MAR.)	1. (Flow sheet)/ (MAR.)	1. (Flow sheet)/ (MAR.)
Knowledge Deficit R/T Surgical Procedure and Discharge Planning	Increased Knowledge R/T Postoperative Care & Discharge Planning			
1. Assess knowledge/instruct/evaluate re: • Pain relief • Preventive postoperative measures.	1. Verbalize understanding &/or Demonstrate: • Preventive postoperative measures & pain relief	1.	1.	1.
2. Review plan of care, including possible discharge date and follow-up plan.	2. Verbalize understanding of plan of care, discharge date & time, & follow-up plan.	2. (Discharge summary)	2. (Discharge summary)	2. (Discharge summary)

MAP009 (10/98)

SAINT VINCENTS HOSPITAL AND MEDICAL CENTER
MULTIDISCIPLINARY ACTION PLAN
POSTOPERATIVE DAY 1
Procedure: Carotid Endarterectomy

MD: _____

RN: _____

Date: _____

MAP DOES NOT REPLACE **MD** ORDERS		NOTES
Tests/Procedures/ Treatments:	Nursing assessment q8hr 6A-2P-10P Notify MD if T>101° HOB ↑ 30° Incentive spirometer 10 × q1hr while awake.	
Medication:	Percocet 1-2 tab PO q3-4 hr PRN pain. ASA 325 mg. PO qd. Initiate usual prescription medications.	
Activity:	Ambulate ad lib.	
Nutrition:	Cardiac prudent diet.	
Consults:		
Patient Education:	Assess, instruct, and evaluate re: • Carotid endarterectomy instructions. • Discharge and follow-up plan of care.	
Social Work:	Psychosocial assessment and intervention, and D/C plan, as indicated.	
Case Management:	Probably for discharge today if outcomes attained. Evaluate individual patient/family needs. Initiate referrals and consults, as indicated.	

MAP009 (10/98)

Saint Vincents Hospital and Medical Center
Multidisciplinary Action Plan
Postoperative Day 1
Procedure: Carotid Endarterectomy

MD: _____

RN: _____

Date: _____

PATIENT PROBLEM AND NURSING INTERVENTIONS	EXPECTED PATIENT OUTCOME &/OR DISCHARGE OUTCOME	ASSESSMENT/EVALUATION		
Alteration in Body Systems	Complications will be Prevented/Minimized			

1. Nursing Assessment
   A. *Vital signs & neurovascular check*
   B. *Assess lung sounds & respirations*
 	
   C. *Assess if neck dressing is intact, and/or for the presence of drainage/bleeding*
   D. *Assess and mobility of extremities.*
	A. VS & neurovascular status WNL.
	B. Respirations unlabored & even; lungs clear. Using incentive spirometer; coughing and deep breathing.
	C. Neck dressing dry and intact or suture line exposed.
	
	D. No signs/symptoms of complications.
		1.
		A. (Flow sheet)
		
		B. (Flow sheet)
		
		C. (Flow sheet)
		
		D. (Flow sheet)
			1.
			A. (Flow sheet)
			
			B. (Flow sheet)
			
			C. (Flow sheet)
			
			D. (Flow sheet)
				1.
				A. (Flow sheet)
				
				B. (Flow sheet)
				
				C. (Flow sheet)
				
				D. (Flow sheet)

Alteration in Comfort	Pain R/T Postoperative Period will be Prevented/Minimized			

1. Incisional pain:
   A. *Assess level of pain (use 1-10 pain scale).*
   B. *Administer pain medications.*
   C. *Assess effect of pain medication.*
   D. *Utilize comfort measures and diversional measures.*
	1. Verbalize minimal discomfort after intervention implemented.
	2. Attain identified goal of pain relief.
		1.
		(Flow sheet)/
		(MAR.)
			1.
			(Flow sheet)/
			(MAR.)
				1.
				(Flow sheet)/
				(MAR.)

Knowledge Deficit R/T Surgical Procedure and Discharge Planning	Increased Knowledge R/T Postoperative Care & Discharge Planning			
1. Assess knowledge/instruct/evaluate re: • Carotid endarterectomy instructions	1. Verbalize understanding of discharge instructions.	1.	1.	1.
2. Review discharge follow-up plan.	2. Verbalize understanding of follow-up plan.	2. (Discharge summary)	2. (Discharge summary)	2. (Discharge summary)

MAP009 (10/98)

SAINT VINCENTS HOSPITAL AND MEDICAL CENTER
MULTIDISCIPLINARY ACTION PLAN
Procedure: Carotid Endarterectomy

PROGRESS NOTES:

_____

_____

_____

_____

_____

_____

_____

_____

_____

_____

_____

_____

_____

_____

_____

_____

_____

_____

_____

_____

_____

MAP 009 (9/98)

APPENDIX 7-2

TMC Healthcare Case Management

MISSION STATEMENT

In collaboration with patients, families, and the health care team, case management facilitates enhanced quality of life for patients with complex health care needs, in the most resource-effective manner.

GOALS

1. To protect quality of care while managing utilization and reimbursement.
2. To decrease healthcare costs for defined populations.
3. To increase satisfaction of the customer.
4. To explore the most appropriate care options for and with individual patients and families.
5. To increase compliance with treatment plans.
6. To reduce fragmentation of care.
7. To improve clinical outcomes, whether this is improved health or dignified death.

Courtesy *Tucson Medical Center, Tucson, Arizona.*

CASE MANAGEMENT MODEL

The TMC Case Management Team is composed of nurse case managers (NCMs), social work case managers (SWCMs), and utilization case managers (UCMs). These three groups of specialists, assisted by the case management techs, interact collaboratively to support the mission and goals of case management. There is a core set of case management functions that is shared by all of the members of the case management team, and also specific functions that fall under the unique expertise of each group.

APPENDIX 7-3

CORE CASE MANAGEMENT FUNCTIONS

The case manager will act to:

1. Identify at-risk populations for high-cost, extended lengths of stay, destabilization, and repeat hospitalization.
2. Coordinate resources to ensure that necessary services are provided at the most appropriate level of care and that there is a smooth progression of the patient throughout the system during hospitalization.
3. Initiate a discharge planning process, beginning at or before hospital admission, that ensures safe and comprehensive support for continued health care needs.
4. Anticipate potential delays in the health care process and act proactively to avoid these delays.
5. Identify obstacles to efficiency and good outcomes and intervene to overcome or eliminate these when possible.
6. Reduce redundancy and fragmentation of care by acting as a communication link between the patient, family, members of the health care team, and payers.
7. Gather, interpret, and use data to identify problems and trends and to demonstrate outcomes and cost-effectiveness.
8. Advocate for the patient and family.
9. Educate the patient, family, and interdisciplinary team regarding health care resources.
10. Share skills and expertise with case management team.

SPECIFIC SPECIALTY FUNCTIONS

UCM

1. Perform utilization review for appropriateness of admission and placement.
2. Identify and refer high-risk complex patients for ongoing case management.
3. Function as expert resource for rules/regulations regarding UM.
4. Perform retroactive reviews when requested.
5. Issue denials when necessary.
6. Be a resource for external utilization managers.

NCM

1. Perform nursing case management assessments.
2. Interact with patients, families, physicians, and other health team members to develop proactive plans of care.
3. Evaluate and modify plan according to changing patient needs and clinical data. Document and communicate plan to all team members.
4. Intervene when medical complexity results in fragmented care.
5. Identify and act to eliminate gaps in clinical care. Make appropriate referrals.

SWCM

1. Perform psychosocial case management assessments
2. Develop, implement, and be accountable for a proactive plan of care. Evaluate and modify plan according to changing patient needs. Document and communicate plan to all team members Provide crisis intervention, bereavement counseling, and substance abuse counseling.
3. Function as social work resource for regulatory and legal issues.
4. Intervene when social/economic issues impact healthcare and disposition.

Rev 5/23/1999.
Courtesy *Tucson Medical Center, Tucson, Arizona.*

APPENDIX 7-4

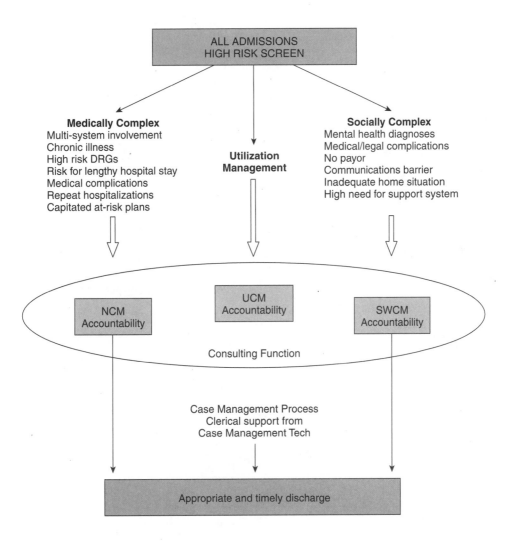

ALL ADMISSIONS
HIGH RISK SCREEN

Medically Complex
Multi-system involvement
Chronic illness
High risk DRGs
Risk for lengthy hospital stay
Medical complications
Repeat hospitalizations
Capitated at-risk plans

Utilization Management

Socially Complex
Mental health diagnoses
Medical/legal complications
No payor
Communications barrier
Inadequate home situation
High need for support system

NCM Accountability

UCM Accountability

SWCM Accountability

Consulting Function

Case Management Process
Clerical support from
Case Management Tech

Appropriate and timely discharge

Rev 5/23/1999.
Courtesy *Tucson Medical Center, Tucson, Arizona.*

Collaborative Models of Case Management

Evelyn Koenig

CHAPTER OVERVIEW

Collaborative models of case management, with interdependence among team members, joint decision-making responsibility, and joint accountability, offer an alternative to one discipline or multidisciplinary models. They assure the ready availability of competencies, knowledge, and skills necessary to comprehensive patient care and to system improvement. They build on the unique strengths of all team members and, when aligned, create solutions better than any one individual can develop in isolation.

EVOLUTION IN CASE MANAGEMENT

Case management is an old concept reborn. Aspects of case management were seen in attempts to care for the poor during the late 1800s. Community-based models of case management have been applied in mental health, social service, and public health settings since that time. Case management has also been used in the insurance industry and in the management of the care of deinstitutionalized mentally ill and developmentally disabled. In the mid-1980s the introduction of the prospective payment system gave impetus to the application of case management concepts in health care settings (Cesta et al., 1998; Cohen & Cesta, 1997; Lyon, 1993).

Case management development in health care was largely a nursing-driven process initiated to support "cost effective, patient outcome oriented care" (Cohen & Cesta, 1997). As managed care spread, case management models proliferated. Many models stressed the need for a multidisciplinary approach, usually under the direction of the nurse case manager. However, as fiscal constraints increased and institutions adopted downsizing as a cost-containment method, some responded by collapsing roles. Nurse case managers often found themselves as sole provider, absorbing aspects of the utilization, social work, and discharge planning roles.

Developing parallel to these more recent trends of single discipline models, downsizing, and role collapse is a growing body of work on collaboration as the most viable method for meeting the pressures of today's environment (Liedtka & Whitten, 1997; Harper & Harper, 1992; Huszczo, 1996). It supports the growing awareness that case management cannot be the function of a single individual (Bach, 1996) and that the nurse case manager will need to develop a collaborative practice with others to better coordinate the delivery of health care (Blancett & Flarey, 1996).

COLLABORATION

Collaboration is a ". . . process of joint decision-making among interdependent parties, involving joint ownership of decisions and collective responsibility for outcomes" (Liedtka & Whitten, 1997). As length of stay decreases, patient complexity increases, and reimbursement systems become increasingly complicated, collaborative models of case management assure the availability of the competencies, knowledge, and skills necessary to the task at hand. With a clear sense of direction, collaborative case management teams can provide higher quality solutions than any one individual working alone or in traditional multidisciplinary relationships.

THE EVOLUTION OF A COLLABORATIVE MODEL

In 1994 Tennessee was faced with the rapid conversion to a Medicaid managed care model. Vanderbilt University Medical Center (VUMC) recognized the need for change to assure a competitive position in the new environment. VUMC costs were significantly higher than local competitors and length of stay was high. The development and initiation of a case management model were seen as important elements in developing a competitive edge and responding to the managed care challenge.

Recognizing the strength brought by a diverse skill mix and the role conflict created by collapsing jobs (Erickson, 1996), case management was seen, from its inception, as the responsibility of a triad of nurse case manager, social worker, and utilization manager (Fig. 8-1). Case management was defined as the process of coordinating patient care across the continuum to assure optimal quality outcomes, patient satisfaction, and appropriate use of resources. Nurses and social workers became partners within this model. While the model recognized and respected the unique skills of each discipline, some sharing of responsibility was also required. The nurse case manager assumed responsibility for clinical coordination, resource utilization, pathway development, and outcome measurement. The social worker provided psychosocial assessment and intervention. High-risk screening and discharge planning were shared between nurse and social worker. Historically lacking in effectiveness, the utilization review function required redesign to make the utilization manager a partner in the triad. Staff was upgraded to licensed or credentialed personnel, and jobs were redesigned to include precertification, recertification, medical record completion, coding, and quality data collection (Erickson, 1996). Each triad was assigned a patient population and assumed responsibility for high-risk screening, assessment, planning/managing and evaluating care, and continuum of care planning. Triads would "run the list" of patients at least daily, dividing the work, reaching joint decisions about assigned responsibilities, and together designing plans of care.

Case management outcomes were impressive. Over a period of 5 years, case management triad efforts helped reduce the gap in charges with local competitors from 39.7% to less than 1% and the average length of stay from 7.1 to 5.2. Case management triads were, in general, functioning well and were providing higher quality solutions than any individual member could develop working alone. The nursing members of the triads, however, began to question their sole responsibility for outcome management. If the triad was responsible for a patient population and outcome management/system improve-

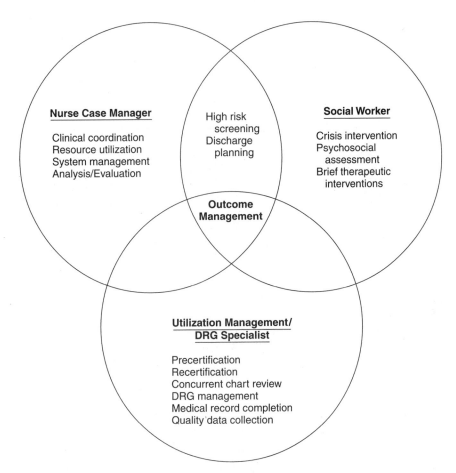

FIGURE **8-1**   Case management triad.

ment was a part of that responsibility, then all triad members should be equally accountable for the work. The triads should become truly collaborative with ". . . collective responsibility for outcomes" (Liedtka & Whitten, 1997). Case management leadership agreed. In a communication to all triad members, team accountability was outlined. "All triad members have responsibility for the work of case management which includes evaluation; evaluation is better with input from different team members; and evaluation is the interdisciplinary collaboration 'walk' " (Erickson, 1997).

Today all members of the case management triad are held accountable as a team for all aspects of case management. They are responsible for assuring their activities fit with the needs of the patient care center (service line) to which they are responsible, using the patient care center business plan as reference. Members continue to screen their patient population using triad-developed high-risk indicators. Patients at risk are assigned, and assessment, care planning/evaluation, and continuum of care planning are provided. The nurse assumes primary responsibility for the clinical coordination of care on the medically complex patients. Physician rounds provide a major forum for the identification of high-risk patients and for recommendations related to care and to resource utilization. Consultation with staff nurses on care plan development also assists in assuring smooth progress across the continuum. The nurse facilitates evidence-based pathway development and revision to enhance consistency and appro-

DRG XXX

	INDICATOR	FY Baseline	1st Quarter	2nd Quarter	3rd Quarter	4th Quarter
D E M O G R A P H I C S	Total admissions	624	75	61	52	
	Admission type					
	Elective	374	48	51	30	
	Emergency	124	15	5	10	
	Observation	0	0	0	2	
	Same day surgery	62	12	2	5	
	Trauma	64	0	3	5	
	Payor mix					
	TennCare	29%	27%	21%	18%	
	Commercial	35%	38%	38%	44%	
	Medicare	25%	27%	25%	25%	
	Self	6%	3%	8%	7%	
	Other	5%	5%	8%	6%	
C O S T	Case mix index	1.4	1.5	1.6	1.7	
	Average LOS	5	5	4	3	
	Charges/Admission	21,000	19,962	18,747	17,213	
	Cost/Admission	11,977	11,660	11,335	11,300	
	Profit/Loss	883	2575	3000	3035	
	Denied days	15	13	15	20	
Q U A L I T Y	Readmits (within 30 days)	16	8	5	3	
	Unrelated	12	6	4	3	
	Related-unavoidable	2	0	1	0	
	Related-avoidable	2	2	0	0	
	Discharge delays	NA				
	Funding		3	1	0	
	Bed availability		1	4	5	
	Patient condition		4	2	6	
	Family issues		1	0	0	
	Other		8	5	3	
	Estimated blood loss	NA				
	Complications (number/type)		4 CSF LEAK	1 CSF LEAK	0 CSF LEAK	
S A T I S F A C T I O N	Patient survey	NA	85% complete	92% complete	95% complete	
	Complaints	NA				
	Patient		3	2	1	
	Physician		5	2	2	
	Other		0	1	0	

FIGURE **8-2** Dashboard sample.

priateness of care. By facilitating discharge of the medically complex patient, the nurse assures that transitions in care are appropriate.

The social worker assumes primary responsibility for the psychosocially complex patients (e.g., those with psychiatric and/or substance abuse problems, family conflict, or lacking resources needed to address care needs). The social worker provides assistance in coordination of care, psychosocial assessment, crisis intervention, brief therapeutic intervention, linkage with resources, and discharge planning for these patients.

The utilization manager assures precertification and recertification for the triad population and continues to provide triad members with information on payer-related issues. The utilization manager also assures that medical record documentation will appropriately support the coding/billing functions.

"Running the list," or the daily discussion of all new and active triad patients, is key to triad function. It is this daily discussion that assures all triad members have an opportunity to contribute to the care of each patient from their own unique perspective.

In addition, each triad has established a case management dashboard, ". . . a system of warning lights and gauges that will allow the case management team to monitor when practice for their assigned population is going well and when there are problems" (Erickson, 1998). Some indicators are common to all case management teams. In addition, each team identifies cost, quality, and patient satisfaction indicators unique to their population (Fig. 8-2). All triad members contribute to the dashboard, and, through trending of the data collected, the triad can identify areas for improvement and design improvement activities.

In a recent assessment of the VUMC case management model, triad members strongly endorsed the collaborative approach. One team member summarized the feelings of many. "We are more powerful as a team than we would be working independently. With complex cases it is impossible for one person to handle all patient/family needs . . . case management enables me to work with someone who has a knowledge base different than mine and they contribute valuable information from their perspective" (VUMC, 1998).

BUILDING A COLLABORATIVE MODEL

Collaborative care models result in a number of positive outcomes, among them the potential to reduce cost while improving quality outcomes, to increase patient satisfaction, and to increase staff satisfaction and commitment (Liedtka & Whitten, 1997). However, health care givers, often involved in multidisciplinary care, rarely work with the interdependence and accountability required by collaboration. A study of 39 Vanderbilt triad members demonstrated that, although experienced in health care, 79.9% of the respondents had never worked in a collaborative model (Kidd & White, 1998). As collaborative care models are rare and require knowledge and skills seldom used or rewarded in traditional health care, preparation for collaborative practice is critical to the model's success.

CREATING THE VISION

Vision is a picture of the future, laid out as a possibility (Whiteside, 1993). It communicates a common purpose and gives coherence to activities. It assists individuals in putting aside differences and working together cooperatively (Senge, 1990). It also helps establish a sense of accountability for system, as well as individual, performance (Liedtka & Whitten, 1997).

A clearly stated vision is a necessary first step in creating a collaborative case management model. It creates a consistent reference point against which the team can measure their performance. The VUMC vision communicates the desired future—case management triads providing leadership to the patient care center in the development and implementation of patient care models that will assure effective coordination of care across the continuum. It defines the desired outcomes—enhanced quality, increased patient and provider satisfaction, and effective use of resources. And it defines the method—a collaborative care model that optimally uses the unique skills of each professional and holds team members

". . . collectively responsible for outcomes" (Liedtka & Whitten, 1997). To keep the vision central, it is incorporated in the scope and standards of practice, is core in orientation, and is reiterated at every opportunity. In this way the vision is the touchstone, the consistent measure of team progress toward the desired future.

BUILDING THE TEAM

The success of the team depends on individual excellence and the ability of the individuals to work together to tap the potential of the whole. It requires alignment, "a commonality of purpose, a shared vision and understanding of how to compliment one another's efforts" (Senge, 1990).

> "Collaborative teams don't just happen when people come together for a meeting. They are created through clear communication and upfront agreements about roles and decision-making that build trust. The agreements that the team begins with will enable it to sustain its focus and achieve its outcomes" (VUMC, 1994).

Team chartering is an efficient, effective method of helping the team define how they will work together. The charter has several elements:

- The purpose of the team
- The scope of the team's work
- Givens or boundaries (those things that cannot be changed)
- Decision-making process and fallback (how decisions will be made and the fallback if agreement cannot be reached)
- Roles (individual and collective responsibilities of team members, including professional roles and roles within the team, such as leadership)
- Norms and ground rules (how members work together)
- Meetings (times and frequency)
- Supports for the team (the supports necessary to ensure success)

Our experience demonstrates that chartered teams function more effectively, as there is commonality of purpose and a defined structure. If the team has problems in functioning, the charter serves as a reference for corrective action. It is also a critical tool in the orientation of new team members.

As collaborative practice requires interdependence, it has also been helpful to assist team members in understanding and valuing individual style. A helpful tool is the Myers-Briggs Type Indicator. Team members complete the inventory and receive an individual interpretation of style preferences. In a group session, all team member preferences are shared and the group learns how individual style impacts the team, the potential inherent in style diversity, and methods to use diverse styles in optimizing team function.

Managing conflict is a major challenge to teams. Each team needs help in ". . . acknowledging and using conflict productively versus suppressing and ignoring it . . ." (Liedtka & Whitten, 1997). The Myers-Briggs tool provides a method for understanding team members' reactions and provides direction in helping people adapt (Barger & Kirby, 1995). The concept of planned renegotiation is also useful. It is a way to provide controlled change by using pinches (indicators of personal discomfort), to anticipate team disruption, and to renegotiate expectations before serious disruption occurs (Sherwood & Glidewell, 1972). The Thomas-Kilmann Conflict Mode Instrument can be useful because it focuses on the individual style used most often in conflictual situations, the adaptiveness of that style, and ways to develop flexibility in matching style to circumstance (Thomas & Kilmann, 1974). Any or all of these tools can be introduced for use by the team.

PREPARING TEAM MEMBERS

Curricula necessary to the preparation of new case management staff have been well-documented (Cohen & Cesta, 1997; Satinsky, 1995; Tahan, 1996). Core content includes the history of case management; case management models; health care trends; payer networks and contracts; systems of reimbursement; case management practice (risk screening, assessment, care planning and evaluation, and continuum of care planning); pathway creation; continuous improvement techniques; and outcomes measurement and management. However, a collaborative model requires that content be reframed to emphasize interdependence and joint accountability.

Orientation begins with the vision for case management and its relationship to the institutional mission and goals. The collaborative aspect of the vision, with its functional interdependence and joint accountability, is emphasized. Information on the characteristics of well-functioning teams is provided. Participants are asked to complete an inventory of their assumptions about teams and those are contrasted to the reality of the collaborative model (Harper, 1992). If individuals are joining a functioning team, they review the team charter to understand its purpose and structure. As the introduction of a new member changes team dynamics, renegotiation of roles may be necessary. Material on conflict management is provided new staff, and they are given the opportunity to practice conflict management techniques. They are also given an understanding of personal style and its impact. Again, if they are joining an established team, they learn how their style complements the team. When core content is presented, it includes reference to the way tasks are carried out in a collaborative model and how joint accountability is measured. Mentors assigned are responsible for assisting in the mastery of case management process and collaborative practice.

EVALUATING THE TEAM

Members of the collaborative teams have both individual and joint accountability. There is individual accountability for the quality of professional practice and for behavior as a team member. There is joint accountability for team functioning and outcomes. Expected outcomes are specific to each team, and a communication loop exists that requires the team to regularly report on its progress and to self-adjust as necessary. Successful individual practice does not result in positive evaluation if the team is failing and this is clearly communicated. Positive evaluation requires individual and team success. This is a unique message to most professionals, necessitating repetition.

SUMMARY

Case management practice continues to evolve. The developing collaborative models provide an alternative to traditional case management models, and outcomes demonstrate the synergy that can develop among members of a well-functioning collaborative team.

References

Bach, D., et al. (1996). Developing a successful hospital case management system. In D. Flarey & S. Blancett (Eds.), *Handbook of nursing case management*, Gaithersburg, MD: Aspen.

Barger, N., & Kirby, L. (1995). *The challenge of change in organizations, helping employees thrive in the new frontier*, Palo Alto: Davies-Black Publishing.

Blancett, S., & Flarey, D. (1996). Case management: The shape of things to come. In D. Flarey & S. Blancett (Eds.), *Handbook of nursing case management,* Gaithersburg, MD: Aspen.

Cesta, T., et al. (1998). *The case manager's survival guide, winning strategies for clinical practice,* St. Louis: Mosby.

Cohen, E., & Cesta, T. (1997). *Nursing case management, from concept to evaluation* (2nd ed.). St. Louis: Mosby.

Erickson, S. (1996, July/Aug). Case management, *Issues and Outcomes,* 6-8.

Erickson, S. (1997). Unpublished presentation.

Erickson, S. (1998). The Vanderbilt model of outcomes management, *Critical Care Nursing Clinics of North America 10*(1), 13-20.

Harper, A., & Harper, B. (1992). *Skill-building for self-directed team members,* New York: MW Corporation.

Huszczo, G. (1996). *Tools for team excellence,* Palo Alto: Davis-Black.

Kidd, K., & White, S. (1998). Unpublished manuscript.

Lenkman, J., & Gribbins, R. (1994). Multidisciplinary teams in the acute care setting, *Holistic Nurse Practice 8*(3), 81-87.

Liedtka, J., & Whitten, E. (1997). Building better patient care services: A collaborative approach, *Health Care Management Review 22*(3), 16-24.

Lyon, J. (1993). Models of nursing care delivery and case management: Clarification of terms, *Nursing Economics 11*(3), 163-169.

Satinsky, M. (1995). *An executive guide to case management strategies, USA,* American Hospital Publishing, Inc.

Senge, P. (1990). *The fifth discipline,* New York: Doubleday.

Sherwood, J., & Glidewell, J. (1972). Planned renegotiation: A norm setting OD intervention. In W. Burke, (Ed.), *Contemporary organization development, approaches and interventions,* Washington, DC: NTL Learning Resources Corporation.

Tahan, H. (1996). Training and education needs of case managers. In D. Flarey, & S. Blancett, (Eds.), *Handbook of nursing case management,* Gaithersburg, MD: Aspen.

Thomas, K., & Kilmann, R. (1974). *Thomas-Kilmann conflict mode instrument,* Xicom, Inc.

Vanderbilt University Medical Center, Center for Patient Care Innovation. (1994). Unpublished material.

Vanderbilt University Medical Center, Office of Case Management. (1998). Unpublished results.

Whiteside, J. (1993). *The Phoenix agenda,* Essex Junction, VT: Oliver Wight Publications, Inc.

Case Management

A Process not a Person

Theresa J. Ortiz, Lynn Rüppi

CHAPTER OVERVIEW

For a successful case management program, the patient, in partnership with many professionals, must engage in a process. Case management or care coordination is not a new concept. Think of a rural physician with limited resources who "manages" his or her patients across their life span. In exchange for their education, on graduation, physicians in many European countries are assigned patients by region or district. In this setting the physician may take on additional roles such as pharmacist, nurse, therapist, or social worker. Home visits are common. Regardless of the structure or where the patient enters the system, the case management process begins with identification of patient needs and risks, development of a plan to address those needs, and monitoring the plan for success. Case management is really a process, not a person. The process has evolved from a simple plan, such as the rural physician who develops a life-long relationship with the patient, to a complex, fragmented arrangement as we try to balance demands from managed care, regulatory agencies, and the sophisticated consumer. Demand for accountability in the case management process will only increase as we enter the next century.

THE CASE MANAGEMENT PROGRAM

The case management model chosen by an institution is determined by many factors. The case management program at University Hospital, a 450-bed tertiary care hospital located in Denver, Colorado, is a partnership between nurse case managers and social workers. The teams started out as unit-based teams, while some have gradually transitioned to population-based teams who follow their patients across the continuum of care.

The evolution of University Hospital's case management program began with the identification of multiple factors, including the hospital's mission and the competitive managed health care market. The hospital's mission includes education, research, and service to the indigent. When designing a case management model in an academic setting, additional factors may need to be considered, depending on the relationship between medical school, physician group practice, and hospital. Balancing the hos-

Table 9-1	WHAT ARE THE MOTIVATING FACTORS FOR EACH GROUP?		
MEDICAL SCHOOL	**PHYSICIAN GROUP**	**UNIVERSITY HOSPITAL**	
How is the hospital reimbursed for the additional costs associated with training?	Physicians trying to balance academic medicine, research, clinical responsibilities, and the reality of managed care.	Competing in a stage 4 managed care market on costs.	
Students must meet minimal requirements for graduation Need to perform required number of procedures, which may not always incorporate utilization management principles.	Physicians develop their own practice patterns. Residents "adopt" the personality of the attending physician.	Reimbursement declining. Need to contain resource utilization.	

pital's mission becomes difficult when the key players are often working toward different objectives. At times their motivating factors may even be in conflict with one another (Table 9-1).

Recognizing that aligning incentives between these three entities was a monumental task, the model was designed to start with what was controllable. Historically, no group other than the utilization review department had been accountable for the utilization of resources and patient length of stay. Staff in general had little understanding of managed care, reimbursement, covered and non-covered benefits, or internal and external resources. In addition, lacking was the concept that case management is a process that includes many disciplines, all of whom have a part in coordinating care.

The optimal situation would be to design a model, hire staff with specific expertise, close the health care system for at least a week to ensure large blocks of training time, and then, when fully prepared, begin the program. In most institutions today, limited budgets, systems constraints, and administrative expectations for quick results do not allow the staff time for adjustment and mastery of new skill sets. The model was piloted in just such an environment. Almost immediately the human barriers to implementation began to surface (Table 9-2).

Data Base Design

As the demand to demonstrate added value in the patient care process increases, case management programs must develop a mechanism to trend system issues (i.e., variances), that impact patient care, resource utilization, length of stay, etc. Data must be formatted so as to identify areas for performance improvement activities, track case manager/social worker productivity, and as a decision-making tool for administration. The case management team data base at University Hospital was designed to capture variations in patient care that prevented a smooth transition through the hospital stay (e.g., a discharge is postponed because a test could not be performed on a timely basis). The foundation for the data base is a data entry sheet completed by the case management teams that identifies and assigns variance days to the responsible party. The responsible party may be a hospital department (e.g., no available operating rooms), a nursing unit (e.g., delay in getting a medication started), a physician (e.g., delay in moving a patient to a lower level of care), or discharge planning (e.g., patient refuses to leave the hospital once he or she is determined to be medically stable). Completing the data entry sheet was an educational experience for most of the case management teams who were not used to tracking outcomes this way. Identifying and assigning variances forced the case management teams to become more proactive in searching for creative funding and placement options.

Table 9-2	HUMAN BARRIERS EXPERIENCED IN IMPLEMENTATION OF THE CASE MANAGEMENT MODEL			
FEAR	**STAFF RESPONSE**	**RATIONALE FOR FEARS**	**LEADERSHIP STRATEGIES**	**OUTCOMES**
Fear of losing my job.	"If I do not go along with this model I will lose my job."	Case management programs nationwide had eliminated or changed roles for social workers and clinical nurse specialists.	Use of a consultant with strong managed care background.	Consultant provided an objective view for program development and was able to solicit cooperation from multiple departments.
Fear of change	"What do I do everyday in this new role?"	New role, new expectations, new job skills, new partner. Feeling of being overwhelmed was real for health care professionals who were very skilled and comfortable in their "old" roles.	Clear structure and accountabilities provided a framework for daily expectations. Job descriptions with performance standards developed. Day-long training session for case management teams.	Took approximately 6 to 9 months for teams to demonstrate team behavior.
Fear of managed care	"I would have gone to business school if I had wanted to deal with finances. I am trained to care for patients."	Fear of managed care in a stage 4 managed care market is a reality. Hospitals in this market were downsizing, consolidating, and/or closing. Lack of under-standing about managed care rules and how to incorporate these into a patient treatment plan were new skill sets that needed to be learned.	"Managed Care 101" training. Training on developing a relationship with a third-party payer.	Teams have become less intimated by third-party payers. Teams see that their role as "financial stewards" for the patient is just as important as their clinical care.

These human barriers, while less tangible, were as much of a challenge to leadership as selecting the right model for the particular setting, developing the right report formats, or refining the data base. *Continued*

Table 9-2	HUMAN BARRIERS EXPERIENCED IN IMPLEMENTATION OF THE CASE MANAGEMENT MODEL—cont'd			
FEAR	**STAFF RESPONSE**	**RATIONALE FOR FEARS**	**LEADERSHIP STRATEGIES**	**OUTCOMES**
Fear of technology	"Why do we have to keep data? I'm a caregiver. People should know that I do a good job."	"What value do your services add to patient care?" This is a question being asked by health care companies as well as administration. Fear of data and technology may be real to health care professionals who have not been exposed to computers, data collection, or evaluation of care provided.	Education stressing "data is your friend." • Technical computer training • Development of tools for data collection • Development of a data base • Development of usable report formats • Education on data analysis • Leadership training in data presentation • Training in the quality improvement process	Teams began to understand their data, began to present it to various committees (i.e. clinical pathway team), and became involved with strategies for improvement.
Fear of being the "bad guy"	"I do not want to be seen as the utilization management police" or "It's not my place to question the physician."	Staff were used to functioning in a clinical role but not in a total patient care coordination role that included attention to financial issues. Understanding that there are limits in providing care and that patients do have responsibilities in their care were new skill sets to be learned.	One-on-one supervision and case review with managers. Relationship building with all health care team members. Focus on the fact that patients are the center of what we do. Education about the "big system" perspective. • Guest lecture from finance discussed how health care dollars are spent in our institution.	Teams developed relationship with business contracting department. Staff became more sophisticated in negotiating for benefit exceptions based on cost analysis.

These human barriers, while less tangible, were as much of a challenge to leadership as selecting the right model for the particular setting, developing the right report formats, or refining the data base.

The case management data base (on Microsoft Access) was designed with a software expert from the financial department and consists of all University Hospital inpatients after DRG assignments have been made. Once the medical records are coded, they are downloaded into the data base. Along with the DRG assignment, demographic data, length of stay, and hospital charges are also included. The program can calculate the cost of a variance by multiplying the average variable direct cost per day of the assigned DRG by the number of days assigned. For example, if the patient's length of stay was decreased by 5 days and the variable cost of the DRG was $500 per day, the facility would potentially save $2,500. This formula may not work for all institutions but was a way to begin showing how variances impact the financial part of providing care for patients. Not all variances are negative; if the case management team intervenes (facilitates a test being done earlier or negotiates for benefits with a third-party payer) and it results in a decreased length of stay, the team receives credit for the intervention.

Specialized reports have been taken to medical quality improvement committees to analyze trends. General monthly summaries are reported to the case managers, social workers, pathway teams, administration, physician, and nursing unit manager. The summaries help each group develop interventions for system areas needing improvement.

Outcomes

The case management program has resulted in a number of positive outcomes (Riippi & Rogers, 1997), including the following:

1. A decrease in the number of patients on the "$20,000 and the $100,000" reports. (These reports list patients whose hospital charges have reached these thresholds.) This means there are significantly fewer dollars outstanding in accounts receivable. This outcome really grabbed the attention of the hospital chief financial officer, who reviewed these reports weekly. When possible, case managers and social workers are placing these patients in more appropriate settings sooner and/or obtaining funding to help these patients access resources. There are now more frequent discharges directly from the ICUs instead of requiring the patient to stay another day in a less acute bed for the purpose of discharge planning.
2. The overall readmission rate has decreased. Case manager social work teams are coordinating follow-up care and return appointments with primary care physicians, clinics, and home care.
3. Emergency department referrals to social workers and case managers have increased, allowing staff to intervene initially and look for appropriate solutions to patients' situations. They now often divert inappropriate admissions. Teams also identified patients who visited the emergency room frequently and developed alternative follow-up plans, thus reducing the frequency of return visits.
4. Improved customer satisfaction is reflected in phone calls and letters, as well as satisfaction surveys. These customers include not only patients but internal customers in other departments and external third-party payer case managers.
5. A significant decrease has occurred over a 3-year period in the monies spent on home care for the indigent. Case management teams were able to work out more cost-effective alternatives for these patients that did not compromise care.
6. Dollars paid to an outside vendor for home infusion services to the indigent decreased from $500,000 to $70,000 the first year the program was piloted. By the third year the spending had decreased to under $30,000. Teams were taught to use an algorithm for possible alternatives to home infusion services. Patients received the same level of service but at times in an alternative setting.

An unexpected bonus to the implementation of the case management program was the networking that has developed. There is now increased collaboration on cases, and patients are moving more smoothly between units and services.

STAGES OF PROGRAM DEVELOPMENT FROM THE HUMAN PERSPECTIVE

Stage 1

As the program was implemented, weekly interdisciplinary meetings were held, consisting of nurse case managers, social workers, home care coordinators, and at times third-party payer case managers. At this point staff were working in dyads as teams, but true team behavior had not yet developed. Nurse case managers and social workers sat on opposite sides of the room, receiving information on the technical aspects and expectations of the new program. At this point inservice training was provided on topics such as medical necessity and level of care criteria, high-risk screening, Medicare and Medicaid regulations, etc. Staff were learning their accountabilities, competency expectations, etc. They listened, but clearly had not yet internalized the process. Questions were basic, technical in nature, and displayed a high level of anxiety. Questions about third-party payers were phrased to indicate staff viewed the third-party payer as the bad guy. Staff did not yet display creativity in options for patients. Often they would advocate for whatever the physician had requested, not yet evaluating whether the request was appropriate or whether there were quality cost-effective alternatives. At the end of meetings, people left immediately without much interaction.

Stage 2

Staff began to implement the model and started to accept that they will have a partner. Beginning compliance with requirements appeared, but teams still required extensive one-on-one supervision. Next appeared the predictable power struggles over role definition. While job descriptions delineated separate duties, some areas of responsibility were gray, forcing each dyad to negotiate a working relationship. Most teams worked out acceptable arrangements without intervention. One or two required mediation. The individual personalities of team members caused each dyad to have its own team personality. Most teams blended well and were able to demonstrate flexibility in working out role assignments.

Stage 3

Teams began to develop a consistent daily routine. The need for supervision on cases decreased to occasional on complex cases. Teams began to consult with internal institutional resources, for example, consulting with the wound care nurse to help a patient improve faster or consulting with the pharmacy to enable a patient to obtain a drug on the correct insurance formulary. Less input from leadership was necessary. More creative planning for cases, incorporating benefit management, financial concerns, patient clinical needs, and psychosocial needs, began to appear. Teams now began to solicit input from all disciplines, such as physical or occupational therapy, speech, and respiratory therapy as well as the physician and incorporate their input into the plan. However, at this stage, when they were presented with data about their team/unit, they were unclear as to how to utilize and analyze. "This is a nice report. Now what am I supposed to do with it?" was often the response.

Stage 4

Cooperation emerged within teams, and they began to function as true working partners, even completing some cross training with each other. This was in sharp contrast to the initial stages where staff were quite territorial about their job duties. Teams now tolerated more shades of gray in role definition, allowing for greater cooperation. Most teams adapted to using the strengths of each partner. The comfort level of approaching physicians proactively for discharge plans versus waiting for a physician recommendation increased tremendously. Questions in meetings became more sophisticated, indicating a new level of knowledge and skill sets and demonstrating a broader system perspective.

Participants began to analyze their data for the purposes of improvements in contrast to the attitude, "I don't want this data to make me look bad." Data were presented to groups outside the team, for example, at a clinical pathway or medical staff quality meeting.

Stage 5 (Current)

As the insurance industry demands evolve, the need for a gradual metamorphosis of the model also has emerged. Continued evaluation of institutional and patient needs has become crucial. The speed at which this needs to occur again sends the team back through the cycle of adjustment to change, but at a higher level of expertise. The model begins to expand from a program to a systemwide way of thinking, incorporating other key players in decision making and development. Case management becomes truly not a person but a process.

Strategies for Implementation or "What Did We Learn Along the Way?"

Any new program is a work in progress, and as much was learned along the way about what didn't work as what was successful.

What Didn't Work?

1. Raw data. In the early stages of data base development, monthly reports were created that summarized all activity for each team. The lengthy data were not in a user-friendly format and were difficult to read, let alone interpret. Over time, the data were formatted into meaningful reports that each team could use to make improvements.
2. Expecting staff to change procedures without a built-in accountability piece. As the program developed, procedures, protocols, and expectations also developed. As a change in protocol became necessary, it would be reviewed with staff and they would verbalize understanding. It was assumed then that since we had laid out our expectations, staff would implement the changed protocol. Later it was discovered that staff actually had difficulty incorporating the changes into their routine unless there was a method of accountability. For example, staff were asked to orchestrate brief multidisciplinary conferences on all patients who stayed longer than 7 days. The purpose was for the team to develop a patient-specific plan to help move the patient to the next lower level of medical care as appropriate. While staff agreed in theory that this was a good idea, as the day got busy, this task was often overlooked. It was not until we instituted a form for documentation that could also be used for auditing purposes that we began to see compliance. The meetings began to be held regularly, resulting in better team planning for patient care.
3. Long presentations to administration. In the beginning, elaborate presentations were prepared demonstrating detail on significant programmatic outcomes. Meetings at upper administrative levels are so tightly packed with agenda that the point of the presentation was rarely reached before the allotted time expired. We learned that the presentations needed to be short, to the point, and "pack a punch." Key outcomes were prepared for the presentation, with background information available only if asked.

What Did Work?

In retrospect, several strategies assisted administration to understand the validity and positive cost-effective program outcomes. There were also several that helped to break down the human barriers and resistance to change.

SELECTIVE USE OF EMAIL. A summary email of important program outcomes sent to key administrators received more feedback than many other strategies. The email listed in bullet form the specific program outcomes.

AWARDS LUNCHEONS. Twice a year a luncheon was held to celebrate the successes of the program. Awards were given for various team successes. Cases selected for recognition were complex, requiring teamwork, creativity, and skill to work toward a quality cost-effective patient outcome. Each team awarded received a certificate. In addition to providing recognition for a job well done, it provided a learning tool to demonstrate complex problem solving, as well as humor. For example, the "best travel agent" award was presented to the case manager who was able to negotiate with an employer for an airline ticket for a stroke patient who couldn't get home. "Most Dollars and Days Saved" was awarded to the neonatal case management team (physician, case manager, social worker, staff nurse, and parents) who worked with the payer in negotiating an early discharge for a premature baby. The payer was able to substitute additional home visits, allowing for the parents to care for their baby at home instead of at the hospital. This saved 3 weeks of hospitalization and improved care for the baby by being at home.

INVITING KEY ADMINISTRATORS TO THE AWARDS LUNCHEON. Inviting administrators to these luncheons helped bring home the point that the program was making a difference in patient care as well as proving to be cost effective. They had a better feel for what the teams accomplished each day.

SYSTEM ACCOUNTABILITY AND CONSISTENT STRUCTURE AND FEEDBACK. This was by far the most labor-intensive part of program startup. Assisting teams to learn the technical aspect of the job as well as make the internal changes necessary to work as a team proved to be a crucial aspect of program development. Setting up how staff team behaviors could be measured, rated, and audited was time consuming but helped change behavior most effectively. Management time was spent on lots of one-on-one supervision on difficult cases, chart audits, feedback and encouragement, helping staff compare data month-to-month, etc.

MODELING BEHAVIOR. At first each team required leadership presence at their quarterly meetings to model how to analyze and present their data. Eventually the case managers were able to assume the leadership function.

Anticipated Further Development

The program began as unit-based teams in order to get the system up and running and assure all patients received services. The program is in process of moving to a more population-based model that will serve inpatients and outpatients, providing for better continuity of care. The logistics of such a model are difficult. How does one team provide inpatient and outpatient care when outpatient clinics are spread all over the city? How do patients receive services who do not fit into one of the team case-managed populations? An additional sophistication in the use of data and outcomes is anticipated. The data were first used to change internal system issues. Hopefully the case management program will partner with the business contract development office. The data should be useful in procuring contracts for the health care institution.

With each change in the model, it is anticipated that the teams will move back into the stages of resistance to change. However, while the process of resistance to change remains the same, staff should deal with it at a less traumatic level because they are at a more sophisticated stage of team development.

Key Factors in Program Success

1. Pay strong attention to the human dynamics, as they are as crucial to program success as the model you choose. Human dynamics are the most labor-intensive part of new program development. It took 6 to 9 months before consistent behavior change occurred on the part of the teams.
2. The model must include consistent ongoing structure, accountability, and feedback to staff. Newly hired staff must be brought up to the same skill level as experienced staff.
3. Personnel skilled in data base design are crucial. A full-time person was available to enter data, develop report formats, and analyze the data.
4. Develop baseline data with measurable outcomes to justify program viability.
5. Market your program to your administrators, as well as internal and external customers.
6. Celebrate your successes to administration and to staff.

. . . . and remember case management is a process, not a person.

Reference

Riippi, L., & Jackson, S. (1997). Case management finds success in a university hospital. *QRC Advisor, 13* (No. 10):7-9.

The Colorado Psychiatric Health Case Management Model

An Innovative Approach to Client-Centered Care

Bari K. Platter, Kay Vaughn, Bonnie Cox Young

CHAPTER OVERVIEW

Managed care's emphasis on providing rapid reintegration of psychiatric clients into the community has forced psychiatric hospitals to develop more efficient care delivery systems. Although Colorado Psychiatric Health faculty have written extensively about provision of inpatient psychiatric treatment in the age of managed care, the body of knowledge concerning brief, cost-effective psychiatric hospital treatment is extremely limited. Furthermore, literature regarding the development of psychiatric case management models is practically nonexistent.

This chapter will discuss how Colorado Psychiatric Health has successfully decreased length of stay while maintaining high-quality care. Ethical considerations, philosophical and theoretical approaches, orientation and training, variance issues, and customer satisfaction will be reviewed. Thoughtful integration of brief therapy approaches, family preservation techniques, and assertive community treatment combined with our strong belief that client input is essential to successful treatment have led to the development of a comprehensive, holistic model of case management.

INTRODUCTION

Although ideas regarding the concept of case management have been present for decades (Tahan, 1998), the advent of managed care in the 1980s has been a catalyst for the development of case management models (Baker & Giese 1992; Ford et al., 1995; Gournay, 1995). In this era of managed care oversight, mental health systems have had to respond with major reform (Hatfield, 1996; Quinn, 1993; RESPONSE, 1998). The literature regarding psychiatric case management is scant and does not outline a comprehensive model that addresses the complexity of psychiatric clients (Baker & Giese, 1992; Erkel, 1993; Marschke & Nolan, 1993; Quinn, 1993; Thomas, Dubousky, & Cox-Young, 1996; Thomas et al., 1996). Because of managed care's insistence that clients be quickly reintegrated into the community, inpatient psychiatric staff can no longer exclusively focus on the micro system of the hospital (Krmpotic,

1992). Development of effective relapse and discharge plans has been one step toward addressing length-of-stay and quality-of-care issues. Another important piece has been the development and use of a treatment plan that drives treatment forward and helps emphasize variances in clinical care (de Woody & Price, 1994; Goode, 1995; Hofmann, 1993).

Historically, economic concerns and societal views about the environment in which psychiatric clients should be treated have influenced the delivery of mental health services (Bodgett, 1993). Currently, the emphasis of mental health treatment is in keeping the client in the community and out of the restrictive and costly environment of the hospital. Since mental health systems have not clearly articulated an inpatient case management model, a comprehensive model includes orientation, training opportunities, and the development of professional standards (Gibson et al., 1994; Trinidad, 1993). In addition, competency demonstration, continuum of care design, and treatment plan development are equally important (Gourney, 1995; Thomas et al., 1995). The literature advocates for input from consumers regarding evolution of the case management model (Higgins, 1994; Lamb & Stempel, 1994; Sherman & Porter, 1991; Van Dongen & Jambunathan, 1992). Incorporation of customer satisfaction data is a component of addressing the need for frequent and continual evaluation of newly developing case management models (Vaughn, Webster, Orahood, Cox-Young, 1995; Vaughn, Cox-Young, Webster, Thomas, 1997; Webster, Vaughn, Webb, Playtev, 1995).

Recent literature also notes the need to discuss theoretical models of case management (Smith, 1994; Wadas, 1993; Williams, 1992). Nursing theory emphasizes the relationship between the caregiver and the client and adds a therapeutic element that can be incorporated into a successful case management model. Thoughtful decision making concerning the underpinnings of theory that guide clinical practice must address the client as central. Montgomery and Webster (Montgomery & Webster, 1994) believe that brief forms of psychiatric care are congruent with nursing's metaparadigm. Brief therapy theories, assertive community treatment models, and family-centered interventions form the theoretical base of a holistic case management model. Ethical dilemmas of managing care must be addressed when developing a case management model (Banja et al., 1997; Curtin, 1996; Montgomery & Webster, 1993, 1994). Basing clinical decisions solely on cost containment is unethical. Case managers must position themselves to advocate for quality of care issues while speaking the language of business concerns of managed care companies. This type of treatment must be highly individualized so the client and family are actively involved in the treatment planning process (Vaughn et al., 1997).

The Colorado Psychiatric Health (CPH) Case Management Model includes a philosophy where the provision of efficacious and quality care is provided within the framework of not a day too long and not a day too short. This chapter will outline an innovative model of inpatient psychiatric case management that bridges the gap between the hospital and the community. This model specifically addresses the scope of practice, training, orientation, support, communication skills, treatment plan development, and macro management of the larger, real world environment of clients. Thoughtful integration of brief therapy approaches, family preservation techniques, and assertive community treatment models are deliberately combined to articulate a theoretical conceptualization of the CPH Case Management Model (Berg, 1991; De Shazar, 1991; Hollaway, Oliver, Collins, Carson, 1995; Karpel, 1986; Lachance & Santos, 1995; Olsen, Rickles, & Travlik, 1995; Steine Test, 1980; Test, 1992).

EVOLUTION OF THE CPH CASE MANAGEMENT MODEL

Early on, CPH recognized the need to respond to the demands of third party providers to offer efficient hospitalization (Webster et al., 1995). With the demand for shorter lengths of stay, CPH leadership realized that we would have to make changes in our philosophy, purpose, and the roles of multidisciplinary team members (Harper, 1988; Santos & McLeod-Bryant, 1991; Vaughn et al., 1995). The ethical dilemma we faced was to provide efficient care without sacrificing quality. As other psychiatric hospitals struggled to shorten lengths of stay while continuing to use longer-term therapy modalities, we, on the other hand, explored theories that envisioned the client as the center of clinical decision making. By reviewing the literature, we ascertained that solution-focused therapy, assertive community treatment, and family preservation models were most congruent with treating the client by focusing on their strengths and real world concerns (Berg, 1991; Stein & Test, 1980; Vaughn et al., 1997). In developing our continuum of care model, we applied principles of solution-focused therapy, assertive community treatment, and family preservation models to acute inpatient services (Vaughn et al., 1997). As length of stay continued to decrease and acuity increased, we quickly realized that close clinical coordination was essential to successful outcomes (Baker & Giese, 1992; Thomas et al., 1996). The role of the case manager (CM) was developed: a clinical coordinator, responsible for driving treatment forward, maintaining a solution-focused approach with clients and their families, efficiently involving ancillary providers in treatment, documenting treatment plans and progress, and developing and maintaining close working relationships with third party providers (Figure 10-1).

Due to fragmentation of the mental health system and the complexity of our clients, we decided to assign a CM to work with each hospitalized client. It was important for us to conceptualize the case

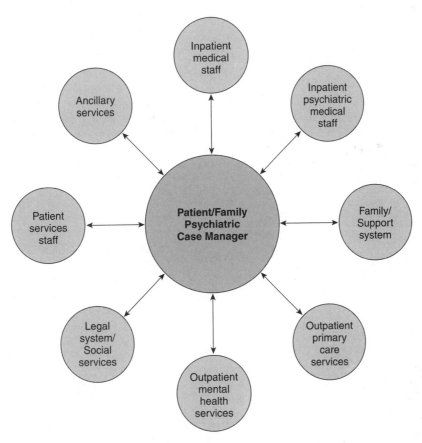

FIGURE **10-1** CPH case management model.

manager role in a way that was congruent with the CPH Continuum of Care Model (Figure 10-2). In the CPH Continuum of Care Model, there is a seamless provision of services from inpatient to community settings (Vaughn et al., 1997).

The CPH Case Management Model was structured to ensure that the CM is able to smoothly guide the client and family through the care continuum (Vaughn et al., 1997). Unlike other case management models, we visualized the scope of this role as encompassing both internal inpatient and outpatient treatment as well as external community systems of care. Consistent with the assumptions of brief therapy, the CPH conceptual framework of the continuum of care includes the value of identifying the client's highest level of functioning, of establishing treatment goals that incorporate what's working in the client's life, and, most importantly, of returning to the community as the paramount goal of hospitalization.

When the CPH Case Management Model was first conceptualized, CPH leadership discussed the parameters of the job description of the CM. Issues that led to development of the CM role included inconsistencies in the quality of treatment plans and a breakdown of communication between the treatment team and line staff. Since nurses are trained in the formulation of psychosocial/biomedical treatment plans and have direct knowledge of formal and informal communication patterns on inpatient psychiatric unit, we determined that a nurse would best fill the role of CM. Social workers were also determined to be important members of the treatment team, coordinating family work and discharge planning. Therefore, when the CPH Case Management Model was first implemented in 1990, each treatment team consisted of a nurse CM, a social worker, and an attending psychiatrist. The case load of one treatment team included approximately five to eight inpatients. Nurse CMs and social workers managed two treatment teams, responsible for the care of a total of 10 to 16 patients.

The nurse CM's role included development of the treatment plans and implementation with the line staff; communication with ancillary services, such as occupational therapy, physical therapy, and pharmacy; coordination of follow-up appointments for medical problems; and utilization review. The social worker's role was limited to providing family intervention and coordinating discharge planning. Social workers were discouraged from participating in discussions of milieu issues, and nurse CMs did not discuss family systems issues. The nurse CM and the social worker met several times each day for clinical updates. Although there was consistency in the provision of care in this model, both the nurse CMs and the social workers were dissatisfied, seeing the model as fragmented and compartmentalized. The

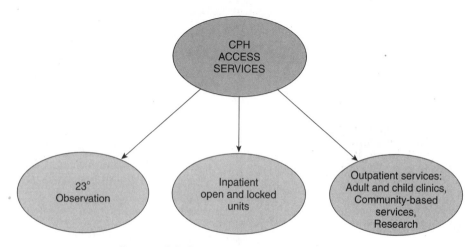

FIGURE **10-2**   CPH continuum of care model.

social workers complained that because they did not know many important details of the patient's treatment, it was difficult to keep the family and outpatient providers updated about the patient's progress. Nurse CMs felt left out of discussions about family and support system issues. As the psychiatric and medical acuity continued to increase, both groups experienced the system as inefficient and unsatisfactory.

To increase efficiency, positive outcomes, and job satisfaction, CPH leadership asked the nurse CMs and the social workers to make a list of job responsibilities. It quickly became apparent that the social worker's scope of practice was limited. The social workers, all experienced in inpatient psychiatry, were quite capable of competently performing many of the duties of the nurse CMs. Conversely, many of the nurse CMs had extensive experience with family and support system work. After many months of negotiating responsibilities, CPH leadership decided that the roles of the nurse CM and the social worker could be combined to form the role of psychiatric CM. In this way, each psychiatric CM would have expanded responsibility for one treatment team (five to eight patients and their families) instead of two teams, as in the previous model.

To ensure a smooth transition from a model with the team consisting of a nurse CM, social worker, and attending psychiatrist to the new model of a psychiatric CM and an attending psychiatrist, both nurses and social workers met weekly over several months. In these meetings, members of each discipline exchanged detailed information about their own duties/responsibilities. When the CMs and leadership felt comfortable with the transition, new teams were formed. Each discipline made a commitment to be available to the other for professional consultation.

Although this chapter will focus on the provision of CM services in the inpatient setting, it is important to recognize that CPH has been able to adapt the CPH case management model to community settings. CPH recently (1994) partnered with a community mental health system to establish the University High Intensity Treatment Team to provide treatment for 80 chronically mentally ill clients. In addition, we had reorganized our outpatient services. A new program, Community Based Case Management (CBCM), had been designed. We strategically organized this program to integrate the CPH case management model with brief therapy–inspired family preservation models. These two outpatient case management models will be briefly discussed.

The University High Intensity Treatment Team (HITT) is a 15-member intensive case management team that provides a full range of therapeutic and rehabilitation services to 100 chronically mentally ill clients (the program originally had 80 clients, but has expanded in response to requests from the mental health community). HITT integrates approaches from the Program in Assertive Community Treatment (PACT) model, brief therapy, and the CPH case management model. CMs, who range in expertise from bachelor's prepared clinicians to a licensed psychologist, work in the community toward social reintegration, medical and psychiatric stability, vocational rehabilitation and decreasing rates of psychiatric hospitalization of their clients (Lachanne & Santos, 1995; Stein & Test, 1980; Test, 1992). Similar to inpatient case managers, HITT case managers coordinate all psychosocial, biomedical, and environmental interventions with their clients. Clinical supervision is also seen as an essential piece of this program. Since most of the case managers are unlicensed and function with delegation from licensed clinicians, it has been imperative to provide close, formal and informal, individual and group clinical supervision. The HITT coordinator, a licensed psychologist and nurse, and the HITT psychiatrist both provide these clinical supervision services. HITT nurses meet frequently with case managers, primarily to assess the client's response to medications, to problem-solve medication compliance issues, and to assess and treat medical issues.

Community-based case management (CBCM) was developed in response to requests from public managed care systems to provide intensive home-based services for their clients. CBCM has integrated approaches in brief family therapy and family preservation with the CPH case management model. This team works with families in their homes, providing case management, psychotherapy, and parenting education. The CMs in this setting, all licensed clinicians, work independently to provide care delivery. Formal group clinical supervision occurs once a week for 2 hours with a psychiatrist and a licensed marriage and family therapist. CBCM clinicians also receive frequent formal and informal individual clinical supervision.

As the CPH continuum of care model evolved, so did the role of the CM. Because CPH conceptualized the CM role to be flexible and dynamic, resistance to change thus far has been minimized (Baker & Giese, 1992; Thomas et al., 1995). CPH leadership recognized that the complexity of this model could lead to role dissatisfaction and poor treatment outcomes. Thoughtful discussions concerning the educational needs of the CM led to the development of a competency-based orientation to the role, continued education and training, and development of ongoing clinical supervision. Although costly to our organization, orientation, training, and supervision programs are strongly supported by our administration. In the next section of this chapter, we will discuss the six components of a successful case management model.

COMPONENTS OF A SUCCESSFUL CASE MANAGEMENT MODEL

Orientation

The process of clinical orientation at CPH is multidimensional. CMs participate in a competency-based, hospital-wide, department, and unit-specific orientation that includes didactic learning experiences and clinical orientation with a trained preceptor. Because CMs are responsible for both communicating the plan of care to the line staff and guiding treatment forward, they must have an understanding of the responsibilities of the line staff and an ability to develop treatment plans that clearly articulate line staff interventions for their patients. To clearly understand the role of line staff, CMs are oriented to milieu management and mental health worker and clinical nurse responsibilities.

Classroom orientation consists of 2 full days of lecture and didactic learning. An overview of CPH patient services programs and our performance improvement model are presented. A clinical nurse specialist with prescriptive authority teaches a 2-hour course about psychotropic medications and administers a competency performance examination to participants. The clinical nurse specialist/educator conducts a 1-hour risk assessment course and a 5-hour brief therapy course (Webster et al., 1995). A mental health worker who has over 15 years of inpatient psychiatry experience teaches a course about lower level interventions in the milieu and behavior management. CMs must demonstrate competency in risk assessment, brief therapy approaches, and behavioral management before orientation is completed.

The clinical nurse specialist/educator meets with each CM orientee before the first clinical orientation day. CM orientees are given a packet called the "Competency Performance Orientation Checklist" (Appendix 10-1). This packet includes competencies, both knowledge and skill-based, that the CM must either understand or demonstrate before the end of the orientation period. The clinical nurse specialist/educator updates the "Competency Performance Orientation Checklist" annually in response to changes in clinical practice and role responsibilities. Areas of competency reviewed in the checklist include utilization of brief therapy approaches, interdisciplinary communication, discharge/disposition planning, group and family therapy, therapeutic relationships, milieu management, policies and procedures, documentation guidelines, and mandatory safety procedures. All of the competencies are reviewed formally in classroom orientation and reinforced in clinical orientation with the assigned clinical preceptor.

The clinical nurse specialist/educator assigns a trained clinical preceptor to provide clinical orientation. During clinical orientation, which lasts 3 to 4 weeks, CM orientees first observe the clinical preceptor on the unit. The clinical preceptor reviews the Competency Orientation Performance Checklist with the CM orientee each morning, developing daily and weekly goals for clinical orientation. Typically, CM orientees begin some independent practice by the end of the first week of clinical orientation. At the end of the clinical orientation, the clinical nurse specialist/educator reviews each section of the completed Competency Orientation Performance Checklist with the CM orientee to ensure that the CM orientee feels comfortable to begin managing a case load. If the CM orientee or the clinical nurse specialist/educator identifies deficits that must be addressed immediately, the clinical nurse specialist/educator can either choose to work directly with the orientee or ask the clinical preceptor to continue clinical orientation. Since the role of CM is so complex, CPH leadership expects that most CMs will work approximately 6 months before they feel a sense of mastery in the position. This expectation is reinforced to new CMs, as many have stated that they feel pressure to "know it all" when clinical orientation ends. To allow new CMs to flourish in this complicated and multifaceted role, CPH leadership has organized extensive clinical supervision for this group.

Clinical Supervision

Since the CMs' role as the hub of the treatment team is crucial for effective treatment, clinical supervision becomes essential for positive treatment outcomes. Historically, patient services staff have not received intense, ongoing clinical supervision, nor has this modality been valued (Pesut & Williams, 1990). Clarity of the supervision model to reinforce competency-based orientation came as CPH leadership recognized the need to provide several modalities of supervision for CMs. Currently, CMs participate in many formal and informal supervision activities. Professional role development, family supervision, and "behind the mirror" supervision will be discussed.

PROFESSIONAL ROLE DEVELOPMENT
To support new CMs in integrating with treatment team members, they meet weekly with the clinical nurse specialist/educator to discuss role development issues. New CMs have struggled to successfully function in this complicated system and have voiced a need to meet with a knowledgeable mentor to discuss emerging role development issues. Areas of discussion include the CPH CM model, CPH continuum of care model, high-risk cases, patient advocacy issues, and customer relations. Since the facilitator of this group is not a direct supervisor, new CMs are more apt to openly discuss barriers to role development. CPH leadership supports this costly intervention, for not to do so causes role ambiguity and may lead to implementation of incongruent philosophies of care. This group meets weekly for 1 hour.

FAMILY SUPERVISION
A key role of the CM is the provision of family and support system intervention. Level of competency in systems interventions varied, depending on the prior training and experience of the CM. Discrepancy in functional levels of the CM led to the need to have formalized supervision that acknowledged the expertise CMs brought to the role, while recognizing that deficits did exist. Because the training needs varied between disciplines, the clinical nurse specialist/educator and the lead social worker met to discuss the goals and format of the supervision.

In the family supervision "Case Presentation Outline" (Box 10-1), the CM's role is structured both to develop a professional case presentation and to facilitate a peer discussion. In the monthly family supervision meetings, CMs have presented a wide variety of cases. Issues have included transcultural in-

---

| Box 10-1 | **COLORADO PSYCHIATRIC HEALTH**
Family Supervision–Case Presentation Outline |

The family supervision presentation is a 30-minute formal presentation followed by a 20-minute peer discussion. The case presentation is to include the following:
1. Warm up
   Why are you presenting this case?
   • Difficult
   • Interesting
   • Negative outcome
   • Positive outcome
2. Literature review
   Present at least one article/book/chapter pertinent to this case.
   Include the following in your presentation:
   • The theoretical framework
   • The main points for the article/book/chapter
3. Analysis of the case
   • Precipitants
   • Goals of the patient, family and support system
   • Clinical assessment
   • Treatment plan and interventions
   • Evaluation
   • Any change in patient, family, or support system goals resulting from the outcome of the case
   • What went well
   • What you would do differently

Courtesy *Colorado Psychiatric Health, University of Colorado Health Sciences Center, Denver, Colorado.*
During the 20-minute peer discussion, participants will:
1. Discuss whether you've dealt with a similar patient, family, or support system.
2. Talk about what approach you took with that family.
3. Describe whether you had a similar or dissimilar outcome.
4. Discuss any feedback you have for the presenter.

tervention, multisystem coordination, countertransference issues, complex medical comorbidity, substance-abusing patients and family members, and how to successfully intervene with families with special needs. Initially, CMs were hesitant to give feedback to their peers. Since clinical supervision has not been consistently valued in inpatient psychiatric settings (Hallberg, 1994), many CMs were not comfortable with and did not understand the concept of giving and receiving peer feedback regarding clinical performance. To model acceptable ways of giving and receiving feedback, the clinical nurse specialist/educator and the lead social worker presented the first two cases in family supervision.

BEHIND THE MIRROR SUPERVISION
Because brief therapy philosophy includes rapid mobilization of client's resources, supervision supporting this philosophy becomes essential in short-term hospitalization. The CM needs expertise in directing clinical care with families, support systems, and inpatient/outpatient staff. Behind the mirror supervision is a process by which CMs are able to receive immediate feedback from their peers and supervisors (Vaughn et al, in press). In behind the mirror supervision, CMs conduct individual interviews with patients and/or families utilizing brief therapy modalities. The literature concerning clinical supervision suggests that the model should reflect the philosophy of patient care delivery (Vaughn et al., in press; Williams, 1992). Therefore supervision is a parallel process whereby the supervision team provides the CM with feedback in the same structured format as used by the CM to give

feedback to the patient/family. This process has been described in detail in previous articles (Vaughn et al., unpublished manuscript).

Multidisciplinary Team

Traditionally, inpatient psychiatric treatment has been coordinated by psychiatrists (Thomas et al., 1995). As third party providers and other external systems have demanded shorter lengths of stay and more consistent communication of the patient's progression, psychiatrists have realized that it is imperative to share and delegate clinical and organizational functions (Baker & Giese, 1992; Thomas et al., 1995; Thomas et al., 1996; Vaughn et al., 1997). Development and implementation of the CPH case management model would not have been successful if the medical staff had not first agreed to change the model of patient care delivery. Thomas et al., (1995) describe the process of redefinition of multidisciplinary team roles. They acknowledge that both attending psychiatrists and trainees initially had difficulty with the transition from a more traditional model of care delivery to the CPH case management model. Their stance, however, is that clear role definition of the CM "insures clinical efficiency" and will ultimately "optimize the use of the psychiatrist's time." Attending psychiatrists are oriented to the CPH case management model by their peers. Support of the model is reinforced when new attending psychiatrists begin working on the units and see the positive effects of collaborative multidisciplinary working relationships. Residents in training and medical students are oriented to the CPH case management model by senior CMs at the beginning of their clinical rotation. Attending psychiatrists and CMs formally and informally reinforce both the CM and resident roles with the residents and medical students during multidisciplinary meetings.

Treatment Plan

Clinical information is formally reviewed with the treatment team in daily multidisciplinary rounds and twice weekly treatment planning meetings. The CM will contact treatment team members informally if there is new clinical information that must be reviewed immediately. The CM is responsible for leading treatment planning meetings and for integrating and documenting all clinical information in the patient's treatment plan. The purpose of treatment planning meetings is to review new clinical information and revise the plan of care. All of the treatment team's patients are presented in 1 hour, giving the treatment team approximately 10 minutes to revise the plan of care for each patient. Indepth discussion regarding the psychodynamic formulation of the case is completed outside of the treatment plan meeting (Baker & Giese, 1992; Thomas et al., 1995).

CMs organize the order in which patients will be presented. CMs contact external providers to negotiate how clinical information will be exchanged. Telephone conferences, treatment update meetings, and discharge meetings are coordinated at the beginning of hospitalization, ensuring external provider participation. Examples of external treatment provider participation include outpatient case managers, group home staff, probation and parole officers, social services technicians, and clergy. The CM is responsible for establishing and maintaining contact with family and community supports. With written permission, CMs make initial contact with family members within 24 hours of the client's admission. Family input is considered essential to successful treatment. Issues that appear to be part of the precipitating events of hospitalization are addressed in family meetings. Patient services staff meet every shift with the client to establish treatment goals and interventions. At the end of each shift, patient services staff document progress toward goal attainment and response to interventions. If the client cannot participate in problem solving because of cognitive impairment, the treatment team will work with the family and community supports to develop goals to expedite restabilization. Patient services staff attend and participate in the treatment planning meeting, bringing up-to-date clinical information.

Treatment plans are structured to provide clear interventions for line staff and the multidisciplinary team. CPH treatment plans are currently in a revision process, led by the treatment plan performance improvement team. This team is chaired by the clinical nurse specialist/educator, and group participants include an attending psychiatrist, patient services managers, a CM, a charge nurse, and a mental health worker.

The first revised treatment plan, "Suicide Attempt/Ideation" (Appendix 10-2), has been implemented on the inpatient units. In the treatment planning meeting, the CM is responsible for completing this form. The first part of the plan includes a brief formulation of the case and the psychiatric and medical diagnoses. The second section of the treatment plan documents measurable goals. Goals are developed with input from the treatment team, line staff, patient, family, and support system (Webster et al., 1994). Next, interventions are addressed. Interventions associated with providing safety (risk assessment and suicide precautions) for the patient and the milieu are listed first. Other interventions include laboratory testing and consultation, medication regimen and administration, medication and illness education, group participation, family and support system interventions, discharge planning issues, and treatment of acute medical issues. The last section of the treatment plan is the outcome section. In this section the treatment team identifies what the functioning level of the patient must be before the patient is discharged. Since CPH provides a continuum of care, including community-based case management (CBCM), the patient may not have to demonstrate baseline level of functioning before discharge.

After the treatment planning meeting is completed, the CM is responsible for ensuring that the line staff implements the interventions outlined in the newly revised plan. Other treatment plan forms that the case manager may use to develop a complete plan of care include the "Behavioral Care Plan" and "Take Care of Yourself" (Appendix 9-3). The Behavioral Care Plan guides the line staff in behavioral interventions aimed at providing the patient with the external structure he or she needs to stay in behavioral control on the unit. The Take Care of Yourself form is completed by the CM with input from the outpatient provider. The outpatient provider gives the CM information about the client's cognitive and functional ability to complete activities of daily living (ADLs). With this information the CM completes the form, giving the line staff detailed information about level of assistance with ADLs and how often ADLs should be completed. Since it is often difficult to assess the client's cognitive and functional ability during a short hospital stay, it is important to provide care that is consistent with the care provided in the community setting. If the level of assistance provided is consistent between inpatient and outpatient providers, the client is less likely to demonstrate symptoms of regression after discharge.

Use of treatment plans is not a new concept; in fact, most medical inpatient units use critical pathways and/or care maps to structure clinical intervention and provide standardized outcome measures (de Woody & Price, 1994; Goode, 1995; Hofmann, 1993; Krmpotic, 1992). In psychiatry, where complex psychosocial and environmental variables influence the client's clinical progress, measuring outcomes and accounting for variances in length of stay is challenging and has not been well documented (Baker & Giese, 1992; Thomas, Dubovsky, & Cox-Young, 1996; Thomas et al., 1996; Thomas et al., 1997).

Variance tracking within mental health systems is sadly at a rudimentary stage of development. CPH has contributed to the development of variance tracking by collecting both inpatient and outpatient outcomes data in conjunction with managed care companies (Baker & Giese, 1992; Thomas, Dubovsky, & Cox-Young, 1996; Thomas et al., 1996; Thomas et al., 1997).

In psychiatric managed care's infancy, CMs partnered with managed care providers to develop utilization review tools that measured length of stay, recidivism, successful suicides, and readmission within 24 hours (Baker & Giese, 1992; Thomas, Dubovsky, & Cox-Young, 1996; Thomas et al., 1996; Thomas et al., 1997). As we developed partnerships with more and more managed care companies, the time expenditure required of CMs to perform utilization review duties began to take away from important clinical responsibilities.

Utilization Review

In June, 1999 a social worker was hired for the specific purpose of completing inpatient utilization review (UR) processes. Before this time CMs were responsible for all authorizations for clients on their caseload. It became evident that the focus of client care was being negatively affected by this UR function. As the UR process became more complicated, it also became more time consuming. Therefore CMs had an increasingly difficult time completing other clinical duties. UR inherently involves a great deal of phone work; therefore unless the CM is readily available to answer phone calls, an inordinate amount of time is spent brokering authorizations for continued treatment. Before changing our UR system the rate of successful authorization for treatment was 50%. Lack of authorizations for treatment created difficulty in hospital billing and collections. On the clinical front, CM documentation suffered and quality of treatment plans was insufficient, secondary to emphasis on the time-consuming task of UR. Another factor that indicated a need to change the UR process was a gradual increase in the average length of stay in the last 3 years (1996-1998) from 7.0 inpatient days to 7.8 inpatient days.

The decision to allocate resources for a UR staff person has had several positive outcomes. The rate of authorization for treatment has quickly risen to 90%, there is increased flexibility in the CM's schedules, the UR process has been connected to our finance department, and there is a more careful review of denial and collection processes. The UR staff person generally works independently, but will consult with CMs when there are complex clinical issues that require additional input for authorization for treatment. This change in our UR system has enabled CMs to refocus their energies on coordinating and managing client care.

We conducted a random chart review (n = 40) 1 month before UR changes and 1 month after UR changes, assessing the presence of adequate treatment plans (2 per 3.5 inpatient days) and CM notes (1 per 7 inpatient days) (Figure 10-3).

This review revealed that the completion of treatment plans increased from 50% to 80% and completion of case management notes increased from 70% to 90% after the UR staff person was hired.

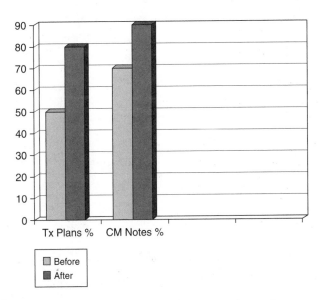

FIGURE **10-3**   Comparison of completion rates of treatment plans and case management progress notes before and after utilization review was separated from case management responsibilities.

Clearly this change in our UR system has contributed to an improvement in CM documentation rates. Other targets for data collection include length of stay, CM job satisfaction, and customer satisfaction.

Customer Satisfaction

Customer satisfaction has long been viewed as an important indicator of quality of care (Goode, 1995; Higgins, 1994; Lamb & Stempel, 1994; Nicols & Zallar, 1995; Ward & Rieve, 1993). In this age of increased managed care, third party providers, and regulatory agency oversight, customer satisfaction data carry more weight (Baker & Giese, 1992). At CPH, we have always maintained that patient satisfaction is the most important indicator of our clinical success. Valuing customer satisfaction meshes solution-focused philosophy with our model of care delivery. In solution-focused therapy, core concepts include the belief that clients have the best answers for their problems and that they should always be involved with formulating treatment goals and evaluating treatment outcomes (Vaughn et al., 1997). We firmly believe that successful evolution of our model depends on client input.

In 1990 we began to gather customer satisfaction data. We used these data to determine educational needs for line staff and program redesign. In 1996 we began to participate in a national patient satisfaction benchmarking program, RESPONSE Healthcare Information Management, Inc. This enabled us to compare our customer satisfaction data with similar psychiatric facilities across the nation. CPH data indicate that across categories we meet or exceed the national benchmark (RESPONSE, 1998) (see Figure 10-4).

As indicated in Figure 10-4, the areas of greatest customer satisfaction were in teamwork among staff, respect and dignity shown, overall quality of care and services, outcome of care, discharge instructions,

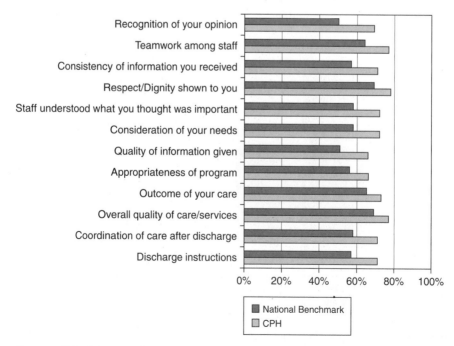

FIGURE **10-4**   Percentage of responses from the "very good" to the "excellent" range.
Data compiled from National Benchmark Report, Psychiatric Hospitals (1998) and RESPONSE, 1998.

and coordination of care after discharge. In completing the customer satisfaction questionnaire, clients are encouraged to provide comments regarding their treatment.

"I realize that most of what needs to be done to help myself needs to come from me." CPH Inpatient, 1998

Clients frequently note how useful the treatment experience has been for them, that the staff gave them confidence to succeed, and that they were involved with treatment decisions.

Customer satisfaction data are regularly reviewed with CMs. This process allows CMs to receive feedback about their role and gives them an opportunity to participate in the dynamic process of performance improvement.

SUMMARY

In this chapter, we have outlined an innovative psychiatric inpatient case management model. We hope that our model adds to the scarcity of information currently available regarding psychiatric case management models. Part of our success has been attributable to the support of CPH leadership, who back expensive orientation, training, and supervision aspects. Theoretical underpinnings that hold the client as central to successful treatment have remained the cornerstone of our success. Evolving treatment plans and UR processes reflect our desire to address our rapidly changing health care system.

Changes in clinical systems are occurring so rapidly that they outstrip the meager empirical data base used to make changes in health care delivery models. Our hope is that psychiatric hospitals will band together to collect essential data regarding clinical variance, clinical outcomes, lengths of stay, and diagnosis-specific critical pathways. Outcome measures are particularly critical because psychiatric inpatient case management is new and relatively unstudied. Formal research projects are required to address the specific needs of various psychiatric populations.

References

Baker, N.J., & Giese, A.A. (1992). Reorganization of a private psychiatric unit to promote collaboration with managed care, *Hospital and Community Psychiatry, 43*(11), 126-129.

Banja, J., Friedman, E., Keffer, J., Meany, M., Mullahy, C. (1997). Ethical accountabilities of case management, *Journal of Case Management, 3*(4), 13-17, 24.

Berg, I.K. (1991). *Family preservation: A brief therapy workbook.* London: BT Press.

Bodgett, B.P. (1993). Case management in mental health. The pendulum still swings, *Journal of Case Management, 2*(3), 96-100.

Curtin, L. (1996). The ethics of managed care: Parts 1, 2 and 3, *Nursing Management, 27*(8,9,10).

de Woody, S., & Price, J. (1994). A systems approach to multidimensional critical paths, *Nursing Management, 25*(11), 47-51.

De Shazer, S. (1991). *Patterns of brief family therapy,* New York: Guilford Press.

Erkel, E.A. (1993). The impact of case management in preventive services, *Journal of Nursing Administration, 23*(1), 27-32.

Ford, R., Beadsmoore, A., Ryan, P., Repper, J., Craig, T., Mujen, M. (1995). Providing the safety net: Case management for people with serious mental illness, *Journal of Mental Health, 1,* 91-97.

Ford, R., Repper, T., Cooke, A., Norton, P., Beadsmoore, A., Clarke, C. (1993). *Implementing case management,* London: Research and Development for Psychiatry.

Gibson, S.J., Martin, S.M., Johnson, M.B., Blue, R., Miller, D.S. (1994). CNS-directed case management: Cost and quality in harmony, *Journal of Nursing Administration, 4*(6), 45-51.

Golonder, L.F. (1999). Consumer voice: From whimper to roar. In E.L. Cohen, & V. De Back (Eds.), *The outcomes mandate. Case management in health care today.* St. Louis: Mosby.

Goode, C. (1995). Impact of a caremap and case management on patient satisfaction, and staff satisfaction, collaboration and autonomy, *Nursing Economic$, 13*(6), 337-348.

Gourney, K. (1995). Changing patterns in mental health care: Implications for evaluation and training, *Psychiatric Care, 2*(3), 93-95.

Gudeman, J.E., Dickey, B., Evans, A., Shore, M.F. (1985). Four-year assessment of a day hospital-inn program as an alternative to inpatient hospitalization. *American Journal of Psychiatry, 142*(11), 1330-1333.

Hallberg, I.R. (1994). Systematic clinical supervision in a child psychiatric ward: Satisfaction with nursing care, tedium, burnout and the nurses' own report on the effects of it, *Archives of Psychiatric Nursing, 8*(1), 44-52.

Harper, G. (1988). Focal inpatient treatment planning, *Journal of the American Academy of Child and Adolescent Psychiatry, 28,* 31-37.

Hatfield, B. (1996). Case management in mental health services: The role of community mental health support teams, *Health and Social Care in the Community, 4*(4), 215-225.

Higgins, R. (1994). User-led case management, *Senior Nurse, 13*(7), 42-46.

Hofmann, P.A. (1993). Critical path method: An important tool for coordinating clinical care, *Journal on Quality Improvement, 19*(7), 235-245.

Holloway, F. (1991). Case management for the mentally ill: Looking at the evidence, *International Journal of Social Psychiatry, 27*(1), 213.

Holloway, F., Oliver, N., Collinas, E., Carson, J. (1995). Case management: A critical review of the outcome literature, *European Psychiatry, 10,* 113-128.

Karpel, M, (Ed.). (1986). *Family resources: The hidden partner in family therapy,* New York: The Guilford Press.

Krmpotic, D. (1992). Successful implementation of case management, *Nursing Connections, 5*(2), 49-50.

Lachance, K.R., & Santos, A.B. (1995). Modifying the PACT model: Preserving critical elements, *Psychiatric Services, 46*(6), 601-604.

Lamb, G.S., & Stempel, J.E. (1994). Nurse case management from the client's view: Growing as insider-expert, *Nursing Outlook, 42*(1), 7-13.

Lehnhoff, J. (1991). Assessment and utilization of patient strengths in acute care treatment planning, *The Psychiatric Hospital, 22*(1), 11-15.

Marschke, P., & Nolan, M.T. (1993). Research related to case management, *Nursing Administration, 17*(3), 16-21.

Montgomery, C., & Webster, D. (1993). Care and nursing's metaparadigm: Can they survive in the era of managed care? *Perspectives in Psychiatric Nursing, 29*(4), 5-12.

Montgomery, C., & Webster, D. (1994). Caring, curing and brief therapy: A model for nurse-psychotherapy, *Archives of Psychiatric Nursing, 8*(5), 291-297.

Nicols, D., & Zallar, M.J. (1995). Care coordination: A new role in a customer-focused healthcare system, *Nursing Case Management, 2*(5), 269-274.

Olsen, D.P., Rickles, J., & Travlik, K. (1995). A treatment-team model of managed mental health care, *Psychiatric Services, 46*(3), 252-256.

Pesut, D.J., & Williams, C.A. (1990). The nature of clinical supervision in psychiatric nursing: A survey of clinical specialists, *Archives of Psychiatric Nursing, 4*(3), 188-194.

Quinn, J. (1993). Case management: As diverse as its clients, *Journal of Case Management, 2*(4), 117.

Rantz, M., & Scott, J. (1997). Promoting self-health management of chronic illness. In E.L. Cohen, & V. De Back (Eds.), *The outcomes mandate. Case management in health care today,* St. Louis: Mosby.

RESPONSE Healthcare Information Management, Inc. (1998). *Patient Satisfaction Survey.*

Santos, A.B., & McLeod-Bryant, S. (1991). Strategies for operational efficiency in a general hospital public inpatient unit, *Hospital and Community Psychiatry, 42*(1), 66-69.

Sherman, P.S., & Porter, R. (1991). Mental health consumers as case management aides, *Hospital and Community Psychiatry, 42*(5), 494-498.

Smith, M. (1994). Case management in the care-healing paradigm, *The New Definition, 10*(2), 1-2.

Solomon, P. (1992). The efficacy of case management, *Community Mental Health Journal, 28*(3), 163-179.

Stein, L.I., & Test, M.A. (1980). Alternative to mental hospital treatment. I: Conceptual model, treatment program, and clinical evaluation, *Archives of General Psychiatry, 37,* 392-397.

Tahan, H. (1998). Case management: A heritage more than a century old, *Nursing Case Management, 3*(2), 55-60.

Taylor, C., & Barnet, R.J. (1999). The ethics of case management. In E.L. Cohen, & V. De Back (Eds.), *The outcomes mandate. Case management in health care today,* St. Louis: Mosby.

Test, M.A. (1992). Training in community living. In R.P. Lieberman (Ed.), *Handbook of psychiatric rehabilitation,* New York: Macmillan.

Thomas, B., & Lovell, K. (1999). Mental health nursing and case management in Great Britain. In E.L. Cohen & V. De Back (Eds.), *The outcomes mandate. Case management in health care today,* St. Louis: Mosby.

Thomas, M.R., House, R., Shore, J., & Cox Young, B. (1995). The impact of economic and health care delivery changes on psychiatric residency training. Adapting to the new realities for clinical services and residency education in managed care, *Proceedings of the AACPD/RTD Conferences.*

Thomas, M.R., Dubovsky, S.L., & Cox-Young, B. (1996). Impact of external versus internal case managers on hospital utilization, *Psychiatric Services, 47*(6), 593-595.

Thomas, M.R., Rosenberg, S.A., Giese, A.A., Dubovsky, S.L., & Shore, J.H. (1996). Shortening length of stay without increasing recidivism on a university-affiliated inpatient unit, *Psychiatric Services, 47*(9), 996-998.

Thomas, M.R., Kassner, C.T., Fryer, G.E., Giese, A.A., Rosenberg, S.A., & Dubovsky, S.L. (1997). Impact of shorter lengths of stay on status at discharge in bipolar mania, *Annals of Clinical Psychiatry, 9*(3), 139-143.

Trinidad, E.A. (1993). Case management: A model of CNS practice, *Clinical Nurse Specialist, 7*(4), 221-223.

Van Dongen, C.J., & Jambunathan, J. (1992). Pilot study results: The psychiatric RN case manager, *Journal of Psychosocial Nursing, 30*(11), 11-36.

Vaughn, K., Webster, D.C., Platter, B., Playter, A., & Webb, M. (Unpublished manuscript.). Solution oriented hospital practice and supervision: Building psychiatric nursing competencies, *Perspectives in Psychiatric Care.*

Vaughn, K., Webster, D.C., Orahood, S., & Cox-Young, B. (1995). Brief inpatient psychiatric treatment: Finding solutions, *Issues in Mental Health Nursing, 16,* 519-531.

Vaughn, K., Hastings-Guerrero, S., & Kassner, C. (1996). Solution-oriented inpatient group therapy, *Journal of Systemic Therapies, 15*(3), 1-13.

Vaughn, K., Cox-Young, B., Webster, D.C., & Thomas, M.R. (1997). Solution-focused work in the hospital. A continuum-of-care model for inpatient psychiatric treatment. In S.D. Miller, M.A. Hubble, & B.L. Duncan (Eds.). *Handbook of solution-focused brief therapy,* San Francisco: Jossey-Bass Publishers.

Wadas, T.M. (1993). Case management and caring behavior, *Nursing Management, 24*(9), 40-46.

Ward, M., & Rieve, J. (1993). Disease management: Case management's return to patient-centered care, *Journal of Care Management, 4*(1), 7-8, 10, 12.

Webster, D.C., Vaughn, K., & Martinez, R. (1994). Introducing solution-focused approaches to staff in inpatient psychiatric settings, *Archives of Psychiatric Nursing, 8*(4), 254-261.

Webster, D.C., Vaughn, K., Webb, M., & Playter, A. (1995). Modeling the client's world through solution-focused therapy, *Issues in Mental Health Nursing, 16*(6), 505-518.

Wehmeyer, M.L. (1993). Sounding a certain trumpet: Case management as a catalyst for empowerment of people with developmental disabilities, *Journal of Case Management, 2*(1), 14-18.

Wetchler, J.L. (1990). Solution-focused supervision, *Family Therapy, 14*(2), 129-138.

Williams, R. (1992). Nurse case management: Working with the community, *Nursing Management, 23*(12), 33-34.

Appendix 10-1

COLORADO PSYCHIATRIC HEALTH DEPARTMENT OF PATIENT SERVICES
Competency Performance Orientation Checklist–
Psychiatric Case Manager

Name:
Competency: Utilizes brief therapy in individual, group, family, and milieu therapy

EVALUATION CRITERIA
1. Verbalizes value system of long- and short-term therapist.
2. States the assumptions of solution-oriented therapy.
3. Verbalizes obstacles and pitfalls to avoid in brief therapy.
4. Reads brief therapy manual.
5. Has 1:1 interactions with patients, families, and support systems using solution-focused therapy and other brief therapy approaches.
6. States factors that contribute to regression in hospitalized patients.
7. Demonstrates use of reframing techniques.
8. States types of interviewing techniques used in solution-focused therapy and other brief therapy approaches.
9. Sets goal with patients, families, and support systems that are client centered, achievable, and measurable.
10. Attends solution-focused therapy and change theory orientation class and demonstrates competency through passing post-test with score of 80% or greater.
11. Attends monthly "behind the mirror" supervision sessions, participating as the clinician and as part of the supervision team.

PRECEPTOR/EDUCATOR			COMMENTS	I HAVE SATISFACTORILY PERFORMED THE ABOVE COMPETENCY
Taught	Performed with assistance	Performed independently		**Orientee** Date **Preceptor** Date

UNIVERSITY HOSPITAL COLORADO PSYCHIATRIC HEALTH
DEPARTMENT OF PATIENT SERVICES
Competency Performance Orientation Checklist–
Psychiatric Case Manager

Name:

Competency: Complies with hospital policies outlining documentation requirements

EVALUATION CRITERIA

1. Completes treatment plan and ensures patient services implementation of treatment plan (including biophysical, psychosocial, and environmental realms).
2. Completes "Behavior Plan" with patient services staff input when applicable; used to address behavioral issues of assigned patients.
3. Completes "Take Care of Yourself" with patient services staff input when applicable; used to address self-care issues of assigned patients.
4. Documentation on the patient record is legible, accurate, and concise.
5. Completes 2-hour RN/LSCW reassessment forms in compliance with "Psychiatric Use of Seclusion and Restraint" policy.
6. Completes risk assessment on the Suicide Risk Assessment and Violence Risk Assessment forms, documents clearly in the chart, and communicates results with treatment team. Repeats this process as indicated, based on patient presentation.
7. Completes case manager section of the discharge plan form. Ensures that an RN has completed the RN section of the form before the patient is discharged.
8. Completes or describes the AMA discharge procedure.
9. Ensures completion of patient teaching standards for medication, diagnosis, and other educational issues.
10. Completes case manager progress note, minimum of 1 per week.

Ensures completion of psychosocial data base (childhood and developmental history, cultural issues, living arrangements, military history sections) and signs encounter form signature log.

PRECEPTOR/EDUCATOR			COMMENTS	I HAVE SATISFACTORILY PERFORMED THE ABOVE COMPETENCY
Taught	Performed with assistance	Performed independently		**Orientee** Date **Preceptor** Date

Courtesy *Colorado Psychiatric Health, University of Colorado Health Sciences Center, Denver, Colorado.*

UNIVERSITY HOSPITAL COLORADO PSYCHIATRIC HEALTH DEPARTMENT OF PATIENT SERVICES
Competency Performance Orientation Checklist— Psychiatric Case Manager

Name:

Competency: Discharge planning

EVALUATION CRITERIA

1. Ensures appropriate transportation is arranged for patient.
2. Clarifies patient's ability to take passes and makes necessary arrangements.
3. Coordinates/leads staffings with outpatient providers.
4. Arranges appropriate psychiatric/medical and other outpatient follow-up.
5. Coordinates/secures appropriate housing at discharge.
6. Educates patient, family, and support system about patient's current medication regimen and ensures that all understand the information presented.
7. Educates patient, family, and support system about how to secure financial resources.
8. Arranges facility transfers as indicated: coordinates completion of EMTALA forms.
9. Ensures completion of paperwork for nursing home placement.
10. Coordinates legal issues, such as legal status on the unit and legal issues in the community.
11. Is a liaison for community resources.

PRECEPTOR/EDUCATOR			COMMENTS	I HAVE SATISFACTORILY PERFORMED THE ABOVE COMPETENCY
Taught	Performed with assistance	Performed independently		**Orientee** Date **Preceptor** Date

Courtesy *Colorado Psychiatric Health, University of Colorado Health Sciences Center, Denver, Colorado.*

UNIVERSITY HOSPITAL COLORADO PSYCHIATRIC HEALTH
DEPARTMENT OF PATIENT SERVICES
Competency Performance Orientation Checklist–
Psychiatric Case Manager

Name:
Competency: Interdisciplinary communication

EVALUATION CRITERIA
1. Demonstrates interdisciplinary communication and coordination with medical staff, students, line staff, occupational therapy pharmacy, family medicine, internal and external consultants, patient representative, and others.
2. Demonstrates and documents appropriate sign-out of cases for planned absences from the unit.
3. Demonstrates appropriate sign-out of cases for unplanned absences.
4. Demonstrates ability to manage complaints related to assigned patients and involves the use of appropriate resources.

PRECEPTOR/EDUCATOR			COMMENTS	I HAVE SATISFACTORILY PERFORMED THE ABOVE COMPETENCY
Taught	Performed with assistance	Performed independently		**Orientee** Date **Preceptor** Date

Courtesy *Colorado Psychiatric Health, University of Colorado Health Sciences Center, Denver, Colorado.*

UNIVERSITY HOSPITAL COLORADO PSYCHIATRIC HEALTH
DEPARTMENT OF PATIENT SERVICES
Competency Performance Orientation Checklist–
Psychiatric Case Manager

Name:
Competency: Establishes therapeutic relationships with patients and families

EVALUATION CRITERIA
1. Reads and signs policy on confidentiality and therapeutic relationships.
2. States principles of therapeutic interactions.
3. Verbalizes difference between therapeutic and social relationships.
4. Reads policy on therapeutic relationships.
5. Reads guideline for staff/patient and family interactions.
6. States how age, race, gender, and culture of patient and family may affect therapeutic relationship.
7. States importance of terminating the therapeutic relationship with the patient and the family when the patient is discharged.
8. Reads adolescent and geriatric manuals and provides age-appropriate care.
9. Attends and participates in monthly family supervision meetings.

PRECEPTOR/EDUCATOR			COMMENTS	I HAVE SATISFACTORILY PERFORMED the ABOVE COMPETENCY
Taught	Performed with assistance	Performed independently		**Orientee** Date **Preceptor** Date

Courtesy *Colorado Psychiatric Health, University of Colorado Health Sciences Center, Denver, Colorado.*

**UNIVERSITY HOSPITAL COLORADO PSYCHIATRIC HEALTH
DEPARTMENT OF PATIENT SERVICES**
Competency Performance Orientation Checklist–
Psychiatric Case Manager

Name:
Competency: Provides and maintains a safe therapeutic environment

EVALUATION CRITERIA
1. States five therapeutic aspects of milieu treatment.
2. Verbalizes difference between traditional inpatient milieu therapy and brief milieu therapy.
3. Verbalizes safety issues in the milieu.
4. Verbalizes hierarchy of interventions in the milieu.
5. Demonstrates use of lower level interventions in the milieu.
6. Verbalizes age-appropriate limit setting in the milieu.
7. Initiates search procedures as indicated.
8. States procedure when patients go AWOL.
9. Attends non-violent crisis intervention (NVCI) and seclusion/restraint class and demonstrates competency by passing the seclusion/restraint test and the NVCI test with scores of 80% or better.
10. Demonstrates safe application of mechanical restraints.
11. Communicates with family and support system about the criteria/procedures for seclusion/restraint and maintenance of a safe milieu.
12. Supports family and support system by maintaining close contact with clinical updates and reassurance when patient is in seclusion/restraint.

PRECEPTOR/EDUCATOR			COMMENTS	I HAVE SATISFACTORILY PERFORMED THE ABOVE COMPETENCY
Taught	Performed with assistance	Performed independently		**Orientee** Date **Preceptor** Date

Courtesy *Colorado Psychiatric Health, University of Colorado Health Sciences Center, Denver, Colorado.*

UNIVERSITY HOSPITAL COLORADO PSYCHIATRIC HEALTH
DEPARTMENT OF PATIENT SERVICES
Competency Performance Orientation Checklist–
Psychiatric Case Manager

Name:
Competency: Co-leads group therapy/family therapy/case conferences

EVALUATION CRITERIA
1. Able to assess and address family dynamics and intervene using brief therapy and systems theory interventions.
2. Formulates the psychosocial focus of the acute care episode with the treatment team.
3. Educates the family and support system about the patient's medications, illness, and treatment needs.
4. Negotiates treatment goals and follow-up plans with the patient, family, and support system.
5. Applies new knowledge in family and support system intervention from monthly family supervision group to clinical practice.
6. Understands expectation of participation in ongoing educational activities that address family and support system intervention.
7. Verbalizes difference between group process and content.
8. Reads guideline on co-therapist before and after group conference.
9. Verbalizes effective and ineffective group therapist language and behavior.
10. Reads group therapy manual.

PRECEPTOR/EDUCATOR			COMMENTS	I HAVE SATISFACTORILY PERFORMED THE ABOVE COMPETENCY
Taught	Performed with assistance	Performed independently		**Orientee** Date **Preceptor** Date

Courtesy *Colorado Psychiatric Health, University of Colorado Health Sciences Center, Denver, Colorado.*

UNIVERSITY HOSPITAL COLORADO PSYCHIATRIC HEALTH
DEPARTMENT OF PATIENT SERVICES
Competency Performance Orientation Checklist–
Psychiatric Case Manager

Name:

Competency: Complies with standards of job description

EVALUATION CRITERIA

1. Verbalizes the three missions of Colorado Psychiatric Health (CPH).
2. Reviews the CPH organizational chart.
3. Reviews the CPH quality management plan and participates in performance improvement projects.
4. Reads and signs job description.
5. Participates in weekly professional role development group with the clinical nurse specialist/educator.

PRECEPTOR/EDUCATOR			COMMENTS	I HAVE SATISFACTORILY PERFORMED THE ABOVE COMPETENCY
Taught	Performed with assistance	Performed independently		**Orientee** Date **Preceptor** Date

Courtesy *Colorado Psychiatric Health, University of Colorado Health Sciences Center, Denver, Colorado.*

UNIVERSITY HOSPITAL COLORADO PSYCHIATRIC HEALTH
DEPARTMENT OF PATIENT SERVICES
Competency Performance Orientation Checklist–
Psychiatric Case Manager

Name:

Competency: Complies with hospital policies and unit guidelines

EVALUATION CRITERIA

1. States purpose of University of Colorado Hospital and Colorado Psychiatric Health policies and procedures.
2. Locates and uses policy manuals.
3. Demonstrates ability to access on-line manuals.
4. Completes policies and procedures test by the end of the first clinical orientation day.
5. Reads Colorado Psychiatric Health Guidelines manual.

PRECEPTOR/EDUCATOR			COMMENTS	I HAVE SATISFACTORILY PERFORMED THE ABOVE COMPETENCY
Taught	Performed with assistance	Performed independently		**Orientee** Date **Preceptor** Date

Courtesy *Colorado Psychiatric Health, University of Colorado Health Sciences Center, Denver, Colorado.*

UNIVERSITY HOSPITAL COLORADO PSYCHIATRIC HEALTH DEPARTMENT OF PATIENT SERVICES
Competency Performance Orientation Checklist–Psychiatric Case Manager

Name:

Competency: Administers prescribed medication safely, accurately, and within hospital guidelines (RNs only)

EVALUATION CRITERIA
1. States side effects of psychotropic medications.
2. Completes medication test with 80% or better (completed in CPH orientation).
3. Documents medication correctly and accurately.
4. Demonstrates or describes procedure for ordering and receiving medication.
5. States dosage range of psychotropic medication for geriatric clients.
6. States procedure for filling prescriptions.
7. Demonstrates safe nursing practice (lock medication cabinets and door to medication room).
8. States indications for orthostatic vital sign assessment (completed in CPH orientation).

PRECEPTOR/EDUCATOR			COMMENTS	I HAVE SATISFACTORILY PERFORMED THE ABOVE COMPETENCY
Taught	Performed with assistance	Performed independently		**Orientee** Date **Preceptor** Date

Courtesy *Colorado Psychiatric Health, University of Colorado Health Sciences Center, Denver, Colorado.*

UNIVERSITY HOSPITAL COLORADO PSYCHIATRIC HEALTH DEPARTMENT OF PATIENT SERVICES
Competency Performance Orientation Checklist–
Psychiatric Case Manager

Name:

Competency: Complies with safety and emergency procedures

EVALUATION CRITERIA
1. States CPH infection control policy (completed in CPH orientation).
2. Locates fire, hazardous material, and disaster manuals.
3. Verbalizes procedure for medical emergencies, fire, bomb threats, psychiatric emergencies, and weather alerts.
4. Locates fire extinguishers and alarms.
5. Locates and describes use of panic buttons.

PRECEPTOR/EDUCATOR			COMMENTS	I HAVE SATISFACTORILY PERFORMED THE ABOVE COMPETENCY
Taught	Performed with assistance	Performed independently		**Orientee** Date **Preceptor** Date

Courtesy *Colorado Psychiatric Health, University of Colorado Health Sciences Center, Denver, Colorado.*

APPENDIX 10-2

Multidisciplinary Treatment Plan

Suicide: Attempt/Ideation

DATE _____   Next Staffing _____

Privileges _____   **Legal status** _____   **ELOS** _____

DIAGNOSIS _____

Focus: Behavior Management: Self-Harm

Related to:

☐ Psychosis ☐ Depression ☐ Panic ☐ Hopelessness ☐ Chronic illness

☐ Terminal illness ☐ Altered cognitive status ☐ Grief/loss _____

☐ Psychoactive substances ☐ _____ ☐ _____

Illustrated by:

☐ Suicidal ideation with a plan _____

☐ Suicide attempt _____

☐ _____

☐ _____

Goals (must be measurable):

☐ Patient will demonstrate ability to manage symptoms.

☐ _____

☐ _____

Interventions

☐ 1. Risk assessment (discipline responsible/frequency) _____

☐ 2. SUICIDE PRECAUTIONS per CPH Guideline 0-3-Psy
   • Assess and document suicidal ideation every shift • Must be RTW and on escape precautions • 15-minute safety checks • Patient searched and placed in hospital gowns • Patient to remain in public areas on the unit during waking • MD note daily regarding continued suicide risk • Controlled items with staff supervision only

☐ 3. Labs/Procedures/Medical Consults:

_____ _____ _____

☐ 4. Medications prescribed (list medications and dosages):

_____ _____

_____ _____

_____ _____

_____ _____

University of Colorado Health Sciences Center
Colorado Psychiatric Health

☐ 5. Administer medications as prescribed and document response
☐ 6. Medication education (as tolerated) to:
    ☐ Patient   ☐ Family   ☐ Outpatient providers   ☐ _____
☐ 7. Patient to receive education or instruction on:
    ☐ Diagnosis   ☐ Symptom management   ☐ Substance abuse
    ☐ Stress management   ☐ _____
☐ 8. Assess/scale current level of hopefulness
☐ 9. Patient to identify ways to increase hopefulness
    ☐ Symptom management plan   ☐ Continue to scale hopefulness
    ☐ _____   ☐ _____
☐ 10. Patient to attend groups as appropriate (list groups):
    ☐ _____   ☐ _____
    ☐ _____   ☐ _____
☐ 11. Administer assessment tools (indicate frequency/discipline responsible):
    ☐ MMSE _____   ☐ Hamilton _____
    ☐ Beck _____   ☐ _____
☐ 12. Assess and document symptoms of psychosis (include confusion, disorganization)
☐ 13. OT consultation (indicate type): _____
☐ 14. Case manager or designee to:
    ☐ Gather collateral data
    ☐ Communicate with outpatient system regarding patient progress and discharge planning
    ☐ Assess and document level of family involvement
    ☐ Document discharge staffing/discharge family meeting _____
    ☐ _____
    ☐ _____
☐ 15. Diet _____
☐ 16. Acute medical issues and interventions _____
☐ _____
☐ _____
☐ _____
☐ _____

Outcomes

The patient demonstrates increased ability to maintain safety, as evidenced by:
☐ Decreased Beck/Hamilton score
☐ Increased GAF
☐ Symptom management plan in place
☐ Increased hopefulness
☐ _____
☐ _____

I have discussed the above treatment plan with my treatment team.

_____   _____
Patient signature   Staff signature

Behavioral Care Plan

Date _____

Warning Signs:

Expectations of Behavior:

Interventions:

Positive Reinforcers:

_____   _____
Client signature   Date

_____   _____
Staff signature   Date

University of Colorado Health Sciences Center
Colorado Psychiatric Hospital
MR#1500.222
3/98 rw

Appendix 10-3

Date: _____

Take Care of Yourself

Levels
1—Independent
2—Prompting
3—With assistance
4—Need 2 for assistance
5—Total care

Level of Assistance

	Frequency	Levels of Assistance	Explanation/Re-Evaluation
Shower			
Meals & fluids			
Deodorant			
Dress			
Mouth care			
Hair care			
Make bed			
Laundry			
Tidy room			
1:1			
Meds			
Group			
Other			

Behavioral Plan:

I understand that I am in the hospital to focus on _____

I agree to do these things to achieve my goal _____

Staff agrees to help me by _____

Client signature _____ **Staff signature** _____

Courtesy of the University of Colorado Health Sciences Center
Colorado Psychiatric Hospital

120

IV

CONTEMPORARY MODELS OF CASE MANAGEMENT

Beyond-the-Walls Case Management

In response to the shift to primary health care interventions and the convergence of wellness and prevention modalities, community-based nursing case management models have literally exploded onto the health care scene. The hallmark of these models is an integrated approach to continuous and seamless health care delivery. Unit IV presents several models that exemplify care of individuals and communities. These models offer up challenges and future ways to make the health care system more effective and enhance the practice of the nurse case manager.

Beyond-the-Walls Case Management

CHAPTER OVERVIEW

Nursing case management approaches have grown in sophistication and diversity as evidenced by their emergence in community-based programs and capitated system arrangements. A beyond-the-walls program offers magnificent opportunities for professional nursing to control and manage health care resources and quality of patient care. Such a program also provides multiple advantages for the coordination and integration of outcomes and costs. The nursing profession's emphasis on the patient strengthens its power base and reconfirms its professional commitment to society.

Beyond-the-walls case management represents yet another example of the versatility and applicability of the case management model. This community-based approach has shown great promise in reshaping nursing practice and health care management. Examples of some of the more prominent models are presented in the next section.

COMPELLING FORERUNNER: NURSING CASE MANAGEMENT ACROSS CARONDELET'S CONTINUUM OF CARE

Cathy Michaels and Gerri Lamb
(adapted for this edition by Elaine Cohen)

Carondelet Health Care—A Network of Nurse Partnerships and Care Coordination Strategies

Over the past 10 years, nursing case management and other nursing partnerships have evolved that prepared Carondelet St. Mary's Hospital & Health Center, Tucson, Arizona for the managed care environment. In 1985, at the onset of nursing case management beyond the walls of Carondelet, this facility began developing nurse partnerships to assist people at varying levels of risk to manage their health care.

Initially, nurse case managers partnered across time and across health care settings with people at high risk. Then nurse practitioners, together with other nurses and disciples, partnered with people at moderate risk in nurse-managed and neighborhood-accessible community health centers. Based on Carondelet's experience of creating and maintaining integrated services of nursing case management and home health, respite, and home infusion therapy (Burns, Lamb, & Wholey, 1996; Michaels, 1991), Carondelet was selected as one of the four national demonstration sites for the Health Care Financing Administration (HCFA)-funded Community Nursing Organization, a risk-adjusted, capitated, nurse-managed ambulatory system of care. In this research program, Carondelet provided nurse partnerships and nurse-authorized services to Medicare enrollees at high, moderate, and low risk. Carondelet offered a system of care coordination and case management.

Evolution

Carondelet's model of professional nursing case management evolved from a decentralized home care program and nursing network that provided a multitude of services in a variety of settings (Ethridge, 1987, 1991; Ethridge & Lamb, 1989). The services available in the original system included acute or inpatient care, long-term extended care, home health care, and hospice, rehabilitation, primary prevention, and ambulatory care (Ethridge, 1991; Ethridge & Lamb, 1989). Nursing case management reduced the fragmentation associated with preadmission assessment, discharge planning, post-discharge follow-up, and hospital readmission (Health Care Advisory Board, 1990). The foundation for this work was partnership based on mutual respect. By helping people to understand the relationship between the choices they made and the consequences of their actions, nurse case managers not only translated the illness experience into learning about self and others but also acknowledged the patient as responsible for outcomes and the nurse for facilitating the process. In this regard, Carondelet nursing case management was one of the first models to relate practice to nursing theory, specifically Newman's Health as Expanding Consciousness (Newman, Lamb, & Michaels, 1991).

Two areas of evaluation predominated: the benefit of partnership and the impact of that partnership on use of hospital services. Qualitative findings supported a strong base in the nurse case manager-client relationship (Lamb & Stempel, 1994; Newman et al., 1991). Quantitative evaluation demonstrated reduced hospital use. The nursing case management process of assessing, coordinating, planning, and monitoring through partnership reflected appropriate use of medical intervention technology, reduced severity of illness when hospitalization was required, subsequent decreases in bed days, and increased accessibility to hospital alternatives (Ethridge, 1991; Ethridge & Lamb, 1989; Health Care Advisory Board, 1990).

Building on the success of this service, Carondelet established a nursing health maintenance organization (HMO) to provide health care and support services to elderly, chronically ill, and disabled individuals within a Medicare Senior Plan Contract (Ethridge, 1991; Michaels, 1991, 1992). If considered high risk, enrollees in this senior plan received integrated, community-focused nursing services, specifically, nursing case management and home health, respite, and home infusion therapy. Enrollees who did not match the high-risk profile were often referred to the Carondelet Community Health Centers for health monitoring, teaching, and care coordination. Overall, hospital bed days for the high-risk senior enrollees were significantly reduced (Burns et al., 1996), and enrollees served expressed high levels of satisfaction.

In 1992 Carondelet was selected as one of the four national sites to establish a Community Nursing Organization. A 3-year program funded by HCFA, the Community Nursing Organization is a research program based on experimental design. Indeed, the first outcome for this program was meeting the enrollment targets of 2,000 in the experimental program called the Healthy Seniors Program and 1,000 in the control group.

Carondelet's initial nursing HMO experience focused on people at high risk for managing their health care; the Healthy Seniors Program offers enrollment to Medicare beneficiaries whatever their risk for managing their health. Hence, nurse partnerships were established for enrollees at low, moderate, and high risk. Building even further on Carondelet's nursing HMO experience, the Healthy Seniors Program is based on a broader array of integrated ambulatory services: community health center, respite, home health, outpatient behavioral health and rehabilitation services, prosthetics, durable medical equipment, respiratory therapy, medical supplies, and ambulance services. This risk-adjusted, capitated, nurse-managed ambulatory system of care for Medicare beneficiaries is slated to end in December 1996 (Lamb, 1995). Although official evaluation is contracted by HCFA, Carondelet is currently exploring program outcomes.

In 1997 Tucson was one of the most heavily penetrated managed care markets in the nation. To provide case management services and other nurse partnerships across Carondelet's full continuum of care, a system of case management evolved to coordinate care for those at high risk. Community-focused or continuum nurse case managers partnered with people at high risk for managing their health concerns across the continuum of care and over time. In general, the people served faced life-threatening chronic illness, such as congestive heart failure and end-stage chronic obstructive pulmonary disease. The community-focused nurse case managers linked with clinical nurse case managers within the hospital (Mahn, 1993). Clinical nurse case managers served patients at high risk during hospitalization, and, like clinical nurse specialists, they had a specialty focus.

Social workers were also available as consultants or as the primary case manager for clients whose situations were confounded by complex shelter, financial, legal, or behavioral issues. Finally, case managers for behavioral health and rehabilitation also offered services to clients needing their specialized continuum of care.

Except for behavioral health, payment for case management services came from the global capitation rate that covered hospitalization and that was negotiated in the contract. Behavioral health services were also capitated but were contracted for separately.

Transition

> "Changing times are invitations for participation"
> — *Anne Wilson Schaef*

Carondelet's model of professional nursing case management has transitioned to fully participate in the many changes occurring in its environment. The pioneers of this model led by example and envisioned a probable future.

It was envisioned that Carondelet would fully implement a risk identification process recently piloted to evaluate a person's risk for managing his or her health care as people shifted into Carondelet's integrated delivery network. Through risk screening and identification of modifiable risk factors, people at high, moderate, and low risk would be identified earlier. Then there would be targeted interventions, framed in terms of primary, secondary, and tertiary prevention and health promotion and based on Carondelet's nurse partnerships, care coordination strategies, practice guidelines, and system of case management. As in the past, Carondelet's goal was to offer service that people believed improved their health and well-being or that brought a peaceful death.

The future will also call for increased integration with primary care providers. For people at moderate risk, especially at the high end, the primary care site was accessible during teachable moments. Targeted intervention may enable people through partnerships with physicians and nurses and other disciplines to stop progression to a higher risk status. As the future builds on experience from the past and the practices of today, Carondelet's goal was constant: through partnership, to offer health services that people believed improved their health and well-being or that facilitated a peaceful death.

Although the practice setting has changed, the principles that Carondelet's model of professional case management imbued have become the foundation and wisdom for the continued development and growth of case management well into the millenium. A more personal and compelling account of the evolution of this model is presented in Chapter 53. The challenges and lessons bear repeating.

References

Burns, R., Lamb, G., & Wholey D. (1996). Impact of integrated community nursing services on hospital utilization and costs in a medicare risk plan. *Inquiry,* 16(1), 1,30-41.

Ethridge, P. (1987). Building successful nursing care delivery systems for the future. In National Commission on Nursing Implementation Project (Ed.), *Post-conference papers second invitational conference.* Milwaukee: W.K. Kellogg Foundation, pp 91-99.

Ethridge, P. (1991). A nursing home: Carondelet St. Mary's experience. *Nursing Management,* 22(7), 22-27.

Ethridge, P., & Lamb, G.S. (1989). Professional nurse case management improves quality, access and costs. *Nursing Management,* 20(3), 30-35.

Health Care Advisory Board (1990). Tactic #6 "home-based" case management. Superlative clinical quality: Special review of pathbreaking ideas. *Clinical quality.* Washington, D.C.: The Advisory Board Company, vol 1, pp 71-74.

Lamb, G.S. (1995). Case management. *Annual Review of Nursing Research,* 13,117-136.

Lamb, G.S., & Stempel, J. (1994, Jan./Feb.). Nurse case management from the client's view: Growing as insider-expert. *Nursing Outlook,* 7-13.

Lamb, G.S. (1992). Conceptual and methodological issues in nurse case management research. *Advances in Nursing Science,* 15(2), 16-24.

Mahn, V. (1993). Clinical nurse case management: A service line approach. *Nursing Management,* 24(9), 48-50.

Michaels, C. (1991). A nursing HMO—10 months with Carondelet St. Mary's hospital-based nurse case management. *Aspen's Advisor for Nurse Executives,* 6(11), 1.3-4.

Michaels, C. (1992). Carondelet St. Mary's nursing enterprise. *Nursing Clinics of North America,* 27(1), 77-86.

Newman, M., Lamb, G., & Michaels, C. (1991). Nurse case management: The coming together of theory and practice. *Nursing & Health Care,* 12, 404-408.

Wilson Schaef, A. (1995) Native wisdom for white minds, NY Ballantine Books, July 23.

Outcomes of Community-Based Nurse Case Management Programs

Jill Scott, Michal Boyd

CHAPTER OVERVIEW

Community-based nurse case management has been effective for individuals with chronic illness. However, measuring success within this complex, relationship-centered delivery model is challenging. Success of the intervention relates to the development of an insider-expert relationship and, hence, the self-management skills. Considering the complexity of this relationship and its influence on the chronically ill person may be enhanced with the use of a health care utilization framework as a means to integrate the multidimensional outcomes that need to be considered as success is evaluated. This chapter considers models of community-based case management, their outcomes, and challenges of measuring the complexities of the insider-expert relationship.

THE CHALLENGE FOR COMMUNITY-BASED CASE MANAGEMENT: THE CHRONICALLY ILL

Chronic illness continues to challenge an acute care–oriented health delivery and payment system (Throne & Robinson, 1989). With the advent of "managed lives" there was hope that concerns related to the health and well-being of the large cohort of chronically ill Americans would be addressed. Capitated systems were heralded as the payment strategy that would direct health care delivery systems to function more holistically in order to decrease costs related to acute health care access (Stahl, 1998; Williams, 1995). The idealistic provider saw opportunity from changes in payment structures. The hope was a new means to motivate health care organizations to focus on health promotion and prevention as well as facilitation of self-management skills. Self-management skills that are facilitated by community-based nurse case managers are designed to decrease the wide variability present within the chronic illness trajectories of many (Scott & Rantz, 1997).

Evaluation of managed care contracts, such as those established in many states by Medicaid, indicate that long-term commitment between payer, providers, and patient continue to put management of chronic illness and promotion of healthful practices as a low priority. Many states have no structured relationships with payers, providers, and patients to facilitate commitment to chronically ill persons for the period of time necessary for the investment to be financially productive for the payer. Development and investment in health care delivery models, such as community-based nurse case management of the chronically ill, requires longitudinal commitment for the "pay-off" to occur.

Ironically, particularly within Medicaid contracts, individuals covered inadvertently sabotage their opportunity for community-based nurse case management by continually changing providers. This behavior undermines the potential for longitudinal relationships so necessary for community-based nurse case management to be successful (Lamb & Stempel, 1994).

Therefore continued examination of the outcomes and populations that community-based nurse case management can and does serve is required. Understanding what should, and does, motivate creation of health care delivery models that enhance self-management skills, such as community-based nurse case management, is essential as the population continues to shift to a larger numbers of elderly and as those with chronic conditions live longer.

This chapter will consider the issues of measurement and determination of success in the community-based care of the chronically ill at an aggregate level and a disease-specific level. In addition, the chapter will consider how historical models and their outcome measures have enhanced our understanding of care of the chronically ill, how community-based nurse case management models have evolved in their delivery of care and the measurement of the outcomes of care, and how we must evaluate and demonstrate success in the care of the chronically ill in the future.

CHRONIC ILLNESS

Chronic illnesses are present across age cohorts. Within each age cohort trajectories and resulting consequences differ. The psychological and physical development and socioeconomic reality of sustained illness have a unique effect on each age cohort. Typically consequences discussed among cohorts relate to psychological and physical development and socioeconomic realities of sustained illness (Lancaster, 1988; Woods & Lewis, 1995). Common chronic illness diagnoses reported in the literature include cancer, diabetes mellitus, cardiovascular disease, chronic obstructive pulmonary diseases, renal disease, arthritis, and neuromuscular disorders (Anderson-Loftin, Wood, & Whitfield, 1995; Hwu, 1995). Also not typically considered are the children with long-term sequelae from prematurity, birth defects, and poor prenatal care.

Chronic illnesses are slow, insidious, irreversible pathological changes. These illnesses require vigilance by the chronically ill person, significant others, and key health care providers to confront the long-term impact on health care, emotional, functional, and financial needs. The effects of chronic illness influence all of human existence (Lancaster, 1988). Lifelong treatment and behavior changes are required for the management of the chronic illness trajectory. Thus the person suffering from the chronic illness must be active in the self-management of his or her chronic illness, further underlining the importance of key health care providers, such as nurse case managers, supporting them within community-based models.

Chronic illnesses have courses that vary and change over time (Corbin & Strauss, 1984, 1988, 1991). According to Corbin and Strauss (1988), the unfolding of any chronic illness may be thought of as traveling a course. It is the trajectory of that course which community-based nurse case management attempts to alter. The course described by Corbin and Strauss (1984, 1989, 1991) is a probable path that the disease progression is predicted to follow. The influences of a chronically ill person's predisposing and enabling attributes directly affects progression of their chronic illness and need for health care resources, particularly community-based health care resources.

Distinctions between the course of a chronic illness and the trajectories of the illness are central to understanding the essence of chronic illnesses and the needs of the patient. Consideration of the trajectory of illness refers not only to physiological unfolding of chronic illness, but also to the total organization of work or self-management and the attributes influencing this work (Strauss, 1975; Strauss et al., 1984). Community-based nurse case management models influence health care utilization through the nurse case manager's influence of the work and self-management required by the chronic illness. Community-based nurse case manager's influence and shape trajectories of chronic illnesses through the building of insider-expert relationships with patients (Lamb & Stempel, 1994; Scott & Rantz, 1997).

Lamb and Stempel (1994) investigated the relationship of the nurse case manager and patient, identifying and describing growing together as insider-experts. The process develops through the affective, cognitive, and behavioral changes brought about by development of a strong, trusting nurse-patient relationship. The result of this relationship is the ability of the nurse case manager to have influence on the chronically ill person and their trajectory of chronic illness. The interpersonal phases of the relationship have been identified as bonding, working, and changing (Lamb & Stempel, 1994). This evolving relationship supports the development of self-management skills to influence the variability of a chronic illness trajectory.

CHRONICALLY ILL PERSONS' UTILIZATION OF HEALTH CARE RESOURCES

Evaluation of those with progressing chronic illnesses as a cohort requiring substantial amounts of health care strongly suggests that the relationship of the person who is chronically ill and the health care system must be considered in the context of a utilization framework. In analyzing the trajectories of the chronically ill, it is critical to consider how and when the health care system is accessed. How and when health care is accessed is a key outcome for consideration in the success of community-based models.

A framework providing integration of key elements related to the population at risk, their attributes, and actual utilization patterns of health care resources provides a context for studying this cohort over time within the context of the larger health care system and all the many variables that influence the delivery of care. Anderson's Framework of Health Care Utilization considers population attributes, health care delivery system attributes, the actual utilization of health care resources, and consumer perception (Aday & Anderson, 1974).

Chronic illness involves complex sets of relationships and structures to support them such as community-based nurse case management. Anderson's Framework of Health Care Utilization facilitates further understanding of the complex relationships among predisposing, enabling, and need attributes within a complex group of patients. Interrelationships among key variables noted above are displayed in Figure 12-1.

Chronically ill persons have a propensity for utilization of health care resources. Predisposing attributes are an abstraction of this concept to the individual level. These propensities are thought to be predictable from individual characteristics before an illness or periods of exacerbation. Many attributes predispose the chronically ill person to utilization of health care resources and can be used within a community-based model to predict those most likely to benefit from nursing case management. Predisposing attributes should be considered as predictor variables of health care utilization (Scott, 1998).

Enabling attributes are abstracted from the proposition that although individuals may be predisposed to the use of health care resources, they must have some means of obtaining resources. Factors typically considered relate to access and economic components of health care (Aday & Anderson, 1974; Wolinsky & Johnson, 1991).

Community-based care models using nurse case managers have proven to be key enablers of care for those who are chronically ill. Community-based nurse case management has demonstrated key outcomes of success related to enabling care with more cost-effective health care utilization. However, many payment models still do not consistently facilitate access to these types of services.

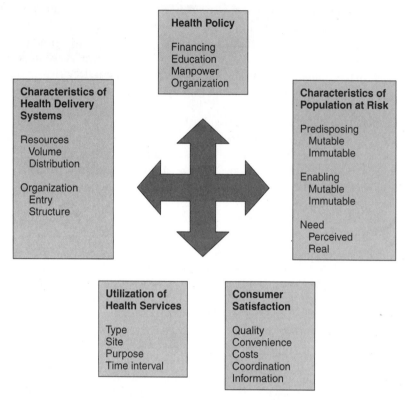

FIGURE **12-1**   An Adaptation of Anderson's Framework of Health Care Utilization.

Predisposing and enabling factors are considered the present reality of the chronically ill person. Predisposing attributes are considered unchangeable. Enabling attributes may be unchangeable, depending on health care resources and financing available to the chronically ill person. Predisposing and enabling attributes are not sufficient in and of themselves to require engagement with the health care system.

The chronically ill person must need to access the health care system. Need typically relates to an inability to self-manage the trajectory of the chronic illness and the certain variability that will be present throughout the progression of the trajectory. Therefore evaluation of the chronically ill and the successful management of their care must consider what predisposing, enabling, and need factors exist within and around the chronically ill person and community-based nurse case manager dyad. These attributes are highlighted in Table 12-1 (Aday & Newman).

Need ultimately creates the immediate cause for accessing the health care system (Wolinsky & Johnson, 1991). Examination of who has historically demonstrated need and how success has and should be measured using community-based nurse case management will be considered through the remainder of the chapter.

Understanding how predisposing, enabling, and need factors relate to health care resource utilization provides insight for the community-based nurse case manager on how to influence these attributes within the context of shaping and managing chronic illness trajectories. Conceptualizing chronic illnesses as a trajectory captures the temporal orientation of chronic illness and the interplay of predisposing, enabling, and need factors. The interplay results in, and places influence on, the use of health

Table 12-1	INDIVIDUAL ATTRIBUTES OR DETERMINANTS OF HEALTH CARE UTILIZATION		
PREDISPOSING	**ENABLING**	**NEED**	
Demographic	Income	Perceived	
Age	Health insurance	Disability	
Gender		Symptoms	
Marital status	Community	Diagnosis	
Past illness	Ratio of health care providers and facilities to population	General state	
Social structure	Type of regular source of health care	Evaluated	
Education	Accessibility of health care	Symptoms	
Race	Compatibility of health care to need	Diagnosis	
Occupation	Presence of community-based services		
Family size		Progression	
Religion	Price of health care services		
Residential mobility	Region of country	Trajectory	
	Urban-rural residence characteristics		
Beliefs			
Values concerning health and illness			
Attitudes toward health care services			

care resources, which is a critical outcome measure for community-based models and nurse case management models. Consideration of chronic illness as a trajectory creates rationales for similarity across chronic illnesses so that evaluating the management and measurement of the multidimensional outcomes can be generalized within the population as it relates to decreasing the variability of the trajectory of illness.

Outcomes related to management of the chronically ill are multidimensional. Quality, cost, and access are often cited as the standard for health measurement and are noted within the Anderson model in Figure 12-1. The following discussion of different models of community-based case management will demonstrate that nurse case management improves quality of care, effectively manages costs, and enhances access (Bower & Falk, 1996).

Although the studies noted will demonstrate many outcomes related to the changes in how resources are used, much is still to be studied related to the qualitative measures of success such as patient and family value related to the support of the trajectory of chronic illness (Papenhausen, 1996) and the value of the development of the insider-expert relationship as it relates to the reduction of stress on the health care team (Scott & Rantz, 1997).

A HISTORICAL REVIEW OF COMMUNITY-BASED CASE MANAGEMENT

Community-based case management can be traced to nursing's early roots in the 1890s when Lillian Wald became one of the first nurses to manage patients in a community setting. She and her colleagues autonomously provided direct patient care and, in addition, organized and mobilized family and community resources. Lillian Wald started the Visiting Nurses Association (VNA) in partnership with the Metropolitan Life Insurance Company. The partnership provided an early measure of success in community-based nursing by demonstrating decreased health care utilization. By 1925 community-based nurse case management provided by the VNA had saved an estimated 43 million dollars (Kersbergen, 1996).

NATIONAL LONG-TERM CARE DEMONSTRATION PROJECTS: "CHANNELING"

During the early 1980s the federal government initiated the National Long-Term Care Demonstration, funded through the Health Care Financing Administration. The demonstration included the Channeling and On Lok programs (Kemper, Applebaum, & Harigan, 1987). Experts in the fields of behavioral health, social work, and health services research initiated this demonstration.

At the time, and still today, these demonstration projects represent some of the most comprehensive assessments of community-based care. The goal of the evaluation was to demonstrate cost containment for the rapidly increasing costs of long-term care with the use of community-based interventions. Although the demonstration projects are considered classic work, because of methodological issues results were not conclusive. However, many valuable lessons were learned for later projects (Christianson et al., 1988; Phillips, Kemper, & Applebaum, 1988).

Of the 10 demonstration projects initiated, five projects focused on measurement related to medical system difficulties because of ineffective or absent information and lack of coordination of services. The interventions within these five projects did not relate to the introduction of case management, but focused on improving information flow and coordination of services, basic case management, and existing community services.

The remaining five demonstration projects provided the same information and coordination of services, but added access to more community resources with additional funding from Medicare and Medicaid. The additional services included such critical elements as in-home care.

The results of these demonstration projects are difficult to interpret because of several issues. First, inconsistent definition of the population and other measures created concerns about generalizability of the findings. Second, case management interventions were poorly defined, and inconsistencies were noted with regard to who was considered the population most likely to benefit from the intervention. Third, inconsistency in group composition was noted. Finally, the studies did not use outcome measures that were keenly sensitive to elucidate the unique contribution of the intervention. These indicators were often defined as the tasks performed, without specific definitions of the clients served, the setting in which they resided, and the distinct services provided by the case managers (Kemper, Applebaum, & Harigan, 1987; Lamb, 1995; Phillips et al., 1988).

One study performed within the Channeling demonstration project did illustrate the impact of case management. Distinct differences were explored between the community-based case management models' function and caseload characteristics. This study (Eggert et al., 1991) noted that community-based case management models that used a more hands-on approach and smaller caseloads did have a reduction in health care expenditures.

EVOLVING MODELS OF COMMUNITY-BASED CASE MANAGEMENT

Community-based case management has been expanding in recent years and is used for a variety of patient populations. These programs have evolved to address client needs and increase quality of care in a changing reimbursement environment. Several different models are presented. Outcome measures are considered within each model as they relate to demonstrating success in the care of the chronically ill.

One of the first community-based nurse case management systems originating from a hospital was the Carondelet St. Mary Professional Nurse Case Management (PNCM) program. This model was developed to decrease hospital lengths of stay in response to Medicare Prospective Payment, which was initiated in 1984. The PNCM worked with individuals in the community along with nurse practitioners based in a system of 20 wellness centers that were located in retirement complexes. Professional nurse case managers bridged the gap between health care settings and followed patients through the hospital, in long-term care facilities, and in their homes. This program was successful in reducing costs through decreased hospital admissions, decreased hospital acuity, and the resulting decreased length of stay, and set the tone for what and how to measure success for the intervention (Ethridge, 1997; Ethridge & Lamb, 1989).

Since the inception of the Carondelet St. Mary's community-based professional nurse case management model, many other hospitals around the country have used it as a prototype for the development their own community-based care programs. Many of the interventions have borrowed from the original Carondelet St. Mary's model and been implemented with some adjustment for a particular setting. However, lack of funding and poor reimbursement have resulted in an inability of many pilot programs to implement the vast network of wellness clinics and integrated care achieved by Carondelet St. Mary's. Despite the struggles to operationalize community-based case management, many programs have achieved impressive outcomes.

One of the first programs developed using the PNCM as a model was at St. Joseph's Medical Center in Wichita, Kansas. In a quasi-experimental study, health care utilization was evaluated pre- and post-case management. This intervention demonstrated a 74% decrease in net Medicare reimbursement, which was defined as the difference between hospital charges and Medicare reimbursement. The study lacked actual cost data for hospitalizations, so the results are somewhat difficult to interpret (Rogers, Riordan, & Swindle, 1991).

A second example of outcomes reported in a community-based nurse case management study was noted from a model in Boulder, Colorado. This model focused on the frail elder population using Boulder Community Hospital. Success of this program was evaluated by examination of the outcome measures of hospitalizations, length of stay, emergency department visits, and physician visits. The study found a 58% decrease in hospital charges for the intervention group when compared to the control group. A significant decrease in emergency department visits was demonstrated between the control and intervention groups. Additionally, the intervention group experienced a 32% decrease in physician visits when compared to the control group (Boyd et al., 1996).

Sund and Sveningson (1998) found similar results through an integrated delivery system incorporating community-based nurse case management as an intervention. This single group pre- and post-intervention study demonstrated the following outcomes: a substantial decrease in hospitalizations (54%), decreased clinic and physician visits (31% decrease), and decreased clinic charges (43% decrease).

Other models of noteworthiness include the Carle Clinic Community-based Case Management Model and the Cooperative Health Clinic. The Carle Clinic Association refers to the nurse case manager as a nurse partner. These nurses work closely with physicians in the clinic to manage high-risk individuals in the community setting. This model is efficient because the physician and nurse partner function as a team in daily contact. The Carle Clinic model provides opportunities for nurse partners to guide the care of individuals across the continuum of health care settings, including ambulatory care, acute care, long-term care, and care in the home.

The model supports coordinated medical intervention and mentoring for the development of self-management skills. Nurses within the model have been creative in their use of the capitated dollar. The nurse partners are able to authorize home repair, transportation, respite services, and home-delivered meals. Availability of these services would be limited in traditional fee-for-service reimbursement systems.

The Cooperative Health Care Clinic of Kaiser Permanente of Colorado implemented a group outpatient visit model providing comprehensive care through an interdisciplinary team approach. This intervention is an efficient method for using an interdisciplinary team. Although this model is mainly used for medical management of the chronically ill, it provides a model in which nurses could easily introduce community-based case management as a supplement. The intervention provides group support, timely medical intervention, education, and information regarding resources. Additionally, longitudinal care needed by the chronically ill is provided. Outcome measures that have indicated success include a decrease in emergency department visits, a decrease in visits to specialists, and a decrease in hospitalization. In addition, the study notes that patients placed more calls to the nurse, visited the nurse more frequently, and engaged with the physician less, providing an outcome measure of appropriate use of the nurse as chronic disease manager (Beck et al., 1997).

In addition to the general models of community-based nurse case management already noted, some models and studies have focused the intervention on a specific population. Many chronically ill populations present unique challenges for the health care team in the management of the trajectory of chronic illness and the development of self-management skills. These unique groups include the mentally ill, those with chronic physical diseases such as congestive heart failure and diabetes, and those with chronic, catastrophic, contagious diseases such as AIDS.

Deinstitutionalization of the chronically mentally ill during the 1950s and 1960s shifted care from the hospital to the community. In response to the needs of this population, mental health professionals created community-based case management programs. An extensive outcome data base exists in the literature regarding the specific outcome measures indicating success as it relates to the care of the mentally ill in the community.

The community-based case management systems that evolved placed the case manager primarily in the role of brokering for community resources and coordinating care. As time progressed, data suggested that there was a need to also integrate the clinical role for the provision of direct care in addition to the brokering and coordinating of care (Mueser et al., 1998).

Two models of community-based models have emerged to support the mentally ill: the Assertive Community Treatment Model and the Intensive Case Management Model. Both models incorporated low patient-to-staff ratios (10:1 rather than 30:1), services in the community rather than mental health centers, 24-hour availability of health care provider support, and the majority of services provided within the organization. Differences in the two models related to who managed the care. The Assertive Community Treatment Model used a team approach of nurses and psychiatrists sharing the caseload (Stein & Test, 1980). The Intensive Case Management Model did not share the caseload among team members, theoretically providing the opportunity for a strengthened relationship between case manager and client (Shern, Surles, & Waizer, 1989; Surles et al., 1992). Both models demonstrated decreased hospitalizations, decreased length of stay, improved housing stability, and independence. Outcomes of the studies also showed an improved quality of life for case-managed chronically mentally ill patients (Meuser et al., 1998).

In addition to the chronically mentally ill, those with long-term chronic physical illness present challenges. The patient with congestive failure is a classic example of a population requiring frequent readmission into the acute care components of the health care system because of high variability within the trajectory of this chronic illness (Kegel, 1995). Many factors have been cited as contributing to rehospitalization of those with congestive heart failure, including a lack of understanding by the patient of the disease process, an inability to self-manage, and inconsistent follow-up care after hospitalization (Vinson et al., 1990). Many patients with congestive heart failure have high variability with the trajectory of their chronic illness and would benefit from community-based case management. The nurse case manager can facilitate the development of self-management skills that decreases this variability.

Rich et al. (1995) used extensive patient assessment by a multidisciplinary team and comprehensive patient education for individuals with congestive heart failure. The intervention included follow-up in the home by nurses to increase the client's ability to self-manage through education and follow-up support. This randomized group comparison study evaluated readmissions as an indicator of decreasing the wide swings in the variability of the illness. The study demonstrated a 33% reduction in hospital readmission when compared to the control group (Rich et al., 1995).

Another chronically ill group that demonstrates a high variability within the trajectory of their illness is the person with diabetes. Not only is variability within the trajectory a challenge, but the long-term sequelae from inaction to the illness early on may have profound consequences. The traditional health care system has been inconsistent in providing the disease management required. Programs are needed that increase monitoring and follow-up to identify potential problems early to reduce the severity of the resulting complications.

Individuals in the community have used an automated voice messaging system to improve the management of diabetes. Patients are identified with poor glucose control or other problems that require more intensive follow-up. An automated voice messaging system calls the patients at their homes and inquires about glucose control and other diabetes-related symptoms to determine what patient education should be provided.

Diabetes nurse educators monitor responses to the calls, and calls are returned to those individuals who require intervention. Preliminary results of enhanced glucose control, early intervention for complications, and acceptance of this technology by patients suggest this is a feasible and innovative alternative to ongoing evaluation and support of patients with diabetes (Piette, 1997).

The need for chronic care of individuals with human immunodeficiency virus (HIV) and acquired immunodeficiency disease (AIDS) has been heightened dramatically by the enhanced availability of drug therapies that have greatly increased life expectancy and the widespread expansion in the number of people infected with HIV. The care of people with AIDS is moving to an integrated system that focuses on health and wellness rather than acute care (Morrison, 1993). Because of the complex physical needs of these individuals, nurse case management has been recommended rather than case management from other disciplines (Green et al., 1987).

In a Robert Wood Johnson demonstration project of case management for people with AIDS, individuals with case management were more likely to report service needs being met than clients without case management (Fleishman, Mr, & Piette, 1991). Outcomes within the study also suggest improved survival for those who were case managed. The results related to mortality were inconclusive, since medical treatment regimens did vary between comparison groups (Sowell et al., 1992).

A second study, the Denver Nursing Project in Human Caring (Schroeder, 1993), provided a nurse-managed outpatient clinic for people with AIDS. Clients of the clinic could elect to enter into a nurse care partnership. This nursing intervention provided care across clinical settings and was particularly helpful when the client was hospitalized. The nurse care partner was a valuable member of the health care team, providing information about the client's wishes and needs. Outcomes from this project demonstrated improved access to cost-effective and high-quality care. Outcomes measured indicating health care savings included decreased hospitalizations, decreased length of stay, decreased cost of outpatient procedures, and increased home care during the dying process (Schroeder, 1993).

COMMUNITY-BASED NURSE CASE MANAGEMENT'S FUTURE: MEASURING SUCCESS

Community-based nurse case management outcomes need additional qualitative and quantitative measurement to provide the multidimensional view required to capture the true impact of the insider-expert relationship. More research is needed on how this relationship impacts self-management skills and the subsequent ability to decrease the variability of an individual's trajectory of chronic illness. Qualitative research is providing insight into patients' and families' values. Papenhausen (1996) found through interviews that these values include decreased physical disability, increased perception of social satisfaction, improved symptom management, decreased severity of illness, and increased general self-efficacy. More studies are required to enhance our understanding of what is valuable to patients and families and how their roles can be enhanced in the management of chronic illnesses.

Quantitative measures must continue to be refined to more accurately reflect the impact of nurse case management's ability to decrease the variability of those with wide swings within their trajectory of chronic illness. Large-scale data mining efforts are needed within national data bases such as Health Care Financing Administration billing data to facilitate additional understanding of what key predisposing, enabling, and need factors best predict wide variability within those chronic illnesses. This understanding will facilitate more effective targeting of the chronically ill persons that would most benefit from community-based nurse care management interventions.

Finally, triangulation of studies related to community-based case management is required to understand the interplay of reducing health care consumption, improving reported well-being and satisfaction of chronically ill persons and their families, and how to measure consistent demonstrations of self-management skills that stabilize the variability of the chronic illness trajectory. Studies should also consider the influence of community-based case management on the functioning and satisfaction of the health care team (Scott & Rantz, 1997). Community-based case management can and does make a difference. The challenge? Prove it!

References

Aday, L.A., & Anderson, R. (1974). A framework for the study of access to medical care. *Health Services Research, 9*(3), 208-220.

Anderson-Loftin, W., Wood, D., & Whitfield, L. (1995). A case study of nursing case management in the rural hospital. *Nursing Administrative Quarterly, 19*(3), 33-40.

Anderson, R., & Newman, J. (1973). Societal and individual determinants of medical care utilization in the United States. *Millbank Quarterly, 51*(1), 95-124.

Beck, A., Scott, J., Williams, P., Robertson, B., Jackson, D., Gade, G., & Cowan, P. (1997). A randomized trial of group outpatient visits for chronically ill older HMO members: The cooperative health care clinic. *Journal of the American Geriatrics Society, 45,* 543-549.

Bower, K.A., & Falk, C.D. (1996). Case management as a response to quality, cost, and access imperatives. In E.L. Cohen, (Ed.), *Nurse case management in the 21st century.* St Louis: Mosby.

Boyd, M.L., Fisher, B., Davidson, A.W., & Neilsen, C.A. (1996). Community-based case management for chronically ill older adults: A comparison study. *Nursing Management, 27*(11), 31-32.

Christianson, J.B., Applebaum, R., Carcagno, G., Phillips, B. (1988). Organizing and delivering case management services: Lessons from the national long term care demonstration. *Home Health Care Services Quarterly, 9*(1), 7-27.

Corbin, J.M., & Strauss, A. (1984). Collaboration: Couples working together to manage chronic illness. *Image: Journal of Nursing Scholarship, 26*(4), 109-115.

Corbin, J.M., & Strauss, A. (1988). *Unending work and care.* San Francisco: Jossey-Bass Publishers.

Corbin, J.M., & Strauss, A. (1991). A nursing model for chronic illness management based upon the trajectory framework. *Scholarly Inquiry for Nursing Practice: An International Journal, 5*(3), 156-174.

Eggert, G.M., Zimmer, J.G., Hall, W.J., & Friedman, B. (1991). Case management: A randomized controlled study comparing a neighborhood team and a centralized individual model. *Health Services Research, 26*(4), 471-505.

Ethridge, P. (1997). The Carondelet experience. *Nursing Management, 28*(3), 26-28.

Ethridge, P., & Lamb, G. (1989). Professional nursing case management improves quality, access and costs. *Nursing Management, 20*(3), 30-35.

Fleishman, J.A., Mr, V., & Piette, J. (1991). AIDS case management: The client's perspective. *Health Services Research, 26*, 447-469.

Green, J., Singer, M., Wintfeld, N., Schulman, K., & Passman, L. (1987). Projecting the impact of AIDS on hospitals. *Health Affairs, 6*, 19-31.

Hwu, Y.J. (1995). The impact of chronic illness on patients. *Rehabilitation Nursing, 20*(4), 221-225.

Kegel, L.M. (1995). Advanced practice nurses can refine the management of heart failure. *Clinical Nurse Specialist, 9*(2), 76-81.

Kemper, P., Applebaum, R., & Harigan, M. (1987). Community care demonstrations: What have we learned. *Health Care Financing Review, 8*(4), 87-100.

Kersbergen, A.L. (1996). Case management: A rich history of coordinating care to control costs. *Nursing Outlook, 44*, 169-172.

Lamb, G.S. (1995). Case management. *Annual Review of Nursing Research, 13*, 117-135.

Lamb, G.S., & Stempel, J.E. (1994). Nurse case management from the client's view: Growing as the insider-expert, *Nursing Outlook, 42*(1), 7-13.

Lancaster, L.E. (1988). Impact of chronic illness over the life span. *American Nephrology Nurses Association, 15*(3), 164-168.

Mueser, K.T., Bond, G.R., Drake, R.E., & Resnick, S.G. (1998). Models of community care for severe mental illness: A review of research on case management. *Schizophrenia Bulletin, 24*(1), 37-74.

Morrison, C. (1993). Delivery systems for the care of persons with HIV infection and AIDS. *Advances in Nursing Research, 28*(2), 317-333.

Papenhausen, J.L. (1996). Discovering and achieving client outcomes. In E.L. Cohen, (Ed.), *Nurse case management in the 21st century.* St. Louis: Mosby.

Phillips, B.R., Kemper, P., & Applebaum, R.A. (1988). The evaluation of the National Long Term Care Demonstration. *Health Services Research, 23*(1), 67-81.

Piette, J.D. (1997). Moving diabetes management from clinic to community: Development of a prototype based on automated voice messaging. *Diabetes Educator, 23*(6), 672-680.

Rich, M.W., Beckham, V., Wittenberg, C., Leven, C.L., Freedland, K.E., & Carney, R.M. (1995). A multidisciplinary intervention to prevent the readmission of elderly patients with congestive heart failure. *The New England Journal of Medicine, 333*(18), 1190-1195.

Rogers, M., Riordan, J., & Swindle, D. (1991). Community-based nursing case management pays off. *Nursing Management, 22*(3), 31-34.

Schraeder, C., & Britt, T. (1997). The Carle Clinic. *Nursing Management, 28*(3), 32-34.

Schroeder, C. Nursing's Response to the crisis of access, costs, and quality in health care. *Advances in Nursing Science, 16*(1):1-20, 1993 Sep. (26 ref).

Schroeder, C., & Maeve, K. (1992). Nursing response to the crisis of costs and quality in health care. *Advances in Nursing Science, 16*(11), 1-20.

Scott, J. (1998). A study of health care utilization among chronically ill rural older adults. In review.

Scott, J., & Rantz, M. (1997). Managing the chronically ill in the midst of the health care revolution, *Nursing Administrative Quarterly, 21*(2), 55-64.

Shern, D.L., Surles, R.C., & Waizer, J. (1989). Designing community treatment systems for the most seriously mentally ill: A state administrative perspective. *Journal of Social Issues, 45*, 105-117.

Sowell, R.L., Gueldner, S.H., Killen, M.R., Lowenstein, A., Fuszard, B., & Swansburg, R. (1992). Impact of case management on hospital charges of PWA's in Georgia. *Journal of the Association of Nurses in AIDS Care, 3,* 24-31.

Stahl, D.A. (1998). Growth through capitation and physician practice management. *Nursing Management, 29*(1), 14-16.

Stein, L.I., & Test, M.A. (1980). Alternative to mental hospital treatment: I. Conceptual model, treatment program, and clinical evaluation. *Archives of General Psychiatry, 37,* 392-397.

Strauss, A. (1975). *Chronic illness and the quality of life.* St. Louis: Mosby.

Strauss, A., Corbin, J., Fagerhaugh, S., Glaser, B.G., Maines, D., Suczek, B., & Wiener, C.L. (1984). *Chronic illness and the quality of life* (2nd ed.). St. Louis: Mosby.

Sund, J., & Sveningson, L. (1998). Case management in an integrated delivery system. *Nursing Management, 29*(1), 24-25.

Surles, R.C., Blanch, A.K., Shern, D.L., & Donahue, S.A. (1992). Case management as a strategy for systems change. *Health Affairs, 11,* 151-163.

Throne, S.E., & Robinson, C.A. (1989). Guarded alliance: Health care relationships in chronic illness. *Image: Journal of Nursing Scholarship, 21*(3), 153-157.

Vinson, J.M., Rich, M.W., Sperry, J.C., Shah, A.S., & McNamara, T. (1990). Early readmission of the elderly patients with congestive heart failure. *Journal of the American Geriatrics Society, 38*(12), 1290-1295.

Williams, D.B. (1995). Case management without walls: Breaking down traditional barriers among organizations. *Inside Case Management, 1*(10), 1-3.

Wolinsky, F.D., & Johnson, R.J. (1991). The use of health services by older adults. *Journal of Gerontology, 46*(6), S345-S357.

Woods, N.F., & Lewis, F.M. (1995). Women with chronic illness: Their views of their families' adaptation. *Health Care for Women International, 16,* 135-148.

Integrated Case Management Model

Mary Lu Gerke

CHAPTER OVERVIEW

Nursing case management is a patient delivery system that evolved out of the primary nursing model. The focus of case management is to use the professional nurse as the agent who integrates care, cost, and quality (Zander, 1985). Like an amoeba, environmental pressure influences nursing case management to change composition, shape, and structure. The ever-changing patient needs, professional roles, and health care systems create space for nursing case management to flow into unexplored territories. Mergers, downsizing, and reengineering have created an opportunity to strategically position nursing case management as the mechanism to assure care to all patients across the continuum. The external force of redesign and integration influenced the evolving form of the Differentiated Case Management Model at Gundersen Lutheran.

The core of nursing case management at Gundersen Lutheran was based on the work of two projects, "Facilitating ADN Competency Development" and "Defining and Differentiating ADN and BSN Competencies." These two projects' outcome was the Differentiated Case Management Model, operationalized in 1990 at the acute care setting, Lutheran Hospital. The model continued to evolve in the acute care setting but was not extended to the ambulatory or home care settings until 1997 when Gundersen Clinic and Lutheran Hospital began the integration process.

This process enabled our organization to clearly see the possibility of providing nursing case management across the continuum. Up to this point, few of the acute care case managers actualized care planning across the continuum. Many of them dreamed of providing a continuum care plan for patients, but physical walls and governing structures impeded their attempts. The clinic and home care systems did not have a case management model in place, but instead practiced in the team or total patient care model.

Integration of systems, models, and people, although difficult in many ways, provides an opportunity to use diverse eyes for seeing new ways of creating and evolving. The merger promoted the evaluation of case management in all three settings: acute care, ambulatory care, and home care. Additionally, it opened the opportunity to build the differentiated case management model across all systems and settings. Weaving new relationships and partnerships, nursing case management is nurtured by integration, growing, changing, and strengthening.

▌DIFFERENTIATED CASE MANAGEMENT MODEL

National Development

Differentiated case management was developed through the work of two major projects sponsored by the Midwest Alliance in Nursing (MAIN) and funded by the W.K. Kellogg Foundation: "Facilitating ADN Competency Development" and "Defining and Differentiating ADN and BSN Competencies." These two studies developed between 1980 and 1984. Service and education together developed a differentiated scope of practice for the BSN and the ADN through competency statements. Dr. Peggy Primm led the task force toward defining competencies in three major areas of care: provision of care, communication, and management of care. Job descriptions were then formatted and several sites selected to test the model (Primm, 1986). In the differentiated case management model, there are two roles established for professional nursing staff: the case manager role and the case associate role. The case manager role is designed to be accountable for the independent scope of practice and focused on health and human response. The case associate role is designed to be accountable for the dependent scope of nursing practice and focused on the technical aspects of care. Together the two roles deliver the full scope of nursing practice to each patient. Each role holds the essence and the full scope of practice of professional nursing. Therefore both participate in all aspects of care, such as admission assessment and preparation for discharge. The difference lies in the focus and depth of each role. The case manager focus is integration and orchestration of the health care team throughout the hospital length of stay, and the case associate focus is on the day-to-day patient assessment, care, teaching, and evaluation.

Application of Differentiated Case Management

In 1988 Lutheran Hospital embarked on a journey of redesign. With the advent of rapid changes in social structures, technology, and health care, the primary nursing model lacked the depth and breadth to meet the changing needs of patients and systems. We hoped we would be able to discover a new patient care delivery model that would support the new consumer of health care and at the same time maintain financial strength. "With health, human response, and quality of life as new imperatives to integrate into each individual's care, the way in which nursing care was organized and delivered clearly required a fundamental change" (Johnson, Friend, & MacDonald, 1997). Professional colleagues and literature searches helped the organization to commit to the differentiated case management model. The underlying belief of the differentiated nursing model is that "each nurse is expert in their role, each role is mutually valued, and collaborative practice utilizing both roles is the whole of nursing" (Larson, 1992). These beliefs fit with the vision of the Lutheran Hospital nursing department.

Differentiating the roles meant redesigning the professional nursing framework. A task force of grassroots staff and leadership participated in developing professional nursing job descriptions and performance appraisals for two registered nurse (RN) roles. This was no small task, since the existing clinical ladder consisted of four levels of RN staff. Therefore eight complete job descriptions and performance appraisals were developed. Countless hours of inservice training and educational sessions were scheduled for 700 RNs as well as licensed practical nurses (LPNs), nursing assistance, and ancillary services staff. After the educational sessions the RNs were asked to complete a factoring tool that assisted them and their nursing directors to dialogue and decide which role, case manager or case associate, best matched their practice. Physicians were educated through their noon conferences and in a one-to-one dialogue. By the end of 1990, Lutheran Hospital practiced in a differentiated case management model.

By 1992, experience with differentiated case management highlighted areas of the model that needed clarification and strengthening. The rehabilitation unit put into place a pilot that further differentiated the two roles of case manager and case associate. In the original model, professional nurses practiced as a case manager with some of the patients and as case associate with other patients during the same shift. This led to confusion and lack of clarity in both roles. The pilot placed professional RN staff into either a case manager or a case associate role that they would practice 100% of the time. Because the case manager was no longer given a patient assignment for direct care, the case associates were assigned more patients with an LPN or nursing assistant colleague to attend to the daily care of the patients. This freed case managers to attend to the individualized care planning for patients. Further change required further education in the areas of delegation and teamwork. Trust and respect for each other's work became core to successfully meeting the needs of patients and families. The case managers primarily work day and evening hours and meet with other health care providers daily to discuss the individual needs of their patients for the acute care stay and the discharge plan. Over a 2-year period, this variation of the differentiated case management model spread to all patient care areas of the hospital. With the job descriptions updated, professional nurses were refactored into a case manager or case associate role. Some patient care units required few case managers, while other patient care units needed several. The decision on the number of case managers required is determined by data such as length of stay, patient populations, and severity of illness on the specific unit.

The case managers meet monthly to discuss practice issues, development of their role, and barriers to their work. Some of the case managers managed the patient care from unit to unit. However, this was not standard practice, inconsistencies became apparent, and, as in any evolutionary system, evaluating and revising are the norm.

Implementation of a Professional Roles Model

In 1996 a task force was formed to evaluate and revise the clinical ladder system at Lutheran Hospital. After a brief review, the task force decided to move from a clinical ladder system to a professional roles model. The new mode used Patricia Benner's 1984 work, *From Novice to Expert,* as a resource and guide. The task force decided to change the title of case manager to care manager and case associate to care associate. Three job descriptions and performance evaluations were developed for the care associate: essential (beginner), proficient, and expert/leader. The care manager job description and performance evaluation were similar in the communication and leadership criteria to the case associate expert/leader criteria but differed in the patient/family criteria. The care associate's focus continues to be the standard technical care, and the care manager continues to focus on the independent individual patient care plan across the episode of illness. (See Appendix 12-1 for job descriptions and competencies of the care manager and care associate.)

The professional role model moved the nursing department to a new way of seeing work. Benner's theory helped the nursing staff understand that differences in practice can and do enrich the care provided for patient and family. Nurses wrote three exemplars reflecting their practice as professionals. With guidance from Benner, Tanner, and Chelsa's book, *Expertise in Nursing Practice—Caring Clinical Judgment and Ethics,* the exemplar assists in assessing the practice level of the nurses. Each nurse presented the exemplars along with the performance appraisal to the unit's peer review committee. This session served as a means to discover, with the individual nurse, where practice has evolved to on the continuum from novice to expert. The process of moving from a clinical ladder system to a professional roles model assisted in evaluating the role of the care manager and raising questions about the purpose and meaning of nursing care management across the continuum. From the very beginning there was good intent to work across the continuum but concerns and barriers continued to block the success of delivery care across the systems.

Barriers to Integrate Nursing Case Management Across the Continuum

There are several models of nursing case management. However, few models have successfully been able to stretch across the ambulatory, acute, and home care settings. Some barriers to building a structure for integrating nursing case management are as follows:

- A perspective by health care providers and society that health care and disease management are owned by the provider, not a mutual partnership between patient and provider
- Health care institutions not governed as a integrated system with poor articulation between the providers of acute care, ambulatory care, and home care
- Different reimbursement and regulations dependent on the location of the treatment or service and which provider is delivering the treatment or service
- Educational curriculums segregated according to ambulatory, acute, or home care settings instead of the focus on primary, secondary, and tertiary care in any setting
- Management structures that place managers leading only a section of the continuum because of physical or economic barriers
- Inability of staffing patterns, budgets, and numerous structures to span the continuum

INTEGRATION OF A CLINIC, HOSPITAL, AND HOME CARE AGENCY

In 1998 Gundersen Clinic and Lutheran Hospital merged. The Lutheran Home Care agency was a branch of Lutheran Hospital and therefore part of the system. The merger brought forth a system composed of regional clinics; regional hospitals and affiliated hospitals, a home care agency, a main clinic of 280 physicians, and a 400-bed acute care hospital. The merging and integration of organizations and systems are now common around the world. Yet we still deal with coping and rebuilding new relationships and organizations from these mergers.

Margaret Wheatley and Myron Kellner-Rogers in their book, A *Simpler Way,* state, "Systems are fluid relationships that we observe as rigid structures. They are webby, wandering, nonlinear, entangled messes . . . systems create pathways, communication flows, causal loops" (Wheatley & Kellner-Rogers, 1996). The work of integration has indeed been a tangled web. Nevertheless, out of the chaos there is blooming the opportunity to reach a wholeness we have not been able to grasp or even dream about in the old structures.

Defining Integration

Integration means "to form, coordinate or blend into a functioning or unified whole, to unite with something else, to incorporate into a larger unit and to end the segregation of and bring into common and equal membership in society or an organization" (Webster, 1988). This definition should strike at the core of nurses, since one tenets of the essence of nursing is the persistence and passion to promote the wellness and *wholeness* of human beings. Therefore, in seeking wholeness integration of nursing case management across the continuum is a natural evolution. Nursing has always integrated the body, mind, and spirit into a holistic approach. Now it is our path to integrate that whole human system throughout the manmade acute, ambulatory, and home care systems.

In reading Florence Nightingale's *Notes on Nursing,* many things have changed but some things have not. Nightingale fought the battle of educating others to understand that nursing is a distinct profession, separate but connected to medicine. More importantly, Nightingale wanted nurses and others to understand the sacredness and importance of the nurse-patient relationship. Her definition of nursing, "Nursing creates an environment to assure that the patients not only be well, but to use well all of their being," was a call to nursing to integrate the parts and to understand the importance of the patient's wholeness. We have now reached into our humanism and understood that mankind is an integral part of the whole and that the environment and all creation affect each other. One element cannot exist separately, for we are all connected; we are all the same stuff. Complementary and alternative therapy is a manifestation of that concept and intent. As nurses we embrace these concepts and appreciate them. Application of our values and beliefs will drive toward integrating patient care to wholeness.

Another level of integration is now our challenge—the work of integrating the care by a nurse for the same patient over the continuum. Nursing can stop the segregation of the patient's health care. Patient care often has different care standards depending on the setting where care is delivered: ambulatory, acute, or home care. We are the link between these settings, not solely by a paper trail, but also by our sacred connectedness and relationships with our patients. We can manifest the essence of nursing embracing a new and different society, a health-centered society with wellness as the core. Collaborating with the mechanistic illness models avails us the opportunity to create a system that provides a holistic care system.

Bringing Two Models Together

Hospital and clinic systems integration started in 1997. It is vital to *understand* that the practice models of team and total patient care gave birth to primary nursing and case management models and that bringing the models together is the goal. Current health care systems have moved toward a case management model. This urges the organization to use the good components of the models currently in the clinic and hospital but also to move beyond what either one has in place. The differentiated case management model in the hospital is evolutionary and needs to expand beyond the walls of the acute care setting.

Establishing trust and respect is the grounding for *understanding* to be a priority. "Understanding takes time. Understanding is a process, not an event, and it is not possible unless we are willing to take the time and effort to stay with it" (Schaef, 1998). The seeking to understand each other as we co-create the new case management model takes patience and persistence. Implementing a new patient care model causes structures, job descriptions, and roles to change to support the model. The clinic and hospital structures, job descriptions, roles, and a multitude of support frameworks are very different as a result of different patient needs and environments.

A task force composed of both ambulatory nurses and hospital care managers developed to work on building a differentiated case management model that spans all settings. The establishment of a position for director of case management promotes the work of building nursing care management across the continuum. This individual will head the task force and work with numerous subgroup specialties to build an integrated patient care model. The first work of the main task force is looking at all the roles of professional nurses in all settings. Many roles exist, and this work will indeed need understanding and patience.

The work is in progress, but some areas have already moved toward successful integration. One departments is the obstetrics service line. Hospital care managers and clinic nurses have developed a care management role that starts with seeing the mom in the clinic three times, continues through the hospital event, and then ends after two follow-up calls and at least one follow-up clinic visit. During the prenatal visits, the care manager works with the parents to complete the individualized care path for the birth. These care paths are on-line so they are readily available in the clinic and hospital. Patient satisfaction has always been very good in this area but is even more positive since the integration of the hospital and clinic care managers became a reality.

In the general surgery area department of the clinic, a care manager follows all patients with breast cancer through the ambulatory, acute, and home care settings. The patients develop a relationship with the nurse built on trust and partnering principles. This alleviates some of the fear and anxiety, establishes a consistent care plan, reduces duplication of baseline assessments, and creates a patient advocate to help navigate a complex health care system.

An area of care management new to Gundersen Lutheran is in the area of infusion therapy. One care manager shares her exemplar:

> I was asked to place a midline catheter on a hospice patient. Upon arriving at the home of the patient to place the midline catheter, the husband smiled with delight to discover that I was going to place the catheter. He reminded me that I had put an IV in his wife when she was in the hospital. He was grateful that someone with that level of expertise was able to come to his or her home. The placement of the catheter went without any complications and both patient and husband were content when I left their home. I found out later that the patient had died the next day. It was a good feeling for me to know that her last day had been a comfortable, peaceful day.

Many areas in the clinic are just starting the process of integration. Some of the interesting obstacles to overcome are as follows:

- Nursing roles that are attached to a physician care provider
- Confusion of nursing assessment responsibilities versus technical skills that could be delegated to medical assistance
- Information systems that are not adapted to facilitate integrated documentation and communication links
- Resistance to implementing a new way without having the model and system completely defined and tested
- Merging a primarily day operation with a 24-hour operation
- Personnel structures of pay and benefits that are not completely integrated
- Need for further education regarding each other's settings and operations

BUILDING RELATIONSHIPS AND PARTNERSHIPS

Nursing case management builds on the partnership and relationship principles of trust, respect, support, communication, and commitment. These principles can be used to build all types of partnerships, not only partnerships with our patients. "Forming a partnership relationship requires time and effort. It means spending time with each other, sharing feelings and perceptions, discussing important values, putting into place the structure for the relationship" (Manion, Sieg, & Watson, 1998). When dealing with an integrated nursing case management system, dual application of these principles occurs, involving the patient and family partnership with the health care provider, and the health care provider with the rest of the health care team.

Trust

The element of trust is core to successful partnership development. The patient and family develop trust in the care provider through dialogue and being present with the care provider. When the care manager is not fully present and rushes through the appointment, the patient and family lose the opportunity to establish a trusting relationship with a care provider. The care manager must provide the component of patient's advocate. To accomplish that measure, time and trust go hand in hand. The care managers working across the continuum need to be expert in establishing trust. Self-reflection on one's own integrity and trust in the team must be part of partnership building, as must a firm belief that each member of the team has the ultimate goal of quality patient care.

Respect

Mutual respect for each other is key in all relationships and partnerships. Lack of respect breeds misunderstanding, leads to poor communication, and inhibits growth and creativity. Respecting the diversity of each individual creates a sense of collective individualism. This element is not easy to attain, since it calls for each person to fully listen and seek to understand the other person's point of view. Frequently, the health care provider sees the patient's viewpoint as less important or valuable than his or her own. The health care provider might believe the patient lacks the scientific knowledge to make complex decisions. The patient brings the expertise of knowing "self." The patient is the only expert on what values and beliefs are key to his or her recovery or coping of an illness; he or she is the only expert that can bring wholeness and health. Many of us have witnessed the patient's point of view and attitude relationed to the outcome of a health care event. Who knows better the needs of an individual than the individual himself? We are guides to offer the alternatives and options to the patient but not to make the health care decision for him. The importance of understanding diversity and respect is paramount to successful integration and partnership relations.

Support

Offering support for each other authentically creates an environment of caring. Supportive behaviors and communication are vital, in the easy times as well as the times of conflict and confusion. In the role of patient advocate, a nurse offering a caring and understanding ear is sometimes all that is necessary. With colleagues this is just as important because it fosters the establishment of the oneness of the health care team. Frequently, the hectic pace we have set builds a maze in front of us, causing confusion and frustration for both provider and patient. Being too busy is an excuse for short, irritated responses and poor listening. Sadly, we all use this excuse and intimately feel the ramifications of a complex world. When this atmosphere is present, there is little or no support offered to either patients or colleagues. By embracing the importance of spending time with each individual, we can improve efficiency and effectiveness and meet the patient's demands.

Communication

Of all the elements of partnership and relationships, communication stands as the cornerstone. No element can build a strong, honest, and whole relationship more than good communication. The art of dialogue needs practice and patience. Honest, authentic messages and fully present listening are essential elements in patient and family care. It is vital to use communication skills that strengthen our connectedness to each other, to our patients, and to their families. Without strong communication, we get lost in the overabundance of information we have available about health care and about our patients. The information and data we collect are useless without connecting the information to each individual's uniqueness and values. Information and data may be our greatest tools or our greatest burdens.

Commitment

Being fully passionate and persistent in developing a partnership relationship with patients and families across the continuum requires a commitment to the human community. Obstacles and barriers—some built by our own egos, by other health care colleagues, or by governmental structures, rules, and agencies—get in the way. Without commitment to the patient and family, nursing lacks the integrity to follow through on the promise as a profession to provide care to society.

SUMMARY

Developing nursing case management is a process, not an outcome. It is a model that creates structures, tools, standards, and paths to accomplish the goal of healing and promoting wholeness. I see no end to the evolution of nursing case management. The amoebic motion of nursing case management will continue growing and constricting as societal pressures and forces affect the model. Integration of this model across the continuum is well on its way, but is the next step the creation of a patient management model that establishes the nurse as a steward and integrator for the health care community? Maybe so.

References

Benner, P. (1984). *From novice to expert,* Menlo Park, Calif.: Addison-Wesley Publishing Co.

Benner, P., Tanner, C., & Chelsa, C. (1996). *Expertise in nursing practice—caring clinical judgment and ethics,* New York: Springer Publishing Co.

Gerke, M.L., & Proksch, M.K. (1995). *Socialization into the differentiated nursing roles of case manager and case associate.* Unpublished master's thesis, Department of Nursing, Winona State University, Winona, Minn.

Johnson, B., Friend, S., & MacDonald, J. (1997). Nurses' changing and emerging roles with use of unlicensed assistive personnel. In S. Moorehead (Ed.), *Nursing roles evolving or recycled?* Thousand Oaks, Calif. Sage Publications.

Larson, J. (1992). The healing we: A transformative model for nursing. *Nursing & Health Care, 13,* 5.

Manion, J., Sieg, M.J., & Watson, P. (1998). Managerial partnerships: The wave of the future, *Journal of Nursing Administration, 28,* 4.

Nightingale, F. (1992). *Notes on nursing,* Philadelphia: J.B. Lippincott.

Primm, P.L. (1986). Entry into practice: Competency statements for BSN and ADNs, *Nursing Outlook, 34,* 3.

Schaef, A.W. (1998). *Living in process,* New York: Ballantine Publishing Group.

Webster, M. (1988). *Webster's ninth new collegiate dictionary,* Springfield, Mass., Merriam-Webster Inc. Publishers.

Wheatley, M.J., & Kellner-Rogers, M. (1996). *A simpler way,* San Francisco: Berrett-Koehler Publishers.

Zander, K. (1985). Second generation primary nursing: A new agenda, *Journal of Nursing Administration, 15,* 3.

APPENDIX 13-1

Job Descriptions and Competencies of the Care Manager and Care Associate

RN CARE MANAGER

	SELF-AWARENESS	PATIENT/FAMILY CARE	RELATIONSHIPS
VALUE	Remains respectful of and committed to: • Role • Own abilities • Experience • Knowledge/learning • Professional practice • Self-confidence • Motivation • Growth and development • Humility	• Profession of nursing • Care delivery continuum • Potential power within patient/family • Patient's own healing power • Patients' health continuum • Patient/family interpretation for their own quality of life • Patients rights • Ethical care	• Mission • Effective teamwork • Expertise of others • Integrity of individuals/teams • Multiple perspectives • Ongoing education, change, and growth • Mentoring • Proactive communication
KNOWLEDGE	Demonstrates consistent understanding of: • Self • When to involve others • Importance of self-care • Boundaries/limitations • Presence • Impact of attitude	• The nursing process • Family dynamics • Teaching theory • Motivation for patients • Impact of patient/family on community • Health care options/trends and resource management • The unexpected and the big picture • Patient/family response to health status • Empathy, compassion, and presence • Coping mechanisms • Systems theory • Assumes responsibility for the assessment and care of patients appropriate to the age of the patients served in the assigned service area	• Change process • Group process • Learning styles • When to risk • Potential impact of attitude on the team • Roles/resources for information/problem solving • Boundaries of individuals and the team • Mentoring • Capacities of team members, when greater expertise may be required

Continued

RN Care Manager—cont'd

Skill	Self-Awareness	Patient/Family Care	Relationships

Consistently and intuitively demonstrates:	• Self-direction and motivation
	• Open and objective perceptions
	• Integration of past/present experiences
	• Accountability for decisions
	• Self-care
	• Time management
	• Independent thinking
	• Self-reflection
		• Resource utilization for optimal, cost-effective care
		• Active listening, connecting, and communicating in patient terms
		• Advocacy
		• Nursing process:
		  • Assess functional health status
		  • Develop mutual goals
		  • Individualize care planning
		  • Evaluate response to care plan
		  • Assess individuals' learning needs
		  • Implement teaching strategies
		  • Plan and coordinate discharge needs
		• Assess need for follow-up
		• Response to ethical challenges
		• Reasoning based on experience
		• Management of multiple tasks simultaneously
		• Resourcefulness—accessible—available—aware
		• Comforting, distracting, being with, relieving pain
		• Obtains and interprets information in terms of the patient's needs that are age specific and carries out treatments
		• Demonstrates a knowledge of normal growth and development
			• Active listening
			• Open dialogue
			• Conflict resolution
			• Utilization of others' expertise
			• Application of knowledge from one situation to another
			• Accountability
			• Flexibility and objectivity
			• Focusing energy in a positive constructive direction
			• Commitment to follow through
			• Risk taking
			• Negotiation—stepping in/back as the situation demands
			• Assertiveness
			• Persistence
			• Persuasion
			• Facilitation of learning for others
			• Investigation of alternatives and shared rationale

RN Care Associate (Essential)

	Self-Awareness	Patient/Family Care	Relationships	Communication
Value Remains respectful of:	• Growth and exploration • Self-perception • Own value clarification	• Essence of nursing • Care delivery system • Patient vulnerability, rights, and choices	• Team concept • Expertise of other disciplines • Multidisciplinary approach • Differentiation in nursing practice • Mission of unit	• Effective communication • Being open and non-judgmental
Knowledge Demonstrates increasing understanding of:	• Self-care • The importance of others' perceptions • Objective feedback • Knowing self and why you are here • Importance of not projecting own value system • Personal/professional limits	• Core nursing skills and practice • Pathophysiology of disease • Concepts of family dynamics • The need for empathy and compassion • Differentiated nursing roles • Assumes responsibility for the assessment and care of patients appropriate to the age of the patients served in the assigned service area	• The elements of a team • The importance of being an effective team member • The roles of other disciplines • The nursing role within the patient care delivery system • Mission of nursing department and organization	• The elements of facilitative communication • Nonverbal language

Skill
 	
Progressively demonstrates ability to:
	• Accept and listen to feedback on feelings/behaviors and reactions to situations
	• Share knowledge
	• Question the unknown
	• Understand and accept values of self and others
		• Perform core nursing process and skills
		• Organize and prioritize patient needs
		• Function in the team and assist patients in achieving mutual goals
		• Evaluate and give feedback on patient's response
		• Manage time
		• Teach
		• Obtains and interprets information in terms of the patient's needs that are age specific and carries out treatments
		• Demonstrates a knowledge of normal growth and development
			• Function in a team
			• Know when and how to recognize and use appropriate disciplines
			• Delegate
				• Recognizes self and others' perceptions and their impact
				• Exhibit effective listening, verbal, nonverbal, and written skills:
				  • Non-blaming
				  • Respectful
				  • Honest
				  • Courteous
				  • Good eye contact
				  • Clear messages
				• Provide concise reports and documentation

RN CARE ASSOCIATE (LEADER/EXPERT)

	SELF-AWARENESS	PATIENT/FAMILY CARE	RELATIONSHIPS
VALUE Remains respectful of and committed to:	• Own abilities—relies on clinical judgment for decisions • Experience • Knowledge/learning • Professional practice • Concern for patient as a person as central to practice • Self-confidence and self-responsibility • Humility • Motivation • Growth and development	• Profession of nursing • Care delivery continuum • Moral and caring practices—doing things for the right reason • Potential power within patient/family • Patient's own self-healing power • Patient's interpretation for own quality of life • Ethical resource utilization	• Change and growth • Expertise of others • Mission of the nursing department/organization • Integrity of individuals/teams • Multiple perspectives • Mentoring • Proactive communication
KNOWLEDGE Demonstrates consistent understanding of:	• Self • Others' skills and knowledge • Boundaries • Presence • Impact of attitude	• Nursing process, caring, and teaching theory • Practical knowledge of particular patient population • Warning signs, subtle changes • The unexpected and the big picture • Different roles of differentiated case management • Patient response to pathophysiology of disease • When technology has become excessive and intervenes appropriately • Empathy, compassion, and presence • The ongoing need for health and well-being • Coping mechanisms • Assumes responsibility for the assessment and care of patients appropriate to the age of the patients served in the assigned service area	• Change process • Group process • Learning styles—strengths and weaknesses of others • When to risk • Resources for problem solving • Capacities of team members, when greater expertise may be required • Timing and pace of whole unit • Stepping in and stepping back as the situation demands • Boundaries of individuals and the team • Mentoring • Creating an environment for effective teamwork

SKILL

Consistently and intuitively demonstrates:

- Self-direction and inner motivation
- Awareness of personal limits
- Open and objective perceptions
- Integration of past/present experiences
- Accountability for decisions
- Self-care
- Time management
- Independent thinking
- Self-reflection

- Nursing process—skilled, innovative performance linked with judgment, timing, and anticipation of future events
- Practical reasoning based on experience
- Organization, prioritization, analysis of data to meet individual needs
- Management of multiple tasks simultaneously
- Thinking in action
- Fluid, seamless performance of difficult tasks under time pressure
- Resourcefulness for patient/family: accessible—available—aware
- Reading patient's response, adjusting for individual needs, desires, wants in both clinical and human dimensions
- Comforting, distracting, being with, relieving pain
- Allowing patient/family to explore care options and respectfully advocates for their decisions; guided by patient response and desired outcomes
- Ability to identify moral issues and to foresee ethical implications of clinical interventions and seek organizational response
- Ability to design systems to support caring practices and create supportive space
- Connecting and communicating in patient terms
- Resource utilization for cost-effective care
- Obtains and interprets information in terms of the patient's needs that are age specific and carries out treatments
- Demonstrates a knowledge of normal growth and development

- Respect, dignity, personhood, the integrity of close relationships
- Advocacy
- Caring relationships guided by patient response
- Openness to exceptions in the usual level of involvement to allow vital caring work to occur
- Utilizing expertise of others—working with others so no one is overburdened and all resources are used
- Resourcefulness—for unit/organization: available—aware—accessible
- Application of knowledge from one situation to another
- Accountability
- Flexibility and objectivity
- Response to ethical challenges (able to take strong positions with health team to get what patient needs)
- Focusing energy in a positive constructive direction
- Active listening
- Commitment to follow through
- Risk taking: negotiation—assertiveness—persistence—persuasion
- Facilitation of learning for others
- Investigation of alternatives and shared rationale
- Open dialogue
- Conflict resolution

RN CARE ASSOCIATE (PROFICIENT)

	SELF-AWARENESS	PATIENT/FAMILY CARE	RELATIONSHIPS	COMMUNICATION
VALUE Remains respectful of and committed to:	• Self • Personal/professional limits • Diversity • Own philosophy regarding quality of life/ethical issues • Reflective learning • Learning from others	• Essence of nursing • Quality individualized care • Care delivery system • Patients rights and choices • Alleviation of pain and suffering • Caring • Cost-effective care	• Mutual respect of team members • Expertise of all disciplines • Team working as a whole • Mentoring	• Process of facilitative communication: 　• Truth 　• Openness 　• Productive outcomes 　• Respect of others 　• Understanding
KNOWLEDGE Demonstrates consistent understanding of:	• Self as a resource • How self is perceived • Personal limits • Own emotions & internal reactions • Self-motivation • Personality traits • Response to diversity • Advocacy • Self-care	• Nursing Code of Ethics & Practice Act • Roles in differentiated case management • Broad range of nursing skills • Significance of signs and symptoms • Complexities of patient's condition • Typical progression of illness and recovery • Pathophysiology of disease process • Family dynamics and importance of support people in healing process • Empathy and compassion • Ongoing need for health and well-being • Assumes responsibility for the assessment and care of patients appropriate to the age of the patients served in the assigned service area	• Various roles of the team members • Limits within the team • Mutual goals and plan of care established with patient • Mission of nursing department and organization • Ongoing need for change and growth • Impact of attitude on team	• Elements of facilitative communication • Variety of learning styles

SKILL

Consistently and effectively demonstrates:

- Independence in practice
- Attentiveness
- Sensitivity to own feelings and external elements that affect those feelings
- Active role in advocating and collaborating for quality of life issues
- Self-care
- Time management

- Nursing process:
- Accurate assessment and problem identification
- Planning/anticipating likely events
- Mastery of difficult technical tasks and multiple demands
- Combining standardization with professional judgment
- Data interpretation to identify complex needs
- Competent clinical judgment
- Organizing, prioritizing, analyzing data to meet needs
- Evaluation and feedback on response, adjusted for individual needs
- Teaching
- Advocacy
- Collaboration
- Obtains and interprets information in terms of the patient's needs that are age specific and carries out treatments
- Demonstrates a knowledge of normal growth and development

- Team collaboration
- Utilization of team members (consults/refers)
- Delegation of responsibility
- Integrity
- Flexibility
- Adaptability
- Commitment
- Professional behavior
- Preceptorship

- Communication in understandable language
- Listening and allowing input
- Sharing and teaching ideas
- Conflict management
- Manner that is approachable, interactive, sees both sides, positive, assertive
- Nonjudgmental interaction

Parish Nursing as Community-Focused Case Management

Nancy J. Brown, Joan K. Magilvy

CHAPTER OVERVIEW

Parish nursing, an emerging nursing practice role set in communities of faith, provides an example of beyond-the-walls case management. Parish nursing is a community-based practice closely related to traditional public health nursing practice in its population focus, emphasis on health promotion and disease prevention, broadly conceptualized and holistic perspective of health, concern for healthier communities, and provision of care to diverse populations in nontraditional settings. In this chapter the authors will provide an overview of parish nursing and show how this new model of care is responding to and impacting the changing health care environment, as well as improving the health of congregations/communities. Parish nursing represents a different model of case management. An example or case study to exemplify the differences between case management in parish nursing and other models of case management will be presented.

A CHANGING HEALTH CARE ENVIRONMENT

Parish nursing is a community-based model of case management well suited to the dramatic and rapid changes in health care delivery. A shift in the health care system has resulted from the health care reform movement and complex economic pressures on health care institutions and providers. The emphasis on community-based, population-focused primary health care reflects a movement from our current engagement with high-tech, institution-based care. These health care system changes are forcing a re-examination of health policy, the organization and location of health care services, the goals of health care delivery, and the intended outcomes of care.

While the shift to community-based services is positive and congruent with consumer wishes, the development of new health care services does not always incorporate a broad, holistic definition of health. This definition would take into account the whole person and recognize the physical, mental-emotional, sociocultural, environmental, and spiritual influences and variables integrated into whole-person health. In addition, from a community- or population-focused perspective on the clients of nursing practice, whole-family, whole-community, and population health would be defined equally broadly. Parish nursing is a community-based practice compatible with the consumer-initiated drive toward holistic, readily accessible, affordable, acceptable health care and needed health care system change.

Consistent with the nature of this health reform movement, nurses and faith communities are exploring innovative models of care congruent with the principles of primary health care. The principles of primary health care delineated at the 1978 World Health Organization Alma Ata Conference include universal access to affordable, comprehensive, coordinated, and continuous health care services provided in the context of, and in partnership with, family and community (WHO, 1978). Parish nursing can impact both the cost and quality of health care. It can foster a relationship between public health and people in communities by increasing the emphasis on health promotion, disease prevention, and care management, reducing fragmentation, emphasizing individual responsibility, and increasing access to care (Magilvy & Brown, 1997; Schank, Weis, & Matheus, 1996).

Parish nursing is an exemplar case management model that reflects the redefinition of health and communities. Concurrent with the health systems changes, the literature points to an increased recognition of the role of faith and spirituality in health and healing (Marty, 1990; McFarling, 1999; McIntosh, 1997). Grounded in shared visions, partnerships, and expansion of health care to a community-based, consumer-oriented delivery system, parish nursing further recognizes the importance of spirituality in health and positive health outcomes.

PARISH NURSING: THE ROLE, SETTING, AND CONTEXT

Many problems facing our current health care delivery system, such as fragmentation of care, rising health care costs, limited access to primary care, and a lack of input from consumers, are being addressed, at least in part, by implementation of parish nursing. Set in communities of faith (churches, synagogues, mosques, or temples), parish nursing is an innovative model of community-based health care focused on health promotion, disease prevention, and care management, emphasizing self-care and individual responsibility.

Faith communities are recognized as effective sites for community-based or population-focused programs because they are accessible and provide a comfortable environment for people to learn about and discuss their health needs or concerns (Magilvy & Brown, 1997). According to Grace (1999), the Kellogg Foundation has become "increasingly convinced of the power of *community* as a positive influence on the health and well-being of people, and often, at the center of the community is the church. . . ." Grace continues, "The development of parish nursing has resulted in the church becoming an increasingly important force influencing the health and well-being of people" (p. xv). Congregations are perfect for addressing many of the health-related objectives of *Healthy People 2000* (USDHHS, 1991), in particular, prevention and accessibility—major goals of the report. Foege and Katz (1990) point out that "primary control over the nation's health prospects lies with the personal decisions each of us makes daily" (p. 9). Foege and Katz go on to point out that our focus needs to be on helping people make better decisions about their health and health behaviors, cleaning-up the environment, and making prevention available to all. These are precisely the kinds of activities undertaken by parish nurses. The authors of *Healthy People 2000 (USDHHS, 1991)* suggest that churches and other religious organizations have the potential to make significant contributions to health promotion and disease prevention efforts, but that this resource is largely untapped (USDHHS, 1991). However, interest in parish nursing, health ministry, and faith-health partnerships is increasing, as noted by the numbers of books and articles on the topic (e.g., Gunderson, 1997; Joel, 1998; McDermott & Burke, 1993; Solari-Twadell & McDermott, 1999; Weis, Matheus & Schank, 1997). The International Parish Nurse Resource Center reports increased attendance at regional and national parish nurse meetings and at basic preparation courses for parish nurses. In addition, a number of professional organizations (APHA, ANA) are developing interest groups centered on faith and health and/or parish nursing/health ministry. An estimated 3000 parish nurses are presently providing primary health care services to persons of all ages and faith traditions, in both rural and urban settings (Weis, et al., 1997).

Parish nurses respond to the holistic health care needs of people of all ages who congregate in self-defined communities. Viewing faith communities as intentional communities, parish nurses work with people where they live and worship and define health as holistic—an integration of physical, emotional, social, and spiritual well-being. As a member of the pastoral care team, the parish nurse provides care to individuals, families, and the congregation/community through health assessment, screening, education, counseling, referral, support, advocacy, and the coordination of volunteers.

Granger Westberg, the "father" of parish nursing and a "driving force behind the whole person health movement," views nurses as the translators or bridges between the language of science and the language of religion, between people and the health care system, and between the congregation and the healing mission of the church (Grace, 1999, p. xv). Helping persons understand their physical condition, whether ill or well, and assisting them to take control of the management of their health is (should be) of primary importance in health care. Unfortunately, all too often the emphasis is on the wonders of technology and our ability to "fix" things (Grace, 1999, p. xvi).

The goals of a parish nurse program are to identify congregational health needs and plan appropriate programs; promote the health and well-being of members; promote lifestyle change and individual and congregational responsibility for health; improve access to and utilization of needed health services; increase involvement in health care; improve quality of life; increase client satisfaction with care; and facilitate community partnerships and promote healthier communities. (Magilvy & Brown, 1997; McDermott & Burke, 1993; Solari-Twadell, 1999; Striepe, 1989; Westberg, 1987, 1990). The parish nurse functions in many ways as a traditional public health nurse (PHN) in a faith community setting. For many years the generalist PHN carried a caseload of families in a designated geographic community or neighborhood. She or he made home visits; ran wellness clinics; offered information and referrals to community resources; participated in school nursing activities; taught health promotion to individuals, groups, and the community; and did individual and family counseling for issues such as end of life or chronic illness care. These activities are consistent with the case management model. The parish nurse, as case manager, carries out many of these activities with individuals and families in the congregation and in outreach to the neighboring community.

Parish nursing is practiced in four different institution- and congregation-based models. In the institutional models, paid and unpaid, the institution (hospital, school of nursing, home care agency, health management organization, or other community agency) employs, supports, and supervises the parish nurse, and the church/faith community contracts or affiliates with this institution for services. In the second form, the congregational models, paid and unpaid, a congregation develops a parish nurse program and employs or initiates another type of agreement with a parish nurse who provides services to the congregation. In both models volunteer nurses often work to supplement the services provided by the parish nurse. Some programs also use trained lay health promoters to extend the services provided. As the practice of parish nursing has expanded, variations on these two models have developed.

CASE MANAGEMENT IN PARISH NURSING: A DIFFERENT MODEL

While there are many variations of case management models, the goals of all are to provide quality, cost-effective services or to reduce health care costs while maintaining quality (Cohen & Cesta, 1997).

The goals often relate to reducing hospitalization and, when hospitalization does occur, to reducing the length of stay. The goals of case management in parish nursing must be viewed with a slightly different lens.

Goals and Philosophy of Case Management in Parish Nursing

The goal of case management in parish nursing is to improve the quality of life of members and constituents of a particular faith community. Moreover, parish nurses play a major role in assisting individuals to integrate spirituality and health in their everyday lives, a goal not usually viewed as part of traditional case management. Part of improving quality of life in this situation is providing accessible, high-quality, primary health care focused on health promotion and disease prevention, which should in the end also help to reduce health care costs, even though that is not a primary goal.

The philosophical differences between case management in parish nursing and other types of nursing case management are subtle but must be considered. They are differences of degree rather than differences of substance. First, parish nurses work in partnership with clients (individuals, families, and communities) and would not normally see themselves as the manager, but as being engaged in a partnership in which both the client and the nurse are managing the care with input from a broader interdisciplinary team. A goal of this partnership would be to assist clients in taking more responsibility for their health and health care, knowing that the nurse will not always be present when health care decisions are being made. By providing clients with the tools for appropriately managing their own care, parish nurses participate in improving the quality of life of their clients and engage clients in the process of ensuring quality in health care and controlling or reducing health care costs. Second, the focus of parish nursing is on noninvasive primary health care (prevention, health promotion, education, counseling, and referral) rather than on providing hands-on care.

Roles of the Case Manager in Parish Nursing

While variations exist in nurse case manager roles across settings, some areas of common ground are observed in the different roles. According to Cohen and Cesta (1997) the three case manager role dimensions most commonly identified across settings are the clinical role, the managerial role, and the financial/business role. In parish nursing case management the emphasis is on primarily the clinical and managerial role dimensions (Box 14-1).

The *clinical role* in parish nursing case management consists of doing holistic assessments of clients (individuals, families, and the congregation), developing nursing diagnoses, developing an individualized plan of care in collaboration with the client and other stakeholders, implementing the plan of care, and evaluating outcomes. The intervention might consist of promoting wellness, preventing disease, facilitating illness management, and providing support to members and families during health care transitions (e.g., identifying appropriate resources, facilitating a discussion of available options, promoting client and family involvement in decision making, reducing fragmentation, and assuring continuity of care). Because of their unique position in the community, parish nurses may identify processes that are not working well for clients and collaborate on clinical improvement efforts within the broader system (Solari-Twadell & McDermott, 1999).

The *managerial role* is much more informal in parish nursing case management than in other types of case management. Parish nurses do not normally work in institutional case management positions and therefore have no official role as a case manager. They practice instead in more of an advocacy role, providing case management in collaboration with members and constituents of the faith community they represent. Again, the primary goal is to improve quality of life by improving access to and quality

Box 14-1	CASE EXAMPLE

Sandy, the congregation-salaried parish nurse in a large urban Protestant congregation, related this story that exemplifies the case management role of a parish nurse:

Lillian is a 92-year-old retired school principal who lives alone in the home her husband had built for them when they married. A widow of 4 years, she has no children, siblings, or living relatives. Her primary sources of support are her church community and two unrelated godchildren, one of whom grew up next door to her. Even before her husband's death, Lillian had selected these two godchildren, both in their 40s, to assist her to make important life and health care decisions and to serve as her surrogate family.

Sandy first met Lillian 3 years ago when she became the congregation's parish nurse. Lillian was in fairly good health at that time and participated actively in congregation life. She was a member of the women's sewing group, regularly attended Sunday worship, and participated in several other activities. Sandy's first interaction with Lillian was around the time of the first anniversary of her husband's death. During a routine blood pressure screening, Sandy assessed high blood pressure and discussed possible reasons with Lillian. They soon determined that the death anniversary might have contributed to the problem. Sandy referred Lillian to her family physician and then began more frequent monitoring when Lillian visited the church parish nurse office. She also provided Lillian with counseling, support, and home visits periodically over the subsequent several years. Sandy assessed that the church community and religion were very important parts of Lillian's life. She had many friends in the congregation who visited her frequently, took her out to dinner, and volunteered to provide assistance as needed.

Recently, over the course of several routine home and office visits, Sandy noticed that Lillian's health was declining. She began to explore Lillian's thoughts about possible housing and care options. Staunchly independent, Lillian refused to consider assisted living or any other alternatives to remaining in her own home. One evening when they had gone out for dinner together, Sandy noticed that Lillian was exhibiting signs of sundowner syndrome and mild confusion. She became quite concerned and began to monitor Lillian more closely.

Early the next week, Sandy made a home visit and found Lillian to be ill and somewhat confused. Refusing to seek treatment that evening, Lillian allowed Sandy to return the next day. At that time Lillian was very ill and barely responsive. Sandy presented Lillian with two options: receive immediate medical treatment at the hospital, or invite someone to stay with her until the next morning when she could go to her doctor's office. With patient discussion and trust built on their long-term relationship, Sandy finally convinced Lillian to go to the emergency room. She was hospitalized immediately with a severe bladder infection and complications requiring lengthy hospitalization and rehabilitation care.

Throughout the week before hospitalization, Sandy repeatedly asked if she could get in touch with Lillian's godchildren, but she did not want to bother them and refused to give Sandy the telephone numbers. However, once hospitalized Lillian became aware of her current level of disability. She arranged for the two godchildren and Sandy to meet in her hospital room. Sandy was pleased to see the warm relationships Lillian had developed with the two adults. Lillian had designated one to assist with management of financial affairs and the other to assist with other decision making and support. Later Lillian expressed sadness to Sandy that the godchildren were not active in a faith community. She commented that nevertheless they were two very loving people whom she had selected purposefully to provide the support she anticipated needing in her later years.

Sandy sensed that the godchildren had many questions and were unaware of what resources Lillian might need. They made a mutual decision to hold a family conference shortly after hospital discharge. Lillian had a home care referral and received intermittent visits from several nurses, aides, and rehabilitation staff in the first few days. However, she soon "fired" all of the helpers and insisted she could manage on her own. Sandy arranged the family conference soon after this decision.

Continued

> Box 14-1 ▶ **CASE EXAMPLE—cont'd**
>
> Sandy arrived at Lillian's home that evening prepared with a list of discussion questions, issues that might need decisions, and potential resources available in the church and larger community. The family conference allowed all of the people who cared about Lillian to show their commitment to her. The conference facilitated decision making that supported her desire to remain as independent as possible in her own home. At the meeting Lillian agreed to wear an electronic emergency notification pendant. She also agreed to hire a woman from the congregation to assist with housekeeping and other chores. The godchildren would continue to help with managing finances, visiting, and other supportive activities. Everyone seemed grateful for the opportunity to join in discussion and problem solving.
>
> Her faith community welcomed Lillian back from the hospital, and she continues to attend church when she is able. Her pastor, other congregation members, and Sandy visit her at home frequently, and at present her health status is stable. Lillian has told Sandy that she remains satisfied with her choice to delegate her godchildren as her primary supporters and she is grateful to Sandy and the congregation for their love and help.
>
> Sandy's *care management* has contributed to Lillian's independence and quality of life. She has empowered Lillian to integrate her spiritual, physical, and emotional health and coached the family through important health decisions. Sandy's knowledge of local resources enabled her to coordinate care and make appropriate referrals to essential health care providers and services. She also assisted the congregation to minister to Lillian as they were able. In conclusion, with the support of her parish nurse, Lillian has been helped to clarify her goals; today she remains in her own home and maintains her connection with her church and family.

of health care, rather than to control or reduce (directly) health care costs. Finally, parish nurse case managers do not act as "gatekeepers of the interdisciplinary team" (Cohen & Cesta, 1997, p. 199). Instead, they communicate and collaborate with those team members on behalf of their clients.

The *financial/business role* dimension is something over which parish nurse case managers have little control. Indirectly, however, they do impact the cost of care by assisting clients in reducing duplication and/or fragmentation of services, by educating clients regarding the importance of early intervention, and by assisting clients to assume greater responsibility for their health and health care. While parish nurse case managers have little to do with maintaining appropriate resource allocation and determining appropriate length of stay, it is imperative that they be familiar with all types of payment systems (prospective payment, managed care, third-party reimbursement) so they can be of greatest help to their clients.

Skills of the Case Manager in Parish Nursing

The skills needed by the parish nurse case manager are basically the same as the skills required of any other nurse case manager. Cohen and Cesta (1997) stress that the nurse case manager must be clinically competent; highly skilled in communication, negotiation, working with teams, decision making, and conflict resolution; and knowledgeable about managed care and other health care financing mechanisms. In addition, the parish nurse case manager must be committed to working in partnership with clients, to facilitating the empowerment of clients to become managers of their own health and health care, and to assisting clients to integrate faith and health in their lives. From this and the previous descriptions of expertise required to fulfill the roles, it is clear that parish nursing is advanced nursing practice (Magilvy & Brown, 1997). Therefore the master's level of educational preparation would be congruent with this advanced practice role. This preparation is also very consistent with the master's or nursing doctorate educational level required for advanced practice nurses in other case management roles.

CASE MANAGEMENT WITH THE COMMUNITY AS CLIENT

Parish nursing provides innovative opportunities for nurses to work in partnership with neighborhoods, urban/suburban communities, and rural communities in a positive outreach of building on community strengths to promote healthier communities. Although community-based health care is not a concept new to nursing practice, the community as the client of nursing practice deserves increased emphasis. Community is a multifaceted level of nursing client reflecting a population or collective of individuals including special populations, such as people identified as underserved, vulnerable, and at risk (Magilvy, Brown, & Moritz, 1999). The term *community* can be applied to cities, towns, villages, urban or suburban neighborhoods or barrios, and schools, as well as to churches and other faith communities. Numerous environmental contexts, such as physical, sociocultural, political, and economic, influence the health of a community (Magilvy et al., 1999). The health of a community is conceptualized broadly to fit the diversity of people within the community. O'Malley (1997) speaks of a new vision of health care necessary to improve the health of the community, with a community-based emphasis on achievement of human potential, connectedness, and a sense of community.

Gunderson (1997) advocates faith communities or congregations creating relationships with their external community to improve the overall health and quality of life in that community. Congregations, led by pastoral staff, including parish nurses, can accomplish this goal in various ways. Congregations can create relational systems for frail community members and create helping roles that facilitate people to volunteer in service to others in need. Congregations may create networks and systems of collaboration to address needs not met by our complex health care system and infuse other community structures with healthy social expectations. Congregations in partnership with communities can make otherwise invisible people visible to the community (Gunderson, 1997). These examples demonstrate community-focused case management and the advanced practice role of nurses in partnership with community.

In rural communities, nursing research has demonstrated the strong connections of residents, especially older adults, to their faith community (Brown, Congdon, & Magilvy, 1996; Magilvy, Congdon, Martinez, Averill, & Davis, in press). In rural areas the church is often a center of community life and spiritual connection for families and persons of all ages. Acknowledging the difficulties of distribution and access to health care services and stigmatization of mental health services in small communities, the church is a safe, accessible, and acceptable place to engage in health promotion activities (Brown et al., 1996). Parish nurses in these small communities work with families in case management of chronic illness and end of life concerns, connecting them with resources and bringing the congregation's spiritual and tangible support to the members in need. Congregation-sponsored health fairs, educational offerings, and support groups engage the entire community in promoting the community's health. In some communities, parish nurses in different congregations integrate the activities of several churches and community agencies to provide community-wide caregiving and other voluntary services.

In conclusion, parish nurses in rural as well as urban communities are providing community-focused case management that impacts the health and quality of life of residents. Community-focused parish nursing is an innovative case management model that potentially contributes to quality and cost-effective outcomes. However, the lack of research on outcomes of parish nursing makes evaluation of the contributions to community health very difficult to measure.

EVALUATION OF PARISH NURSING

While some attempts to evaluate the practice of parish nursing are being made, a systematic approach to evaluation is lacking in the literature. Indicators of quality parish nursing case management practice and outcomes are needed. To evaluate parish nursing practice, one would need measures appropriate to the individual, family, congregation, and community level of client. Data collection instruments for use in a parish nurse practice are at an early stage of development and are aimed primarily at the individual and family units of analysis. The NANDA, NIC, NOC, and OMAHA system instruments have been adapted for use in planning, implementing, and evaluating parish nursing interventions for individuals and families (Burkhart, 1998; Denton, 1992). A need is strongly indicated for the development of instruments to measure outcomes of parish nursing programs in terms of improving health at the congregational and community levels. Congregational assessments are used to identify needs, satisfaction with, and utilization of parish nurse services. Community partnerships and relationships mentioned previously are important aspects of building healthier communities, but measures of the degree to which partnerships exist and community health is improved are lacking.

Parish nursing case management interventions could produce outcomes such as improved access to diverse health care services and more appropriate utilization of health care resources. Community members would actively participate in primary, secondary, and tertiary prevention programs offered by various community organizations, such as mental health agencies, hospice, violence prevention programs, farm safety seminars, and nutritional programs. Exploration of the outcomes of parish nursing programs and community partnerships should enable evaluation of the impact of parish nursing on the quality and cost of health care in the community. A need is indicated for extensive nursing research in these areas.

References

Brown, N.J., Congdon, J.A., & Magilvy, J.K. (1996). An approach to care management for rural older adults. *New Horizons 5*(27), 7.

Burkhart, L. (1998). *Parish nurse documentation applying NANDA, NIC, and NOC: Creating common communication between nursing specialties.* Park Ridge, IL: International Parish Nurse Resource Center.

Cohen, E.L., & Cesta, T.G. (1997). *Nursing case management: From concept to evaluation, ed. 2.* St. Louis, Mosby.

Joel, L.A. (1998). Parish nursing: As old as faith communities. *American Journal of Nursing 98*(8), 1-3.

Denton, J. (1992). Parish nursing and the Omaha system. In K.S. Martin, & N.J. Scheet (Eds.), *The Omaha system: Applications for community health nursing.* Philadelphia: WB Saunders.

Foege, W.H., & Katz, M. (1990). The 1990 objectives: A progress report. In M. Marty (Ed.), *Healthy people 2000: A role for America's religious communities.* Park Ridge, IL: Carter Center and Park Ridge Center.

Grace, H.K. (1999). Forward. In P.A. Solari-Twadell & M.A. McDermott (Eds.), *Parish nursing: Promoting whole person health within faith communities.* Thousand Oaks, Calif.: Sage.

Gunderson, G. (1997). *Deeply woven roots.* Minneapolis, Fortress Press.

Magilvy, J.K., & Brown, N.J. (1997). Parish nursing: Advanced practice nursing model for healthier communities. *Advanced Practice Nursing Quarterly 2*(4), 67-72.

Magilvy, J.K., Congdon, J.A., Martinez, R., Averill, J., & Davis, R. (In press). *Caring for our own: Health care experiences of rural hispanic elders. Journal of Aging Studies.*

Magilvy, J.K., Brown, N.J., & Moritz, P. (1999). Community-focused interventions and outcomes strategies. In A.S. Hinshaw, S. Feetham, & J. Shaver (Eds.), *Handbook of clinical research.* Thousand Oaks: Sage.

Marty, M.E. (1990). Health, medicine and the faith traditions. In M. Marty (Ed.), *Healthy people 2000: A role for America's religious communities.* Park Ridge, IL: Carter Center and Park Ridge Center.

McDermott, M.A., & Burke, J. (1993). When the population is a congregation: The emerging role of the parish nurse. *Journal of Community Health Nursing 10*(3), 179-190.

McFarling, U.L. (1999, Saturday, Jan. 23). The power to heal. *San Jose Mercury News: Religion & Ethics,* pp. 1E-3E.

McIntosh, P. (1997, Nov./Dec.). Why doctors say faith is powerful medicine: Not just for the mind, for the body, *Remedy,* pp. 26-30.

O'Malley, J. (1997). Emergence of healthier communities. *Advanced Practice Nursing Quarterly, 2*(4), v-vi.

Schank, M.J., Weis, D., & Matheus, R. (1996). Parish nursing: Ministry of healing. *Geriatric Nursing 17*(1), 11-13.

Solari-Twadell, P.A. (1999). The emerging practice of parish nursing. In P.A. Solari-Twadell, & M.A. McDermott, (Eds.), *Parish nursing promoting whole person health within faith communities.* Thousand Oaks, Calif.: Sage.

Solari-Twadell, P.A. & McDermott, M.A. (1999). *Parish nursing: Promoting whole person health within faith communities.* Thousand Oaks, Calif.: Sage.

Solari-Twadell, P.A., Djupe, A.M., & McDermott, M.A. (1990). *Parish nursing: The developing practice,* Oak Brook, IL: International Parish Nurse Resource Center.

Striepe, J.M. (1989). *Nurses in churches: A manual for developing parish nurse services and networks* (2nd ed.). Park Ridge, IL: National Parish Nurse Resource Center.

U.S.D.H.H.S. (1991). *Healthy people 2000: National health promotion and disease prevention objectives* (DHHS Publication No. PHS 91-50213). Washington, DC: Government Printing Office.

Weis, D., Matheus, R., & Schank, M.J. (1997). Health care delivery in faith communities: The parish nurse model. *Public Health Nursing 14*(6), 368-372.

Westberg, G.E. (1987). *The parish nurse,* Park Ridge, Ill.: National Parish Nurse Resource Center.

Westberg, G.E. (1990). *The parish nurse.* Minneapolis: Augsburg Fortress Press.

World Health Organization (1978). *Report of the international conference on primary health care.* Alma Ata, Russia: WHO.

A Faculty Case Management Practice in a College of Nursing*

Sharol F. Jacobson, Margo MacRobert, and Mary Allen Carey

CHAPTER OVERVIEW

Since 1995 the University of Oklahoma Health Sciences College of Nursing has been an accredited case management provider to the state of Oklahoma. As far as we know, we are the only university to have such a form of faculty practice. In this chapter we will describe the process by which we identified and instituted this service, our use of it for faculty practice and student learning, and the ongoing and emerging issues that mark its continuance.

THE ORIGIN OF THE CASE MANAGEMENT SERVICE

The faculty of the University of Oklahoma College of Nursing (OUCN) made major curriculum revisions in the mid-1990s to prepare students better for the evolving changes in the profession and the health care job market. Our deliberations supported the need for four significant changes. First, students needed more experiences in the community and clients' homes and with the aged, the chronically ill, and the disabled. Second, students needed greater familiarity with managed care, Medicare, and Medicaid and more active involvement in the wise use of limited resources. Third, they needed more experience working on interdisciplinary teams and with the management of care across sites and levels of acuity. Fourth, they needed more consistent integration of research and health promotion into their learning in relation to emerging trends in health care and nursing practice (Jacobson et al., 1998).

Achieving general faculty support for these principles was relatively easy. Determining how the needed experiences could be provided and in what proportions was much more difficult. Student data indicated a strong desire for more, not less, practice in acute care settings and strong resistance to more experience with the elderly and the chronically ill. Many faculty expressed a lack of personal experience in the community with elderly or chronically ill populations and with managed care systems and voiced concern about their ability to guide students in these areas. A perennial community barrier was the shortage of sufficient practice sites with nursing role models and nursing control to provide the desired learning.

*Portions of this chapter were adapted from A Faculty Case Management Practice Integrating Teaching, Service, and Research by S.F. Jacobson, M. McRobert, C. Leon & E. McKennon, Nursing Health and Perspectives, Vol. 19, No. 5, pp. 220-223. Used with permission.

A concurrent, contextual faculty issue was the nature and importance of faculty practice. Although OUCN was an early leader in defining faculty practice as part of faculty workload and in defining a practice plan for compensation (Smith, 1980), historically only about 10% of faculty (mostly psychiatric nurses) engaged in what would be consistent with contemporary views of faculty practice as linked to revenue generation and student experience. However, the advent of certification and its accompanying need for practice, the start of a nurse practitioner program, the expectations by university administration that faculty would generate revenue, and the burgeoning literature on nursing centers and clinics revived interest in faculty practice at OUCN and its potential for student experience.

A possible solution to our curriculum and practice debates came with the state's entry into managed care. In 1995 the state legislature created the ADvantage program, a Medicaid-funded program providing home and community-based services to frail elders and adults over age 21 years, to be managed by the Long Term Care Authority of Tulsa (LTCA). Analysis of the ADvantage program philosophy by a core of faculty found it to emphasize involvement of clients in service planning, interagency and interdisciplinary collaboration, health promotion as well as maintenance, use of family and community resources to supplement state funds, and separation of case management from provision of actual health care. These themes were highly compatible with our nursing values and needs for new student experiences and faculty practice. In September 1995, following faculty deliberation and creation of a business plan, the college became an accredited case management provider to the Oklahoma ADvantage Program. Our goals were to provide a quality, visible nursing service to Oklahomans; a nurse-controlled experience for futuristic undergraduate and graduate education; a needed site for faculty practice and learning; a source of revenue for the college; and eventually, a site for research, thus integrating the missions of the university (Jacobson et al., 1998).

THE ADVANTAGE PROGRAM OF OKLAHOMA

The ADvantage Program was developed to implement Oklahoma's 2176 Medicaid waiver. Its goal is to assist, in a cost-effective manner, clients with nursing home–level needs to remain in their homes with the formal services needed to do so. These services include case management, skilled nursing, personal care, homemaking, specialized medical equipment and supplies, prescription medications, home-delivered meals, environmental modifications to make the home safe and accessible, adult day care, various therapies, and respite for family caregivers. There were six original case management (CM) providers to ADvantage, including Eldercare, for-profit home health agencies, a community mental health center, and OUCN. We were the only provider based in a university, with all registered nurse (RN) case managers (CMs) and with all RNs holding master's or doctoral degrees. Within the conceptualization of case management models proposed by Conti (1999), our service is most closely related to the broker model. In Austin's typology of case management (Austin, 1992), our service is closest to the service management model, as we operate within clearly specified fiscal limits and purchase services on our clients' behalf.

The training of CMs begins with 7 days of instruction by the LTCA staff. CMs first become certified in the use of the client assessment tool that is completed by state health department nurses before client selection of a CM provider. Next they work through the entire CM philosophy and process using lecture, discussion, and role-playing. Following the management of five full cases under the supervision of LTCA staff, they are certified by LTCA and are allowed to carry ADvantage clients.

The actual CM process begins when LTCA notifies the CM provider that a new client has been screened for eligibility and has selected us as the CM provider. Faculty may be assigned to cases by the CM director or may volunteer for cases according to their expertise. The CM then contacts the client and makes a home visit to validate or update the original client assessment. Next, the CM schedules an interdisciplinary team meeting with the client, family, key informal support persons, an RN from the home health agency, and other formal providers, such as physicians or Medicare. At this meeting participants discuss and agree on the general plan of care. The CM then develops a service plan with goals, action steps, outcomes, and an expenditure plan that fits within the capitated rate of $12,000 per year. After approval by the client and LTCA, the CM implements the plan with the interdisciplinary team, monitors the client throughout the year, and evaluates and modifies the plan as needed.

Launching the Faculty Case Management Venture

Despite commitment to curricular redesign and faculty practice in some form, many faculty were not enthusiastic about the college becoming a full-time service provider to a state agency. The 24-hour, 7-days-a-week responsibility to clients and an external employer represented a major discontinuity with the traditional rhythm of academic life and traditional faculty practice. Dissenting faculty pointed out, quite correctly, that few descriptions of faculty practice in the literature involved everyday, round-the-clock service and that 24-hour coverage was not the norm for existing CM services. (In 1998 Mullahy (1998) identified 24-hour coverage as a trend but still not common.) How, faculty asked, could such coverage be provided when CM activities were to be performed in addition to regular teaching responsibilities? The fear that the CM venture would devalue acute care skills for students or the faculty teaching in critical care resurfaced. Concerns about job security and issues of academic freedom were raised for faculty who were unwilling or unable to acquire experience in this practice arena. Questions about the relative emphasis on the need for a new form of student experience versus the need for revenue generation and whether students would be exploited if they participated in an activity for which faculty received additional pay circulated overtly and covertly. Nevertheless, a core of seven graduate and undergraduate faculty volunteered to be trained as CMs and to develop student learning experiences in the program. The director of research also completed the training as an aid to future development of research on case management.

Dr. Patricia Forni, Dean of the College of Nursing, provided strong administrative support for the program. A faculty member with experience in administration, community health, and managed care was designated as the CM coordinator. Her visibility and legitimacy were enhanced by her appointment to the College Administrative Council and the Partnerships and Innovative Care Models Council. Secretarial support, office space, and equipment were provided. Teaching assistants were hired to relieve faculty taking CM training, and faculty were reimbursed for travel to training sites. A portion of the college's reimbursement from LTCA was used to pay CMs for mileage, in addition to their hourly rate. Faculty CMs also received merit points for service at their annual evaluations.

The period of training faculty as CMs and launching the service was neither smooth nor short. The CM coordinator position had to be filled three times in the first year. Turnover of faculty CMs was high initially because of dislike of the activity, frustration with the state bureaucracy, or competing demands from teaching assignments. Of 21 faculty trained as CMs in the first year, only 10 continued. Twice in the early months of the program we were unable to accept clients because of a shortage of CMs. We now emphasize that CM training is a practice commitment to the college and we require faculty CMs to carry at least 20 clients.

Use of the CM Program for Student Learning

Student experience in the CM program started in fall 1997, the second anniversary of the CM service. Two faculty offered 16 weeks of CM experience as a community clinical option for seniors; six responded. In Spring 1998, 14 undergraduates chose case management for their leadership experience. To date, 48 undergraduates have had CM experience. We currently offer clinical experience in case management to senior students in the community and leadership courses and to juniors in the disabilities course.

Four graduate students have also had learning experiences in case management. Two in the clinical specialist track chose it as a clinical practicum site and worked with the CM coordinator to develop a quality management program. Two from the administration/management track carried out required synthesis projects in case management, such as preparing a business plan for comprehensive case management, defined as a combination of case management and home health care.

Student learning has exceeded all faculty expectations: "They see teams and coordination like they've never seen it before with the nurse CM as the linchpin. They are accomplished users of the telephone. They know the nature and cost of all the assistive equipment. They see the patient's physical environment and get steps repaired and ramps built. They've internalized the roles of advocate, planner, and coordinator far more than I've seen them do in the hospital (Jacobson et al., 1998).

The effects of the CM experience continue when students return to inpatient settings. They are vocal about explaining how patients' needs could be adequately met in the community "without using up all their Medicare days." Their hospital discharge planning reflects much greater awareness of what is needed at home and what is available through the community. They recognize opportunities for health promotion among the chronically ill and disabled and that there are dynamic and critical episodes within chronicity (Jacobson et al., 1998).

Faculty also noted positive effects on the student-teacher relationship. In contrast to teaching in agencies where the faculty and students were guests and outsiders, "In CM, the students see me, a nurse, working in a college-controlled nursing setting. I perform in front of them and with them. I get more respect and more collegiality with students than I've ever known before (Jacobson et al., 1998).

A graduate faculty member in the administration/management track reported: "This is exactly the type of clinical exposure administration students need—not site or specialty-bound and not hierarchically organized. It's good for them to be reminded of just how cost-effective expert nursing is . . . to think about what background is really needed for good case management and what's worth paying for. And this program and role are still so fluid yet, they get a real sense of grappling with the future (Jacobson et al., 1998).

Faculty Experiences With the CM Program

PERSONAL SATISFACTION AND PROFESSIONAL GROWTH

Faculty CMs report great personal satisfaction with their work. They can see that their efforts have made important differences in client lives. Simply keeping patients in their homes where they wish to be is immensely satisfying. They have enjoyed more dramatic successes with clients other CM agencies had given up on, such as a young quadriplegic Indian man who overcame depression and alcoholism, obtained his GED, and enrolled in college.

Developing their interviewing, negotiating, and telephone skills has been gratifying. Getting clients what they really need within the budgeting constraints of ADvantage or advocating successfully to override the budget limits in a particular case are personal and professional triumphs. Faculty without prior knowledge of community resources, managed care, and reimbursement systems now feel confident about their ability to guide student learning in these areas.

INTERACTIONS WITH PHYSICIANS

Despite fears that physicians would view us as threats to their autonomy, faculty interactions with physicians have been almost entirely positive. Physicians in general and rural physicians in particular have been appreciative of what CMs are doing for their patients and have been willing to learn about community resources. They have expressed pleasure at working with nursing faculty as CMs because they believe that their patients are getting the benefits of the latest nursing knowledge. Some CMs state that they and the nursing profession experience more respect from physicians in the CM context than they have been awarded in acute care settings.

ETHICAL ISSUES IN CASE MANAGEMENT

Long-term case management has been characterized as an "ethical minefield" in which issues of quality and cost, regulation and personal and professional integrity, and ethical theories or perspectives clash (Barnett & Taylor, 1999; McAuley, Teaster, & Safewright, 1999). During the third year of the case management service, the frequency and complexity of ethical issues facing CMs led to the creation of a case management ethics committee. The membership consisted of the director of case management, two senior CMs, and faculty members who teach ethics courses. The committee meets on an ad hoc basis to deal with very complex situations with no apparent or optimal solution. These situations most frequently involve suspected mental illness of the client or family members providing informal support, suspected abuse or neglect, situations where the CM believes the client must be removed from the home but neither the client or the family will agree, or a combination of these circumstances. The committee has also dealt with cases where clients have had multiple case management providers and multiple CMs from within provider agencies and who have pushed us—the last available CM provider—to the point where the CM wishes to discuss the option of discontinuing services to the client. The ethics committee meetings have also served as a site for student learning for students in the policy and ethics course in the graduate program.

In regard to the perennial tension between client advocacy and gatekeeping responsibilities, a recent article (McAuley et al., 1999) contrasting regulatory system approaches and feminist ethics has been helpful. Briefly, the regulatory system approach used by social service agencies and programs originated in organizations designed to produce products. It values uniformity, order, certainty, and logical reasoning leading to reduction of case (human) circumstances to checklists and tallies. Circumstances that do not fit the official instrument or plan are ignored or considered irrelevant in the interests of values-neutral decision making, unbiased application of the rules, and accountability to the organization. In contrast, the feminist ethics that underlie nursing emphasize listening to all voices in decision making, the importance of caring and of meeting needs in an individualized manner, and acceptance of emotion and intuition as elements of decision making in addition to logical reasoning. Both models are, and should be, visible in CMs to varying degrees, as total reliance on one model would bring its faults into bold relief. We agree with the authors that the critical needs in case management are achieving a respected voice for feminist ethics in public programs and establishing an appropriate and flexible balance between the two approaches. At stake is the *care* in managed care.

EDUCATIONAL AND EXPERIENTIAL PREPARATION FOR CASE MANAGEMENT

Our experience with case management has provided much opportunity to reflect on the educational and experiential background that makes a good CM. We realize that people of diverse backgrounds are functioning successfully as CMs, that certifying standards exist for CMs of many origins, and that interdisciplinary partnerships can work well (Mullahy, 1998).

Our clients, by their very eligibility for the ADvantage Program, are of very low income (an average of $513 per month), have at least two primary diagnoses (including HIV/AIDS and actual or potential mental health problems), and already meet the standards for admission to nursing homes, as shown by a mean risk assessment score of 108.6, where 106 indicates high risk for institutionalization (Long Term

Care Authority of Tulsa, 1999). Comorbidities and polypharmacy predispose them to rapid change and decline. Their medical problems and needs for monitoring are so complex that the lack of a nursing knowledge base is detrimental to most of them. All CMs can supply examples of walking in on clients in acute medical or psychiatric emergencies or clients in whom subtle changes, which only a nurse would recognize, required immediate care. The scarcity of, or distance to, inpatient and emergency services for our rural clients makes the ability to make a prompt nursing judgment even more essential. It is far easier for nurses to acquire knowledge of community resources and reimbursement guidelines than for non-nurses to obtain the necessary clinical knowledge themselves or to secure timely consultation. We also believe that client needs require a minimum of baccalaureate preparation in nursing and that master's preparation in a clinical specialty is optimal and should become the standard. Furthermore, RNs with advanced preparation and faculty appointments have internalized the concept of lifelong learning and readily see the need for continuing education, which Mullahy (1998) identifies as a deficiency for some CMs.

Desirable experience for nurses before case management can best be described as broad. Ideally, prospective CMs should have several years of experience in more than one clinical area, in more than one type of treatment facility, and with patients of all ages. Experience in home health or community health is a major asset. At least some CMs in a service require knowledge of Medicare and Medicaid regulations and home health procedure and the ability to impart that knowledge to CMs without it. Superior oral and written communication skills and the ability to adapt them for different people or circumstances are essential. Because the family dynamics issues that CMs encounter are very draining and because conflicts between the client and team or between team members are inevitable, CMs need exceptional physical and emotional stamina.

Our best CMs are able to work in situations that are ambiguous, where there are no black-and-white answers or perfect solutions, and where there is often a need to switch mental gears and change plans and activities quickly. Novice nurses are usually unable to do this or are not comfortable doing this.

Of course CMs with ideal backgrounds are scarce, and CM supervisors, like those in acute care facilities, must develop less experienced or more narrowly experienced nurses as CMs. Our director has observed some common difficulties faced by new CMs. One circumstance that shocks people with experience only in hospitals is that the equipment and supplies always available in the hospital must be *found* in the case management situation. The role transition from being the person who gives the hands-on care to being a consultant, advisor, and facilitator of care is a major adjustment for some. Finally, a full appreciation of the autonomy of the client in the CM situation is a novel experience for many.

The case management supervisor also makes the CMs aware that burnout is a job hazard in this specialty. One advantage of the faculty CM service is that our CMs are not isolated, and observation by or interaction with sympathetic or knowledgeable others is always available. The faculty CMs also report that, after gaining a sense of proficiency in the CM role, their teaching responsibilities actually provide a buffer from the intense involvement with some clients.

CASE MANAGEMENT IN RURAL SETTINGS

Our clients are located in both rural and urban counties, giving us an opportunity to reflect on this dimension of case management. Demographically rural CM clients have been described as elderly, extremely hardy individuals who delay seeking health care longer than urban residents and are therefore sicker on entry into the CM system. They tend to be poorer than urban clients, to be more isolated, and to live in dilapidated housing, sometimes without electricity, telephones, or indoor plumbing. Their independence and self-reliance may predispose them to resist assistance from outsiders, making case management a sensitive issue for them. Service providers are fewer in rural areas but informal support systems for neighbors are often more common (Parker et al., 1991).

These characteristics are often true of our rural clients. However, the statewide publicity given to the ADvantage program and the fact that it aims to keep people in their homes as long as possible have worked to desensitize case management as an issue. Also, nurses are highly respected in rural areas, and we have benefited by being members of this trusted profession. At times, not being from the immediate community has been an advantage in that we are seen as safe confidants and not as people who will gossip about clients. Therefore we have not encountered the suspicion or distrust of urban health professionals described as characteristic of rural clients (Parker et al., 1991). If anything, our rural clients are more appreciative of our efforts and services than our urban clients.

Although there are fewer service providers to choose from, the stability and commitment to clients among home health aides from rural agencies has actually been higher than that among aides from urban agencies. Perhaps in the rural counties jobs are scarcer, so aides have fewer job alternatives and therefore tend to do better work and be more dependable.

Distance and mileage to clients' homes are time and money issues for our service. Our CMs drive 400 to 800 miles per month just in their part-time CM responsibilities. Although they are reimbursed, we have had to seek permission to pay a lower rate than the state allows to keep this budget component in check. Also, we often spend considerable time locating pharmacies who will deliver orders free to rural clients.

LOOKING BACK AND AHEAD

Adjusting to the demands of the case management service on the faculty has often been more a game of catch-up than of anticipation. After a slow start we experienced explosive growth in our client load caused by the demise of two of the original CM providers. In just 3 months, our caseload soared from 180 to 325 clients. The need to meet client needs immediately meant that the CMs coped without having time to think about how to adjust faculty assignments as the practice volume increased. The director of case management found herself with overall responsibility for the care of over 300 clients, a personal caseload of 25 clients, and supervision of faculty and nonfaculty CMs. One of the original CMs has now been designated as her official assistant, and the teaching loads of both CM supervisors will be decreased to recognize their practice responsibilities.

This increased client base, plus the inability to enlist sufficient numbers of faculty CMs, led to another change in the original structure of our service. We hired nine nonfaculty nurses (five with baccalaureate degrees and four with masters' degrees) as part-time CMs. Most were obtained from home health agencies and work for us on their own time. We could not continue without them, but we are no longer entirely a staff of *faculty* CMs.

A CM Track in the Graduate Program

In Fall 1999 OUCN offered a CM focus within the clinical nurse specialist (CNS) track. Students desiring CM preparation take the course in financial management currently taken by students in administration/management. This course includes content on the financing of managed care approaches. The core course, "Policy and Ethics in Health Care," and the concepts courses in the CNS track added content relevant to case management. One of two required clinical practicum courses is devoted entirely to case management and provides 288 hours of CM practice.

Case Management and the Research Mission of the University

Use of the CM service for research is still a goal. We are also open to multi-site collaboration with external investigators.

SUMMARY

Although the current faculty CMs are devoted to the program and wish to continue it, we realize that it will not enjoy the faculty-wide support we had originally hoped for, either for faculty practice or for student experience. Although some faculty have been impressed by the national interest in the service and the recruitment of a division director (author Allen-Carey) as a clinical specialist CM has reduced some criticism, the program is likely to remain controversial. We are heartened, however, by the quickness with which most students recognize the advantages of CM experience to them. Their comments about really understanding continuity of care, integrating all their nursing knowledge just before writing the NCLEX, CM as a showcase for professional and advanced practice, and CM as an area for entrepreneurship are extremely reinforcing.

Above all, the ADvantage program is maintaining indigent elderly and disabled Oklahomans in their homes and is saving Oklahoma taxpayers money—approximately $32,000,000 per year in 1998 (Long Term Care Authority of Tulsa, 1999). We are very proud that we have helped to bring the benefits of case management and the resources of the College of Nursing to our citizens.

References

Austin, C.D. (1992). Have we oversold case management as a "quick fix" for our long-term term-care system? *J Case Mgmt 1*, 61-65.

Barnett, R.J. & Taylor, C. (1999). The ethics of case management: Communication challenges. In E.L. Cohen, & V. De Back (Eds.), *The outcomes mandate: Case management in health care today* (pp 328-338). St. Louis: Mosby.

Conti, R.M. (1999). The broker model of case management. In E.L. Cohen, & V. De Back (Eds.), *The outcomes mandate: Case management in health care today* (pp 122-131). St. Louis: Mosby.

Jacobson, S.F. et al. (1998). A faculty case management practice: Integrating teaching, service, and research. *Nurse Health Care Perspectives 19*, 220-223.

Long Term Care Authority of Tulsa (1999, Jan.) *ADvantage Waiver Status Report.* Tulsa: Author.

McAuley, W.J., Teaster, P.B., & Safewright, M.P. (1999). Incorporating feminist ethics into case management programs. *J Applied Gerontology 18*, 3-23.

Mullahy, C.M. (1998). *The case manager's handbook,* (2nd ed). Gaithersburg, Md: Aspen.

Parker, M. et al. (1991). Case management in rural areas: Definition, clients, financing, staffing, and service delivery issues. In A. Bushy (Ed.). Rural nursing (pp 29-40) (vol. 2). Newbury Park, Calif: Sage.

Smith, G.R. (1980). Compensating faculty for their clinical practice. *Nurse Outlook 28*(11), 673-676.

A Model of Emergency Department Case Management

Developing Strategies and Outcomes

Carolee Whitehill

CHAPTER OVERVIEW

Significant public health issues impact the provision of services in the emergency department (ED): restrictions in access to care, the growing uninsured population, financial limitations, overcrowding, and staffing constraints, including physicians, resident positions, and the pressure to replace licensed nurses with unlicensed caregivers. Substantial attention is given to the concern of "inappropriate" ED visits, particularly by payor sources. This concerning belief assumes patients are making poor judgments when the ED is potentially providing a safe refuge by addressing a health care need not being met elsewhere.

A MODEL OF EMERGENCY DEPARTMENT CASE MANAGEMENT

Emergency Care Issues

The high volume of patients treated within emergency care facilities provides a unique opportunity not only to address acute clinical care, but also to offer appropriate education, screening, and health care resources within the context of the patient's specific needs and desires. Although overall goals of case management programs are similar, designing programs for the ED require a unique approach. Unlike traditional hospital or community case management programs, which allow for thorough and repeat assessments, family contact, time for discharge planning, and the potential for long-term follow-up, the emergency environment is episodic and spontaneous. The patient contact involves rapid assessment, usually limited to the immediate event, appropriate acute interventions, and an expeditious disposition process. As emergency department case management programs evolve, it is important for the ED to identify its place in the continuum of care. What are patients' needs regarding clinical care, disposition, follow-up arrangements, education, and resources? Who are the partners the ED staff can contact to integrate patient services? Are the linkages made on an individual patient level or by developing system-wide programs? In addition, providers of emergency care need to develop outcome measurements to determine the impact of emergency treatment, risk screening, and cost effectiveness and quality of care (Cairns et al., 1998).

Finding a Focus

Surrounded by a multitude of fragmented health delivery systems while treating high volumes of patients who often have complex needs, it may be difficult to initiate a clear plan of action in developing a case management program for the ED. Start by asking questions regarding patients, systems, and caregivers. This process may help focus on priority concerns.

Does the department have high-acuity, high-cost patients? Significant chronic care population? Long patient length of stay? Quality of care issues? High volume of nonurgent patients? Patients who have difficulty accessing health care resources? Significant uninsured population? Clear expectations among the ED team? Efficient coordination of services between inpatient and outpatient sites? Adequate communication with primary care providers? Reimbursement denials? A need to search for cost savings? A growing capitated payor population? Patient satisfaction that needs improving? Individual patients with special needs? Repeaters or re-admissions to the hospital? Patients who are noncompliant with discharge instructions?

Although this is just a sampling of potential case management issues, together they impact quality of care, efficient and cost-effective use of resources, access to care, and integration of services. When addressed, they may improve continuity of care and the health status of patients, which are the ultimate goals of ED case management programs.

A Model of ED Case Management

Current and evolving ED case management programs may be organized into four prominent areas (Figure 16-1):

Primary care programs
Population-based programs
Admission and discharge planning
Individual patient plans

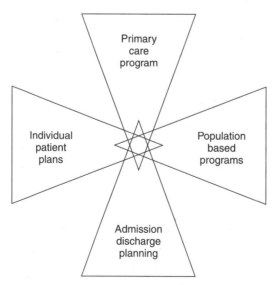

FIGURE **16-1**   ED case management.
(Copyright, 1999 Carolee Whitehill.)

This model serves as a tool to assist in program design and to identify issues, goals, strategies, and outcomes within the context of each area. The center star represents goals that are potentially shared among the programs and patients who may benefit from more than one program. Case managers may develop selective programs based on the priority issues within the facility and the distinctive needs of the patient population. ED case management programs are not developed in isolation, but by building alliances with providers in and out of the hospital setting.

Frustration regarding "frequent visitors" or repeaters is common among ED staff. As a group these patients have very diverse needs, resources, and reasons for using the ED. It is recommended that recidivism be evaluated within each program area to analyze and develop options appropriate to the specific patient or group of patients.

PRIMARY CARE PROGRAMS

Issues

ACCESS

United States government reports state that across the nation the acuity mix for emergency departments is 17% emergent, 40% urgent, and 43% nonurgent (General Accounting Office, 1993). Significant attention is being given to the nonurgent and a portion of the urgent population with the prevailing assumption that these visits are inappropriate and costly.

However, if there is an acute care need, patients may not be able to access their primary care office for urgent issues because of busy provider schedules. Patients may be told to wait a day(s) or to seek care in an ED or urgent care clinic. Payors strongly attempt to minimize ED visits, citing high cost as a detriment. Some patients use the ED for convenience; it is available 24 hours a day, 7 days a week without appointments. Many patients lack the flexibility with work schedules to attend appointments during weekday hours.

Patients are expected to determine the need for emergency care. In a study of 1190 ambulatory patients in an urban public hospital, the majority of whom were uninsured, patients were asked if they needed to be seen immediately, with 89% responding positively. However, according to a physician acuteness rating, 56% did not require care within 24 hours (Baker, Stevens, Brook, 1995). Patients and providers are given conflicting messages. Although the federal government passed a law stating patients have a right to access emergency services if their condition warrants immediate assistance as judged by any prudent layperson, payors continue to limit reimbursements to providers based on the findings of emergency treatment.

In examining factors that lead patients to use the ED for nonurgent care, Padgett and Brodsky (1992) found the most common reason was that patients reported no other care was available. In addition to lack of primary care resources, the authors report that psychiatric co-morbidities, socioeconomic stressors, and lack of social support influence patients' decision making. This reliance on the ED as a "safety net" for patients has been described as providing "almshouse" services, such as warmth, rest, clothing, food, shelter, and relief from social distress (Malone, 1998).

EDs continue to provide a health care safety net for the medically underserved in the United States. A study designed to identify the willingness of ED and private practitioners to see medically indigent patients found that the majority of EDs recommended a patient come to the ED when he/she called to request care regardless of insurance status. However, 62% of private practitioners' staff reported they were not taking new patients when the patient identified he or she had no insurance, whereas only 35%

were not taking new patients when the patient identified having insurance (Iserson & Kastre, 1996). It has also been found that access to primary care services for the medically uninsured is affected by the area in which they live and state and local policies, which vary widely across the country (Cunningham & Kemper, 1998).

COST

Emergency departments operate predominately on a fixed budget based on historical workloads. Providers are available 24 hours a day, 7 days a week. It is a widely accepted belief that diverting nonurgent patients from emergency departments to physician offices would result in significant cost savings. That belief is being challenged. Williams (1996) reports the marginal costs, defined as the extra costs of an additional ED visit, as $25 for a nonurgent visit. Diverting patients to a physician office would result in relatively low savings. Actual charges for the visits are often higher to compensate for overall poor reimbursements of care provided (Williams, 1996).

It is also widely assumed that emergency care consumes a large portion of the health care dollar. Data suggest that less than 2% of national health expenditures occurred in EDs and limiting access to this care would not result in substantial cost savings (Tyrance, Himmelsteine, & Woolhandler, 1996).

Therefore the purpose in designing primary care programs is to identify patients who would benefit from primary care services and match available resources to patients needs. Improving the health status of the population is the primary goal, rather than demonstrating a cost savings.

Goals

The goals for primary care programs are not designed to remove the ED from a health delivery resource or to eliminate it as a "safe refuge" for the population. Rather, the goals should encourage ED providers to more thoroughly evaluate the specific needs and desires of a patient and match these needs with available resources. These resources are offered with respect to insurance benefits with sliding scale or lower cost options for the uninsured. Goals for primary care programs might include the following:

- Identify and maintain current resources for primary care services, health screenings, health education, psychosocial assistance, and community resources; match patient needs to available resources to improve the patient's health status.
- Act as a liaison to improve communication between the ED and primary care providers.
- Decrease overcrowding, minimize waiting time, and increase patient satisfaction.

Strategies and Outcomes

RESOURCES AND EDUCATION

Primary care service needs of the ED patient population should be assessed. *What percent of the population is without primary care services? What resources are available for the insured and uninsured? Are the patients with primary care services knowledgeable about access and appropriate use? Do primary care providers receive summary notes of their patient's ED treatment?* Once the patient's needs and available resources are identified, patient and staff education becomes the priority.

Many patients need education regarding the benefits of primary care services: disease screening, health education and maintenance, prevention services, chronic disease management, medication monitoring, consistency and continuity of the provider, and extended follow-up. These services are not routinely provided in the ED. In addition, patients need access education: encouragement to call the provider 24 hours a day for health care advice, keep appointments even if feeling well, and call after the ED visit for a follow-up or new appointment.

Not all patients perceive the need for primary care services. It is important to determine the needs of the patients regarding ongoing continuity of care and the patient's incentive for compliance. There are several subgroups of patients whose resources might be more individualized. Patients with chronic illnesses or conditions should be strongly encouraged to obtain primary care services as their health status and quality of life can be improved and their disease more successfully managed through regular primary care. Patients who have significant psychosocial stresses such as poverty, homelessness, mental illness, substance abuse, or domestic violence often use the ED because their needs are not being met elsewhere. Although primary care may be indicated for a medical condition, arranging social service intervention, counseling, addiction services, financial assistance, and community resources are the priority concerns.

There remains a subgroup of patients who are generally young or middle aged and healthy who use the ED for urgent health care needs. Some of these patients do not perceive a benefit of primary care and only access health care when they are ill or injured and prefer the convenience of the ED. Perhaps these patients would benefit from education regarding the recommended disease screenings (i.e., Pap smear, mammography, prostate, colon cancer, cholesterol, etc.). It may be advantageous to offer patients without insurance benefits resources for low-cost, sliding scale services available in the area.

Outcomes regarding the success of patients obtaining new primary care services, compliance with follow-up appointments, and feedback regarding appointment availability can be helpful in adjusting resource education. In addition, monitoring the efficiency of forwarding ED visit documentation to primary care providers is an appropriate outcome measurement.

HOSPITAL-BASED CLINICS

Many EDs have initiated fast track or urgent care clinics to assist with patient flow in the department. These clinics are focused on providing efficient care to nonurgent and stable urgent patients with the goals and outcomes of decreasing wait time, overcrowding of the ED, and improving patient satisfaction.

If there are limited resources for the medically underserved in the area, and the ED is the regular provider of care the uninsured population, it may be beneficial to develop a hospital-based primary care clinic. If significant programs are developed with the goal of decreasing nonurgent patient volume in the ED, decreases in the low acuity triage categories may be useful as an outcome measurement.

POPULATION-BASED PROGRAMS

Issues

As health care policy is evolving, there is an increased emphasis on managing the health needs of populations rather than individuals. Among the most innovative ED programs are those focused on targeted population groups. Disease management programs evaluate health care needs of patients with a specific chronic condition or shared indicator such as age and develop a plan of care that addresses clinical needs, health maintenance and educational needs, resource utilization, and continuity of care with the purpose of improving the patient's health status. Although the primary focus of the ED is and will continue to be to provide emergent/urgent clinical care, by extending relationships with other providers, emergency caregivers are offered a great opportunity to expand the integration of health care services for targeted patient populations. Strengthening partnerships between the ED and primary care providers, acute care services, specialists, community resources, home care agencies, extended care facilities, alternative medicine providers, and payors will allow a more integrated, efficient, and resourceful health care delivery system to evolve.

Estimates suggest 10% to 15% of ED patient visits result from exacerbations of chronic illnesses. Managing chronic care patients is often cited as the most successful method to decrease costs of preventable care in the ED (Advisory Board Company, 1993). In addition to acute care services to treat illness exacerbations, patients need information for accessing primary care services and education resources for managing their own disease.

One might select a patient group that accounts for a high volume or high cost to the institution, significant re-admission rate, or a population that receives inconsistent care. Examples of population-based groups appropriate for disease or group management programs in the ED are as follows:

- Diabetes
- Asthma
- CHF
- Trauma
- Chest pain
- COPD
- Sickle cell disease
- HIV/AIDS
- Elderly
- Pediatrics

Goals

The goals for population-based programs involve patient issues beyond the immediate ED visit. Therefore some of the goals are attained in conjunction with interventions from other providers.

- Coordinate services to provide patient access to appropriate and cost-effective primary and specialty outpatient care, health education, and community resources.
- Improve quality of life indicators and patient's health status.
- Decrease repeat ED visits of targeted population because of a decrease in number of illness exacerbations.
- Provide an organized, efficient, and consistent multidisciplinary approach to care for a targeted population.
- Decrease hospital or ED length of stay.
- Decrease cost of care.

Strategies and Outcomes

RISK ASSESSMENT

One approach to developing a population-based program is initiating risk assessments to identify patients who are at risk for high service utilization and who might benefit from selective services. In Clough's (1996) review of risk assessment research, five indicators were determined to identify patients at risk for high use of health care services: (1) previous service utilization, (2) perceived health, (3) type and number of conditions, (4) type and number of medications, and (5) age (Boult et al., 1993; Connelly et al., 1989; Levkoff et al., 1985; Wasson et al., 1987).

Lowenstein et al. (1998) studied 923 patients to determine the prevalence of chronic disease risk factors and injury-prone behaviors among an ED population. Examples of the results are as follows:

- Of women over the age of 50 years: 42% had no PAP in the previous 2 years and 14% never had mammography

- 23% of patients had positive CAGE screens for problem drinking
- 38% reported no access to primary health care services
- 53% reported they did not wear seat belts regularly
- 20% had contemplated or planned suicide at least once in their lives
- 17% of women had been assaulted at least once in the preceding year

The researchers suggest ED providers use screening data to target patients in need of counseling, prevention, and referral services.

A risk assessment program was initiated at University Hospital in Denver, Colorado in the ED for patients with diabetes. The purpose of the program was to identify patients in need of (1) primary care services, (2) diabetes self-care education, (3) specialty care (eye, endocrine, podiatry, or vascular), or (4) social service or home health care. The primary goal was to advocate patient access to appropriate and cost-effective primary and specialty outpatient care, health education, and community resources. In addition, outcome goals to be evaluated were to improve the health status of targeted population (hospital-wide goal) and to decrease ED/urgent care clinic visits of the targeted population with a corresponding decrease in costs related to that care.

The target population was patients who identified a medical history of insulin or non-insulin-dependent diabetes. A convenience sample of 114 patients was contacted by phone during August through November 1997 and, as part of a courtesy follow-up call, asked additional risk assessment questions. Resource and referral information was provided as indicated as well as education on accessing and using primary care services.

Visits to the ED and urgent care clinic for the population group during the prior 12 months were calculated. ED and urgent care visits for the 12 months following the risk assessment were tracked, indicating a decreased visit rate of 46% overall. Based on average direct costs for the diabetic patients in the ED, the cost avoidance for the decrease in repeat visits was calculated at $13,300 for avoided outpatient ED visits and $135,087 for avoided admissions. It is important to note that with the exception of supply costs, most of the ED costs are "fixed." Unless programs result in a significant decrease in ED volume, personnel costs will not vary. Therefore it may be more appropriate to consider the savings a "cost diversion" for staff to focus on critical patients, improvement of patient flow, decreased wait time, and improvement of patient satisfaction.

CLINICAL PATHWAYS

An alternative approach for population-based programs is developing clinical pathways to provide an organized method to manage an acute episode of illness or injury. Clinical pathways assist in identifying and attaining outcomes-based, efficient, and consistent care to a targeted population. They are an evolution of protocols, algorithms, and standards of care that have been in existence for a number of years. What makes clinical pathways inherently unique from past management tools are that they:

- Are interdisciplinary (identify who, does what, when)
- Contain a time component (hours or phases; for example, triage, assessment, intervention, disposition)
- Measure specific outcomes (clinical, functional, system process, financial, patient satisfaction)
- Monitor variances to the outcomes (patient/family, caregiver, internal system, external system)

Outcomes may be measurements of reference points along the process of patient care, not just at the end point. Clinical pathways are not standing orders, but rather guides, that should be varied when indicated.

A number of published resources exist for clinical pathways for ED patients: asthma (Pins & Swanson, 1993), myocardial infarction, or chest pain (Ison 1991, Nelson 1993), a variety of pathways published by Emergency Nurses Association (Cosby et al., 1996), and several through the American College of Emergency Physicians.

Inpatient hospital pathways are generally focused on a specific diagnosis or an elective procedure. In the ED, focusing on presenting signs and symptoms (i.e., abdominal pain, chest pain, altered mental status) or systems process (i.e., criteria for laboratory and radiology testing) may be more appropriate. A mechanism that may improve compliance with clinical pathways is to develop the pathway as a documentation tool (Veenema, 1994).

ADMISSION AND DISCHARGE PLANNING

Issues

The traditional admission and discharge planning responsibilities of the case manager in an acute hospital setting may be extended into the ED. This role allows for early assessment and intervention for selected patients.

Goals

The goals for admission and discharge programs might be:

- Act as a liaison for hospital and community case managers to improve continuity of care.
- Ensure and expedite appropriate patient disposition: evaluate admission criteria, level of care, and alternative placements.
- Coordinate appropriate and efficient use of services and resources.
- Evaluate systems concerning admission and discharge processes to ensure compliance with regulations, efficiency, and integration of resources.

Strategies and Outcomes

INDIVIDUAL PATIENT APPROACH

If the department has case management resources available during the times of heavy ED volume, attention to individual patients is greatly beneficial. For patients destined for admission to the hospital, one can address:

- Admission to appropriate level of care, inpatient versus observational status, admission versus transfer to rehabilitation or extended care or discharge patient with home care.
- Contact the primary care provider.
- Determine if the patient qualifies for an inpatient clinical pathway or research protocol.
- Expedite plan for hospital case manager or social worker.
- Provide family support.
- Initiate insurance notification and out of network issues.

Brewer and Jackson (1997) reported a savings of $20,000+ over 6 months as a result of deferred inpatient admissions for patients whose care was manageable with home care assistance. Perhaps when an ED case manager is not available to assess an admitted patient, the ED charge nurse or primary nurse could contact the appropriate inpatient case manager or social worker with specific concerns.

For those patients who will be discharged from the department, the case manager might address:

- Evaluate options for follow-up plan: home care, community services, primary and specialty care, transportation, and medical equipment with respect to benefits.
- Assure compliance with transfer policies.
- Determine if patient qualifies for outpatient clinical pathway or research protocol.
- Contact primary care provider.
- Monitor compliance of follow-up care arranged.
- Complete laboratory and radiology follow-up.
- Provide financial assistance.
- Provide family support.

Traditionally, these interventions represent short-term patient involvement after an episode of acute illness. For those selected patients who may benefit from long-term follow-up, a more formal individualized plan may be indicated along with expanded monitoring.

Dubay (1997) described a unique referral nurse role that followed up on selected discharged patients from a Level II trauma center. Outcome goals were to improve continuity of care and decrease unnecessary repeat visits to the ED. From 30 to 50 patients were identified daily and contacted after discharge. Selection criteria included those with a questionable discharge diagnosis and home health referrals, as well as contacting patients to monitor compliance with physician follow-up. Patients could also call the referral nurse to clarify discharge instructions. In addition, this nurse also screened laboratory results and radiology discrepancies.

SYSTEMS APPROACH

If the staff in the ED currently fulfill admission and discharge functions, or if case management services are limited, perhaps a more pertinent approach may be to focus on systems issues. Ask the following questions:

How well has the organization integrated inpatient and outpatient services to ensure continuity of care? Is the ED linked to inpatient clinical pathways? What are the eligibility criteria for observation status and what is the compliance? What is the denial rate from payors for charges? Are denials due to level of service decisions or documentation issues? Is the department compliant with EMTALA regulations? What are the trends with frequent re-admissions? Is patient "choice" in post-discharge service arrangements being offered and documented? Can the uninsured population access care recommended in the discharge instructions? Does the cost of care for a particular patient group "match" with the contracts negotiated by the business office? These issues are system-wide concerns, and it is imperative that the ED is represented during their resolution.

INDIVIDUAL PATIENT PLANS

Issues

There are patients who "fall out" of the previously described programs and who may benefit from individualized interventions. These patients may have specialized clinical needs for which ED visits are expected; it is useful to have guidelines to provide consistent care. Or they may possess significant psychosocial stresses such as substance abuse, homelessness, poverty, mental illness, or domestic violence that contribute to a pattern of noncompliance with follow-up arrangement, frequent ED visits, or both.

The presence of these patients often causes distress among the staff because of the inability to provide an efficient resolution.

Goals

Goals for individual patient plans might be:

- Develop guidelines to provide consistent care to identified patients by integrating information from all involved providers.
- Advocate access and appropriate use of primary care and community resources.
- Decrease unnecessary utilization of the ED by patients who are frequent visitors.
- Improve quality of life indicators.

These are general goals and will not pertain to every patient's plan. For example, a patient with significant clinical pathology may continue to have frequent ED visits; the goal would be to provide consistent care for that patient.

Strategies and Outcomes

REFERRALS

At University Hospital in Denver, Colorado individual patient referrals are forwarded to the nurse case manager by nurses and physicians. The patient's records are reviewed, including past 12-month ED visit history and hospital admission rate, current providers of care are contacted for advice, the social worker or emergency psychiatric services are contacted as indicated, and a discussion with the patient and pertinent family members occurs.

The plan may be as simple as more individualized patient/family education in accessing health care resources and completing follow-up calls to encourage compliance. If indicated, a clinical protocol is developed in conjunction with providers of care to ensure continuity and a consistent approach to the patient in the ED. Involvement with other case managers within the patient's provider sites is solicited. These protocols are only guidelines and will be adjusted according to the patient's presentation and response. The protocols are reviewed and revised at least once a year. Although the goal of decreasing ED visits may or may not be a part of the plan, patient visits are monitored and primary care providers receive dictated ED notes. Often the providers of patients who have been frequent visitors will be more flexible in accommodating the patient for unscheduled, urgent events. To date, based on 12-month follow-up, there has been a 55% decrease in repeat ED visits of the patients for whom that was a goal.

As a note of caution, occasionally a primary care provider has requested that the ED staff "refuse" to see a patient. These providers need to be educated that all EDs must provide at minimum a medical screening examination as dictated by EMTALA regulations, and refusing to treat a patient is not a legal option.

PARTNERSHIPS WITH COMMUNITY CASE MANAGERS

Developing partnerships among case managers in other health care settings may improve the continuity of care. A community case management program followed 21 adult patients identified with frequent ED visits and hospital admissions and with difficulty managing a chronic illness. Reported outcomes at 6 months indicated a 52% decrease in hospital admissions and 30% decrease in costs (Sund & Severingson, 1998). A similar program managed 38 chronically ill or frail patients in the community. Cost outcomes indicated a resource savings of $226,089 under a nurse case management system compared to resource utilization before case management (Rogers, Riordan, & Swindle, 1991).

CHALLENGES AND OPPORTUNITIES

ED case managers are on the horizon of a great opportunity to expand outreach to the inpatient and community setting. The health care market is increasingly difficult for patients to manage; ED staff have the ability to assist large volumes of patients with access to care, public health education, and individualized resources. Partnerships must be developed within health care delivery systems to share resources and information, avoid duplication of services, and improve continuity of care (Smith & Brooks, 1999). Any of the strategies and outcomes related to enhancing the delivery of care to patients or system improvements would be recognized as continuous quality improvement programs. The emerging roles of ED case managers will encompass many responsibilities and processes: access, advocacy, education, resource, referral, liaison, evaluation, monitor outcomes, program design, and partnerships.

References

Advisory Board Company (1993). *Redefining the emergency department; five strategies for reducing unnecessary visits.* Washington, D.C.

Baker, D., Stevens, C., & Brook, R., (1995, March). Determinates of emergency department use by ambulatory patients at a urban public hospital. *Annals of Emergency Medicine, 25*(3), 311-316.

Boult, C., Dowd, B., McCaffery, D., et al. (1993). Screening elders for risk of hospital admission. *Journal of the American Geriatric Society, 41*(8), 811-817.

Brewer, B., & Jackson, L. (1997, Dec.). A case management model for the emergency department. *Journal of Emergency Nursing, 23*(6), 618-621.

Cairns, C., Garrison, H., Hedges, J., et al. (1998). Development of new methods to assess the outcomes of emergency care. *Annals of Emergency Medicine, 31*(2), 166-171.

Clough, J. (1996). Risk identification: Management versus avoidance. In E. Cohen, (Ed.), *Nurse case management in the 21st century* (pp 168-180). St. Louis: Mosby-Year Book, Inc.

Connelly, J., Philbrick, J., Smith, R., et al. (1989). Health perceptions of primary care patients and the influence on health care utilization. *Medical Care, 27*(3, suppl), 99-108.

Cosby, C., Kozeny, D., O'Neal, A. et al. (1996). *Case management; a dynamic process.* Park Ridge, Ill., Emergency Nurses Association.

Cunningham, P., & Kemper, P. (1998, Sept.). Ability to obtain medical care for the uninsured. *JAMA, 280*(10), 921-927.

Dubay, D. (1997, Oct.). Emergency center follow-up program. *Journal of Emergency Nursing, 23*(5), 455-456.

General Accounting Office (1993). Emergency departments: Unevenly affected by growth and change in patient use. Washington D.C.: United States General Accounting Office.

Iserson, K., & Kastre, T. (1996). Are emergency departments really a "safety net" for the medically indigent? *American Journal of Emergency Medicine, 14*(1), 1-5.

Ison, A. (1991, April). Nursing case management: An innovative approach to care in the emergency department. *Topics of Emergency Medicine, 13*(3), 35-46.

Levkoff, S., Wettle, T., Coakley, E., et al. (1985). Predictors of service utilization by medicare hmo enrollees. *HMO Practice Research, 2*(2), 58-65.

Lowenstein, S., Kozial-McLain, J., Thompson, M., et al. (1998, Aug.). Behavioral risk factors in emergency department patients: A multi-site survey. *Academic Emergency Medicine, 5*(8), 781-787.

Malone, R. (1998, Oct.). Wither the almshouse? Over-utilization and the role of the emergency department. *Journal of Health Politics, Policy and Law, 23*(5), 795-832.

Nelson, M. (1993, April). Critical pathways in the emergency department. *Journal of Emergency Nursing, 19*(2), 110-114.

Padgett, D., & Brodsky, B. (1992). Psychosocial factors influencing non-urgent use of the emergency room. *Social Science Medicine, 35*(9), 1189-1197.

Pins, C., & Swanson, M.E. (1993, Dec.). A suburban community emergency departments' adaptation of case management. *Journal of Emergency Nursing, 19*(6), 503-509.

Rogers, M., Riordan, J., & Swindle, D. (1991, March). Community based nursing case management pays off. *Nursing Management, 22*(3), 30-34.

Smith, T., & Brooks, A.M. (1999). Redefining quality. In E. Cohen Ed, *The outcomes mandate: Case management in health care today* (pp. 198-206). St. Louis: Mosby-Year Book, Inc.

Sund, J., & Sveningson, L. (1998, Jan.). Case management in an integrated delivery system. *Nursing Management, 29*(1), 24-25.

Tyrance, P., Himmelsteine, D., Woolhandler, S. (1996, Nov.). U.S. emergency department costs: No emergency. *American Journal of Public Health, 86*(11), 1527-1531.

Veenema, T. (1994, Aug.). The ten most frequently asked questions about case management in the emergency department. *Journal of Emergency Nursing, 20*(4), 289-292.

Wasson, J., Sauvigne, A., Balestra, D., et al. (1987). Capitation for medical care. *Medical Care, 25*(10), 1002-1005.

Williams, R. (1996, March). The costs of visits to emergency departments. *The New England Journal of Medicine, 334*(10), 642-646.

ADDRESSING HEALTH CARE DELIVERY THROUGH CASE MANAGEMENT

Public Policy Implications

The day to day work of the case manager is greatly affected by public policy, particularly at the Federal and state levels. Conversely, case managers are in a position to affect public policy as it impacts on health care legislation and the delivery of patient care services. Up-to-date knowledge of legislative changes can assist case managers in their role as patient advocate. Unit V provides a framework for understanding current legislative issues in terms of their broad effects on health care reimbursement and their application at the patient level. Knowledge of both perspectives is imperative for the successful case manager.

Patient Demographics Affecting Health Care

CHAPTER OVERVIEW

Recent shifts in the nation's demographics are causing substantial changes in the delivery of health care. Both the growing elderly population and the acquired immunodeficiency syndrome (AIDS) epidemic have prompted health care workers to look for alternatives to the traditional approaches of acute patient care and have fostered the growth of integrative models such as case management. The prevalence of chronic illness and disability associated with demographic changes is also influencing public health policy as we shift our resources from acute to chronic care.

Enacted legislation has provided for the civil rights and liberties of individuals with chronic illness and has supported much-needed community-based, long-term health care delivery systems. Many businesses and corporations have begun to develop programs and services that will help them adapt to the long-range social, economic, and health care implications of the growing number of elderly and those with AIDS.

AGING PATIENT POPULATION

The U.S. Department of Health and Human Services (DHHS) (1990) predicts that by the year 2020, 7 million Americans will be older than age 85 years. Estimates reveal that by 2050, one in four Americans will be age 65 years or older (Freudenheim, 1996). There is no doubt that the older adult group represents the fastest growing section of the U.S. population. This increase in the number and percentage of older individuals primarily results from advances in research, technology, and preventive treatments that have markedly reduced the mortality associated with cancer, cardiovascular disease, diabetes, stroke, and hypertension (National Center for Health Statistics, 1985; Olshansky, 1985).

Rogers, Rogers, and Belanger (1989) found a correlation between dependency and age. Their study indicates that with an increase in age there is a corresponding rise in functional dependency related to basic activities of daily living. Furthermore, once dependency sets in, the likelihood of returning to an independent status decreases. An example of this is that although women have a longer life expectancy than men, much of that time is spent in dependent situations, which increases the morbidity of this population group (Manton, 1988; Schneider & Brody, 1983).

The DHHS estimates of years of healthy life showed a decline in health-related quality of life despite increases in life expectancy (U.S. Department of Health and Human Services, 1995a). Statistical projections show that by the year 2044, 7.3 million people will have dependent lifestyles (Rogers et al., 1989). Another projection indicates that by the year 2040, the elderly population will account for 45% of health care expenditures (Callahan, 1987).

With advanced age there is also a proportionate growth in the incidence of chronic diseases, mental disability, and degenerative illnesses. These factors, along with increased dependency and disability, intensify the need and demand for health care services (Freudenheim, 1996; Goldsmith, 1989; Guralnik, Yanagishita, & Schneider, 1988; Shi & Singh, 1998a).

It is estimated that by the year 2040, 2.8 million people, age 85 years and older, will require institutional care (Guralnik et al., 1988). These data indicate that the aging population will have a significant effect on long-term and skilled nursing care.

Increased longevity and its concomitant effects have encouraged new approaches to the delivery of health care services and development of noninstitutional systems of care. Nursing case management, managed care programs, community-based home care, and chronic care networks that include hospitals, nursing homes, residential community services, and care management (White, 1999) are some examples of alternative approaches to meeting the health care needs of the elderly. These approaches lend themselves to scrutiny and analysis related to cost-effectiveness and the value and quality of services delivered.

In an extensive review of home- and community-based long-term care programs, Weissert, Cready, and Pawelak (1988) found that there were greater total expenditures and no statistically significant cost savings related to home- and community-based care. In fact, an analysis of the effectiveness of various programs showed that even though there were reductions in admissions to institutional care settings, these findings were significant for only a small group of patients who had an obvious need for home-based care. This group consisted of the disabled, chronically ill, and frail elderly.

The study showed, however, that within this patient population, preadmission assessment and screening of those individuals at risk for institutionalization effectively reduced nursing home use. This finding was supported in studies that evaluated the effectiveness of community-based programs in preventing hospitalization. It is known that more specific identification and evaluation of patient requirements of care decrease the need for and length of inpatient treatment and hospitalization (Eggert & Friedman, 1988; Potthoff, Kane, & Franco, 1997).

A recent study conducted by Naylor et al. (1999) demonstrated that focused discharge planning and care management of hospitalized elderly patients helped reduce readmissions, increased time spent out of the hospital, and decreased cost of care. Success factors highlighted by the authors of this study pointed to clinical interventions by advanced practice nurses on patient care–related events the move beyond disease management models and look at primary health problems, comorbidity, and other health and social issues that are common in the elderly patient population (Boling, 1999; Naylor et al., 1999).

One major benefit of community- and home-based care was found in its beneficial and significant effect on the psychosocial well-being and satisfaction of patients and care providers. The community- or home-based care proved better at meeting the patients' needs for physical and social activities as well as medical, mental health, and educational requirements (Weissert, 1985). In an extensive study conducted by Burns, Lamb, and Wholey (1996), the value of integrated community nursing services for elderly people in a health maintenance organization (HMO) was substantiated. The result showed that this integrated community program was associated with reduced hospital costs, preventable admissions, and intensive care visits. Services provided included continuity of care, management of patients across organizational settings, and high-risk screening and identification (Burns et al., 1996).

Another study, conducted by Roos, Shapiro, and Tate (1989), indicated that only 5% of the elderly are extensive users of health care in the inpatient acute care and nursing home settings. The expenditures associated with this care are higher during the individual's last year of life. However, 45% of the elderly population make large demands on the health care system, and these demands entail greater expenditures.

One recommendation for decreasing the chance of hospitalization is to provide the elderly with a geriatric specialist. Early assessment and evaluation by such a specialist might help reduce the incidence of hospitalization, which in turn decreases costs. In addition, continuous monitoring of discharged patients through home care, community-based care, long-term care, and primary preventive services can be cost-effective and aid in the transition to a more independent lifestyle (Stuck, Aronow, Steiner, et al., 1995).

It is clear that to plan effectively for future health care needs of the elderly and disabled population, changes in the delivery of health care services and benefits are needed. Resources are now being shifted from acute care and long-term institutional care to home care, community-based services, respite centers, nurse-run HMOs and care centers, case management, and rehabilitation programs (Dimond, 1989; Hollinger & Brugler, 1991; Manninen & Baines, 1998; Maraldo & Solomon, 1987; Marshall, 1999; Shi & Singh, 1998a). Many alternatives to nursing home services have become available for older people who require long-term care. Popular choices include home care, congregate housing, assisted living, continuing care retirement communities, and adult day care (Booth, 1999; Greenwald, 1999; Shi & Singh, 1998a). In addition, some nursing homes have engaged in transforming themselves to improve the quality of life and care for their residents (Drew & Brooke, 1999). As advocated by Shi and Singh (1998a), long-term care must be integrated within the entire health care delivery system to maintain a seamless transition between different types of health care settings and services.

To maintain control of some of the long-range economic and social implications, major business groups and corporations have developed and offered resources and referral services to employees who have caretaking responsibilities for elderly and dependent family members (Buchsbaum, 1991; Peterson, 1992). Called eldercare, these programs provide a range of services, including counseling, family leave plans, position reinstatement, flexible work schedules, automated office arrangements that make it possible for employees to work at home, subsidized health care benefits, and reimbursement for adult day care. Websites have also been developed that provide information and assistance regarding funding for care referral sources, provider lists, and research findings (Field, 1999).

The benefits of such an approach include decreased work-related conflicts; lowered costs associated with recruitment, training, and absenteeism of personnel; and increased productivity, loyalty, and commitment to the organization. Referral services have also helped decrease the costs of health services associated with deferred spending, out-of-pocket expenses, lost time, and stress (Buchsbaum, 1991; Peterson, 1992).

Increasing costs, aging baby boomers, and new government regulations have raised challenges with regard to the solvency of Medicare. Estimates show that by the year 2030 the projected Medicare eligibility will approach 20% of the U.S. population (Leone, 1997). Although strategies abound in saving Medicare from further spending reductions in the wake of the Balanced Budget Act (BBA) of 1997, the provision of health insurance coverage for the elderly has become the key issue in many political arenas. This challenge will have reverberations well into the next century and involve measures aimed at offering long-term care (LTC) insurance policies as employee benefits and making LTC premiums fully tax-deductible (Gleckman, 1999). Other initiatives include prescription drug subsidies and allowances for transportation and housekeeping services to keep individuals in their home environment (Garrett, 1999; Shapiro, 1999).

HUMAN IMMUNODEFICIENCY VIRUS (HIV) INFECTION

Surveillance data from the Centers for Disease Control and Prevention show that over one-half million Americans have contracted AIDS and that 62% of these persons have died. HIV infection is currently considered the leading cause of death in men age 25 to 44 years and the third leading cause of death in women of the same age group (U.S. Department of Health and Human Services, 1995b).

There is substantial evidence that the rapid spread of HIV will increase hospitalizations and use of more complex health care resources.

Federal spending for HIV is in medical care, education and prevention, research, and assistance programs (Shi & Singh, 1998b). Current estimates place total medical care costs of HIV at $119,000 per person (Aday, 1993). This estimate includes the cost of hospitalization, home health care, hospice, and outpatient care as well as costs related to disability and chronicity.

Studies show the initial length of hospitalization averages 30 to 60 days, with cumulative acute care treatment lasting up to 170 days (Hardy et al., 1986; Sedaka & O'Reilly, 1986). On average, a person with AIDS is hospitalized three to four times. These hospitalizations occur in the early and late stages of illness (Scitovsky, Cline, & Lee, 1986).

Because AIDS is chronic, debilitating, and terminal, it places a substantial burden on the health care system (Benjamin, 1988). Continuum of care approaches that provide home care, community-based services, hospice, disease management, and case management are alternatives to hospitalization (Case Management Advisor 1998; Shi & Singh, 1998b).

Various strategies have been considered to improve accessibility to AIDS care settings. Hospitals have created designated AIDS units where registered nurses coordinate, plan, and evaluate the delivery of care (Chow, 1989; Fox, Aiken, & Messikomer, 1990). Some institutions, such as the San Francisco General Hospital, have implemented comprehensive care programs through multidisciplinary, collaborative efforts with outpatient and community-based services, and home care agencies (Volberding, 1985). These initiatives, along with improvement in treatment and management protocols, have worked toward decreasing the length of stay for AIDS patients, thereby affecting the overall care and cost-effectiveness of this group (Fox, 1986).

The effectiveness of ambulatory and community-based programs for AIDS care is being evaluated in many federal, state, and private foundation-sponsored projects (Benjamin, 1988; Fox, 1986). The programs could reduce cost by reducing the need for inpatient hospital care resources and services.

Hospice care is another promising alternative for AIDS treatment. Using a multidisciplinary team approach, the hospice setting provides for the psychosocial needs of both the patient and caregiver (Benjamin, 1988). The emphasis of hospice care is on reducing time spent in institutional care and eliminating the need for acute medical intervention.

Studies done by Mor and Kidder (1985) on the cost-effectiveness of hospice care show savings related to decreases in inpatient length of stay and use of hospital resources. Such decreases possibly result from the shift in caregiving responsibility to the patient's community, family, and significant others.

Case management presents an additional option for planning nonacute care services and interventions for individuals with AIDS. Capitman, Haskins, and Bernstein (1986) and Spitz (1987) demonstrated the effectiveness and efficiency of a well-integrated case management system. Their studies show that through comprehensive targeting and planning and integration of inpatient, ambulatory, and community-based services, the medical and social needs of AIDS patients can be met. Case management also provides flexibility in service options and reduces the inappropriateness, overuse, and inefficiency associated with hospital and medical care of the chronically ill (Schramm, 1990). Other hospital-based nursing case management models dedicated to AIDS care have also been effective in delivering less-expensive quality care (American Nurses Association, 1988).

Since AIDS presents enormous acute and long-term care needs, business firms have begun to develop and provide employee education and assistance programs, counseling services, nondiscriminatory employment policies, and flexible work schedules. Corporations have also begun to comply with federal, state, and local infection control guidelines (McDonald, 1990; Mello, 1991).

The passage of the Americans with Disabilities Act (ADA) in 1992 has also helped to ensure the rights of HIV- and AIDS-infected people in the workplace. The benefits and entitlements under this act include opportunities for employment, access to public services, accessible transportation, and a mechanism of communication with employers to support nondiscriminatory policies, confidentiality, and ongoing education (Feldblum, 1991; LaPlante, 1991). The Medicaid waiver program and the Ryan White Comprehensive AIDS Resource Emergency (CARE) Act are additional initiatives that work toward providing treatment and care coordination for individuals with HIV and AIDS (Shi & Singh, 1998b; Summer, 1991).

Innovative case management models have emerged in developing countries such as East Africa to care for people with AIDS. These models are grounded in the principles of primary health care and have demonstrated enhanced individual and community health outcomes (Ivantic-Doucette & Maashao, 1999). These case management models serve as exemplars and point to the basic fact that attention to a community's primary health care needs of access to care and interventions driven from within communities and with community participation are crucial to success (Ivantic-Doucette & Maashao, 1999).

References

Aday, L. (1993). *At risk in America: The health and health care needs of vulnerable populations in the United States.* San Francisco: Jossey-Bass Publishers.

American Nurses Association (1988). *Nursing case management.* Kansas City, Mo.: American Nurses Association.

Benjamin, A.E. (1988). Long-term care and AIDS: Perspectives from experience with the elderly. *The Milbank Quarterly, 66*(3), 415-443.

Boling, P. (1999). The value of targeted case management during transitional care. *Journal of the American Medical Association, 281*(7), 656-657.

Booth, C. (1999, Aug. 30). Taking care of our aging parents. *Time,* 48-51.

Buchsbaum, S. (1991). Sending "care" packages to the workplace. *Business and Health, 9*(5), 56-69.

Burns, L.R., Lamb, G.S., Wholey, D.R. (1996). Impact of integrated community nursing services on hospital utilization and costs in a Medicare risk plan. *Inquiry, 33,* 30-41.

Callahan, D. (1987). *Setting limits: Medical goals in an aging society.* New York: Simon and Schuster.

Capitman, J.A., Haskins, B., & Bernstein, J. (1986). Case management approaches in community oriented long-term care demonstrations. *Gerontologist, 26,* 398-404.

Case Management Advisor. (1998, Oct.). Case management leads to success in HIV/AIDS managed care. *Case Management Advisor, 9* (10), 177-179.

Chow, M. (1989). Nursing's response to the challenge of AIDS. *Nursing Outlook, 37*(2), 82-83.

Drew, J.C., & Brooke, V. (1999). Changing a legacy: The Eden alternative nursing home. *Annals of Long-Term Care, 7*(3), 115-121.

Dimond, M. (1989). Health care and the aging population. *Nursing Outlook, 37*(2), 76-77.

Eggert, G., & Friedman, B. (1988, suppl.). The need for special interventions for multiple hospital admission patients. *Health Care Financing Review,* 57-67.

Feldblum, C. (1991). Employment protections. *The Milbank Quarterly, 69*(suppl. ½), 81-110.

Field, A. (1999, Nov. 22). The best old-age home may be at home. *Business Week,* 180-182.

Fox, D. (1986). AIDS and the American health policy: History and prospects of a crises of authority. *The Milbank Quarterly, 64,* 7-33.

Fox, D. (1989). Policy and epidemiology: Financing health services for the chronically ill and disabled, 1930-1990. *The Milbank Quarterly, 67*(suppl. 2, part 2), 257-287.

Fox, R., Aiken, L., & Messikomer, C. (1990). The culture of caring: AIDS and the nursing profession. *The Milbank Quarterly, 68*(suppl. 2), 226-256.

Freudenheim, D. (1996). *Chronic care in American: A 21ˢᵗ century challenge.* Princeton, NJ: Institute for Health and Aging.

Garrett, M. (1999, Nov. 22). Health divides the candidates. *U.S. News & World Report, 24.*

Gleckman, H. (1999, March 29). A golden (years) opportunity. *Business Week,* 181-182.

Goldsmith, J. (1989). Radical prescription for hospitals. *Harvard Business Review, 89*(3), 104-111.

Greenwald. J. (1999, Aug. 30). Elder care: making the right choice. *Time,* 52-56.

Guralnik, J., Yanagishita, M., & Schneider, E. (1988). Projecting the older population of the United States: Lessons from the past and prospects for the future. *The Milbank Quarterly, 66*(2), 283-308.

Hardy, A., Rauch, K., Echenberg, D., Morgan, W., & Curran, J.W. (1986). The economic impact of the first 10,000 cases of acquired immunodeficiency syndrome in the United States. *Journal of the American Medical Association, 225,* 209-211.

Hollinger, W., & Brugler, K. (1991). Managing resource use. *Healthcare Forum, 34*(6), 45-47.

Ivantic-Doucette, K. & Maashao, G. (1999). Huduma Kwa Wagonjwa: An African perspective on case management. In E. Cohen & V. De Back (Eds.), *The outcomes mandate: Case management in health care today* (pp. 276-285). St. Louis: Mosby, Inc.

LaPlante, M. (1991). The demographics of disability. *The Milbank Quarterly, 69*(suppl. ½), 55-77.

Leone, R. (1997). Why boomers don't spell bust. *The American Prospect, 30*(1), 68-72.

Manninen, R. & Baines, B. (1998). Medical management in the Medicare population. In P.R. Kongstvedt & D.W. Plocher (Eds.), *Best practices in medical management,* pp. 623-636. Gaithersburg, Md.: Aspen Publications.

Manton, K.G. (1988). A longitudinal study of functional change and mortality in the United States. *Journal of Gerontology, 43*(5), 153-161.

Maraldo, P., & Solomon, S. (1987). Nursing's window of opportunity. *Image, 19*(2), 8386.

Marhsall, B.S. (1999, Nov./Dec.). Case management of the elderly in a health maintenance organization: The implications for program administration under managed care. *Journal of Healthcare Management, 44*(6), 477-493.

McDonald, M. (1990). How to deal with AIDS in the workplace. *Business and Health, 8*(7), 12-22.

Mello, J. (1991, Sept.). Getting to know about AIDS. *Business and Health, 9*(9), 88-89.

Mor, V., & Kidder, D. (1985). Cost savings in hospice: Final results of the National Hospice Study. *Health Services Research, 20,* 407-421.

National Center for Health Statistics. (1985). *Vital Statistics of the United States, 1980.* 2(pt. A., mortality). DHHS pub. no. (PHS) 85-1101. Washington, D.C.

National Center for Health Statistics. (1987). Use of nursing homes by the elderly, preliminary data from the 1985 National Nursing Home Survey, by E. Hing. *Vital and Health Statistics,* no. 135. DHHS pub. no. (PHS) 87-1250. Washington, D.C.

Naylor, M., Brooten, D., Campbell, R., Jacobsen, B., Mezey, M., Pauly, M., & Schwartz, J. (1999). Comprehensive discharge planning and home follow-up of hospitalized elders: A randomized clinical trial. *Journal of American Medical Association, 28*(7), 613-620.

Olshansky, S.J. (1985). Pursuing longevity: Delay vs. elimination of degenerative diseases. *American Journal of Public Health, 75,* 754-757.

Peterson, H. (1992, Feb.). Eldercare: More than company kindness. *Business & Health, 10*(2), 54-57.

Potthoff, S., Kane, R., & Franco, S. (1997). Improving hospital discharge planning for elderly patients. *Health Care Financing Review, 19,* 47-72.

Rogers, R., Rogers, A., & Belanger, A. (1989). Active life among the elderly in the United States: Multistate Life-table estimates and population projections. *The Milbank Quarterly, 67*(3-4), 370-411.

Roos, N., Shapiro, E., & Tate, R. (1989). Does a small minority of elderly account for a majority of healthcare expenditures? A sixteen-year perspective. *The Milbank Quarterly, 67*(3-4), 347-369.

Schneider, E., & Brody, J. (1983). Aging, natural death, and the compression of morbidity: Another view. *New England Journal of Medicine, 309*(14), 854-855.

Schramm, C. (1990). Health care industry problems call for cooperative solutions. *Healthcare Financial Management, 54*-61.

Scitovsky, A.A., Cline, M., & Lee, P.R. (1986). Medical care costs of patients with AIDS in San Francisco. *Journal of the American Medical Association, 256,* 3103-3106.

Sedaka, S., & O'Reilly, M. (1986). The financial implications of AIDS. *Caring, 5*(6), 38-44.

Shapiro, J. (1999, Nov. 22). Giving doctors the final word. *U.S. News & World Report,* 20-24.

Shi, L., & Singh, D. (1998a). *Delivering health care in America: A systems approach.* Health Services for Special Populations (Chapter 11), pp. 426-440. Gaithersburg, Md.: Aspen Publication.

Shi, L., & Singh, D. (1998b). *Delivering health care in America: A systems approach.* Long Term Care (Chapter 10), pp. 344-391. Gaithersburg, Md.: Aspen Publication.

Spitz, B. (1987). National survey of Medicaid case management. *Health Affairs, 6,* 61-70.

Stuck, A., Aronow, H., Steiner, A., et al. (1995). A trial of in-home comprehensive discharge assessments for elderly people living in the community. *New England Journal of Medicine, 333,* 1184-1189.

Summer, L. (1991). *Limited access: Health care for the rural poor.* Washington, D.C.: Center on Budget and Policy Priorities.

U.S. Department of Health and Human Services. (1990). *Healthy People 2000.* Washington, D.C.: DHHS.

U.S. Department of Health and Human Services. (1995a). *Healthy People 2000: Midcourse review and 1995 revisions* (p. 6). Washington, D.C.: DHHS.

U.S. Department of Health and Human Services. Centers for Disease Control and Prevention. (1995b). *HIV/AIDS surveillance report: U.S. HIV and AIDS cases reported through December 1995, 7*(2), 1-39.

Volberding, P.A. (1985). The clinical spectrum of the acquired immunodeficiency syndrome: Implications for comprehensive patient care. *Annals of Internal Medicine, 103,* 729-732.

Weissert, W.G. (1985). Seven reasons why it is so difficult to make community-based long term care cost effective. *Health Services Research, 20*(4), 423-433.

Weissert, W.G., Cready, C., & Pawelak, J. (1988). The past and future of home- and community-based long term care. *The Milbank Quarterly, 66*(2), 309-388.

White, M. (1999). Eligibility in the ever-changing continuum of care. *Annals of Long-Term Care, 7*(3), 113-114.

The Business of Health Care and the Prospective Payment System

CHAPTER OVERVIEW

Changes in consumer behavior, along with various government and private industry strategies, have started to change the health care delivery environment. Programs are being developed to increase access to care and to evaluate and monitor cost-effective outcomes. National health reform initiatives address universal access to care by working for changes in insurance coverage and benefits, reimbursement regulation, and alternative care arrangements. Quality and cost are also addressed through managed care and capitated payment approaches. Long-term care services are being sponsored both publicly and privately.

Collaboration among health care providers for policy formation and implementation, public and private support for health care planning and outcome research, and further development of alternative care delivery and clinical resource models are among the crucial factors needed to develop an accessible, effective, and socially responsive health care system.

COST CONTAINMENT—THE ADVENT OF THE PROSPECTIVE PAYMENT SYSTEM

The incentives promoted by the prospective payment system not only affect the efficiency, safety, and quality of health care in the inpatient setting but also have a direct relationship to the cost containment efforts present in managed care arrangements (Jones, 1989; Sloan, Morrisey, & Valvona, 1988). Increased enrollment in HMOs and other prepaid, coordinated health care plans, restructuring of the physician fee and payment schedule to provide incentives for the delivery of primary care services, the national drive for health care reform, and competition among alternative delivery systems to improve cost-effectiveness and quality all influence prospective payment initiatives (Enthoven & Kronick, 1989a, 1989b; Ginsburg & Hackbarth, 1986; Swoap, 1984; Waldo, Levit, & Lazenby, 1986; Wilensky, 1991).

Prospective payment has also promoted a more efficient use of health care resources and encouraged the study of outcomes to evaluate accessibility, management, and economic effectiveness of care (Jones, 1989; Sloan et al., 1988).

The economic effect of rising health care costs has taken its toll on the private sector through increases in group health insurance premium rates and changes in the structure of employee health care benefits. Mullen (1988) and Traska (1989) reported that employers experienced rate increases of 15% to 29% in their efforts to cover health care costs. According to the Hewitt Associates' survey, the double-digit inflation was due to an estimated 21.5% increase by insurance carriers in medical benefit costs (Hewitt Associates, 1989). Increases in premiums were driven primarily by rises in the cost, volume, and variations in health services and were fostered by medical technological change, an inadequate reimbursement system, demographic changes of an aging population, acquired immunodeficiency syndrome (AIDS), and chronic illness (Kramon, 1989; Welling, 1990).

The issue of escalating health care costs has entered both the political and economic arenas and has prompted furious debates in the public and private sectors over the provision of basic health care services (Hospitals, 1992). Advocates for a national health care policy have locked horns with those who support the rationing of health services. Attempts have been made by Congress to institute a national health insurance plan to ensure equal access to care (Altman & Rodmin, 1988; Reinhardt, 1987a, 1987b). Legislative mandates and congressional bills that would provide health care coverage have been introduced as a means of rationing care through regulation and achieving control over government expenditures. State-mandated benefit laws offer a broad range of service coverage and access to mental health and substance abuse care, prenatal care, mammography, cancer screening, and major organ transplants (Brown, 1988; Davis, 1985; Dwyer and Garland, 1991; Eckholm, 1991; Frieden, 1991; Tallon, 1991; Thorpe, 1991; Traska, 1989).

Major health care reform for America began in 1993 with the introduction of the *Health Security Act* (HR3600, 1993), a President Clinton initiative. For almost a year the administration sought information about the existing health care system through task forces, committees, and town meetings directed by the First Lady, Hillary Rodham Clinton. This data collection process stimulated discussions nationwide about the present and future health care systems. The momentum created by a national discussion on health care reform gave the change process a life of its own, separate from the administrative and legislative agendas. Health care providers, health care agencies, and state governmental agencies began to design new systems based on a shifting paradigm—even before federal laws were enacted. The basic premise of the new paradigm, which continues to unfold, is a focus on health and care replacing or augmenting the old paradigm of illness and cure (DeBack & Cohen, 1996).

Many special interest groups have joined forces to propose reform in the current health care system. One such group, the American Medical Association, supports an employer-based health care plan, and another group from organized nursing has endorsed a proposal titled *Nursing's Agenda for Health Care Reform*. The latter plan supports a consumer partnership with the health care provider regarding decisions about care; access to primary health care services via community-based settings; allocation of more resources to chronic and long-term care; increased access to nonphysician providers, such as nurse practitioners; wellness and prevention classes, public and private sector review and financing of health care; and managed care and case management arrangements (National League for Nursing, 1991).

Changes in payment structure have taken place in almost every sector of the health care industry. Private corporations and insurance providers have adopted many different strategies aimed at cost containment. Various efforts have focused on the redesigning of health insurance plans and policies, shifting the direct financial burden of health care expenditures to the federal government and individual payers. This approach includes the following: a single-payer plan, which is a government-financed plan that insures all individuals; introduction of copayments and deductibles applied to health care services; cost sharing, in which employees share the costs of health care by paying for the care of convalescing patients and hospice care for the terminally ill; catastrophic health plans, which provide coverage for high-cost illnesses; second opinions for surgical interventions; and primary prevention and stress management programs aimed at controlling smoking, alcohol use, and hypertension (Brown, 1988; Frieden, 1991; Gilman & Bucco, 1987; Herzlinger & Calkins, 1986; Herzlinger & Schwartz, 1985; Peres, 1992).

As an effective strategy for controlling health care costs, major corporations have also encouraged participation in comprehensive, capitated rate plans, such as health maintenance organizations (HMOs) and preferred provider organizations (PPOs). In these managed care plans, providers set an amount to cover all of their enrollees' health care needs. A percentage of that payment is put into a risk pool as insurance against unexpected expenditures. Providers assume a certain element of risk in exchange for the opportunity to benefit from lower costs, an integrated care system, and management savings (Brown, 1988; Christensen, 1991; Hicks, Stallmeyer, & Coleman, 1992; O'Connor, 1991).

Another initiative, called *managed competition,* finances health insurance coverage through large businesses. The employer is required to purchase insurance or pay a payroll tax for a public (government) sponsor. This system promotes competition among private insurers and ensures quality improvement standards (Enthoven & Kronick, 1989a, 1989b; Garland, 1991). All these health care delivery arrangements focus on both primary and secondary prevention, thereby increasing positive health outcomes and reducing costs (Hospitals, 1988; Luft, 1978, 1982; Rosenberg, Perlis, Lynne, & Leto, 1991; Sloss et al., 1987).

Another response to the problems of financing health care benefits is assuring the employer's involvement in managing the delivery of health care services. Providers are developing and participating in corporate health care programs that monitor cost and use of health care services. Those services that are monitored include preadmission testing, which has been shown to reduce inpatient stays, utilization review, monitoring of catastrophic illness and injury through medical case management programs, and mandatory employer-sponsored health insurance that would extend both private and public employer-sponsored health insurance coverage through various financial arrangements (Aaron, 1991; Brown, 1988; Dalton, 1987; Dentzer, 1991; Herzlinger, 1985; Herzlinger & Calkins, 1986; Herzlinger & Schwartz, 1985; Peres, 1992). Such monitoring programs have helped reduce and eliminate medical inefficiency and have improved the effectiveness of care delivery.

Businesses have also begun to form health care coalitions that purchase health care services and offer them at a discount to their members. These coalitions guarantee accessible health care services, cost-effective delivery, and quality care. Some of the services provided by the coalitions include workers' compensation, inpatient and outpatient programs, primary prevention and treatment, and case management services (Bell, 1991).

CONTEMPORARY APPROACHES TO COST CONTAINMENT

Regulatory attempts to contain health care costs continue to grow through various managed care strategies. The Health Care Financing Administration (HCFA) initiated a reimbursement method for outpatient procedures called ambulatory patient groups (APGs). APGs are for the ambulatory setting as DRGs are for inpatient services, and reimburses for the cost of providing outpatient procedures or visits. APGs reimbursement, however, does not cover the professional or physician cost elements (HCFA, 1996; Shi & Singh, 1998). Ambulatory payment classification (APC), an offshoot of APG's is a more refined reimbursement strategy recently implemented by HCFA.

Skilled nursing facilities will also be under a prospective payment system initiative. Called resource utilization groups (RUGs), this approach mandated by the Balanced Budget Act (BBA) of 1997, differentiates nursing home patients by their levels of resource use, that is, principal diagnosis and activities of daily living (ADLs) (Shi & Singh, 1998).

The Medicare program itself is predicted to become bankrupt by this century and is targeted for major cutback initiatives (Rabinowitz, 1996). The BBA is legislation that was initiated in 1997 to reduce payments to providers by $116 billion over a 5-year period starting in 1998 and extending to 2003. Its intent is to keep Medicare solvent through 2007.

The effects of BBA, however, have been devastating and have reached into the coffers of hospitals, physicians, home care, skilled nursing facilities, and Medicare beneficiaries (American Organization of Nurse Executives, 1999; McGinley, 1999). Some of the unintended consequences have resulted in closures of several home care facilities and nursing homes, making patient placements difficult. In addition, appropriate follow-up care has suffered, making access to continuum of care services problematic.

Relief in terms of a $16 billion Medicare bill was advocated. Overall, the provisions of the bill may give back funds to institutions affected by the Medicare payment reductions and hopefully restore access to care (American Hospital Association, 1999).

NON-NURSING CASE MANAGEMENT MODELS

The primary focus of the case management model is to improve patient outcomes and control costs through the organization and coordination of health care services. The underlying economic premises of case management depend on the linkage to managed care strategies developed by the private sector and insurance provider groups. Managed care programs became popular when private corporations and industry affiliations took an active part in maintaining control over soaring health care expenditures (Federation of American Health Systems Review, 1988).

Medical case management has become an effective way for private industry groups to maintain control over the use and costs of health care and to develop effective management and intervention methods (Califano, 1987; Dentzer, 1991; Katz, 1991). Case management identifies procedures used excessively that involve extended hospital stays and evaluates uncoordinated health care delivery systems, which promote duplication and fragmentation of services. Medical case management controls both the demand for and the supply of health care by identifying potential high-cost cases (appropriate targeting); by coordinating and channeling the delivery of care among providers, patients, insurers, and agencies that may be involved; and by evaluating and managing the patient's existing benefits plan to cover needed services (Dentzer, 1991; Henderson, Bergman, Collard, Souder, & Wallack, 1987; Henderson & Collard, 1988).

Until recently, the cost-effectiveness of the case management method has not been implicitly justified. Past research investigations were concerned with process and structured measures of efficiency. Such investigations sought to discover whether the use of a physician as a case manager or an HMO as an insurer and provider of care actually reduced health care expenditures and increased quality assurance (Austin, 1983; Manning, Liebowitz, Goldberg, Rogers, & Newhouse, 1984).

In 1986 researchers at the Bigel Institute for Health Policy Studies at Brandeis University undertook a major study to evaluate medical case management for catastrophic illnesses. Funding from The Robert Wood Johnson Foundation (Henderson et al., 1987) supported this 2-year project. Specifically the project involved the evaluation of a case management program offered by a predominantly private insurance group and was representative of other case management arrangements offered by other major insurers (Henderson et al., 1987; Henderson & Collard, 1988; Henderson & Wallack, 1987).

Patient case load was identified by five diagnostic categories, which included the high-risk infant, head trauma, spinal cord injury, cancer, and AIDS (Henderson et al., 1987; Henderson & Wallack, 1987). Cost criteria were developed that incorporated the economic rationale of limiting inappropriate use of high-cost procedures and unnecessary ancillary resources. The factors contributing to high costs that were evaluated included patient length of stay that exceeded predefined limits, evidence of complications indicated by the primary and secondary diagnoses, a repeat admission within a set time frame, and total patient charges exceeding a certain limit (Henderson & Wallack, 1987).

Cost-effectiveness was determined when the case management program was initiated and implemented an alternative plan that decreased the patient's length of stay in the hospital, facilitated patient transfer to a less costly facility, and decreased expenditures associated with home care services (Henderson et al., 1987).

Case management responsibilities in this study were assigned to registered nurses who were accountable for the assessment, care planning, monitoring, and evaluation activities. A case management plan was developed that incorporated the input of the physician provider and used appropriate resources to meet the individual needs of the patient and family (Henderson & Collard, 1988). Henderson and Collard found that the successful implementation of the case management plan required the cooperation of the attending physician. For the most part, case management was seen as a comprehensive plan for ensuring patients would receive health care services that would not ordinarily be reimbursable.

The Brandeis study found that use of the medical case management model significantly reduced costs. Several factors contributed to the effectiveness of this program:

- Early patient identification and intervention assure access to the most appropriate and least restrictive care.
- Appropriate resource use helps maintain cost-effective care.
- Alternative treatment programming and benefit management allow for flexibility in the payment structure.
- Directing of the case management approach to specific patient groups helps achieve significant gains from services.
- A cooperative and supportive relationship develops between the care provider and case recipients.
- Interpretable, standardized reporting mechanisms help relate program objectives to patient care delivery.
- Case management integrates the case planning process with resource allocation based on a patient classification system or DRG methodology.
- A computerized information system allows for continuous data monitoring and analysis (Henderson et al., 1987; Henderson & Collard, 1988; Weisman, 1987; White, 1986).

CASE MANAGEMENT AND CATASTROPHIC ILLNESS

The case management model used depends on the patient population it serves. Such adaptability makes it possible to match a particular patient's needs with the appropriate case management approach. For example, the primary care case management model, when used for treating chronically ill patients, may require the addition of medical or social case management services (Merrill, 1985).

Although no one model of case management is applicable in all circumstances, medical case management programs recently have been adapted for use in the management of care associated with catastrophic illness or injury (Brown, 1988; Henderson & Wallack, 1987). Traditionally, care of those with catastrophic illnesses has been expensive because of a lack of coordination and fragmentation of services. Duplication of patient services and failure to work out alternative care arrangements have also added to the cost of treating catastrophic illness (Henderson & Collard, 1987). The medical case management model focuses cost-containment efforts on a small percentage of the patient population that includes frequent users of hospital and medical technology services (Rosenbloom & Gertman, 1984; Zook & Moore, 1980). Zook and Moore identified two types of catastrophic cases that used a considerable amount of health care resources. The first group consisted of unanticipated illnesses such as spinal cord injury, head trauma, neonatal complications, cancer, cardiac disease, and stroke. The second type of catastrophic illness includes chronic medical or psychiatric conditions.

The rationale behind using the medical case management model with catastrophic illness is based on a study by the Health Data Institute of the medical care patterns of major businesses in the United States. This investigation showed that in more than 1 million episodes of hospital care between 1980 and 1983, there were consistent patterns of high-cost illness. This study revealed that a large proportion of health care costs were attributable to only 5% to 10% of health-insured individuals (Rosenbloom & Gertman, 1984). Because catastrophic illness occurs less frequently than ordinary ailments, cost-containment efforts should be directed to some of these high-cost illnesses. The Health Data Institute study indicates that medical, social, and financial consequences of catastrophic illness and injury can be controlled through a systematic effort characteristic of the case management approach.

References

Aaron, H. (1991). Choosing from the health care reform menu. *The Journal of American Health Policy, 1*(3), 23-27.

Altman, S.H., & Rodmin, M.A. (1988). Halfway competitive markets and ineffective regulation: The American health care system. *Journal of Health Politics, Policy and Law, 13*(2), 323-339.

American Hospital Association. (1999, Nov.). *AHA News Wire.* AHA website: www.aha.org.

American Organization of Nurse Executives. (1999, Aug.). AONE Policy Briefing: Balanced Budget Act Relief. Chicago: AONE.

Austin, C.D. (1983). Case management in long-term care: Options and opportunities. *Health and Social Work, 8*(1), 16-30.

Bell, N. (1991). From the trenches: Strategies that work. *Business and Health, 9*(5), 19-25.

Brown, R. (1988). Principles for a national health program: A framework for analysis and development. *The Milbank Quarterly, 66*(4), 573-617.

Califano, J. (1987). Guiding the forces of the health care revolution. *Nursing and Health Care 8*(7), 400-404.

Christensen, L. (1991). The highs and lows of PPOs. *Business and Health, 9*(9), 72-77.

Dalton, J. (1987). Alternative delivery systems and employers. *Topics in Health Care Financing, 13*(3), 68-76.

Davis, R.G. (1985). Congress and the emergence of public health policy. *Health Care Management Review, 10*(1), 61-73.

DeBack, V., & Cohen, E. (1996). The new practice environment. In E. Cohen (Ed.), *Nurse case management in the 21st century* (pp. 3-9). St. Louis: Mosby.

Dentzer, S. (1991, Sept. 23). Agenda for business: How to fight killer health costs. *U.S. News and World Report,* 50-58.

Dwyer, P., & Garland, S. (1991, Nov. 25). A roar of discontent: Voters want health care reform now. *Business Week,* 28-30.

Eckholm, E. (1991, May 2). Rescuing health care. *The New York Times,* A 1, B 12.

Enthoven, A., & Kronick, R. (1989a). A consumer-choice health plan for the 1990s, part I. *New England Journal of Medicine, 320*(1), 29-37.

Enthoven, A., & Kronick, R. (1989b). A consumer-choice health plan for the 1990s, part II. *New England Journal of Medicine, 320*(2), 94-101.

Federation of American Health Systems Review (1988, July/Aug.). Special report: The facts of life about managed care. Author, 20-49.

Frieden, J. (1991). Many roads lead to health system reform. *Business and Health, 9*(11), 38-66.

Garland, S. (1991, Oct. 7). The health care crises: A prescription for reform. *Business Week,* 59-66.

Gilman, T., & Bucco, C. (1987). Alternate delivery systems: An overview. *Topics in Health Care Financing, 13*(3), 1-7.

Ginsburg, R.B., & Hackbarth, G.M. (1986). Alternative delivery systems and Medicare. *Health Affairs, 5*(1), 6-22.

Health Care Financing Administration (1996). Overview of the Medicare program. *Health Care Financing Review: Medicare and Medicaid Statistical Supplement 5.*

Henderson, M., Bergman, A., Collard, A., Souder, B., Wallack, S. (Draft, May 1, 1987). *Private sector medical case management for high cost illness.* Brandeis University Heller Graduate School Health Policy Center, Waltham, Mass.

Henderson, M.G., & Collard, A. (1988). Measuring quality in medical case management programs. *Quality Review Bulletin, 14*(2) 33-39.

Henderson, M.G., & Wallack, S.S. (1987). Evaluating case management for catastrophic illness. *Business and Health, 4*(3), 7-11.

Herzlinger, R.E. (1985). How companies tackle health care costs: Part II. *Harvard Business Review, 63*(5), 108-120.

Herzlinger, R.E., & Calkins, D. (1986). How companies tackle health care costs: Part III. *Harvard Business Review, 64*(1), 70-80.

Herzlinger, R.E., & Schwartz, J. (1985). How companies tackle health care costs: Part I. *Harvard Business Review, 63*(4), 68-81.

Hewitt Associates. (1989). *Salaried employee benefits provided by major U.S. employers.* Lincolnshire, Ill.: Hewitt Associates.

Hicks, L., Stallmeyer, J., & Coleman, J. (1992). Nursing challenges in managed care. *Nursing Economics, 10*(4), 265-275.

Hospitals (1988, April 5). Managed care: Whoever has the data wins the game. *Hospitals,* 50-55.

Hospitals (1992, Jan. 20). Health care reform a priority in the legislative years. *Hospitals,* 32-50.

Jones, K. (1989). Evolution of the prospective payment system: Implications for nursing. *Nursing Economics, 7*(6), 299-305.

Katz, F. (1991). Making a case for case management. *Business and Health, 9*(4), 75-77.

Kramon, G. (1989, Jan. 8). Taking a scalpel to health costs. *The New York Times,* pp. 1, 9.

Luft, H.S. (1978). How do health maintenance organizations achieve their savings? Rhetoric and evidence. *New England Journal of Medicine, 298*(11), 1336-1343.

Luft, H.S. (1982). Health maintenance organizations and the rationing of medical care. *The Milbank Quarterly, 60*(2), 268-306.

Manning, W.G., Leibowitz, A., Goldberg, G., Rogers, W., & Newhouse, J. (1984). A controlled trial of the effect of a prepaid group practice on the use of services. *New England Journal of Medicine, 310*(23), 1505-1510.

McGinley, L. (1999, May 26). As nursing homes say 'no,' hospitals feel pain. *The Wall Street Journal.* B1-B4.

Merrill, J.C. (1985). Defining case management. *Business and Health, 3*(5-9), 5-9.

Mullen, P. (1988, Dec. 27). Big increase in health premiums. *Health Week, 2*(26), 1, 26.

National League for Nursing (1991). *Nursing's agenda for health care reform.* New York: NLN.

O'Connor, K. (1991). Risky business: HMOs and managed care. *Business and Health, 9*(6), 30-34.

Peres, A. (1992). Business must act now to shape reform. *Business and Health, 10*(1), 72.

Rabinowitz, H. (1996). Health policy and the future of health care reform. *Journal of the American Board of Family Practice, 9*(1), 37-40.

Reinhardt, U.E. (1987a, Jan. 11). Toward a fail-safe health-insurance system. *The Wall Street Journal.*

Reinhardt, U.E. (1987b). Health insurance for the nation's poor. *Health Affairs, 6*(1), 101-102.

Rosenberg, S., Perlis, H., Lynne, D., & Leto, L. (1991). A second look at second surgical opinions. *Business and Health, 9*(2), 14-28.

Rosenbloom, D., & Gertman, P. (1984). An intervention strategy for controlling costly care. *Business and Health, 1*(8), 17-21.

Shi, L., & Singh, D. (1998). *Delivering health care in America: A systems approach.* Cost, Access, Quality. (Chapter 12), 443-488. Gaithersburg, Md.: Aspen Publication.

Sloan, F., Morrisey, M., & Valvona, J. (1988). Effects of the Medicare prospective payment system on hospital cost containment: An early appraisal. *The Milbank Quarterly, 66*(2), 191-220.

Sloss, E.M., Keeler, E.B., Brook, R.H., Operskalski, B.H., Goldberg, G.A., & Newhouse, J.P. (1987). Effect of a health maintenance organization on physiologic health. *Annals of Internal Medicine, 106*(1), 130-138.

Swoap, D. (1984). Beyond DRGs: Shifting the risk to providers. *Health Affairs, 3*(4), 117-121.

Tallon, J.R. (1991). A report from the front line: Policy and politics in health reform. *The Journal of American Health Policy, 1*(1), 47-50.

Thorpe, K. (1991). The national health insurance conundrum: Shifting paradigms and potential solutions. *The Journal of American Health Policy, 1*(1), 17-22.

Traska, M.R. (1989). What 1989 holds for health benefits. *Business and Health, 1*(1), 22-30.

Waldo, D.R., Levit, J.R., & Lazenby, H. (1986). National health expenditures, 1985. *Health Care Financing Review, 8*(1), 1-21.

Weisman, E. (1987). Practical approaches for developing a case management program. *Quality Review Bulletin, 13*(11), 380-382.

Welling, K. (1990, June 11). The sickening spiral: Health-care costs continue to grow at an alarming rate. *Barron's,* 8.

White, M. (1986). Case management. In G.L. Maddox (Ed.), *The encyclopedia of aging* (pp. 92-96). New York: Springer Publishing.

Wilensky, G. (1991). Treat the causes, not the symptoms of the health care cost problem. *The Journal of American Health Policy, 1*(2), 15-17.

Zook, C.V., & Moore, F.D. (1980). High-cost users of medical care. *New England Journal of Medicine, 302*(18), 996-1002.

Patient Mix and Cost Related to Length of Hospital Stay

CHAPTER OVERVIEW

Prospective payment systems have influenced the development of innovative care delivery models by placing limits on the use of hospital resources. Because the length of time an individual spends in the hospital affects the appropriation of services and costs involved in that care, the number of hospitalized days becomes an important variable in assessing and measuring the institution's financial outcome.

The effects of care delivery models on health care services provided an important strategy for evaluating system effectiveness, efficiency, and quality. The coordination and integration required for case management are two reasons why such a health care delivery model maximizes the use and allocation of available resources and services.

Nursing case management methods provide indicators that help assess the effectiveness of patient care delivery. By focusing on the coordination and integration of inpatient services, nursing case management can impact the patient length of stay (LOS) while keeping it within medically appropriate boundaries.

With the implementation of DRG strategies, patient LOS has become an overall indicator of a hospital's financial performance and cost-effectiveness. Numerous variables that have an effect on the cost and LOS have been identified. This chapter reviews and analyzes studies related to patient length-of-stay variables.

The chapter is divided into three general categories: (1) patient demographics, such as age and gender variables; (2) related variables, such as diagnosis and comorbidity, discharge planning, patient care delivery systems, and nursing intensity and workload (a critique of the nursing intensity and workload studies is provided); and (3) nonclinical variables that affect patient LOS, such as day-of-the-week admission (weekday versus weekend) and organizational factors.

PATIENT DEMOGRAPHICS

Certain patient characteristics, such as age, were reported to be important in judging the postoperative recovery time of patients undergoing surgical procedures, such as a hernia repair or a cholecystectomy

(Kolouch, 1965). Although the reasons for a correlation between age and length of surgical convalescent time were not provided, the finding was anticipated because of the close association between age, chronicity, hospital-induced infections, age-related risk factors, patient dependency needs, and increased time required for postoperative healing.

In this study, however, age did not account for all the variations in average LOS reported by surgical case mix. Other variables existed that were not subject to control, such as postoperative surgical complications, patient rehabilitation time, method of payment (i.e., third-party, Blue Cross, or charity), and type of hospital (i.e., teaching or nonteaching).

In another study by Marchette and Holloman (1986), age was the significant variable in prolonging the LOS of cerebrovascular accident (CVA) patients. On average the CVA patients were older and had the longest hospital stays. Again, as in the Kolouch (1965) study, age did not account for all of the diversity attributed to LOS. Other intervening variables, such as severity of illness, discharge planning, and social consults, also affected the average LOS of the hospitalized patients.

Posner and Lin (1975) studied the age variable in association with predicted LOS for medical patients. In this study, age was evaluated in terms of its effects on comparable diagnoses. The study also evaluated the effect of various hospital settings (voluntary or municipal) on the length of patient stay. It was found that the hospital LOS was not exclusively affected by the age of the patient. Wide variations were found in LOS within age groups even when diagnostic categories and hospital variables were controlled.

The unreliability of age as a predictor of hospital LOS was confirmed in another study by Lave and Leinhardt (1976). This study placed emphasis on case-mix factors and variables that related to the patient's medical condition and that contributed to changes in the patient's LOS.

Both Lave and Leinhardt (1976) and Marchette and Holloman (1986) looked at the effect of gender on patient LOS. Findings showed that male patients have shorter lengths of hospital stay than female patients and that single women have the longest stays. Several explanations of these findings were offered. First, because women live longer than men, women will experience more hospitalizations. Second, single women have longer stays because they less often have adult family members available to care for them. Although all these findings are associated with longer than average hospital stays, the effect of patient gender could not be validated. Lave and Leinhardt (1976) advised that although patient demographic variables may be statistically significant in some situations, such variables may have minimal effect on the overall variability of the patient's LOS.

CLINICALLY RELATED VARIABLES

The patient's primary diagnosis, number of surgical procedures, and number of secondary diagnoses were factors that had a significant effect on patient LOS (Lave & Leinhardt, 1976; Lew, 1966; McCorkle, 1970; Ro, 1969). These variables were found to account for 38% of the variation in LOS, with primary diagnosis alone accounting for 27% of the variability in patient LOS (Lave & Leinhardt, 1976). Patients diagnosed with acute myocardial infarction had the longest hospital stays, whereas patients with hyperplasia of the prostate had shorter lengths of stay. The findings indicate that patients with urgent or emergent status had longer hospital stays. In addition, the poor health of such patients on admission and the unscheduled nature of these admissions resulted in delays and inefficient mobilization of hospital services.

In two earlier studies, Riedel and Fitzpatrick (1964) and Mughrabi (1976) concluded that the primary diagnosis and the concomitant levels of severity are the most important factors contributing to the length of a patient's hospitalization. Additional studies indicated that comorbidity and related complications resulted in significantly longer lengths of stay (Berki, Ashcraft, & Newbrander, 1984; Grau & Kovner, 1986).

In an investigation conducted by Marchette and Holloman (1986), discharge planning (nurses' and social workers') was found to affect patient LOS. This study demonstrated a decrease of 0.8 day of hospitalization for those patients who received discharge planning early in their hospital stays. Conversely, the LOS increased by 0.8 day for those patients who received discharge planning later in their hospitalization. In addition, a decrease of 2 days of hospitalization was shown because of nurses' discharge planning activities with patients diagnosed with CVA. This finding demonstrates that the effect of discharge planning is indicative of individual patient diagnoses (Cable & Mayers, 1983).

Timely social service planning and early referral programs were shown to shorten a patient's LOS. Factors associated with changes in patients' Medicaid status, a lack of alternate care resources, failure of medical staff to complete transfer and referral forms, and other confounding variables delayed patient discharge (Altman, 1965; Boone, Coulton, & Keller, 1981; Schrager, Halman, Myers, Nichols, & Rosenblum, 1978; Schuman, Ostfeld, & Willard, 1976; Zimmer, 1974).

The nursing case management model for patient care delivery has been recognized for its significant effect on decreasing patient LOS (Zander, 1988). Through the coordination and monitoring of resources needed for patient care, ischemic stroke patients' LOS was reduced by 29%, and adult leukemia patients' LOS decreased from an average of 6 to 8 weeks to 32 days.

Rogers (1992) makes a distinction between the way that beyond-the-walls (BTW) and within-the-walls (WTW) models affect LOS:

> Both models involve nurses in relatively autonomous positions that use a holistic nursing approach, "system savvy," collaboration to coordinate professional care team functions, and individualized care planning to achieve reductions in resource utilization while enhancing actual, as well as perceived, quality of care. The reduction in patient anxiety and increased patient compliance when they are more involved in the process and assured that someone they know is watching over things is attested to almost daily. These translate to reduced demands on nursing time during a given stay and in reductions in the actual length of stay.
>
> Beyond this, our experience has been that enhanced transit through the course of a stay and improved discharge planning, particularly with acute cases, takes days off of the end of the stay. This phenomenon is a hallmark of the WTW model.

On the other hand, the forte of the BTW models is care of the chronically ill. The impact of these models on LOS tends to be on the beginning of the stay. This occurs because the BTW nurse case managers know their patients' patterns and disease processes very well. They tend to get these patients into the hospital earlier in an exacerbation than they previously were. Being admitted "less sick" tends to keep these patients out of high-cost emergency and critical care departments and keep the overall LOS down. This phenomenon was noted by Ethridge and Lamb (1989) and alluded to by Rogers, Riordan, and Swindle (1991). St. Joseph Medical Center in Wichita, in an unpublished internal management analysis, has since documented an overall reduction in the admission acuity for their BTW patients.

A major problem with studies relating to patient care delivery systems is the lack of uniformity and sophistication in defining costs. Variations exist as to what factors should be included in direct and indirect cost categories. Some studies included supplies and equipment, while other investigations allocated costs based on overhead expenses from ancillary and support services and general hospital operations. In some studies, nursing costs included the professional services of registered nurses. In other studies, nursing costs included all of the costs of providing nursing care to hospitalized patients (Edwardson & Giovannetti, 1987). Further research is needed to determine the applicability of cost accounting approaches to nursing models of care with the expected clinical and financial outcomes.

Nursing intensity, which is the amount of nursing care provided per patient day, along with various nursing interventions and staffing levels, was cited as reducing LOS and costs associated with hospitalization. In an investigation done by Halloran (1983a, 1983b), nursing diagnoses were used to classify patients according to their nursing care requirements and to describe the time spent by professional nurses in caring for patients. Nursing diagnoses describe patient conditions and problems that require nursing intervention. It was found that a predominantly registered nurse staff, versus a staffing mix of registered nurses, licensed practical nurses, and nursing attendants, decreased costs associated with patient care. The investigation showed that an all-registered-nurse staff would be more likely to deal with total patient needs than a staff composed of various skill mixes. Halloran also proposed that nursing care costs should be identified and defined according to nursing diagnoses (unit of service) instead of the medical diagnosis-related group (DRG) currently in use.

In another study, Halloran and Kiley (1984) proposed a nursing information system model that allocated staffing and resources using nursing diagnoses. This process was based on a nursing workload unit of analysis that calculated costs using a patient classification system for staffing. The reason for using a patient classification system was that such a system made it possible to measure the nursing workload and allocate costs to distinguish the costs of nursing care services from the cost of the hospital's room and board rate.

As outlined by Edwardson and Giovannetti (1987), the patient classification system makes it possible to calculate the hours of care used during a patient's hospitalization. Once the number of patient care hours is identified, this number is translated into a dollar amount. Patients are then classified into DRG categories, and nursing care costs for patients are aggregated and analyzed.

Although patient classification systems offer a more reliable representation than traditional methods of identifying the nursing care needs of patients (i.e., global averages, such as the average amount of care required per day by the typical patient), there are still some inherent problems. As identified by Giovannetti (1972) and Edwardson and Giovannetti (1987), the problems associated with this system include the inadvisability of comparing a patient classification system developed in one hospital with that in another because of the differences in treatment modalities, architectural structure and design of the inpatient units, and standards and policies of the institution. Some of the factors used to weigh the categories are subjective, which results in problems of reliability. Furthermore, methods of validating the system and workload indexes are not transferable. Despite these difficulties, the method of staffing by workload index has been generally accepted by health care institutions across the country.

An investigation done by Halloran and Halloran (1985) found that nursing diagnoses were accurate for predicting nursing workload and quantity of nursing care. In addition, nursing diagnoses contributed to some of the variation in patient LOS. It was suggested that nursing instead of medical needs kept patients in the hospital. Nursing diagnoses that dealt with the patient's psychosocial needs and self-care requirements were significant in increasing nursing workload. In another study, nursing workload activities correlated with 77% of the patient's length of hospitalization. These findings imply that variations in LOS within specific DRG categories can be explained by the clinical management of patient care by nurses (Halloran & Kiley, 1986).

Ventura, Young, Feldman, Pastore, Pikula, and Yates (1985) found that nursing interventions associated with health protection activities for patients with peripheral vascular disease significantly decreased the patient's LOS and lowered hospitalization costs, which were based on a fixed per diem rate. Mumford, Schlesinger, and Glass (1982) and Devine and Cook (1983) demonstrated that psychological and educational interventions (i.e., patient teaching related to pain prevention and complications) with postsurgical patients reduced the LOS and improved patient recovery time.

Flood and Diers (1988) identified the effect of professional nurse staffing levels on LOS. According to the study, decreased nurse staffing levels could lead to a reduction in productivity and inadequate patient care, resulting in longer hospitalization. Patients whose case mixes included gastrointestinal hemorrhages and CVAs and who had been located on a unit with significant staffing shortages were found to have longer LOS intervals, 3.8 and 4.14 days, respectively, when compared with patients on a unit that had adequate staffing levels. The increase in LOS was attributed to patient-related complications and nosocomial infections and resulted in the use of high levels of nursing care resources.

However, the findings of the Flood and Diers study are speculative because many of the variables associated with patient LOS, for example, primary diagnosis, comorbidity, medical complications, and discharge planning factors, had not been controlled. Because these variables were not controlled, the study is not adequate for showing a significant correlation between nurse staffing levels and LOS.

The results of the nursing intensity and workload investigations support the premise that patient care requirements, nursing interventions, and level of staff affect the delivery of care. However, other variables that have a profound effect on the delivery of nursing care services were not accounted for. Some of these variables were identified by Edwardson and Giovannetti (1987) and include service standards of the institution, physician practice patterns, nature and extent of support services, adequacy of the physical plant, and quality-of-care indexes. The last variable would have to be studied with various mixes of staffing personnel to determine the efficacy of patient care delivery.

The general findings of the nursing intensity and workload studies take on a different perspective when viewed in light of the investigations done by the Prospective Payment Assessment Commission (ProPAC). ProPAC was established as an independent advisory board to the Department of Health and Human Services (HHS) and Congress to report on issues surrounding the impact of the prospective payment system on health care delivery and finance. ProPAC's responsibilities include annual recommendations to HHS regarding appropriate changes in Medicare payments for inpatient hospital care and changes in the relative weights of DRGs. ProPAC is also required to report to Congress its evaluation of any adjustments made to DRG classifications and weights (Price & Lake, 1988).

ProPAC focused its research efforts on the DRG allocation method as it related to the intensity of nursing care. The nursing intensity and workload studies done over the last few years established that inaccuracies existed in the allocation of DRG weights to nursing costs. In the past, nursing service in health care institutions was calculated as part of the room and board rate and did not directly affect patient charges. Variations in the patient's nursing care and attributable costs were strictly related to the patient's LOS and routine and intensive care levels (Cromwell & Price, 1988; Young, 1986).

Accounting for the amount of time spent and for the type of care delivered by nursing is one problem generated by the nature of the services offered. Defining nursing care through a patient classification system became one way of alleviating this difficulty. Matching the type of care a patient will need with a specific category on the patient classification instrument and then determining the amount of nursing resources needed for that patient category provided the foundation for establishing the costs of nursing services and developing a basis for charges to patients. The patient classification system was used as an instrument to measure the severity level of patients (in terms of nursing workload) as well as variations in nursing care. However, studies have shown that because of systematic errors (i.e., quantity of care and level of care are both objective and subjective estimates), a lack of cross-institutional comparability and generalizability, and lack of ongoing validity and reliability, patient classification systems were not accurate resources for determining the cost of nursing services (Dijkers & Paradise, 1986). In addition, the wide variations in the methods used in the numerous nursing intensity studies question the appropriateness and applicability of using nursing patient classification systems to account for DRG-specific nursing intensity values (Price & Lake, 1988).

In view of these limitations, a major research effort directed by ProPAC to provide national adjustments of DRG weights based on nursing intensity variations was abandoned (Cromwell & Price, 1988; Price & Lake, 1988). Recommendations from ProPAC for further research included the following:

- Developing nursing intensity adjustments for selected DRGs on a case-by-case basis
- Documenting nursing intensity variation with DRGs over a patient's LOS by identifying factors related to patient complexity, changes in staff volume, and skill mix
- Establishing uniformity among patient classification systems
- Establishing the cost base used to allocate DRG weights

ProPAC also said that the effects of nursing intensity on DRG weights would be greater if applied to all routine and department costs rather than just direct nursing care (Cromwell & Price, 1988; Price & Lake, 1988).

A recent study by Blegen, Goode, & Reed (1998) demonstrated that the total hours of care from nursing personnel were associated directly with medication errors, incidence of decubiti, patient complaints, and mortality. The study indicated that as the proportion of registered nurses to patients increased, rates of unfavorable outcomes decreased. This research validates that nurse staffing ratios compared with patient outcomes is another dimension of quality care that impacts LOS.

NONCLINICAL VARIABLES

Lew (1966) studied how the day of the week that a patient was admitted affected the average LOS. Patients who came in for medical admissions on Sunday had the lowest average LOS, 10.83 days, and those admitted on Friday had the highest average LOS, 13.81 days. For surgical patients, those admitted on Wednesday had the lowest average LOS, 9.88 days, and those admitted on Friday had the highest average LOS, 11.85 days. When medical and surgical admissions were combined, those patients admitted on Friday had the highest average LOS and those admitted on Sunday had the lowest average LOS. Reasons for the variations in the lengths of weekday stay were attributed to the availability of resources—such as personnel, operating rooms, equipment, and procedures—and services needed for the care of the patient.

Day-of-the-week variables were found significant in studies conducted by Lave and Leinhardt (1976) and Mughrabi (1976). However, these variables did not account for a large portion of the variation in average LOS.

Institutional practices related to management, patient care delivery, and use of facility resources (e.g., laboratory, radiology) were among the many variables that affected LOS. Becker, Shortell, and Neuhouser (1980) identified managerial and organizational factors that had significant effects on overall patient LOS. In this study, reductions in patient LOS and increases in the quality and efficiency of services were attributable to the following variables:

- Administrative and clinical managers' awareness of traditional outcome measurements of patient care (i.e., LOS, infection and mortality indexes, and preventable complications) compared with other hospitals
- The degree of professional autonomy related to hospital operations and clinical decision making
- Interdisciplinary as well as interdepartmental collaboration and accountability for the efficient use, coordination, and monitoring of hospital resources, including nursing services, radiology, and laboratory

Decreased length of hospital stay facilitated by interdepartmental coordination and integration of patient services was achieved by regularly scheduled meetings among radiology, nursing service, and laboratory personnel.

Another study, conducted by Berki, Ashcraft, and Newbrander (1984), showed that with certain DRG classifications, patient LOS variations were related to use and consumption of hospital services. Increases in laboratory and radiology services were found to be associated with longer LOS periods in those DRG categories, such as diabetes and arthritis, that required intensive use of ancillary services. Other DRG categories, for example, eye disease, which requires reattachment of the retina and repair of the cornea, increased nursing service intensity and resulted in decreased patient LOS.

References

Altman, I. (1965). Some factors affecting hospital length of stay. *Hospitals, 39*(7), 68-176.

Becker, S., Shortell, S., & Neuhouser, D. (1980). Management practices and hospital length of stay. *Inquiry, 17,* 318-330.

Berki, S., Ashcraft, M., & Newbrander, W. (1984). Length of stay variations within ICDA-8 diagnosis related groups. *Medical Care, 22*(2), 126-142.

Blegen, M., Goode, C., & Reed, L. (1998, Jan./Feb.). Nurse staffing and patient outcomes. *Nursing Research,* 43-50.

Boone, C., Coulton, C., & Keller, S. (1981). The impact of early and comprehensive social work services on length of stay. *Social Work in Health Care, 7*(1), 1-9.

Cable E., & Mayers, S. (1983). Discharge planning effect on length of hospital stay. *Archives of Physical Medicine and Rehabilitation, 64*(2), 57-60.

Cromwell, J., & Price, K. (1988). The sensitivity of DRG weights to variation in nursing intensity. *Nursing Economics, 6*(1), 18-26.

Devine, E., & Cook, T. (1983). A meta-analytic analysis of effects of psychoeducational interventions on length of postsurgical hospital stay. *Nursing Research, 32*(5), 267-274.

Dijkers, M., & Paradise, T. (1986). PCS: One system for both staffing and costing. Do services rendered match need estimates? *Nursing Management, 17*(1), 25-34.

Edwardson, S., & Giovannetti, P. (1987). A review of cost accounting methods for nursing services. *Nursing Economics, 5*(3), 107-117.

Ethridge, P., & Lamb, G. (1989). Professional nursing case management improves quality, access and costs. *Nursing Management, 20*(3), 30-35.

Farren, E., (1991). Effects of early discharge planning on length of hospital stay. *Nursing Economics, 9*(1), 25-30.

Flood, S., & Diers, D. (1988). Nurse staffing, patient outcome and cost. *Nursing Management, 19*(5), 34-43.

Giovannetti, P. (May 1972). *Measurement of patient's requirements for nursing services.* Paper presented to the National Institute of Health Conference, Virginia.

Grau, L., & Kovnor, C. (1986). Comorbidity one length of stay: A case study. In F.A. Shaffer (Ed.), *Patients and purse strings: Patient classification and case management* (pp. 233-242). New York: National League for Nursing.

Halloran, E. (1983a). Staffing assignment: By task or by patient. *Nursing Management, 14*(8), 16-18.

Halloran, E. (1983b). RN staffing: More care less cost. *Nursing Management, 14*(9), 18-22.

Halloran, E., & Halloran, D. (1985). Exploring the DRG/nursing equation. *American Journal of Nursing, 85*(10), 1093-1095.

Halloran, E., & Kiley, M. (1984). Case mix management. *Nursing Management, 15*(2), 39-45.

Halloran, E., & Kiley, M.L. (1986). The nurse's role and length of stay. *Medical Care, 23*(9), 1122-1124.

Kolouch, F. (1965). Computer shows how patient stays vary. *The Modern Hospital, 105*(5), 130-134.

Lave, J., & Leinhardt, S. (1976). The costand length of a hospital stay. *Inquiry, 13,* 327-343.

Lew, I. (1966). Day of the week and other variables affecting hospital admissions, discharges and length of stay for patients in the Pittsburgh area. *Inquiry, 3,* 3-39.

Marchette, L., & Holloman, F. (1986). Length of stay variables. *Journal of Nursing Administration, 165*(3), 12-19.

McCorkle, L. (1970). Duration of hospitalization prior to surgery. *Health Services Research, 5,* 114-131.

Mughrabi, M.A. (1976). The effects of selected demographic and clinical variables on the length of hospital stay. *Hospital Administration in Canada, 18,* 82-88.

Mumford, E., Schlesinger, H., & Glass, G. (1982). The effects of psychological intervention on recovery from surgery and heart attacks: An analysis of the literature. *American Journal of Public Health, 72*(2), 141-151.

Posner, J., & Lin, H. (1975). Effects of age on length of hospital stay in a low income population. *Medical Care, 13*(10), 855-875.

Price, K., & Lake, E. (1988). ProPAC's assessment of DRGs and nursing intensity. *Nursing Economics, 6*(1), 10-16.

Riedel, D., & Fitzpatrick, T. (1964). *Patterns of patient care: A study of hospital use in six diagnosis.* Ann Arbor: The University of Michigan Graduate School of Business Administration.

Ro, K.K. (1969). Patient characteristics, hospital characteristics and hospital use. *Medical Care, 7*(4), 295-312.

Rogers, M., Personal communication. (Aug. 1992).

Rogers, M., Riordan, J., & Swindle, D. (1991). Community-based nursing case management pays off. *Nursing Management, 22*(3), 30-34.

Schrager, J., Halman, M., Myers, D., Nichols, R., & Rosenblum, L. (1978). Impediments to the course and effectiveness of discharge planning. *Social Work in Health Care, 4*(1), 65-79.

Schuman, J., Ostfeld, A., & Willard, H. (1976). Discharge planning in an acute hospital. *Archives of Physical Medicine and Rehabilitation, 57*(7), 343-347.

Ventura, M., Young, D., Feldman, M.J., Pastore, P., Pikula, S., & Yates, M.A. (1985). Cost savings as an indicator of successful nursing intervention. *Nursing Research, 34*(1), 50-53.

Young, D. (1986). ProPAC: Future Directions. *Nursing Economics, 4*(1), 12-15.

Zander, K. (1988). Nursing care management: Strategic management of cost and quality outcomes. *Journal of Nursing Administration, 18*(5), 23-30.

Zimmer, J. (1974). Length of stay and hospital bed misutilization. *Medical Care, 12*(5), 453-462.

Case Management Legislation

National Attempts to Provide Efficient Health Care

CHAPTER OVERVIEW

Because the prospective payment system gave hospitals the incentive to shorten length of stay, strategies using case management are being developed to focus on postdischarge planning and community-based long-term care. Case management has also demonstrated its applicability as a resource in the development of health legislation and policy in regard to the delivery of patient care. The usefulness of case management is an integral part of the administration and management of health care and is also a vital cost-containment measure.

HISTORICAL LEGISLATION

In 1992, 37 states had Medicaid provisions for case management. Legislation for governing the practices of case managers and for developing national certification and specific state requirements was also considered (National Case Management Task Force Steering Committee, 1991-1992; Sager, 1992).

Case management has been integrated into many of the federal and state policies associated with the delivery of health care and social support services. The overall goal is to reduce the use and costs of expensive treatments. Case management is used in these situations to reduce institutionalization, increase and monitor access of needed services, and expand alternative community resources such as home and long-term care (Boling, 1992; Capitman, 1986; Kane, 1985; Strickland, 1992).

Case management has also been a major component in several federally funded demonstration projects.

The Triage demonstration project provided case management and health care services outside the traditional Medicare benefits. These services include adult day care, companion homemaking services, counseling, transportation, pharmaceuticals, and access to residential care. To be eligible for these services, persons had to be age 65 years or older; had to have medical, social, and financial problems and a failing support system; and had to be at risk for institutionalization. Case management services were provided by a professional team consisting of registered nurses, physicians, and social workers (O'Rourke, Raisz, & Segal, 1982).

People eligible for the Wisconsin Community Care Organization included those individuals who were at risk for institutionalization as determined by the Geriatric Functional Rating Scale. This scale rated individuals' ability to perform functional and cognitive activities.

Services included companion and home health aide services, medical supplies and equipment, transportation, respite care, and skilled nursing care (Applebaum, Seidl, & Austin, 1980; Seidl, Applebaum, Austin, & Mahoney, 1983).

The On Lok demonstration project provided case management to dependent and elderly individuals eligible for skilled nursing or intermediate nursing home care. Acute care services, including hospitalization, were provided in addition to other services, including adult and social day care, dental care, home health care, optometry, and occupational and pharmaceutical services. Case management is provided by registered nurses, physicians, social workers, physical and occupational therapists, and dietitians (Zawadski, Shen, Yordi, & Hansen, 1984).

The New York City Home Care program offered services to chronically ill and elderly individuals residing in the New York City area. The program provided homemaker and personal care, transportation assistance, and various medical therapies (Sainer et al., 1984).

The Long-Term Care Channeling Demonstration Project provided case management services to dependent and chronically ill individuals. Services included mental health counseling, homemaking, personal care, supportive services, such as adult foster care and day care, skilled nursing, transportation, medical therapies, and equipment (Applebaum, Harrigan, & Kemper, 1986; Kemper et al., 1986; Wooldridge & Schore, 1986).

Those who were eligible for Access, Medicare's long-term care demonstration project, included all individuals age 18 years or older and Medicare beneficiaries older than age 65 years who needed long-term, skilled nursing care. Services included case management, skilled nursing and home care, and Medicaid-waived services. Waived services included community health nursing, home health aide, medical and nursing consultations and therapies, personal care, equipment and supplies, respite care, and transportation (Berkeley Planning Associates, 1987; Eggert, Bowlyow, & Nichols, 1980).

LEGISLATION SUPPORTING THE DELIVERY OF CASE MANAGEMENT SERVICES

Despite the defeat of health care reform measures proposed at the start of the Clinton administration, several legislation and health care reform proposals have pointed to principles of managed or coordinated care for providing a framework for cost-effective health care delivery. By focusing on case management and long-term care, an alternative to costly hospital and institutional care can be found. These legislative proposals have sought to reduce unneeded care and the use of expensive inpatient services through preventive and primary care interventions. They have also supported comprehensive community-based services and initiatives to improve overall health status and prevent inappropriate hospitalizations (Blankenau, 1992; Pollack, 1992; Strickland, 1992; Wagner, 1991).

Targeted populations included, among others, the chronically ill elderly, young and middle-age individuals with chronic illness and disabilities, the uninsured, and the impoverished. It was also suggested that resources be directed to reducing infant mortality and improving maternal health status (Darman, 1991; Hospitals, 1992a; Wagner, 1991).

Managed care has played a major role in proposals to expand Medicare and Medicaid. The social health maintenance organization (SHMO) is a national managed-care demonstration program initiated in 1985 to provide and finance long-term care services for the elderly. The program includes four nonprofit sites and has recently been approved by Congress for six additional locations. Sponsored by the Health Care Financing Administration (HCFA) in cooperation with the Health Policy Center of Brandeis University, this initiative uses case management and integrated service delivery as key features at each of the demonstration sites. The SHMO is recognized as one of the only national demonstration projects to successfully integrate acute and chronic care using existing funding resources (Abrahams, 1990; Abrahams, Macko, & Grais, 1992; Paone, 1996; Yordi, 1988) and one in which such care can be delivered within a capitated system.

Managed Medicaid legislation, passed in 1987, makes recommendations for a flat payment for Medicaid beneficiaries in need of medical and long-term care. This plan reduces hospital stays and excessive use of services, increases affordable access, and strengthens community-based services and resources (Hospitals, 1992b; McNeil, 1991; "Medicaid-Mandated Managed Care," 1992).

Another example of how the concept of case managed care is used is with the legislation of the CHAMPUS (Civilian Health and Medical Program of the Uniformed Services) Reform Initiative (CRI). This plan extends coverage under a case managed structure for military dependents and retirees younger than age 65 years (Burke, 1992). It also helps reduce health care expenditures and increase access by encouraging the use of military medical services and facilities (Burke, 1992).

Tricare, introduced as an alternative to CHAMPUS, is structured to be a more efficient, cost-effective system of delivering care. It offers three options for medical care: (1) services can be obtained from a government-approved network; (2) users can choose their own medical providers; and (3) inpatient care can be obtained at an out-of-network facility (CHAMPUS, 1995).

Of the major reform plans introduced in the 102nd Congress, six addressed long-term care policies and legislation. It is important to note that these health reform proposals were ground-breaking legislation for case management.

The 1990 Pepper Commission Proposal, developed by the Bipartisan Commission on Health Care, suggested extending Medicare's long-term care initiatives to all disabled individuals. Under the proposal, which was introduced in the Senate by Senator Jay Rockefeller (D-W.Va.), eligibility would be determined by state, local, or federally funded agencies and based on standardized assessments of the beneficiary's resources and support systems.

It was proposed that case managers be used to evaluate and monitor the services provided. Benefits were to include comprehensive home- and community-based services that involve skilled nursing; physical, occupational, and speech therapies; personal care; homemaker services; adult and social day care; respite care for caregivers; hospital care; primary and preventive care; and support counseling (Darman, 1991; Harrington, 1990; Pepper Commission, 1990).

Coverage structure would have incorporated a play or pay plan requiring employers to provide health insurance to employees and their dependents or pay into a public tax plan. A provision was made in this plan for the phasing in of small businesses. Federal and state financing was to have been made available to cover home- and community-based care programs and nursing home care.

Quality of care issues were addressed through standardized practice guidelines, outcomes research, and peer review. Overall costs for this proposal included $24 billion for home care and $18.8 billion for nursing home care (Darman, 1991; Frieden, 1991).

The Long-Term Home Care Act (HR 2263), introduced by Senator Claude Pepper (D-Fla.), proposed to provide coverage for the chronically ill or disabled elderly and children younger than 19 with cognitive and functional impairments. It also included individuals with severe functional disabilities.

Benefits included skilled nursing care, homemaker and personal care services, physical, occupational, speech, and respiratory therapies, medical supplies and equipment, caregiver education, support and counseling, and adult day care. Eligibility determination was to be made by a long-term care management agency or private nonprofit agency along with the individual's physician.

Patient care management was to be provided through case management agencies that did not have affiliations or control interest in the referral facilities. Estimated costs for this plan were $8.9 billion (Darman, 1991).

The Elder Care Program (HR 3140), proposed by Representative Harry Waxman (D-Calif.), was to provide for Medicare beneficiaries and disabled individuals. Eligibility determination was to be made by community assessment and review agencies that were restricted in affiliation and ownership to community or nursing care facilities.

Home and community-based services were to include adult day care, skilled nursing, homemaker, and personal care services, medical and social services, diagnostic tests, medical supplies and equipment, caregiver education and training, and physical and occupational therapy. Estimated costs ranged from $50 billion to $60 billion in 1992 (Darman, 1991; Hospitals, 1992a).

Life Care (S2163/HR4093), sponsored by Senator Edward Kennedy (D-Mass.) and Representative Edward Roybal (D-Calif.), proposed extending eligibility to the chronically ill older than age 65 years or younger than age 19 years, all disabled and dependent individuals, and people with a life expectancy of 1 year or less.

Federally funded case management agencies were to determine eligibility and provide patient management. Benefit coverage was to include up to the first 6 months of nursing home care with extended nursing home coverage provided through a federal long-term care insurance program.

Proposed financial structure included Medicaid and income-related subsidies. Services provided included skilled nursing, adult day care, primary and preventive care, transportation to health and social care facilities, respite care, institutional or noninstitutional care, nutrition and dietary counseling, and physical, occupational, and speech therapies. The estimated cost of such a program was $20 billion (Darman, 1991; Harrington, 1990; Hospitals, 1992a).

Similar to Life Care, the Comprehensive Health Care Plan (HR 4253), proposed providing for the chronically ill older than 65 or younger than 19. The plan also was to provide for Medicare-eligible disabled individuals of all ages and insure those with a life expectancy of 1 year or less.

Eligibility and patient care were to be determined by federally funded case management agencies. Benefits were to include nursing home coverage and income assistance programs.

Home- and community-based services were to include skilled nursing; physical, occupational, and speech therapies; homemaker services; medical and social work care; transportation; adult day care and respite care; and counseling services. The estimated cost of this plan was $258 billion, which included universal health care and preventive and long-term care provisions (Darman, 1991).

MediPlan (HR 5300), sponsored by representative Pete Stark (D-Calif.), suggested that Medicare benefits be extended to chronically ill and disabled individuals of all ages. This plan also included primary and preventive care for children in addition to well-baby care.

It was proposed that eligibility determination and patient management be conducted by case management agencies, which were to have provider and ownership restrictions. A full range of home- and community-based services were to be provided, including skilled nursing; counseling services; medical supplies; adult day care; physical, occupational, and respiratory therapies; medical and social services; caregiver education and training; homemaker and personal care services; and prescription-drug coverage.

The plan's financing structure incorporated payroll tax increases and state contributions. The estimated cost of such a program was $120 billion, which included universal health care provisions and long-term care arrangements (Darman, 1991; Frieden, 1991; Hospitals, 1992a).

Additional legislative initiatives have indicated case management as an integral component of health care delivery and policy formation. This plan was one of several state assembly and senate bills developed in California that would have affected case management (Kowlsen, 1991). An overview of three such bills follows.

California Assembly Bill 1341 was to provide for a 3-year demonstration project to provide case management to children at risk for abuse and neglect. Case management services were to be provided by public health nurses. The goal of this project was to reduce shelter or foster care placement and decrease emergency room visits and hospitalizations among children.

California Senate Bill 1108 established the Primary Care Case Management Advisory Board as part of the California Department of Health Services. It also provided for the delivery of case management services for Medicaid-eligible individuals to promote and increase accessibility to affordable health care resources.

California Assembly Bill 14 would have ratified primary health care coverage to all individuals. Cost-containment strategies were to include managed care principles such as case management.

References

Abrahams, R. (1990, Aug.). The social/HMO: Case management in an integrated acute and long-term care system. *Caring Magazine*, 30-40.

Abrahams, R., Macko, P., & Grais, M.I. (1992). Across the great divide: Integrating acute postacute, and long-term care. *Journal of Case Management, 1*(4), 124-134.

Applebaum, R., Seidl, F.W., & Austin, C.D. (1980). The Wisconsin community care organization: Preliminary findings from the Milwaukee experiment. *Gerontologist, 20*, 350-355.

Applebaum, R.A., Harrigan, M.N. & Kemper, P. (1986). *The evaluation of the national long-term care demonstration: Tables comparing channeling to other community care demonstrations.* Princeton, N.J.: Mathematica Policy Research, Inc.

Berkeley Planning Associates (1987). *Evaluation of the Access: Medicare long-term care demonstration project. Final Report.* Berkeley, Calif.

Blankenau, R. (1992, Jan. 6). Health-reform bills top 1992 agendas of Hill health leaders. *AHA News.*

Boling, J. (1992). An American integrated health care system? Where are we now? *The Case Manager, 3*(3), 53-59.

Burke, M. (1992, Jan. 20). Armed services are marching toward managed care alternatives. *AHA News, 28*(3), 6.

Capitman, J.A. (1986). Community-based long-term care models, target groups, and impacts on service use. *Gerontologist, 26*(4), 389-397.

CHAMPUS (1995, March 13). *CHAMPUS user's guide* (pp. 1-28). Author (special section to Army Times, Navy Times, and Air Force Times).

Darman, R. (1991, Oct. 10). *Comprehensive health reform: Observations about the problem and alternative approaches to solution. Presented to the House Committee on Ways and Means.* Washington, D.C.: Executive Office of the President, Office of Management and Budget.

Eggert, G., Bowlyow, J., & Nichols, C. (1980). Gaining control of the long-term care systems: First returns from the access experiment. *Gerontologist, 20*, 356-363.

Frieden, J. (1991). Many roads lead to health system reform. *Business and Health, 9*(11), 38-66.

Harrington, C. (1990). Policy options for a national health care plan. *Nursing Outlook, 38*(5), 223-228.

Hospitals (1992a, Jan. 20). Health care reform a priority in the new legislative year. 32-50.

Hospitals (1992b, March 20). Managed care in the 1990s: Providers' new role for innovative health delivery. 26-34.

Kane, R. (1985). Case management in health care settings. In M. Weil & J. Karls (Eds.), *Case management in human service practice* (pp. 170-203). San Francisco: Josey Bass Pub.

Kemper, P., Brown, R., Carcagno, G., Applebaum, R., Christianson, J., Carson, W., Dunstan, S., Grannemann, T., Harrigan, M., Holden, N., Phillips, B., Schore, J., Thornton, C., Wooldridge, J., & Skidmore, F. (1986). *The evolution of the national long-term care demonstration: Final report.* Princeton, N.J.: Mathematica Policy Research, Inc.

Kowlsen, T. (1991, Oct.). California dreaming. *Washington Health Beat*, 28-29.

McNeil, D. (1991, Nov. 17). Washington tries to sort out health insurance proposals. *New York Times*, 2.

Medicaid-mandated managed care. (1992, June). *Nursing & Health Care, 13*(6), p. 288.

National Case Management Task Force Steering Committee (1991-1992, Feb. 9). *Work summary and survey of case management toward medical case manager certification.* Little Rock, Ark.: Systemedic Corporation.

O'Rourke, B., Raisz, H., & Segal, J. (1982). *Triage II: Coordinated delivery of services to the elderly: Final report.* Volume 1-2. Plainville, Conn.: Triage, Inc.

Paone, D. (1996). Hospitals. In C.J. Evashwick (Ed.) *The continuum of long-term care: An integrated systems approach.* (pp. 25-42). Albany, NY: Delmar Publishers.

Pepper Commission (1990, March 2). *Access to healthcare and long-term care for all Americans.* Washington, D.C.: U.S. Bipartisan Commission on Comprehensive Health.

Pollack, R. (1992, Jan. 13). Hospitals ready for reform of national health care system. *AHA News.*

Sager, O. (1992). Certification: From need to reality. *The Case Manager, 3*(3), 81-84.

Sainer, J.S., Brill, R.S., Horowitz, A., Weinstein, M., Dono, J.E., & Korniloff, N. (1984). *Delivery of medical and social services to the homebound elderly: A demonstration of intersystem coordination: Final report.* New York: New York City Department for the Aging.

Seidl, F.W., Applebaum, R., Austin, C., & Mahoney, K. (1983). *Delivering in-home services to the aged and disabled: The Wisconsin experiment.* Lexington, Mass.: Lexington Books.

Strickland, T. (1992, April, May, June). Profile [Interview with Gail R. Wilensky, Deputy Assistant to the President for Policy Development]. *The Case Manager, 3*(2), 72-81.

Wagner, L. (1991, Dec. 9). Cost containment: Carrot or the stick? *Modern Healthcare,* 36-40.

Wooldridge, J., & Schore, J. (1986). *Evaluation of the national long-term care demonstration: Channeling effects on hospital, nursing home, and other medical services.* Princeton, N.J.: Mathematica Policy Research, Inc.

Yordi, C. (1988). Case management in the social health maintenance organization demonstration. *Health Care Financing Review* (annual supplement), 83-88.

Zawadski, R.T., Shen, J., Yordi, C., & Hansen, J.C. (1984). *On Lok's community care organization for dependent adults: A research and development project (1978-1983): Final report.* San Francisco: On Lok Senior Health Services.

The Managed Care Market

Nurse Case Management as a Strategy for Success

Tina Gerardi

CHAPTER OVERVIEW

Managed care has become the primary health care policy in the United States. Coupled with capitation—fixed per member–per month payments—managed care is supposed to solve all of the U.S. health care problems, from rocketing health care costs to perceived shortcomings in health care quality. Remarkably there is little consensus, especially among the public, as to just what managed care actually is. Nurse case managers must understand managed care if they are to navigate the health care delivery system to meet the complex needs of their patients. This chapter describes the basics of managed care and interprets concepts as they relate to the current marketplace. The role of case management as a strategy for success in the managed care market is also discussed.

WHY MANAGED CARE?

Before World War I, hospitals were only for the most seriously ill patients. Babies were born at home, and family doctors made house calls. The center of care was the home, and financing was pay-as-you-go. Costs were relatively low, since medicine was not that sophisticated. Also, most people could not afford high fees. Only the very wealthy could afford a specialist.

After World War II, antibiotics made advanced surgery and long-term survival possible. New technologies made hospitals the centers of care, where patients came to see specialists. The federal government, through the Hill-Burton Act in 1946, subsidized hospital construction, which led to a hospital construction boom. With the passage of the Medicare and Medicaid bills in 1965, health care became an industry. The incentives were to fill beds and perform more procedures, and hospitals competed to have the best and most advanced facilities, creating a "technological race." Meanwhile, because most of the public were covered by some sort of indemnity insurance coverage, they were insulated from the true cost of care.

The traditional fee-for-service reimbursement system encouraged overutilization. With this type of reimbursement, hospitals and health care providers were reimbursed for each service provided; therefore the more you ordered or provided, the more you were paid. In the 1960s, health industry leaders began to recognize the potential of prepaid group practice plans as mechanisms to contain the dramatic rise in health care costs. The federal government provided the impetus for expanding the number of prepaid health plans through legislation enacted in 1973. The term *health maintenance organization (HMO)* was coined during the Nixon administration.

Soaring insurance premiums in the 1980s caused businesses to reexamine the system for delivering and financing health care. Commercial insurance plans sought to protect their revenue base by writing narrower policies and raising group premiums based on the experience of one individual in the group. Use of services was discouraged by high deductibles and copayments. Staff were hired to review and approve individual cases to reduce inappropriate services. The diagnosis-related group (DRG)–based payment, a fixed rate for specific diagnoses or procedures, was also introduced as a means of controlling escalating health care costs. The utilization review programs and DRG system have been unsuccessful in reducing health care costs.

The predecessors of the HMO include organizations that mutualized costs and provided direct health care services for Venetian seaman in the thirteenth century, for British seamen in the sixteenth century, and for American merchant seamen in 1798. Kaiser-Permanente, the major prototype of the HMO, traces its origins to the 1930s. It developed from a system serving workers building the Los Angeles Aqueduct in 1933, construction workers and their families at the Grand Coulee Dam project in eastern Washington in 1938, and, on a larger scale, Kaiser shipyard employees in and around Portland, Oregon, and San Francisco, and employees of the Kaiser steel plant at Fontana, California, during World War II. The system was open to the public in 1945. Organized consumers formed the Group Health Cooperative of Puget Sound in 1946, and the Health Insurance Plan of Greater New York was organized in 1947.

Several advantages were identified as these organizations emerged:

- Assured availability of and access to services through integrated group practices
- Evolution and creation of prepaid insurance plans
- Budgeting for provision of services
- Incentives for health maintenance and preventive health services
- Assurance of quality care through the group practice of physicians offering multiple specialties

To control escalating health care costs, payment systems and cost control measures have been discussed, and managed care programs have been reexamined by both the business community and health economists. Managed care is not a new idea, but it will definitely have new implications, particularly for nursing.

HOW DOES MANAGED CARE WORK?

Patient care has somehow always been "managed." In many cases, human illness has been managed by the patient and family alone. At other times it has been managed for the patient and family by the health care professional (a gatekeeper) accountable for coordinating all patient health care services and also supplying certain aspects of the patient's health services.

Managed care in its broadest form currently refers to any health care delivery system in which a party other than the health care giver or the patient influences the type of health care delivered. A managed care provider takes the risk for the patient's health care. In this way, rather than simply approving or denying the health benefit, the managed care provider will intervene to provide what it considers to be appropriate health care for the patient.

A montage of managed care organizations has evolved in response to the steady rise in health care costs as a percentage of our gross domestic product (GDP) (see Fig. 21-1). Health spending as a share of the GDP is estimated to increase from 13.6% to 16.6% from 1999-2007. Society has decided that the current growth of health care as a proportion of the GDP is more than it is willing to pay. Our average health benefits have increased in a similar vein. According to the Comparative Performance of U.S. Hospitals, the average cost per employee for annual health benefits in late 1998 was approximately $4,000, as compared to $600 in 1976. In the mid-late 90's managed care was viewed as an answer to the problems of increasing price, decreasing access, and uncertain quality. In response to these escalating costs, purchasers of health plans, mainly local businesses, have embraced the tenets of managed care and have made arrangements with HMOs or independent managed care companies.

According to the Comparative Performance of U.S. Hospitals, the percentage of hospitals with arrangements with HMOs increased from 48% in 1986 to 98% in 1996. In traditional fee-for-service plans an individual encounter between a covered individual and the health care system is compensated for by the insurer, if the encounter represents a covered benefit of the patient's plan, subject to deductibles or other contractual reductions in benefits. If the patient does not have insurance coverage or the encounter is not a covered benefit, the patient is liable for the bill. The patient chooses the health care professional or hospital to provide the service based on his or her own criteria. On the other hand, the managed care organization generally presents the patient with a list of health care professionals from which to choose the one to supply a covered benefit. Many managed care plans have specified times during which patients can change health care professionals; therefore once a provider is chosen, it may be difficult to change. Depending on the plan, the patient may be required to see a primary care provider who will be responsible for making all assessments and determinations as to health care needs. Referrals must be initiated by the primary care provider. The patient is likely to have a fixed copayment or fee for every visit, regardless of its complexity, and will probably not need to file insurance papers or be responsible for any other payment. Hospitalizations are likely to be covered entirely with the exception of certain medically unnecessary amenities. Prevention visits such as immunizations, well-baby visits, Pap smears, and mammograms are likely to be covered benefits, with a copayment.

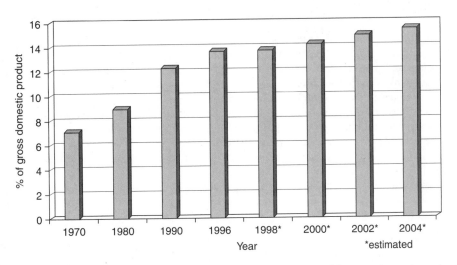

FIGURE **21-1**   The increase of health care expenses as a percentage of the gross domestic product.
From U.S. Department of Health and Human Services, 1997.

Traditionally, health care providers were physicians and hospitals. Physicians saw patients in their offices and in hospitals or clinics. Managed care has introduced a large number of additional people to the health care delivery system. Many managed care organizations have begun to depend on physician assistants and nurse practitioners to provide services, especially in the areas of primary care. In the "good old days" the choice of hospital was made predominantly by the physician. In a managed care environment the choice is almost entirely made by the payor according to contractual arrangements negotiated for the entire plan. This makes the hospital a provider as well, since many of the covered benefits are provided as part of hospital services. These include home health nursing, pharmacy, physical and occupational therapy, respiratory therapy and ventilator management and dietary counseling to name a few.

To understand the cost control changes to the health care marketplace, we must first understand the traditional methods for managing health care costs and current managed care structures. Early managed care programs under the guidance of the professional standards review organizations (PSROs) attempted to control costs through cost sharing, education, second opinions for surgery, and incentives to use lower-cost sites of care such as ambulatory surgery. These early plans also assumed that physicians would modify their behavior based on information alone. Unfortunately, none of these early strategies controlled the continuing escalation of costs. However, the key characteristic of the most effective managed care plans was identified: control of cost and utilization. The cost, use, and appropriateness of services rendered by providers are tightly controlled. Providers are selected who are able to provide cost-effective care.

HMOs, preferred provider organizations (PPOs), and indemnity forms of insurance once were distinct products for providing health care benefits. Today the distinctions are disappearing as each product takes on characteristics of the other. Other common managed care structures include exclusive provider organizations (EPOs), independent practice associations (IPAs), and point-of-service (POS) plans. Definitions for each of these plans will be provided in an attempt to clarify this managed care alphabet soup.

HMOs are organized health care delivery systems responsible for both the financing and the delivery of health care services to an enrolled population. There are five common models of HMOs:

1. In **staff model** HMOs the physicians are employed by the HMO to provide covered services to the health plan enrollees. They are usually paid a salary with some bonus or incentive based on performance and productivity.
2. In the **group practice model** HMO the HMO contracts with a multispecialty physician group practice to provide all physician services to the HMO's members. The physician group is technically independent but depends significantly on the HMO contracts for patients. An example of this type of model is the Permanente Medical Group under the Kaiser Foundation Health Plan.
3. In a **network model** a network contracts with more than one group practice to provide physician services to the HMO's members. An example is the Health Insurance Plan (HIP) of Greater New York, which contracts with many multispecialty physician group practices in the New York City area.
4. In the **independent practice association (IPA) model** the HMO contracts with an association of physicians to provide services to its members. Physicians are members of the IPA for purposes of the HMO contract but retain their practices separately and distinctly from each other.
5. **Direct contract models** contract directly with individual physicians to provide services to their members. In direct contracting arrangements the employer contracts directly with the provider to provide health care services, thus eliminating the insurer.

An IPA is an association of individual independent physicians or small physician group practices formed for the purpose of contracting with one or more managed health care organizations. The attractiveness of an IPA structure to HMOs and other managed care organizations is the IPA's ability to provide a large panel of providers and accept payment on a capitated basis.

PPOs are entities through which employer health benefit plans and health insurance carriers contract to purchase health care services for covered beneficiaries from a selected group of participating providers. These providers may include hospitals, physicians, IPAs, or physician-hospital organizations. Most often PPOs negotiate on a basis of discounted fee-for-service charges, all-inclusive per diem rates, or payments based on DRGs. A major difference between PPOs and HMOs is the patient's ability to choose a non-PPO member for covered services, subject to a higher level of deductible and copayment.

EPOs are structured like PPOs but behave much like HMOs in their limitation of choice of providers. HMOs are carefully regulated by specific HMO statutes in the states in which they operate, whereas EPOs are insurance products subject to less rigorous insurance laws.

POS plans contain features of PPO and HMO arrangements. Under POS plans, primary care physicians are reimbursed through fixed per member–per month payments (capitation) or other performance-based reimbursement methods. The primary care provider acts as a gatekeeper for referral and institutional medical services.

Health care providers are responding to the changing market and expansion of managed care products, which place greater emphasis on value, access, and quality of care. Responses to the market include provider's developing organizations that accommodate coordinated care and shared reimbursement. For example, an integrated health care delivery system provides coordinated care that allows participating providers, using economies of scale, to increase productivity, enhance the scope and quality of services, and reduce the administrative burden associated with those services. The goal of a mature, integrated health care delivery system is to become a provider organization that is seamless in its ability to deliver a broad range of health care services. Direct contracting is another financial arrangement that is gaining in popularity in the more mature markets. In direct contracting arrangements the employer contracts directly with the provider to provide health care services, thus eliminating the insurer. The benefits to the provider in this type of arrangement are a known volume of beneficiaries and increased cash flow directly from the employer to the provider, generally on a monthly basis. The employer realizes decreased health care benefit costs and added value of working directly with the provider to realize specific services for their employee population.

RESPONSES TO MANAGED CARE

Provider responses to managed care varied from "bar the doors," to "respond only if pressured," to "let's reach out to the business community and begin strategic planning for these integrated services." The physician community appears to be most affected by the multiple changes in health care. Individual physicians have seen their autonomy and their often unique relationship with patients and families usurped by managed care companies. The individual physician in a solo practice cannot survive under either traditional managed care or any managed competition model. The cost of operating a small business is too high compared to the access to information and the discounted purchasing and discounted contracting provided by a managed care company or required by a health purchasing cooperative. Managed care places new organizational demands on physicians, such as restricted referral and hospital panels, increased bureaucratic overhead from many types of plans, and an inability to refer out difficult patients. Many physicians view managed care with fear and loathing. Loss of autonomy is the most common fear. As more nurse practitioners are becoming providers in the managed care environment, they may also experience these feelings of loss of autonomy. However, most nurses are experiencing increased opportunities in the managed care arena. Many managed care companies are seeing nurse practitioners and nurse midwives as cost-effective providers of primary care services and are increasing their provider panels to include these health professionals.

Physicians have led attempts to reduce medical costs since the introduction of PSROs in the 1960s. But physician costs account for only about one fifth of the total health care dollar expenditure. They do, however, as gatekeepers control the expenditure of many resources such as diagnostic tests and procedures. Until the late 90s, physician income had not been greatly affected by health care reform. As primary care providers increased their control of specialist care, however, physician income declined. In response to the pressure to reduce overall costs, physicians have organized into managed care organizations, have worked with hospitals in the development of clinical pathways, and have supported clinical case management in both the acute and community setting.

As 1998 came to a close, many managed care organizations were looking at the concept of the primary care provider as gatekeeper. Many organizations were rethinking the role of the specialist as gatekeeper for certain illnesses. They believed that certain diseases such as diabetes, asthma, and chronic pulmonary disease may be most cost-effectively managed by a specialist who is familiar with the effects of the disease on the entire body, rather than a primary care provider who may not be as knowledgeable of state-of-the-art treatments and medications. Although there is no consensus on the role of the primary care provider versus the specialist, the gatekeeper function may no longer be in the sole domain of the primary care provider.

Since the inception of DRGs in 1983, hospitals have been forced to focus on outcomes, utilization, and cost. For this reason, hospitals were better prepared than physicians for managed care. Physicians were not directly affected by DRGs because as private physicians they were reimbursed for services rendered in the hospital. Providers, such as hospitals, who accepted the managed care trend as reality, took a proactive approach to managed care. HMO contracting, network development, integrated service delivery, and the formation of independent managed care organizations have proliferated across the country. Resource allocation in the areas of inpatient care, outpatient care, and continuing care services are being evaluated and analyzed by individual providers as well as by networks. The goal is to be able to deliver seamless health care to specified populations. Inpatient utilization has dramatically decreased as managed care has penetrated certain markets.

Federal and state governments embraced the tenets of managed care and actively promoted Medicare and Medicaid managed care programs. Under these programs, Medicare and Medicaid recipients are enrolled in managed care programs in which they have a primary care provider from the managed care organization or HMO. In theory, they will receive the same access, quality, and cost that other members receive. This attempt by the government to reduce costs associated with caring for these distinct populations was under considerable scrutiny in late 1998-1999. The large for-profit health insurance companies and the Health Care Financing Administration (HCFA) found that many of the Medicare and Medicaid managed care programs were underfunded and unable to provide the services advertised to beneficiaries. In late 1998 several large companies withdrew from participating in Medicare and left many elderly individuals without health insurance. HCFA's total count as of October 1998 was that 507,727 Medicare beneficiaries would lose their current health plan coverage effective January 1999. The hardest hit state was Florida, followed by New York, California, Texas, Maryland, Washington, Ohio, Nevada, and Massachusetts.

These issues with managed Medicare and Medicaid bring to light other issues that are plaguing managed care providers as we begin the new millennium. There are increasing calls from grassroots consumer groups to hold managed care companies liable for bad outcomes of care, especially for individuals who are harmed by denials of care. The care issues being debated in 1998-1999 include the following:

- Liability of managed care providers
- Access questions, including choice of primary care provider, access to specialty care, and emergency care
- Timely claims decisions, including grievance and appeals provisions
- Privacy of medical information

Although there is an impact from managed care throughout the health care industry, there is specific impact on the operational areas of a facility. Providers have seen an increased need for discharge planning, social services, patient education, and a medical record that will follow the patient across multiple settings in a delivery system. The clinical impact has been evidenced by increased emphasis on length of stay reductions, evaluations of medical practice patterns with the purpose of reducing variation, the development of clinical pathways, and the implementation of case management. Although initially these clinical impact areas were mainly in the acute care institutions, the impact has spread to home care, subacute care, long-term care, and other continuing care services.

NURSE CASE MANAGEMENT IN A CHANGING ENVIRONMENT

Nurse case managers assist in creating and help to administer a network of services for their patients. The role of case manager was created solely to negotiate for, organize, and evaluate the need for using various resources for patient care. Traditionally case managers have operated between the realities of costs or covered services and the perceptions of patients' needs. The role of the case manager supports and embellishes the concepts of managed care.

Many professionals, as well as patients and families, can coordinate multiple services. The increased emphasis on discharge planning and social services highlights the need for professionals in these disciplines to coordinate these aspects of patient care both efficiently and effectively. However, the more complicated the services become or the more unable the patient or family becomes to coordinate care, the more an official case manager may be needed.

Nurse case managers traditionally have been based in conventional care settings (hospitals, hospices, clinics), dealing with episode-based management. Case managers sequence and organize services from many departments within the organization and are accountable for good financial and clinical outcomes. Nurse case management within the managed care environment has expanded to continuum-based case management in which accountability continues for good financial and clinical outcomes. The coordination of services and resources for the individual with complex needs continues indefinitely while the individual is covered by the managed care organization. In other words, the nurse case manager maintains a relationship with the individual after the disease or episode-specific problem has been resolved. In community health, nurses traditionally have practiced health promotion and disease prevention rather than cure and illness. This prevents the escalation of a person's health condition into a more serious condition. Community health nurses practice collaborative and comprehensive care rather than short-term intervention and episodic care. This integration of health services and health care delivery effects a more efficient use of health care services. Thus the community health care nurse can be an effective nurse case manager. In view of this, managed care programs have a unique opportunity to recognize the value of nursing both economically and in the provision of comprehensive care.

The nurse case manager must understand the contract the managed care organization or HMO has with the provider. This information is valuable in negotiating discharge and other care options for the patient. For example, if the managed care organization has a capitated or per diem financial arrangement with the provider, the organization is more willing to support less expensive settings for care delivery, such as home care, subacute care, or nursing home care. However, if the same provider has a DRG payment arrangement with the managed care organization, the organization may be less likely to support home care or a transitional care option until the patient has received inpatient services to cover the DRG prospective payment. In other words, home care may not be approved to expedite discharge, even though it is a covered benefit, until the patient has reached the DRG length of stay in the inpatient setting. In this instance the nurse case manager will need strong negotiation skills coupled with knowledge of the managed care financing system to advocate for the best quality care option for the patient.

As the nurse case manager identifies conflicts between managed care organization financing and quality of care issues, they should be brought to the attention of the provider administration. This information can be tracked and used in future contract negotiations with the managed care organization.

Nurse case managers are taking the lead in developing clinical pathways, practice guidelines, and outcomes measurements. Their knowledge of the health care environment and complex patient needs, coupled with their education and training, have given them the opportunity to lead multidisciplinary teams to develop cost-effective models of care that achieve positive patient outcomes and increased practitioner and patient satisfaction.

There are tremendous opportunities for nurse case managers in community-based practices where they assist individuals in managing both their health and their illnesses. Nurse case managers, who traditionally have dealt only with acute care, are now following up individuals beyond the walls of the facility into the clinic, home, and long-term care facility and assisting in coordinating services to keep them well. These practitioner-based models require sound financial and clinical judgment, as well as keen physical and psychosocial assessment skills. Some case management practices focus more on interaction with the individual by telephone rather than in person. Many managed care organizations prefer the telephone approach because of the decrease in overhead costs; however, it is impossible to measure the cost of losing the in-person interaction with the patient and family. Traditionally, nurse case managers have believed that in identifying patient needs, nothing compares with the opportunity to use all their senses in a complete face-to-face, patient or family assessment. This assessment, coupled with sound financial and resource management of the individual's health benefits, will result in the goals of managed care: high-quality, accessible care at the lowest possible cost. Nurse case management should never be considered a replacement for accountability in each professional discipline at the direct care level; for complex cases, however, there is no substitute for an effective nurse case management program.

Health care has seen a paradigm shift over the last decade of the 20th century. We are moving from a health care system built on a paradigm of unpredictable, acute simple disease to a focus on a paradigm of predictable, chronic complex illness that would favorably impact our ability to measure and manage quality care. According to the Centers for Disease Control's National Center for Chronic Disease Prevention, chronic illness accounts for 90% of all illnesses and 70% of all deaths; it is the single most rapidly growing component of health care; and it is the greatest financial exposure for employers, business alliances, and managed care organizations. Case management may be moving toward an integrated lifetime care approach where a continuum of care is required that includes preventive, acute, psychological, rehabilitative, educational, and self-management interventions to meet both complex health and psychosocial needs of patients and families. This approach, again, supports the role of the nurse as the case manager. Nurses are educated to actively collaborate with individuals with complex, rare, or multiple risk factors. Nurses have a rich history in promoting preventive health and wellness services, with a focus on the patient's lifetime health care needs and concerns, as defined by the patient. As we look to the future, nurse case managers are well prepared and positioned to move into the role of the lifetime care manager.

Nurse case management also provides an excellent opportunity for the profession to increase public awareness of the role and image of nursing in the health care delivery system: to educate the consumer, the provider, and the payer as to the expertise of the nurse case manager, the registered professional nurse, and the advanced practice nurse. As one looks to the future, nursing research must validate the positive effect of nurse case management on health care costs, access to services, quality of services, and customer satisfaction.

References

Barth, S.M. (1997). Integrating payer and provider risk through capitation. *Managed Care Quarterly, 5*(1), 19-24.

Blendon, R.J., et al. (1993). Physician's perspectives on caring for patients in the United States, Canada, and West Germany. *New England Journal of Medicine, 328*(9), 621-627.

Deloitte and Touche, LLP and HCIA, Inc. (1995). *The comparative performance of U.S. hospitals: The sourcebook.* Baltimore: Author.

Fuchs, V.R. (1990). The health sector's share of the gross national product. *Science, 247,* 534-538.

Garcia, L.B., Safriet, S., & Russell, D.C. (1998). *Healthcare financial management, 52*(7), 52-57.

Gaynor, M., & Vogt, W.B. (1997). What does economics have to say about health policy anyway? A comment and correction on Evans and Rice. (Commentary). *Journal of Health Politics, Policy and Law, 22,* 475-496.

Ginzberg, E. (1996). The potential and limits of competition in health care. *Bulletin of the New York Academy of Medicine, 73,* 224-236.

Grimaldi, P. (1998). Medicare's new capitation method. *Journal of Health Care Finance, 24*(4), 7-21.

Healthcare Underwriters Mutual, HUM Healthcare Systems, & PSS—Physician Sales & Service, Inc. (1996). *Managed care & capitation: Preparing for success.* Papers presented at a conference in Lake Placid, New York, May 9 & 10, 1996.

Kavaler, F., & Zavin, S. (1992). Health care for seamen in the port of New York. *New York State Journal of Medicine, 92*(8), 353-358.

Kennedy, K.M., & Merlino, D.J. (1998). Alternatives to traditional capitation in managed care agreements. *Healthcare Financial Management, 52*(4), 46-50.

Kongstvedt, P.R. (Ed.). (1993). *The managed health care handbook* (2nd ed.). Gaithersburg, Md.: Aspen.

Kongstvedt, P.R. (Ed.). (1995). *Essentials of managed care.* Gaithersburg, Md.: Aspen.

Marmor, T.R. (1998). Forecasting American health care: How we got here and where we might be going. *Journal of Health Politics, Policy and Law, 23,* 551-571.

Menkin, H. (Ed.). (1997). *Handbook of managed care terminology.* Albany, N.Y.: CHPS Consulting.

Nelson, H. (1997). *Nonprofit & for-profit HMOs: Converging practices for different goals?* New York: Milbank Memorial Fund.

Phelps, C.E. (1997). *Health economics* (2nd ed.). Reading, Mass.: Addison Wesley Longman, Inc.

Reinhardt, U.E. (1995). Turning our gaze from bread and circus games. *Health Affairs, 14*(2), 33-36.

Saward, E.W., & Fleming, S. (1980). Health maintenance organizations. *Scientific American, 243*(4), 47-53.

Sonnefeld, S.T., et al. (1991, Fall). Projections of the national health expenditures through the year 2000, *Health Care Financing.*

Financing Health Care in the U.S.

Economic and Policy Implications

Richard W. Redman

CHAPTER OVERVIEW

The financing of health care in the United States has evolved into a model unique among major industrialized countries in the world. The market-driven economy of the U.S. is clearly reflected in the way that health care is paid for. In addition to these market features, the American value of individual rights prevailing over those of community good also is evident in health care. American citizens demand the right to choose their health care provider and the types of services they want in the same way that they make all other consumer choices. While this "right to choose" has been challenged somewhat during the era of managed care, individuals still are willing to pay additional money where possible to maintain their freedom of choice. These unique American values have contributed to the way health care system financing has evolved.

This chapter provides an overview of how the major financing mechanisms in the United States have evolved as well as an examination of the total amount of national resources allocated for health care services. Issues and trends in the financing of health care delivery are also presented. As will be seen, the financing mechanisms and the projections for the future provide an excellent foundation for the role of the nurse case manager as the coordinator of resources for the delivery of quality services efficiently and effectively.

FINANCING MECHANISMS FOR HEALTH CARE

Over the second half of the 20th century the financing of the American health care system has undergone tremendous change. The fee-for-service payment mechanism, where purchasers of care paid for each health care service or product, has been replaced for the most part by managed care. Even traditional indemnity insurance programs, such as Aetna and Metropolitan, and government insurance programs, such as Medicare and Medicaid, have adopted the principles and practices of managed care. These practices include programs such as second opinion, hospital precertification, and case management for groups with high-cost diseases and conditions.

"Managed care" refers to both an organization that coordinates the purchase and/or delivery of health care services and a set of techniques used to ensure the efficiency and effectiveness of the use of health care services. The health maintenance organization (HMO) is often seen as the prototype for a managed care organization, although in reality it is only one of many organizational forms. Managed care techniques, increasingly used by any type of health care provider or purchaser, include financial incentives for providers, health promotion and risk reduction programs, early identification of disease, disease management programs, and utilization management.

At the beginning of the 20th century, hospitals were not the center of the health care system. In fact, the health care system's abilities to meet the major challenges of the day, e.g., infectious diseases, were minimal. Most services were provided by physicians in their offices or to people in their homes at low cost. After World War II the level of sophistication of health care interventions and technologies available began to gradually change. With that came increased cost of health services and an unrelenting demand on the part of the American public for whatever treatment the health care system could provide.

The payment mechanisms for health reflected this evolution and change in consumer demand throughout the century. From 1920 to 1950, different financing mechanisms developed to meet the needs of consumers for purchasing health care services. The first Blue Cross program was developed in 1929. Several HMOs were also developed during this period, primarily to meet the needs of various groups of industrial employees. These early HMOs are still evident today and include Kaiser (founded in 1937 in California), Group Health Association (founded in Washington, DC in 1937), and Group Health Cooperative of Puget Sound (founded in Washington in 1947) (Fox, 1996).

The government became a major purchaser of health care when the Medicare program was implemented in 1965. This was followed shortly after by Medicaid, a program jointly funded by the federal and state governments. These programs enabled many who did not have access previously to seek health care services. This time period is often seen as the beginning of a 40-year period of unprecedented growth in health care, both in terms of types of services and therapies available, and the continual increase in costs to provide those services. As the third party payment system evolved, the individual consumer was not directly responsible for payment of the health care services. This dynamic contributed to ever-increasing demand for services, often without awareness of their cost.

Until the early 1980s, most health care was paid for on a fee-for-service basis. It was referred to as retrospective payment because the bill for health care services was determined after all needed services were provided. This type of payment mechanism is now viewed as having served as an incentive for providers to deliver whatever the patient required or demanded, since it would be paid for by the purchaser, often an insurance company or governmental agency. During the 1970s, a period of high inflationary growth in all sectors of the American economy, health care costs skyrocketed. As a means to control health care inflation, several cost-containment and cost-limiting programs were introduced. First, voluntary mechanisms were employed; eventually they became mandated programs. These programs concentrated on the hospital sector because this increasingly was the most expensive component in the health care system. Eventually, the programs focused on physician services as well (Abbey, 1996; Fisher & Welch, 1999; Fox, 1996).

In the 1980s a new payment mechanism was introduced. Prospective payment systems were implemented for hospital care. Diagnosis Related Groups (DRGs) were implemented, first by Medicare and then quickly by other payer groups, with fixed payments attached for each DRG. This resulted in a major change in incentives for providers, who had become quite adept at functioning under the retrospective payment incentives. Under prospective payment, hospitals now had incentives to control the utilization of resources and the length of stay to minimize expenditures. If a hospital spent more to care for a patient than would be reimbursable under the fixed payment system, the hospital had to absorb the loss.

During the 1980s the principles and techniques of managed care also began to be employed by indemnity insurance groups. Examples include the requirement of second opinion programs for elective surgery and the use of case management programs for high-cost diseases and conditions. Large employer groups also became much more involved in purchasing health care for the benefit packages of their employees. Often employers pointed out that the health care system was operating inefficiently and they stated they declined to absorb the annual inflation in health care services that they had to purchase for employees. Employers began to introduce utilization review programs. In addition, they became very interested in the competitive pricing available through managed care providers. The rapid growth in managed care throughout the United States is generally attributed to large employer groups who turned rapidly to this form of health care financing as a cost-effective approach to meeting the health benefit needs of their employees.

CURRENT LEVELS OF EXPENDITURES

The United States spent $1.1 trillion on health care in 1997—approximately $4000 for each citizen. Private funding for health care comprised 53.6% of total expenditures ($585.3 billion); public or governmental sources paid for 46.4% ($507.1 billion) (Health Care Financing Administration, 1998, 1999a). The sources of public and private funds and the types of services they purchased can be seen in Table 22-1.

As the data illustrate, hospital and physician expenditures traditionally account for the majority of health care expenditures. However, growth in those categories has slowed in recent years. Expenditures for prescription drugs have increased dramatically because of the availability of new, high-priced drugs, increased consumer demand for the drugs, and an increase in the number of prescriptions filled (Health Care Financing Administration, 1999a).

Health insurance coverage is an important determinant of access to health care services. Individuals without either private or public health insurance coverage are more likely to report unmet needs for health care, less likely to have a usual source of health care, and less likely to receive preventive health care services (Peters, 1998).

The level of funding from public sources has led to debate about whether the U.S. health care system is private or public. In 1996, 43.1% of the U.S. population had health insurance paid for by private-

Table 22-1 ▶ HEALTH CARE EXPENDITURES IN THE UNITED STATES: 1997			
SOURCES OF FUNDS	**PERCENTAGE OF TOTAL**	**DISTRIBUTION OF FUNDS**	**PERCENTAGE OF TOTAL**
Private insurance	31.9%	Hospital care	34.0%
Medicare	19.6%	Physician services	19.9%
Medicaid	14.6%	Nursing homes	7.6%
Other public sources	12.2%	Prescription drugs	7.2%
Out-of-pocket	17.2%	Program administration costs	4.6%
Other private sources	4.6%	Other*	26.7%

*Includes dental and other professional services, home health care, over-the-counter drugs and supplies, and other expenditures for personal health care services.
From Health Care Financing Administration, Office of the Actuary, National Health Statistics Group.

sector employers. An additional 34% had publicly funded health insurance covered by Medicaid, Medicare, insurance resulting from former or current military service, or the Indian Health Service. Approximately 7% purchased their own insurance coverage, and nearly 18% were uninsured (Carrasquillo, Himmelstein, Woolhandler, & Bor, 1999). These data suggest that the U.S. system is still primarily a privately funded system, although the share of health care paid for by public sources is increasing. Private employers as purchasers of health insurance for employee benefit packages remain very influential in the health care marketplace.

ISSUES AND TRENDS

The evolution of the health care financing system and the interplay of the public and private sectors has shaped the health care delivery system as we know it today. Several issues and trends are noteworthy for the foreseeable future. These trends include system inequities, increasing potential for challenging decisions and ethical dilemmas, the increased importance of primary care providers, and renewed interest in population health outcomes.

System Inequities

The market-based financing for health care in the United States has contributed to many of the inequities citizens experience with respect to access to quality health care services. The American system is often described as employer based because nearly all individuals who have access to private health insurance receive that insurance as part of employer benefits packages. Generally, individuals who are not employed either depend on public sources of funding, such as Medicaid, or have no coverage.

In 1997, 18% of individuals between ages 18 and 64 years had no health insurance. Seventy-three percent of individuals had private insurance, 7% had Medicaid or some other type of public assistance, and Medicare covered 2%. Once an individual reaches age 65 years, Medicare coverage is available, so less than 1% of the elderly are uninsured (Health Care Financing Administration, 1999a).

Considerable inequities exist among different groups in society, however. Hispanic adults are much more likely to be uninsured than white or black Americans. In 1997, 34% of Hispanic adults lacked health insurance, more than twice the percent of non-Hispanic white persons without health insurance coverage and almost 60% more than the numbers of African-Americans without insurance coverage (Health Care Financing Administration, 1998, 1999a; Pamuk, Makuc, Heck, Reuben, & Lochner, 1998).

Poor adults are much more likely to be uninsured regardless of race, ethnicity, or sex. Poor white, African-American, or Hispanic men are seven times as likely to be uninsured. Poor white women are eight times more likely than those with high incomes to be uninsured. At each level of income, Hispanics are more likely to be uninsured than either their white or African-American counterparts. Within most income categories, the numbers of African-American individuals without insurance are either slightly higher or similar to white individuals without insurance. Poor African-American women are less likely than poor white women to be uninsured because of their higher levels of Medicaid coverage (Pamuk et al., 1998).

Unless a major change is made in the financing system for health care, it is unlikely that these inequities will change. In fact, they have continued to increase over the last two decades and will likely continue without some type of government intervention. It does not appear that Americans are willing to establish a nationalized health care system, especially if it would compromise choice. Given this fact, it does not appear that a resolution to the growing numbers of uninsured will be forthcoming in the short run.

Importance of the Primary Care Provider

The shift to managed care mechanisms has resulted in the dominance of primary care providers who have assumed responsibility for overseeing the allocation of resources in a managed care system. In a dramatic role reversal, primary care providers have generally risen above specialists in the health care hierarchy. Primary care providers serve as gatekeepers who control access to services and specialty care in the managed care network. Many of these primary care providers are nurse practitioners who work in collaboration with large physician organizations or individual physician associations (IPAs). The functions performed by these primary care providers have been essential in managed care systems. In addition, they have given renewed interest within the medical care system to preventive and health promoting services, the hallmark of primary care providers.

Future Health Policy: Individuals versus Populations and Illness versus Wellness

The U.S. health care system is often criticized because of its overwhelming focus on illness and disease, especially given the amount of resources allocated to these types of services. A preferred approach would be to refocus services and incentives to promote health and reduce present or future risk for developing disease. While it is difficult currently to identify a clear national health policy in the United States, the focus on illness and disease is clear.

Peters (1998) states that U.S. health care policy has been built on a "clinical" model that has provided financial incentives for sophisticated technological excellence. Evidence of this includes the ongoing allocation of large amounts of the total health care dollar to hospital care and related treatments and interventions. Even in the managed care arena, it is often difficult to identify a focus or set of incentives directed toward health promotion. Often the cost savings in managed care are associated with the treatment of disease after it has developed, rather than examining cost savings associated with preventive services (Peters, 1998). An example of this would be the comparative study of breast cancer stage at diagnosis and treatment patterns for elderly women in HMO and fee-for-service settings. The results indicated that HMO enrollees are less likely to have breast cancer diagnosed at later stages than women in fee-for-service settings. While this evidence supports the importance of early detection in managed care environments, it also supports the observation that even managed care groups are often focused on cost-reducing treatments rather than extensive screening programs (Riley, Potosky, Klabunde, Warren, & Ballard-Barbash, 1999).

Kindig (1999) recommends that health policy must move beyond focusing on individuals and begin to emphasize population health as the desired outcome. In fee-for-service and capitated systems, incentives encourage providers to produce fewer hospital days and services along with lower unit prices. However, this focus on individuals fails to place individuals in a social context, ignoring the important contributions to health made by non-medical factors such as socioeconomic status, the environment, and other societal factors. Given that the general indices of health in the United States, such as mortality rates, are still at unacceptable levels, policy needs to focus on the development of incentives and services that will contribute to the overall health of populations (Moskowitz, 1997).

A paradigm shift from individual to population is beginning to appear. Managed care concepts are compatible with this population focus, although the annual turnover in many HMO enrollee groups still operates against a population incentive in the long run. Given the large investment of public funds in purchasing health care, developing policies and programs that serve as incentives for increasing the health of populations will provide improved health outcomes per dollar invested.

Implications of Slower Expansion in Future Health Care Expenditures

As mentioned previously, the U.S. health care system has undergone a 40-year expansion with continual growth and increased spending. This era is often referred to as the Golden Age of Health Care. However, recent statistics suggest that a plateau has been reached in the percentage of gross domestic product (GDP) allocated to health care in the U.S. The share of GDP for health care had been increasing gradually over a 30-year period, reaching a high point of 13.6% for the years 1993-1996. In 1997, however, health spending as a share of GDP fell slightly to 13.5% (Fisher & Welch, 1999; Health Care Financing Administration, 1999a). This plateau and slight decrease provide the first signs that the United States may no longer be able to sustain unlimited growth in expenditures for health care.

The gross indicators of morbidity and mortality are still at undesirably high levels, suggesting there is major room for improvement in the health care system. Yet, we are increasingly faced with difficult choices about how to allocate these fixed or declining resources for health care needs. The dynamics of public health care policy in a fixed state are projected to be very different from those when the health care economy was continually expanding. It is likely that the American public will face difficult decisions, including the possibility of rationing of health care. This type of decision making has been unacceptable to the American public in the past. It also is likely to exaggerate the inequities and maldistribution of health care resources still seen today.

References

Abbey, F.B. (1996). Managed care and health care reform: Evolution or revolution? In P.R. Kongstvedt (Ed.), *The managed care handbook* (3rd ed.). Gaithersburg, Md.: Aspen Publishers, Inc.

Amaradio, L. (Winter 1998). Financing long-term care for elderly persons: What are the options? *J Health Care Finance, 25,* 75-84.

Carrasquillo, O., Himmelstein, D.U., Woolhandler, S., & Bor, D.H. (1999, Jan. 14). A reappraisal of private employers' role in providing health insurance, *New England Journal of Medicine, 340,* 109-114.

Fisher, E.S., & Welch, H.G. (1999, Feb. 3). Avoiding the unintended consequences of growth in medical care: How might more be worse? *Journal of the American Medical Association, 281,* 446-453.

Fox, P.D. (1996). An overview of managed care. In P.R. Kongstvedt (Ed.), *The managed care handbook* (3rd ed.). Gaithersburg, Md.: Aspen Publishers, Inc.

Health Care Financing Administration (1998). Statistical supplement. *Health Care Financing Review.*

Health Care Financing Administration (1999a). *Highlights: National health expenditures, 1997,* http://www.hcfa.gov/stats/nhe-oact/hilites.

Health Care Financing Administration (1999b). *Highlights of the national health expenditure projections, 1997-2007,* http://www.hcfa.gov/stats/NHE-Proj/hilites.

Kindig, D.A. (1999). Purchasing population health: Aligning financial incentives to improve health outcomes, *Nursing Outlook, 47,* 15-22.

Moskowitz, D.B. (Ed.). (1997). *Health care almanac & yearbook,* New York: Faulkner & Gray, Inc.

Pamuk, E., Makuc, D., Heck, K., Reuben, C., Lochner, K. (Eds.) (1998). *Health, United States, 1998 with socioeconomic status and health chartbook.* Hyattsville, Md.: National Center for Health Statistics.

Peters, R.M. (1998). The negative effect of the clinical model of "health": Implications for health care policy. *J Health Care Finance, 25,* 78-92.

Riley, G.F., Potosky, A.L., Klabunde, C.N., Warren, J.L., Ballard-Barbash, R. (1999). Stage at diagnosis and treatment patterns among older women with breast cancer. *Journal of the American Medical Association, 281,* 720-726.

Public Policy, Managed Care, and Case Management

The Emerging Role of the Community Nurse Organization

Patricia Moritz

CHAPTER OVERVIEW

A large measure of the recent policy debate over managed care has been fueled by anecdotal reports of incidents such as emergency room care denials for acute chest pain, "drive-by" deliveries of newborns, women being discharged 24 hours after a mastectomy, and frail elders being sent home 2 days after hip replacement surgery. State and federal legislatures have responded by proposing, and often passing, legislation to regulate managed care organizations. A special Presidential Commission was also established to examine the quality of care in the health care industry, particularly managed care, and the protections available to consumers when they use the health care system. The 32-member commission included two nurses: Mary Wakefield, who directs the Center for Health Policy at George Mason University, and Beverly Malone, President of the American Nurses Association.

MANAGED CARE: A PUBLIC POLICY TARGET

The commission's interim report, *The Consumer Bill of Rights and Responsibilities,* noted seven consumer rights and 13 responsibilities. The consumer rights include information disclosure, choice of providers and health plans, access to emergency services, participation in treatment decisions, respect and nondiscrimination, confidentiality of health information, and access to a fair and efficient process for complaints and appeals. Consumer responsibilities are in such areas as developing healthy habits, becoming involved in decisions, working collaboratively with providers, abiding by a health plan's procedures and internal complaint and appeals processes, and making a good-faith effort to meet financial responsibilities.

The commission's final report, *Quality First: Better Health Care for All Americans,* built on these themes, emphasizing that "the purpose of the purpose of the health care system must be to continuously reduce the impact and burden of illness, injury, and disability and to improve the health and functioning of the people of the United States" (p. 1). In its recommendations the commission called for the formation of public and private entities to partner in articulating areas for health care improvement and strategies for quality measurement and to address access to health care for the 41.7 million Americans who are uninsured, including 10 million children. Specific core aims for improvement in health care include (1) reducing the underlying causes of illness, injury, and disability; (2) expanding research on new treatments and evidence of effectiveness; (3) ensuring the appropriateness of health care services; (4) reducing health care errors; (5) increasing patients' participation in their care; and (6) addressing the oversupply and undersupply of health care resources. This report and its predecessor articulate important areas for policy change and health care improvements that the President and others can challenge Congress and other policymakers to implement. This is an important area for nursing to advance by continuing to be active in its leadership position in health care policy. More extensive detail about these reports is available on the Internet at: ***http://www.hcqualitycommission.gov/.***

In another policy-level response the Agency of Healthcare and Quality (formerly the Agency for Health Care Policy and Research of USDHHS) has funded a consortium of health services research and policy organizations to develop and test the Consumer Assessment of Health Plans Study, or CHAPS (Crofton, Lublin, & Darby, 1999). Among the many surveys of health plans, CHAPS is uniquely designed to take the consumers' perspective, asking questions about health care experiences, identifying information that consumers want and need to know, and ensuring that the information is understandable by a variety of consumers and that the surveys are brief and easy to use. As CHAPS develops, its approach and processes may be incorporated into other consumer assessment systems such as the managed care accrediting group, the National Committee on Quality Assurance (NCQA). Further information about CHAPS can be found at ***www.ahrq.gov/*** and about NCQA at ***www.ncqa.org/.***

UNDERSTANDING THE TERMINOLOGY OF MANAGED CARE

There should be a clear understanding of the most frequently used terms in this policy debate. Managed care organizations (MCO) are public or private legal health care entities that combine two important functions: the provision of health care services and the payment for services provided to the MCOs' members. Because of these dual functions, MCOs have strong incentives to control the use of health care services by their members, the types or kinds of treatments recommended by clinicians providing care to the MCOs' members, and the costs paid for any services provided to their members. Another term used for these organizations is health plans, to distinguish them from insurers and other forms of care delivery services that do not include payment from the same organization. There are various types of MCOs, but one of the earliest and most enduring is the health maintenance organization (HMO), which enrolls about 25% of the population across the United States, with its heaviest concentrations in the Northeast and West (National Center for Health Statistics [NCHS], 1998). The limits of the "formal" health care system, however, are reflected in the 15.6% of the U.S. population in 1996 who had no form of health care coverage, while about 14% ($132.2 billion) of that year's gross national product was expended on health (NCHS, 1998).

MCOs today seem to base their decisions about coverage for services on certain assumptions, which come from an interpretation of the managed care environment, the results of health services research, and their own internal data evaluation systems. Among these are (1) that the utilization of health care can be managed; (2) that individuals seek and therefore consume too many services; (3) that much of the health care provided is unnecessary or not effective; (4) that efficiencies of scale can be achieved and costs for each enrollee lowered; and (5) that profits can be made through controlling service use and through judicious payment for those services. MCOs also have been accused of using overly broad reasons for denial of service coverage, such as the treatment is experimental, the service was not necessary, and pre-approval was not obtained.

Public organizations are distinguished from private organizations based on ownership and tax status. Public organizations are either owned by governmental agencies, such as a city or a state, or are publicly traded corporations that are for-profit, pay taxes, and have shareholders to whom they pay dividends. Private organizations are owned by individuals, groups, or not-for-profit entities, and they may be private corporations that pay taxes. In the health care arena, they may also be mission-focused, religious organization–affiliated, or privately owned by a group of people such as physicians in a specialty offering care only in a specific area such as cataract surgery.

From a policy perspective, public policies are those decisions and rules made at the national, state, or county level by individuals and organizations within the executive, legislative, and judicial branches. Public policies are usually governmental policies. Within the framework of government, public policies are "authoritative decisions" (Longest, 1998, p. 4) intended to influence the actions or decisions of those targeted by the policy. Medicare and Medicaid are two examples of public health care policies that were not originally intended to be connected to managed care but that are so connected today. Medicare is the federal entitlement program providing health care for elders and some disabled people who have paid federal Social Security taxes. Medicaid is a shared federal-state program providing for health services for the eligible poor. Both became law in 1965 as part of federal policy initiatives targeting those persons and groups who were most vulnerable, and both programs now have managed care as an optional or required component of the program.

POLICY LINKAGES OF CASE MANAGEMENT AND MANAGED CARE

The vision of MCOs is focused on the system of care delivery and cost management for large numbers of members, while the vision of those conducting case management is on the individuals receiving care. Case managers provide care coordination by assessing, planning, and organizing health care services within a framework of funds available, guidelines or protocols, and the health status of those who receive their care through managed care. Case managers have a strong advocacy role in that they represent their patients' best interests in coordinating care that is ethical and of value to all stakeholders—patients, their families, health care colleagues, and the involved MCO. Increasingly, case managers also have had to balance competing forces that influence their care delivery—the MCO, the patient, and the medical or nursing practitioner responsible for the overall care provided. This need to balance competing factors has increased the requirement that case managers have a strong clinical background as well as clinical and fiscal management expertise and a knowledge of social and psychological factors, family dynamics, and care management. Registered professional nurses are usually the best-qualified care providers to bring all of these skills and perspectives to the case manager's role.

Managed care had its start in HMOs in the late 1930s, starting with the Kaiser-Permanente program for workers in California (Birenbaum, 1997). With an emphasis on maintaining people's health as well as restoring their health, this new form of health care delivery based on a membership organization and a small common fee strategy was a component of the more recent national health planning reforms designed to increase access, facilitate quality health care, and, over time, increase cost-effectiveness. Current health planning policies are an attempt to bring organization out of the chaos that emerged from the federal Great Society legislation of the 1960s and 1970s, and they include a conscious strategy to move from a focus on illness care to emphasizing prevention, while providing the full spectrum of care. Ideally, this strategy would keep members healthy all their lives, thus increasing longevity and reducing cost over time. Premised on the idea that doing less is doing more, HMOs continue today as an important form of managed care.

A further review of how the U.S. health care system and related health policy initiatives evolved in recent years will suggest how we got to the current state of managed care as we enter the 21st century. With few exceptions until very recently, health policy, driven by decisions at the national level, was public policy. But the failure of the Clinton administration's Health Care Reform policy initiative in 1993 created a vacuum that the market-driven private sector of the health care industry filled by rapidly expanding all forms of managed care. This expansion, however, was targeted primarily at those who could pay for health care coverage and was marketed as a less expensive alternative to fee-for-service coverage. In addition, employer-provided health insurance, long a standard benefit given to workers, was becoming less and less available as employers scaled back benefits to decrease business expenses. As a result, the numbers of those who were employed in the United States without health benefits has been growing for the first time in decades.

These developments, other changes, and the resulting increases in the numbers of uninsured and underinsured people led to increasing applications for Medicaid support. The states, under fiscal pressure from the ever-growing costs of their portion of the Medicaid program, began to move segments of this population into managed care programs. This move was designed to provide health services within the funds available and at the same time put in place several of the techniques used in managed care to control service use and cost. The Medicaid managed care programs were made available in each participating state through various MCOs—for profit, not for profit, and the traditional "safety net" providers, such as public hospitals and clinics and academic health science centers. Before the government opened Medicaid managed care to for-profit as well as not-for-profit MCOs, few of these organizations were interested in having Medicaid clients because payments for services were substantially below those of any other form of coverage and because these clients were considered heavy users of health care services.

MEDICAID AND MEDICARE: THE FEDERAL PRESENCE IN MANAGED CARE

Medicaid, established in 1965 (P.L. 89-97), is a federal-state program of services to poor citizens who meet certain requirements. (Information about this law and others noted in this chapter can be found on the Library of Congress's Internet website at: *www.thomas.loc.gov/*.) The Medicaid program is not an entitlement and has an income and asset test for eligibility for coverage of services. The federal government has certain program requirements that the state governments must provide, but there is flexibility for other provisions. Eligibility for the Medicaid program was substantially affected by the Personal Responsibility and Work Opportunity Reconciliation Act of 1996 (P.L. 104-193), better known as the Welfare Reform Act. This new law ended the automatic inclusion of a key welfare benefit, Aid to Families with Dependent Children (AFDC), with Medicaid eligibility. This situation was further complicated by provisions of the Temporary Assistance to Needy Families (TANF) legislation, which replaced the federal AFDC program with block grants to those states that created work and income support programs with time restrictions. TANF allows families formerly eligible for Medicaid under AFDC to continue that eligibility, but the states have had to develop new procedures to review each client's applications for Medicaid eligibility and to enroll those qualified.

Welfare "reform" occurred because of the continuing growth in welfare costs at both the national and state levels and because, from a policy perspective, many policymakers found the concept of welfare as entitlement unacceptable. Welfare reform, however, did not stem the upward drive of Medicaid costs. To target this problem, states began to apply for waivers from federal requirements, so as to move Medicaid into a managed care format. By the end of the 1990s, many states had established Medicaid managed care programs through which existing MCOs and organizations that traditionally provided health care to the needy would compete for Medicaid recipients. While payments are low under this system, the payments are reliable as long as eligible Medicaid recipients are enrolled. Many of the various providers seek this income source because of the reliability of Medicaid, the growing numbers of uninsured who seek health care services, and the increasing costs for indigent care.

Medicaid managed care is also viewed as a source of support for uninsured and underserved children and youth. Considerable concern developed during the latter part of the 1990s about the growing number of children and youth living in poverty and lacking health care coverage. In addition, the U.S. Congress passed the Child Health Plan that provides matching funds to states that appropriate companion funding. The purpose of this legislation is to assure that children have access to health care services and some means to pay for those services. It also recognizes that children are a national and state asset that must be protected when their parents cannot support such protection.

Medicare, the national health program for elders and some disabled people, was initiated in 1965 and continues as an entitlement to all who pay federal Social Security taxes and meet eligibility requirements in terms of age or clinical condition. Medicare does not pay for all health care, but for selected benefits that have remained relatively constant since it began. Additional supplemental insurance is required for those who want to have coverage for most or all health care services under Medicare. An alteration to the Medicare law in 1986 introduced the Prospective Payment System now used to limit costs of hospital fees by setting maximum charges and time limits for certain diagnoses that fall within diagnostic-related groups (DRG). The concept of DRGs is currently the starting point for an examination of whether a variety of procedures, care strategies, and lengths of time for care in long-term care facilities and subacute care units can be "bundled" into new categories for prospective payment.

Medicare managed care is relatively new, but has already brought added pressure for the types of cost and treatment reductions already imposed on those who are served by the MCOs that offer this form of coverage. In late 1998 a number of MCOs made headlines by announcing that as of January 1999, they would no longer provide coverage to those under Medicare managed care because the announced level of payments for 1999 was too low to provide adequate service and to cover overhead. Medicare is one of the federal government's most expensive entitlement programs and is one that politicians are reluctant to reduce because elders vote more actively than any other age group. With Medicare's and managed care's imperative to manage, if not control, utilization and cost of services to members, it is likely that change and uncertainty will continue as clinicians, health care delivery settings, and consumers continue to adapt or react to policies and management strategies.

CURRENT CHARACTERISTICS OF THE U.S. HEALTH CARE SYSTEM

Change has been the most consistent feature of the U.S. health care system in recent years, and a variety of both complimentary and derogatory descriptors have been used to describe its changing nature. This change occurs at all levels, takes place under all kinds of situations, and affects all providers, payers, and consumers. The system today is market driven even when the system component is not a component of the market. Some of the factors in this change are noted here.

Turbulence and Dynamism in the Health Care Environment

Individual health care providers and systems have not been able to achieve stability in their operating environment for some time. A number of policy strategies at national, state, and corporate levels have been put in place to evaluate the effects of new ideas to constrain or control costs. The movement of market-oriented businesses into the health care industry has introduced new dynamics and uncertainties. The move of the health care system from a not-for-profit operating venue to a for-profit imperative has required considerable rethinking of mission and motivation for profits. On almost a daily basis, health care providers are notified of requirements for changes, business opportunities, or new regulations or certifications, all of which cost time and money.

Health Care Regulation

Health care is highly regulated, especially in long-term care (LTC) segment. Substantial regulation occurs for all segments of the health care industry—acute care, long-term care, ambulatory care, licensing, and the like. This regulation is both private sector and public. For example, in the private sector the Joint Commission on Accreditation for Health Care Organizations (JCAHO) sets standards and carries out accreditation assessments that have the power, if accreditation is denied, to block payments for health services to clients of federal programs. MCOs set standards and corporate goals that members' organizations are expected to achieve or their executives will be replaced. For consumers there is some distrust that the health care industry will provide readily available, high-quality care for a reasonable cost—even with some sort of prodding.

The lack of trust applies to the whole industry, but is most obvious in LTC, which is a potential policy target for managed care and prospective payment bundling of services. Without question, LTC is costly to families and has a high penetration of for-profit providers. In addition, the number of skilled nursing care facilities has been limited, causing a type of informal rationing based on ability to pay. The regulation of the long-term care segment of health care began with a series of exposes about squalid conditions in our nation's nursing homes and an influential report of the Institute of Medicine of the National Academy of Sciences (Institute of Medicine, 1987). This interdisciplinary group of experts, including nurses, determined that a total revamping of LTC was needed and recommended substantial changes. Among the changes called for were an assessment system of residents in LTC facilities (later known as the LTC minimum data set and care plan), new staffing requirements for nursing homes that included 24-hour nursing coverage (whether these were registered or licensed practical nurses became a multi-year controversy), and a substantial number of other requirements. After Congress enacted new laws, it took years to make or even initiate all the provisions.

Health Care Providers' Responsiveness to Financial Incentives

All types of health care providers respond to financial incentives, and the incentives have come in various forms, including both incentives to provide high-quality care and corresponding disincentives to providing care at all. Some types of incentives have been questioned as representing a conflict of interest if responded to by health care providers who also have a duty to provide the most appropriate care that a client or group of clients requires. This is a potential quagmire for managed care, as MCOs have a history of providing both incentives and disincentives to meet MCO goals that may or may not be in the clients' best interests. However, setting rules for types, levels, and costs of care can change provider decisions. It is also believed that if such goals are not stated, providers will act to maximize their incomes regardless of the need or the effectiveness of the services used.

Health Care as a Market-Focused and Market-Driven Entity

An unregulated marketplace in any business sector will focus on value (however defined), with the objective of maximizing profits. There is growing concern—expressed in recent issues of the publications of health professions' organizations—that the overriding emphasis in health care decision making has shifted to a focus on cost-saving and profit-making at the expense of quality of care as the health care industry shifts from a mostly not-for-profit and mission-focused set of institutions to a for-profit and market-focused set of enterprises.

Some have tried to define a balance between quality and cost that represents "value," and others have called for a change in strategic focus from cost-cutting and profit to an emphasis on quality care in a cost-effective modality. Such a strategy was the underlying theme of a conference held in 1995 to examine ways to move from the current situation to one that is more patient care oriented. The report of this conference notes that consumer choice, quality care, accountability for services and practitioners, and public disclosure of evaluation and quality report data are vital elements in assuring a certain level of quality care. In addition, making known the rights that patients forfeit once they sign up as a health plan member, such as their right to sue for malpractice, was considered critically important and should be disclosed before the patient or family joins a health plan (Baer, Fagin, & Gordon, 1996).

Use of Community-Based Alternatives That are not Population Focused

Health care was essentially a set of services provided by hospitals and primary care providers in the mid-part of the 20th century. Into the late 1970s, health policy emphasized providing access to larger segments of our population and increasing the numbers of primary care providers both to increase access and to provide a more health promotion– and disease prevention–focus within service delivery. The 1980s saw a major shift in health policy toward a market perspective, as health care increasingly became viewed as a commody rather than a social good. With this change came a variety of health service delivery mechanisms, still present today, and the organization of health care horizontally and vertically into for-profit or not-for-profit corporations.

Despite a decided trend toward providing health care outside of institutions, there has been no major move to population-focused health care. Whenever a population perspective is taken, it is usually from that of a particular managed care health plan rather than that of a community's population. Today there is an emphasis on integrated health care delivery systems in which patients receive their care in the setting deemed most appropriate and within the fiscal constraints of their health plans. This usually means care in the community outside of an acute care setting and requires an increasing proportion of self-care or family care. This potentially leaves individual health plan participants in a situation where care is in the community, but care coordination is not. This is an important opportunity for nursing case management.

Self-Care and Family Care—The Unspoken Policy Expectation

Health care today relies on the individuals receiving care to take care of themselves or for family members to care for them. Recognizing that health care delivery in the past provided health as well as social and personal care, governmental and corporate policymakers have been making clear that health care is expensive and should only be provided when it is clearly required. Health care today provides the service, the intervention, and then the individual—not the health plan—is responsible for himself or herself. The gap is an expansion of self-care requirements that are usually not proactively articulated in MCO publications. One practice requirements for nurse case managers to sort out is gaining clarity about the health care services available, how they are provided, and under what circumstances. These case managers are also responsible for coordinating care to meet the integrity requirements of both professional responsibility and personal responsibility to the employing or contracting health plan.

Technology: Part of the Solution and Part of the Problem

Technology enables the gathering and analysis of information about multiple aspects of the health care system and services provided, their costs, and their effectiveness as well as appropriateness. Such information is crucial to nursing; without it nursing cannot demonstrate its effectiveness. Many recent efforts have been made to make nursing terms more available in clinical and other databases so that, when searching for information on a topic, nursing information is inherent in the vocabulary and readily available. Cutting-edge technology in the United States with new techniques and devices is available every day. This proliferation in technology is believed to be one of the drivers of health care costs, but it also can help to contain and expand costs. Where is the balance, and how is it achieved?

THE COMMUNITY NURSING ORGANIZATION: CASE MANAGEMENT AS AN ELEMENT OF POLICY

The U.S. Congress has provided a unique opportunity for nursing to demonstrate its effectiveness in case management by mandating the demonstration and evaluation of nurse case management provided in the community. The Community Nursing Organization (CNO) Demonstration presented a wonderful opportunity for nursing to participate in shaping an important part of managed care—care for some the most vulnerable in our society: elders and those with disabilities who are covered by Medicare (Daly & Mitchell, 1996). The inclusion of this innovative approach to providing community nursing and ambulatory care services was mandated by the Omnibus Budget Reconciliation Act (OBRA) of 1987 (P.L. 100-203), which provided a new payment mechanism for Medicare-covered community and out-patient care. Using a capitated payment approach that provides a set fee for each participant, the CNO was designed to change a recognized problem—the lack of a single health care professional to coordinate Medicare community health services—and to replace the multiple payment methods for those services, including predetermined fee schedules, reasonable costs, and prevailing charges. The then-current system was seen by the writers of the legislation as providing inadequate, fragmented, and inappropriate care, leading to increased frailty and possible deterioration in health and function as a result, and possibly contributing to the rising costs of care. The CNO was seen as a way to examine the feasibility of reducing fragmentation while increasing coordination and appropriate use of care. The ability to bridge hospital and home care and to continue successful living at home has long been a major problem for elders requiring multi-service care (Kersten & Hackenitz, 1991). The design was such that nurses practicing in the CNO would have more freedom to prescribe nursing care and coordinate various other clinical services to meet the participants' assessed requirements.

However, there was a 7-year period between the 1987 legislation and the first real demonstration project in 1993. The nation's nursing leadership had worked for years with great tenacity just to get the legislation enacted, and they spent those intervening years working to get the rules written and to get federal agency officials to provide funding for the start-up of the CNOs.

The purposes of the CNO Demonstration, initiated late in 1993, were (1) to test whether a system of capitated community nursing care with nurse-centered decision making and coordination of services could exist as a fully operational, free-standing, and financially viable organization and (2) to determine the effect of membership in a CNO on Medicare beneficiaries' use of services, both CNO-related and others, such as inpatient hospital care. The OBRA of 1987 specified a package of services for the CNO in two parts: mandatory services and suggested optional services that the CNO could chose to offer. Funds for mandatory services were provided by a premium paid by the participants; optional services required an additional payment.

Few of the CNOs in the demonstration chose to offer optional services, which included such items as homemaker services, home health aide services, personal care in the home, adult day care, and respite services. The mandatory services included case management to coordinate health services for a group of participants; intermittent nursing care furnished by or under the supervision of registered professional nurses; physical, occupational, or speech therapy; social and related services supportive of ambulatory care; services of a home health aide; medical supplies and durable medical equipment while under a plan of care; and medical services, rural health clinic services, and ambulance services as required by the location of the CNO.

Each of the four CNO sites brought unique perspectives, organization, and types of services and was building on a history of providing community nursing services. The sites included in the CNO demonstration and evaluation were as follows:

1. Carondelet Health Care (CHC) in Tucson, Arizona, which includes three hospitals, family center, and community centers and is a division of the Carondelet Health System based in Missouri. CHC had nursing case management system in place at the time of the initiation of the CNO (Ethridge, 1997).
2. Visiting Nurse Service of New York in New York City, arguably the largest not-for-profit home health agency in the nation, providing multiple services and products in several boroughs of the city (Storfjell, Mitchell, & Daly, 1997).
3. Carle Clinic in Mahomet, Illinois, a large regional multispecialty medical group with a large nursing component, including advanced practice nurses, and a network of community based clinics that serve predominately rural residents in two states (Schraeder & Britt, 1997; Schraeder, Shelton, Britt, & Buttitta, 1996).
4. Living at Home/Block Nurse Program, St. Paul, Minnesota, a community service that organizes, supports, and supplements existing community resources with a mix of services, including nursing, counseling, transport, personal care, and others, through a program of trained volunteers and nurse support for elders.

All Medicare enrollees residing in a specified catchment area who were receiving benefits under Parts A (hospital services) and B (medical equipment, ambulatory services) with few exceptions (e.g., those receiving hospice care) were eligible to enroll in the CNO. The CNOs' payment system was capitated for each enrollee, meaning that the CNO received a set monthly dollar amount for each enrollee no matter what level of services was used. All care was to be provided under the supervision of a registered nurse, with each enrolled participant having a primary nurse provider responsible for case management and, at times, direct care. The goals for the CNO case management strategy were to promote continuity of care, reduce unneeded care, increase independence and function, prevent hospitalization and institutionalization of clients, promote participant and family involvement in decisions and care, and increase use of appropriate prevention strategies. The foci of this strategy combine multiple aspects of managed care with unique clinical nursing imperatives, such as client and family involvement and increasing independence and function.

Three aspects of the CNOs are important to nursing: (1) the opportunity to initiate and evaluate a community-based nursing strategy that clarifies and enhances nursing role and functions; (2) the expansion of traditional home care and primary care functions into a coherent case management approach that includes both; and (3) the recognition of the importance of increasing access to nursing services. The CNOs provide an environment to demonstrate the effects of nursing coordination, monitoring, and surveillance; teaching and counseling; client-partnered decision making; family-centered approaches; and clinical care that integrates prevention, clinical coordination, service management, and advocacy.

The demonstration and evaluation is the first effort to examine a partially capitated model for the delivery of Medicare services using a model of nursing managed and delivered community and ambulatory services. To obtain some degree of consistency in the approach to documenting management, clinical, and fiscal information, the four CNO sites agreed to partially implement the Omaha nursing classification system for community health nursing (Martin & Scheet, 1992) for the clients in the demonstration. The plan was to have a common clinical language with a consistent set of terms for assessment, interventions, and outcomes used across the four sites so that data used for analyses and comparisons would be more reliable. However, although all sites implemented case management, each site was free to use their judgment in deciding what form of case management they would implement to meet their participants' needs. Unfortunately, this failure to experimentally control the implementation across sites or participants severely limited the demonstration's usefulness in determining and differentiating the effect of case management on evaluation outcomes (Schmitz et al., 1996).

The evaluation was designed to include both quantitative (Medicare enrollment and claims data, CNO service records) and qualitative (interviews, telephone surveys) approaches to determine outcome effects of CNO enrollment on participants. Descriptive data were to be examined and outcomes analyses focused on factors such as access to services, continuity and quality of services, health status, function, quality of life, satisfaction, and mortality. Having only four CNO sites in the demonstration makes it difficult to "distinguish the distinct effects of capitation and case management on . . . outcomes, utilization, or cost" of CNO services (Schmitz et al., 1996, pp. 1-4). There are issues inherent in evaluating a program where the participants whose data will be used in the evaluation self-select into the intervention being examined. However, there are mechanisms for working with this issue, including using comparison groups, which is planned in the evaluation.

Participants receiving care through the CNOs have various levels of health status, function, and illness, making some participants more high risk that others for higher utilization, having multiple co-existing conditions, and raising the overall cost for the CNO. Being able to stratify CNO participants into groups of participants with varying risk factors should enable more accurate findings in the evaluation. The leaders of the CNO sites believe that it is crucial to carry out risk stratification in the evaluation because in their clinical impression, CNOs may be substantially less expensive for the higher risk participants (Lamb, 1999). In addition, clinical evaluation in an active, real-world, changing situation is a challenge for evaluators in meeting specification and consistency requirements for data accuracy and reliability with the use of a single classification system for all four sites assists. It will be some time before the final results of the CNO evaluation are available.

The CNO program was extended by the U.S. Congress into 1998 (Vanderbilt, 1996), which has delayed dissemination of findings. The CNO demonstrations should continue into the 21st century, but their longer-term future is uncertain because of the program's uniqueness and the need for a more permanent policy decision if the program is deemed effective and cost worthy in the CNO evaluation. This extraordinary opportunity to have nursing and its contributions recognized at the national policy levels is a significant indicator of the strength and importance of nursing's role in the nation's health care system. However, we must remember that the leadership and hard work of nurses involved in health policy, managed care, and providing case management to our most vulnerable populations were essential in making opportunities such as the CNO Demonstration available, and enabling nursing to demonstrate its effectiveness.

SUMMARY

Case management is an established and vital component of nursing practice that has been incorporated in varying ways and degrees into the myriad strategies of managed care organizations and programs. Nursing case management most effectively enables providers to meet individuals' health care needs and requirements while also meeting the system demands of managed care—striking the balance among quality, cost, equity, and integrity.

References

Aday, L.U., Begley, C.E., Lairson, D.R., & Slater, C.H. (1998). *Evaluating the healthcare system: Effectiveness, efficiency, and equity*. Chicago: Health Administration Press.

Advisory Commission on Consumer Protection and Quality in the Health Care Industry (1997). *Consumer bill of rights and responsibilities*. Washington, D.C.: Executive Office of the President.

Baer, E.D., Fagin, C.M., & Gordon, S. (1996). *Abandonment of the patient*. New York: Springer Publishing.

Birenbaum, A. (1997). *Managed care: Made in America*. Westport, Conn.: Praeger.

Crofton, C., Lublin, J.S., & Darby, C. (1999). Consumer assessment of health plans study (CHAPS): Foreword. *Med Care, 37*, MS1.

Daly, G.M., & Mitchell, R.D. (1996). Case management in the community setting. *Nursing Clinics of North America, 31*, 527.

Ethridge, P. (1997, March). Historical perspective: The Carondelet experience. *Nursing Management, 28*(3), 26-27.

Institute of Medicine (1987). *The quality of nursing homes*. Washington, D.C.: National Academy Press.

Kersten, D., & Hackenitz, E. (1991). How to bridge the gap between hospital and home? *Journal of Advanced Nursing, 16*, 4.

Lamb, G.S. (1999, March 12). Personal communication.

Longest, B.B. (1998). *Health policy making in the United States*. Chicago: Health Administration Press.

Martin, K.S., & Scheet, N.J. (1992a). *The Omaha system: Applications for community health nursing*. Philadelphia: W.B. Saunders

Martin, K.S., & Scheet, N.J. (1992b). *The Omaha system: A pocket guide for community health nursing*. Philadelphia: W.B. Saunders.

National Center for Health Statistics (NCHS). (1998). *Health, United States chartbook*. Hyattsville, Md.: NCHS.

Schmitz, R.J., Axelrod, E., Goldberg, H., LeBlond, K., Murphy, M., Teitelbaum, M., & Thomas, L. (1996). *Evaluation of the community nursing organization demonstration: Interim report*. Cambridge, Mass.: Abt Associates.

Schraeder, C., Shelton, P., Britt, T., & Buttitta, K. (1996, Summer). Case management in a capitated system: The community nursing organization. *Journal of Case Management, 5*(2), 58.

Schraeder, C., & Britt, T. (1997, March). The Carle Clinic: Case study three. *Nursing Management, 28*(3), 32.

Storfjell, J.I., Mitchell, R., & Daly, G.M. (1997, Oct.) Nurse-managed healthcare: New York's community nursing organization. *Journal of Nursing Administration, 27*(10), 21-27.

Vanderbilt, M. (1996, Nov.-Dec.) ANA succeeds in getting community nursing organization project extended one year. *American Nurse, 28*(8), 15.

VI

THE PLANNING PROCESS
Developing Collaborative Relationships

Relationships are the foundation of any organization and the building blocks of any successful change process. In order to develop successful partnerships within any organization, a commitment to planned change must be made. Unit VI outlines the assessment data needed to affect a successful change to case management. The assessment process must include an analysis of the organization itself as well as the role functions of its members. With that information at the ready, the change agent can begin to design and implement a successful case management system. A sound educational program will also assist the organization in planning for this change and should not be neglected during the planning process. Included in this section are design options for educational programs within any learning organization.

Assessing the System and Creating an Environment for Change

CHAPTER OVERVIEW

Successful implementation of a case management system begins with a solid, well-conceived plan. The first step in creating the plan is to assess the system in which the case management model will be implemented. Human and financial resources should be reviewed. This information helps determine the degree of change that the organization can tolerate and the chances for a successful conversion.

Implementation involves a nine-step process. Target patient populations are identified and matched to nursing units, and the design structure for the units is decided. This new structure involves a change in the staff mix. The next step is the formation of interdisciplinary groups. These groups consist of the case manager, physician(s), social worker, and any other pertinent health care professionals. Benchmarks, which determine how the change will be monitored and evaluated over time, must be selected. Before implementation takes place, pre-implementation data must be collected. The next step involves educating staff, physicians, and other professionals who will be affected by conversion to the case management model. At this stage, training is provided for the case managers. After managers are educated on how the model works, it can be implemented. Finally, evaluation should take place at predetermined intervals. Necessary changes should be made as quickly as possible.

FEASIBILITY OF THE MODEL

Converting to a case management model requires systematic planning. A solid plan that has been well thought out guarantees a higher rate of successful conversion. Without a plan, it is likely that the expected outcome of the model will be lost or that some important elements will be left out.

Administrators have always known that a plan is essential for change in any organization. This philosophy is no less true for nurses attempting to create a major change such as a conversion to a case management model. The first step in any planning process is to determine if the change is not only feasible but also worthwhile. The potential for success and the effect such a change will have on the organization must be evaluated from both a positive and negative perspective. Overall, the change should lead the organization in a positive direction.

ASSESSMENT OF RESOURCES

Assessing resources requires some homework. A thorough analysis of the organization, including its structure and financial status, must be done. Those implementing the change need to determine if the organization is strong enough to withstand the temporary instability that will accompany the change. As with any major change, errors will be made along the way. The complete support of all top administrators and a commitment to the long haul are absolutely necessary. In the beginning the road will be bumpy, and everyone concerned should be aware of this and ready to be supportive every step of the way.

THE COST OF IMPLEMENTATION

A case management system can be implemented with few additional personnel costs for the organization if the change is implemented carefully. For instance, good choices for the pilot program would be units that have current openings or units that have budgeted for an additional person. Such an opening can then be filled by someone qualified to be a case manager. In this way the new position will not incur any costs outside of those already budgeted. This is essential for a plan that must show success before it receives an allotment in the budget. Internal and preexisting resources can then be used for implementation.

If possible, the organization's budget should allow for certain expenditures needed for implementation. These expenditures will probably not be related to personnel costs unless the organization decides to hire a project manager. Costs may be incurred for documentation system changes or for data collection and statistical analysis necessary for measuring success. Additional resources needed include clerical support staff to perform such functions as faxing, photocopying, ordering durable medical equipment (DME), and providing transportation. The use of clerical staff can be an important adjunct to the professional staffing. In some cases the use of clerical support staff may mean that the professional staff can carry a higher caseload.

Today's contemporary case management departments also need to have computerized support in the form of databases, case management software programs, and hardware. Hardware may include laptops, hand- or palm-held computers, scanning capability, and variance collection and analysis capability (Favor & Ricks, 1996).

Both administrative and financial support must be obtained before switching over to a case management system.

INTERNAL MARKETING

Obtaining the support of those in senior management is relatively easy if the administrators already have some familiarity with the model. Senior management may have heard or read about the model and already have realized the need for such a change. Conversely, they may have misconceptions or may be misinformed about the model. Senior management might also object to the change solely because it comes at an inopportune time.

National managed care infiltration has now created an environment in which most forward-thinking organizations recognize that systems must be implemented that truly and consistently control cost and quality. Infiltration may be real or anticipated. In either case, senior administrators must support a conceptual and actual shift to case management. This process is much less difficult than it was even 10 years ago. Status quo is no longer an option, and each organization must determine what changes are needed to support a constantly changing health care environment.

Senior management support is a prerequisite for beginning the change process. The ways change may be attained are as diverse as the management styles of the individuals involved. Making sure that administrators are familiar with those initiating the change, and that they have positive working relationships with them, is essential for success.

Furthermore, the concept of the case management system should be introduced by someone who is familiar with the administrator, the president, the executive vice president of operations, and the chief financial officer. Essentially all executive staff of the organization should be included. Use of an outside consultant to introduce the concept may provide the catalyst the organization needs for change. The individual who introduces the concept to the administrator must have the facts of implementation readily available. Estimated cost, staffing needs, and time frames must be prepared for the first meeting. Expected outcomes, goals, and long-range plans should also be presented. A review of other organizations that have implemented the concept and have had positive results lends credibility to the proposed plan.

It may be necessary to explain the definition of case management from a care delivery perspective if the administrator has no previous knowledge of the model. Emphasis should be placed on how the model benefits all disciplines. Finally, but possibly most important, it is necessary to review the financial implications of conversion. An initiative whose goal is to reduce patient length of stay may be the best-selling feature in today's financial climate. An explanation as to why a nurse may be best suited to monitor this process may take some extra effort. Many people believe that social work, utilization review, or physicians themselves should be the facilitators and coordinators of the care plan. Other initiatives aimed at reducing length of stay may already have been attempted. The failure of these initiatives may help convince administrators to try a new approach. It is important to emphasize that although nursing drives the process, all disciplines must take part in achieving success. The input and participation of all health care providers are essential. The keys to case management's success are its nursing and interdisciplinary approaches.

Within the prospective payment system, length of stay can determine financial success or failure. However, in a discussion of how case management affects a reduction in length of stay, how length of stay affects quality should also be emphasized. The cost/quality ratio as it relates to case management must be reviewed. Any initiative that reduces length of stay without looking at quality and resources is doomed to fail the organization and the patients.

Although length of stay continues to be the clearest and most tangible way to measure financial success, other measures may add additional credibility. If available, a cost-accounting system helps identify reductions in the use or misuse of hospital resources. Other parallel reductions must also be seen. If the length of stay is reduced but the amount of resources is simply collapsed into fewer days, true financial savings are less likely.

In managed care reimbursement systems, shortened length of stay and overall cost reductions remain extremely important. Capitated or per diem managed care rates still require serious and consistent cost reductions.

The support of nursing administration is another vital component. Nurse managers and upper managers must support the concept fully to achieve success. Some suspicion may initially be felt as nursing roles change. The nurse manager may feel threatened by the introduction of another individual who is also managing care on the unit. Other departments most directly involved in the change process, and from whom support is needed, include social work, utilization management, and discharge planning. Initial and on-going support is essential here.

Before the advent of the prospective payment system, flex time, increased severity levels, and technology, the nurse manager carried out many of the role functions associated with case management, such as facilitation and coordination of patient care services. As the nurse manager's role expanded and became more administrative, the nurse had less time to focus on facilitating and coordinating the progression of patient care. It is necessary to emphasize that the new concept will allow the nurse manager to concentrate more on administrative functions, which will in turn mean patients receive a higher quality of care. Reducing the sense of personal threat is essential to effecting a positive change.

Downsizing and restructuring in health care organizations has in many cases eliminated the assistant director of nursing position. There is often no nursing administrator between the nurse manager and the director of nursing. Elimination of this position has placed a greater administrative responsibility on the nurse manager. Add accelerated hospital stays to the equation, and the result is a less than efficient system.

Case managers, if provided with the authority and accountability necessary, can become the clinical eyes and ears for the nurse manager. Additionally, another fallout of the downsizing era has been elimination of many nurse educator positions. Perhaps among the most dangerous of reductions, removal of nurse educator positions has meant that unit-based staff development has suffered. This is particularly true for new staff nurses who need significant and consistent ongoing support. Although traditionally case managers have focused on patient and family education, in downsized environments they may need to incorporate staff education. This may take the form of case conferences or unit-based in-service training geared toward specific clinical issues.

STAFF INTEGRATION

If the nursing chief executive initiated the change to case management, then the staff might already accept the change. In this case, conversation with this group should concentrate on explaining the case management concept thoroughly and the changes it will bring.

The need to educate and fully enlist the support of staff nurses cannot be emphasized enough. If the organization has decided to create the case manager position as a staff position, then staff nurses must be fully aware of the role. The job expectations of the case manager should be clear. If available, the job description should be distributed and reviewed. The role of the case manager in relation to other nursing positions should be made as clear as possible.

As with the introduction of any new position, there may be some initial role blending, role conflict, or both. This can be minimized through open discussion and ongoing review of the role after implementation. Nurses should anticipate that roles and responsibilities will evolve over time. The fluid nature of the position means it can be improved and enhanced as a part of the evaluation process. Some role blending and confusion related to the changing roles of nursing and other disciplines, particularly social work and utilization management, can be expected. Job descriptions must be reviewed and amended to reflect the changing roles of all members of the health care team.

The collaborative nature of the model means that all disciplines must support it. At the top of this list are the physicians. Getting the involvement of both medical physicians and surgeons requires varying techniques, with emphasis placed on the outcomes achievable for their patients. Rogers says, "It is important to use nurses well known to the physicians, who have a history of solid communication, mutual trust, clinical experience, and an overall positive experiential record. This serves to gain the initial support of physicians who might otherwise be resistant" (Rogers, M. Personal communication, 1992.)

For the surgeon who is reimbursed on a case basis, the incentive to discharge the patient more rapidly is a financial one because the discharge of one patient allows for the admission of the next. In addition, surgeons traditionally have treated patients in a protocoled manner. In this setting the applicability of the case management approach is easily understood and appreciated. Because the surgical patient generally runs a predictable course of recovery, care can be planned in an organized way. For this reason, surgeons are probably those most receptive to implementation of the concept.

The medical physician may pose a greater challenge. Within the prospective payment system and most managed care contracts, no financial incentives motivate these professionals to discharge patients more rapidly. Furthermore, it may be more difficult to predict the course of events for a particular medical diagnosis or condition. As the extent of managed care penetration has accelerated, some managed care organizations have begun to implement financial penalties on the physician for hospital days during which an acute care level of service was not rendered. Until recently, only the hospital received a denial of payment from the third party payer for days of service that were below the acute care level. By denying payment to the physician as well as the hospital, the managed care organization is producing incentives for the physician to be responsible and accountable for these non-reimbursable days.

Incentives motivating the medical physician toward an appreciation of the case management approach are probably not based on length of stay improvements unless these length of stay reductions are tied to quality issues. For example, are significant days added to the hospital stay during which little or nothing is being done for the patient? Emphasizing that improved quality of care will result may be one way to enlist physician support. Emphasis on the role of the case manager in assuring, with the multidisciplinary action plan, that the physician's best plan is initiated and followed may also help enlist support.

In some cases other initiatives may be useful. If the institution has several medical diagnoses whose lengths of stay are beyond state or federal averages, these should be targeted for initial intervention. In these cases the chief physician may need to intervene. Essentially a practice guideline would be established that all physicians caring for a particular type of patient would be expected to follow. Whenever possible, active and positive participation is preferred.

Chart review and research are other techniques used to sell a treatment plan for a particular medical condition. Chart review often uncovers various ways to treat a medical problem. Each plan may not be equally effective, financially appropriate concerning resource use, or equally appropriate in terms of length of stay. By using chart review, inappropriate physician and nursing treatment interventions can be enhanced. The way other institutions treat particular types of problems can be used as a resource to determine the best possible treatment plan.

If the organization supports the notion that decreased variation in treatment will reduce costs and improve quality, more aggressive measures may be necessary. For example, if all admitted patients are to be treated under a particular case management plan, then a mandate from the president of the organization may be necessary. If there is a case management plan available for a particular case type, all patients admitted who match that case type should be treated consistently. Regardless of whether the patient is a service or private-pay patient or of whether the attending physician is in full agreement, that practice plan is initiated for that patient. This sort of global support may not be possible without a decree from a top administrator who has the power to demand uniform clinical management.

Standardized treatment plans are a great resource and asset for the resident or intern house staff. In addition, the case manager serves as a skilled resource for the new physician who is rotating through a particular nursing unit and is unfamiliar with the patient's present or past condition. In addition, the case manager helps the house officer elicit quick and accurate information. Ongoing dialogue between the two helps assure that the best plan will be carried out.

Case management cannot be completely successful without the support and cooperation of ancillary departments. It is doubtful that an ancillary department will object to the model, although passive support is not enough to ensure success. To empower the case manager, a contact person in each department should be assigned to whom needs or concerns about patients can be referred.

Some areas play a bigger part than others. For example, the radiology department plays a key role in some length of stay issues. Appropriate scheduling of tests in terms of order and timeliness is crucial to an early diagnosis and treatment. Appropriate preparation also ensures that the patient's movement through the hospital is smooth.

Other ancillary departments, which play a key role in the case management model, are the admitting office, the medical records department, the pharmacy, the laboratory, and the emergency department. Failure to obtain the support and commitment of these departments will create problems during implementation and evaluation of the model.

Clearly, other direct care providers must be fully supportive and committed for the model to be most effective. Key areas for such support include social work, physical therapy, and nutrition. The patient problem or surgery determines the areas most vital at any particular time, but certainly each department should be fully educated and agreeable before implementation.

Most ancillary departments appreciate the opportunity to work collaboratively with other disciplines. Nursing is not the only discipline plagued by frustration because of the divergent directions taken by each group of providers.

PLANNED CHANGE

A plan for implementation provides the foundation for successful change. Each element outlined in this chapter should be evaluated and acted on if appropriate for the institution. Planning for implementation should be carefully thought out and choreographed. The nine-step plan for implementation outlined in Box 24-1 provides the foundation for the plan and identifies subsequent changes. This nine-step process provides a structure for planning any implementation program. Each element is reviewed and every aspect covered during the planning process. The ordering of each step may vary, depending on the institution, and certain steps may occur simultaneously.

Clearly the order is not as important as the actual carrying out of each step. This implementation process should be shared with everyone in the organization as the process is begun. The plan's steps for implementation, the ways in which those steps will be carried out, and the method of evaluation should be shared openly so that all those concerned have a chance to give input.

Box 24-1 ▶ NINE-STEP PLAN FOR IMPLEMENTATION

1. Define target populations for case management.
2. Define target areas.
3. Agree on design structure for areas selected.
4. Form collaborative practice groups.
5. Choose benchmarks.
6. Collect pre-implementation data.
7. Provide advanced skills and knowledge.
8. Implement model.
9. Evaluate model.

Because it will be advantageous to demonstrate some immediate success, selecting where to begin is important. A bad choice may mean failure or the cancellation of plans for adding units or teams to the model.

Step 1: Define Target Populations for Case Management

Target patient populations are selected based on the following factors:

    Volume of discharges
    Variance from length of stay standards
    Variance from length of stay at similar institutions
    Feasibility of developing case management plans
    Potential for control of resource consumption
    Opportunity for improvement in quality of care

If the organization's goal for implementation is to improve quality of care, this may be an additional factor to consider during the selection process. This determination can be made through chart reviews of targeted populations.

Step 2: Define Target Areas

Once the selection of patient populations has been made, these patients are matched to appropriate clinical areas. In some cases the type of patient group selected may not be found in one particular area of the hospital; therefore a *non-unit-based* case management team approach may be more appropriate. Some case management designs that are non-unit-based follow product lines, service lines, disease groups, populations, or across the continuum.

In other cases it will be possible to gather patients from a designated geographic area. The more homogeneous the patient population on a nursing unit, the fewer the resources needed in terms of physicians and case management plans. Thus the model will positively affect a greater number of patients.

Step 3: Agree on Design Structure for Areas Selected

Once the nursing unit, geographic area, or patient type has been selected, the design structure is determined. If a *unit-based* model is being introduced, a determination must be made as to how many case managers will be on the unit. This decision is based on the number of patient beds, the severity of the patients' conditions, the average length of stay, and the available resources. If only one position is available for conversion, this may be the deciding factor. Additional factors to consider include the role functions of the case manager. The three common role functions of a hospital-based case manager include clinical coordination/facilitation, utilization management, and discharge planning. Beyond these core functions the case manager may be responsible for outcomes data collection or research, variance analysis, quality management, or patient education. The more functions that are combined in the role, the smaller the caseload will need to be.

If a *non-unit-based* case management model is being implemented, different factors are considered. Most case management teams have members from several disciplines. Therefore this type of team may require a greater number of resources for implementation. A physician, nurse, social worker, and others must be deployed, which may mean taking them away from other jobs or assignments, thereby requiring a greater financial commitment from the organization. The disciplines represented depend on the particular clinical type being followed by the team. For example, a diabetes team clearly needs a nutritionist and a social worker. Consultants with an affiliation to the team might include a podiatrist or an ophthalmologist.

An additional factor to consider during this step is the integration of beyond-the-walls clinical areas such as clinics, physician offices, and home care, among others. Relationships between the hospital-based case manager and these non-acute clinical areas must be considered in the design. Managed care areas, particularly those with capitated reimbursements, must allot time in the design phase to think about how case management might be structured in these areas (Swindle, Weyant, & Mar, 1994). More detailed information on community-based case management programs can be found in Unit IV.

Step 4: Form Collaborative Practice Groups

In the *unit-based* model the teams have a fluid structure, and the members of the team constantly change. The only constant member is the unit-based case manager. The patient, physician, social worker, and so on change as the professionals assigned to the patient change. For each new patient the case manager must gather a team, identify who is responsible for which aspects of the care plan, and ensure that everyone is working toward the same goals.

In the *non-unit-based* case management model the professional team members remain constant, and the only changing member is the patient. In this model the team members and their respective roles are clearly defined up front, so there is no need to bring the group together.

Step 5: Choose Benchmarks

As discussed in another chapter, choosing the outcome measures or benchmarks is an important step. Benchmarks must be selected as early as possible and certainly before implementation. The method of evaluation depends on the outcome measures chosen and the resources available for tracking the data.

Step 6: Collect Pre-Implementation Data

Once the benchmarks have been selected, the method for data collection is determined. The time frames are documented in advance and the individuals responsible for the various elements identified.

It may be necessary and appropriate to enlist the help of employees from other departments who have access to certain data. For example, a representative from the data support or the medical records department might be assigned the responsibility of monitoring and tracking the length of stay data. A representative from the quality improvement department might be recruited to track quality of care data on a quarterly basis. In some cases, it may even be possible to use students to assist with staff and patient questionnaires. A patient representative might be another good choice to help with patient satisfaction questionnaires.

Regardless of the data being evaluated, baseline data sets must be established before education or implementation of the model. If the staff is being tested via questionnaires, those questionnaires must be distributed and returned before implementation. Some of the data are retrospective; therefore the actual time when the data are pulled together is not as important.

Step 7: Provide Advanced Skills and Knowledge

In Chapter 12 the elements of a good educational program are reviewed and discussed. Employees from all departments must understand the general concepts of a case management system. To attain such understanding, an educational program may be offered, but the extent of such a program depends on the resources available.

The case managers should be provided with as extensive a program as possible. It cannot be assumed that an employee comes to the position with the skills and knowledge necessary to carry out the role effectively. An investment and commitment from the organization for providing advanced skills and knowledge help develop highly effective case managers. The need for education cannot be overemphasized.

To prevent contamination of subjects, educational preparation must follow any pre-implementation data collection. This maintains the integrity of the study sample.

Step 8: Implement Model

Once all the previous steps have been accomplished, the model can be effectively implemented. The date for beginning is clearly communicated. The case management documentation system selected may or may not be in place; although it is desirable, it is not essential. The case manager can begin changing the system immediately after entering the position. Having the case manager begin the changes might be the only practical way because other employees do not have the time or advanced skills necessary to make this change.

The question is often asked, "How do we begin?" The answer to this question is simple—*by beginning*. The transition phase, or the time between announced implementation and a full integration of the change, may be as long as a year or more. Therefore, after completing all pre-implementation steps, the case manager can work in the change gradually. It will take many months for all those involved to adjust to the system.

This time period requires communication with other members of the health care team, letting them know that the changeover has taken place and exactly what that means to them and to the organization. The more open and candid the communication, the more likely the change will be accepted. The beginning is when many organizations falter because they expect much of the change to have already been made. This expectation, however, is not practical. Everyone must understand in advance that the bulk of the changes will be phased in slowly.

Step 9: Evaluate Model

Evaluation of the model involves rigorous data collection and analysis. Unit VI covers the evaluation process in detail. The time frames for analysis are driven by the data elements themselves. Some data, such as length of stay, are collected and analyzed monthly. Other data, such as patient satisfaction, may only need to be tracked every 6 months. Annual tracking of staff satisfaction is sufficient.

In addition to this formal data collection and analysis, an informal evaluation should be ongoing. Those responsible for the model should never forget to query practitioners who work day by day within the model at the patient's bedside. Through discussions with the staff nurses and others, problem areas can be identified and corrective action taken. This ongoing dialogue may continue for 1 to 2 years while the change is being integrated. As the model expands, more and more employees will be affected. Barriers for successful integration continue to appear as the model expands in sophistication and sphere of influence.

References

Favor, G., & Ricks, R. (1996). Preparing to automate the case management process. *Nursing Case Management,* 1(3), 100-106.

Swindle, D.N., Weyant, J.L., & Mar, P.S. (1994). Nurse case management: Collaboration beyond the hospital walls. *Journal of Case Management, 3*(2), 51-52.

Case Management Education

*Preparing for Successful
Implementation*

CHAPTER OVERVIEW

Education is an essential element in successful implementation of a case management model. This chapter reviews the two types of curricula required for implementation of a case management model. The first program, a general orientation to a case management model, is geared to a wide array of health care practitioners. The second program is a 3-day seminar designed to educate and train potential case managers. This chapter provides topical outlines and objectives for each program.

CURRICULUM DEVELOPMENT

Since case management's introduction to hospitals in 1985, implementation has often called for elaborate planning, meetings, time, and commitment. What has been lacking to this point is a formal means of educating the staff nurses, case managers, and other personnel who might be interacting with the case manager.

Although case management theory has been introduced into some undergraduate as well as graduate curricula, those employees already in the health care field probably have not been introduced to the concepts through formal education (American Association of Colleges of Nursing, 1997; Toran, 1998). Therefore education is a key element of success. The length of the institution's educational program will depend on the time that workers can take from their units to attend classroom instruction. For the most part the concepts of case management are relatively new to most employees, so didactic methods are important.

The amount of time set aside for instruction can range from 3 to 6 or more hours. However, the longer the program, the less likely it will be that employees from other disciplines can be included. Although it is crucial that all staff nurses and ancillary nursing personnel attend these introductory sessions, it is also important for members of other disciplines to participate. The number of hours that these employees can be present in the program will depend on the staffing patterns of their departments. Although other disciplines may be committed to the case management model, they may not have the financial or personnel resources to allow workers to leave their jobs for more than 1 hour. For off-peak shifts, participation may be even less possible. It may be necessary to provide different programs of varying lengths to ensure that everyone can attend. The material is important here, not the length of the program.

The topical outline for an introduction to a case management program should contain the following essential elements. Development of the curriculum should reflect all elements and characteristics of the case management process (Fineman, 1996). Other topics might be added, depending on the needs of the organization. The more preparation and education provided to all members of the organization, the greater the chances are for success. Even those departments not directly involved with the program should be invited to attend. Although it may not be immediately obvious, switching to case management will eventually affect areas such as the pharmacy or the radiology department. At the very least, all administrators and executive management should be encouraged to attend. Those involved in operations in the hospital can provide valuable insight into elements required for successful functioning of the model. Other departments—such as medicine, social work, quality improvement, discharge planning, utilization review, the patient representative department, nutrition, medical records, and admitting—are vital to the success of a case management model. Even though some individuals in these departments may be familiar with the case management concept, it is still important to educate them on how case management will be implemented in their organization. Such instruction will help prevent misunderstandings.

MULTIDISCIPLINARY EDUCATION

The content of a program geared to a broad audience must be general enough to hold the attention of a wide range of health care providers, administrators, and operations personnel. This is no easy task. Specific examples of how case management might affect some of these workers will be helpful and should be included in the program.

Begin the presentation with an overview of case management, including the evolution of nursing delivery models, which provides the program's groundwork. Next, explain the relevance of case management in light of today's health care issues. Covering such topics will answer the "Why case management?" and "Why now?" questions. An understanding of the changes in health care reimbursement, downsizing and restructuring, changes in the current patient population, and other health care issues will help the audience see why case management is timely and essential for the continued success of most health care organizations. This framework for discussion will show that case management is not just a nursing project or a nursing problem. Case management needs them, and they need case management.

Empowering the Case Manager

Introducing the case manager and introducing the case management plans are the most essential changes in the implementation of a case management model. Although many, more subtle changes will occur, these are the changes from which all the others will come.

The case manager must be empowered, and one technique for empowering is ensuring that everyone in the organization knows what a case manager does and how the case manager fits into workers' daily routines. If a case manager calls to speak to the patient representative and the patient representative does not understand the case manager's role and function, problems arise.

Table 25-1	GENERAL ORIENTATION PROGRAM CONTENT OUTLINE
OBJECTIVES	**CONTENT**

Define the concepts of case management.	Overview
	   A conceptual framework for case management
	   Evolution of nursing delivery models

Describe the role of the case manager.	Review
	   Job description
	   Job responsibilities
	   Daily operations
	   Relationship to other disciplines

Understand the changing roles of the health care team in case management	Social work Discharge planning Utilization management Physicians

Explain the relationship between the prospective payment system and case management; explain the use of case management plans; review managed care reimbursement.	DRGs
	   Definition/changes in reimbursement/managed care
	   Relationship and link to case management
	   Use of case management plans and their relationship to DRGs/guidelines

Identify the case management outcomes for research.	Research outcomes
	   Improved registered nurse satisfaction
	   Decreased burnout
	   Decreased length of stay
	   Improved patient satisfaction
	   Improved quality of care

Other disciplines' roles must be reviewed and clearly understood. Those who are most immediately affected are the social workers, utilization managers, discharge planners, and physicians. Some of these roles may be downsized, redesigned, or eliminated by the introduction of case management. If these changes have not occurred by the time the educational program begins, there may be resistance or hostility from those employees who fear being affected. Take care to engage these individuals, not alienate them.

Each discipline should understand and appreciate the other disciplines' roles and responsibilities. This mutual respect and understanding facilitates a smoother transition as role functions and responsibilities are reallocated.

Topical Outline

A curriculum that addresses a wide audience can cover an array of topics that are relevant to all employees (see Table 25-1). The following is a list of possible topics:

Define the concepts of case management.
Describe the role of the case manager.
Understand the changing roles of the health care team in case management.

Define the relationship between the prospective payment system and case management.
Review the managed care reimbursement system.
Understand the use of the case management plan.
Identify the case management outcomes for evaluation or research.

Defining the concepts of case management can be extensive or limited, depending on the audience. In the overview, include discussion of previous nursing care delivery models, current health care crises, and health care reimbursement methods in reference to case management. An in-depth discussion of the prospective payment system and managed care reimbursements is essential.

Include also the evolution of the functional, team, and primary models and how these models relate to the case management model. After all, case management combines elements of team and primary nursing models.

Because institutions may implement a unit-based, free-floating, or combined case management model, the subtle variations should be explored and discussed. This discussion should include how the various versions are structured, organized, and implemented.

The changing role of each member of the health care team is an important element of the discussion. Discuss current role functions as well as how roles will change under case management.

Finally, offer a general overview of the expected outcomes of the case management model. The expected outcomes provide a relevant arena from which to set case management goals both for the organization and for individual workers.

A Conceptual Framework for Case Management

Any discussion of case management must take place in a context of cost and quality. Case management provides the process, structure, and outcomes that control the quality of care while reducing cost. An understanding of this framework and overall goals provides the context for the discussions that follow. A review of how case management as a contemporary and interdisciplinary care delivery system can enhance hospital revenues is essential.

Role of the Case Manager

During implementation, many false conceptions of the role of the case manager develop, usually because of a lack of understanding. Professionals from other disciplines may draw their own conclusions concerning what the case manager should or should not be doing. Although some role blending is necessary, education is the main way to avoid role confusion (Kahn et al., 1964).

Distribute the case manager job description during the educational sessions or at least review it. This is the first step in distinguishing the roles and responsibilities of the case manager. Such steps help to ensure that other disciplines will respect the boundaries of the case manager's job description and will not expect the manager to function beyond those boundaries. Some workers may expect case managers to be less influential than their job descriptions indicate. Others may expect duties beyond the scope of their job descriptions. A clear description of the role set forth in the beginning will help minimize misunderstandings (Tahan, 1998).

A clear way in which to define and illustrate the job functions of the case manager is through a description of daily operations along with a description of what the case manager's typical day might be like. It is not uncommon to be asked, *What exactly does a case manager do?* Like many jobs of this nature, the specific tasks are often invisible, intangible, or both. Once again, emphasize the theoretic framework of the model and the expected outcomes.

Reviewing the Health Care Reimbursement Systems

Case management's basic premise is that expected outcomes of care can be achieved within appropriate time frames. A portion of the curriculum should be devoted to reviewing the present health care reimbursement systems. It is around these systems that much of case management is built (Cesta, Tahan, & Fink, 1998). Other points to be covered include how diagnosis-related groups (DRGs) work and how these predetermined lengths of stay determine reimbursement rates.

DRGs are one tool to help determine the goal length of stay for the case management plans. Other benchmarks used are national guidelines such as those of Milliman and Robertson (1997). Define these relationships in detail. Also review other uses of case management plans, including how they are used to maintain quality in an accelerated health care system. Review the links between quality and cost in a case management environment.

The effects of managed care infiltration should provide an additional context for case management. Whether the issue is capitated rates or per diem reimbursements, length of stay and resource allocation remain important. The processes applied through case management are applicable within the context of the prospective payment system or managed care. Include reviews of each in your discussions.

Projected Outcomes

The projected outcomes of the model can be covered next. Outline the general goals of any case management model and the specific goals of the organization. Include topics such as improved quality of care, improved caregiver satisfaction, improved patient satisfaction, decreased length of stay, and decreased resource utilization. Other projected outcomes might include reduction in insurance denials of payment, better turn-around time for tests, treatments, procedures and consults, and variance analysis methods.

Once again, the length and detail of this program must be determined by the audience and the amount of time that can be allotted by the various departments.

CASE MANAGER EDUCATION

Education of case managers requires several days to weeks. It cannot be assumed that nurses newly promoted to the role of case manager can function without training. Individual organizations must decide who is best qualified to provide this education. In some cases, outside consultants or experts in the field may be needed to provide this service.

In a 3-day program, 2 days are devoted to case management concepts and 1 day to leadership/management training. Nurses promoted to case management roles may have had no experience in either managing or case management.

Day One

Explain the differences between leadership and management during the first day (see Table 25-2). Functioning as a case manager requires the use of both skills (Holle & Blatchley, 1987).

Some topics to be covered might be the qualities of a leader, the correlation between administrative style and the nursing process, contingency management theory, and accountability versus responsibility. Although the case manager role is not identifiable as a management position in the traditional sense, it is essential that the case manager understand these concepts and be able to use them to effect the changes necessary for achieving excellent outcomes.

Table 25-2 ▶ CASE MANAGER EDUCATION DAY 1 CONTENT OUTLINE	
OBJECTIVES	**CONTENT**
Define leadership vs. management.	Leadership vs. management Definitions of leadership and management Qualities of a leader Difference between administrative process and nursing process Contingency management (situational management) Accountability vs. responsibility

Describe power and its uses for a case manager.	Definition of power
	    Five sources of power
	    Constructive and destructive uses of power
	    Strategies to obtain power

Identify the change process.	Change theory
	    Three types of change
	        Technical
	        Structural
	        People oriented
	    Lewin's Phases of Change
	        Freezing
	        Moving
	        Exploring
	        Refreezing
	        Implementation
	    Effecting positive change in management
	    Ten conditions that make change acceptable
	    Approaches to decreasing resistance to change

Relate the concepts of power and change.	Relationship between power and change
	    Empowerment
	    Change = empowerment: empowerment = change

The case manager will, at the least, be managing patient care. This will be accomplished through the role's facilitation and coordination aspects. Additionally the case manager will be managing the health care team by assuring that the interdisciplinary plan of care is in place and moving along in a timely fashion. These two elements of the role require excellent management skills. To be maximally effective, these management skills should be coupled with strong leadership skills.

The case manager must be empowered. A portion of this perceived empowerment must be inherent in the individual assuming the role (Bennis & Nanus, 1985). A working knowledge of the theories of power and their relationship to the case manager role should be included in the curriculum. Case managers should understand that their personal power sources are as related to their personal style as those found in the job description. Review strategies for obtaining as well as using power. A positive use of power will enhance self-esteem and bring more effectiveness to the role.

Implementation of a case management model involves both subtle and overt changes. It has been said that change is painful, but just how painful depends on the level of organizational support as well as individual support. Understanding the stages and processes of change can help decrease the difficul-

Table 25-2	**CASE MANAGER EDUCATION DAY 1 CONTENT OUTLINE–cont'd**

OBJECTIVES	CONTENT

Demonstrate effective communication techniques.	Communication
	    Do's and don'ts of effective communication
	    Active listening
	    Assertive vs. aggressive behavior
	        Conflict
	            Source
	            Resolutions
	        Problem-solving strategies

Describe the process of patient education.	Patient education
	    Adult learning principles
	    Strategies for effective teaching and learning

State the legal rights of patients.	Legal rights of patients
	    Patient bill of rights
	    Health care proxy
	    Living will
	    Do-not-resuscitate (DNR) laws
	    Managed care legal issues

Implement discharge planning process.	Discharge planning
	    Collaborative process
	    Assessment and planning
	    Referrals to provide continuity of care
	    Balanced Budget Act

Review utilization management techniques.	Utilization management
	    Assessment review
	    Continued review
	    Appeals process
	    Using criteria

ties associated with change. Whether the organization is large or small, complex or simple, change is never easy and seldom goes smoothly. If the case manager understands this in advance, difficulties can be lessened and ambiguities between case manager and other workers reduced.

The specific theory of change used by the instructor is not as important as conveying the message that the conversion to case management will be bumpy and that some days will not be productive or fulfilling. Nevertheless, the case manager should understand the techniques for effecting positive change and the conditions that make change more acceptable.

Implementation always involves some resistance. A portion of the organization will accept the change immediately; some will be resistant; and others will remain in the middle of the road, reserving judgment until they see the model in action. It will be impossible to win everyone over, and the case manager should understand this. Approaches to reducing resistance to change might be employed to help make the transition as smooth as possible.

Power and change are interrelated concepts. An empowered individual is in a better position to effect change. At the same time, the more change that is effected, the more empowered the individual becomes.

The effectiveness of any leader or manager depends on the styles of communication used. A substantial portion of the curriculum should be devoted to teaching effective communication techniques. One topic that can make a difference in the successful integration of the case manager role is the use of proper verbal and nonverbal communication styles, as well as proper techniques for listening. Active listening can result in positive communication interactions.

Integrated in this should be the technique for assertive communication versus the aggressive communication style, which has been shown to be less effective.

Finally, the case manager should be aware of the various sources of conflict that may come about as a result of the intregration of this role and of the problem-solving strategies that should be used for resolving conflict.

Patient education is one of the three main role functions of the case manager. Therefore the principles of adult learning and strategies for effective teaching and learning should be included in the curriculum. Effective inpatient teaching is an aid to successful recovery at home.

The case manager must serve as a patient advocate, interacting on the patient's behalf with other departments and disciplines. This advocacy role is possibly more important than ever before. Include in the curriculum a discussion of do-not-resuscitate (DNR) laws, living wills, and health care proxy laws and the Balanced Budget Act. A lecturer with expertise in these areas should be recruited.

A portion of the curriculum should cover discharge planning, with an emphasis on collaboration. If the organization has a discharge planning department, the discharge planning process can be reviewed from this perspective. The role of the social worker is important in the discharge planning process, and a social worker should be enlisted to provide insights on how case manager and social worker roles can work together. Many disciplines share the responsibility of assessing and planning for discharge. Reaching out to the community is part of the discharge planning process. As much as possible, the case manager should be made aware of the various community resources available to address patient problems. Some of these referral sources will come to the case manager's attention once the manager begins working in the role, but giving the case manager an overview of some of the resources available is important. Utilization management education should include techniques for performing assessment and continued stay reviews as well as strategies for appealing third party payer denials. Finally, the use of criteria such as Interqual (1998) or Milliman and Robertson (1997) should be explained in detail. The use of case studies here is helpful.

Day Two

On the second day (see Table 25-3), provide an overview and definition of case management. Review the relationship between cost and quality as they relate to case management along with the goals of a case management model. Also include an in-depth historical perspective of the evolution of nursing care delivery models. This will help to put today's case management model in perspective and give it relevance.

Case management is important as it relates to the past and present health care environment. There are numerous relevant health care crises, but some of the top ones might include the nursing shortage and how it affected the evolution of case management, changes in health care reimbursement as related to the prospective payment system, an aging patient population, the AIDS epidemic, and increased technology in health care. Case management has evolved out of the current crises. Presenting case management from its historical perspective will lend relevance to the model.

Cover the prospective payment system in detail because it is this system of predetermined lengths of stay as related to the DRG system that has led to evolution of the concept of case management. Cover the system in its entirety. Discuss the differences between what the state calls an acceptable length of stay

Table 25-3	CASE MANAGER EDUCATION DAY 2 CONTENT OUTLINE

OBJECTIVES	CONTENT
Define the concepts of case management.	Overview of case management 　Definition 　Nine steps to case management 　Goals of case management 　Expected outcomes of case management
Identify issues affecting health care delivery in the 1990s.	Health care crisis 　Nursing shortage 　Changes in reimbursement 　Aging population 　AIDS epidemic 　Increased technology
Explain the DRG reimbursement system.	Fiscal issues facing nursing 　DRGs 　Length of stay
Discuss managed care reimbursement.	Managed care 　HMOs 　PPOs 　Capitation
State the role of case manager and other members of the health care team.	Professional image Case Manager job 　Case manager job description 　Collaborative roles 　　Nursing 　　Physicians 　　Social work
Define case management plans.	Case management plans 　Design 　Documentation 　Relationship to length of stay 　Collaborative tool 　Education 　Quality of care
Document accurately the changes in case management using the case management plan.	Changes 　Length of stay 　Patient/practitioner variances 　Quality of care
Identify appropriate strategies for measuring, evaluating, and assessing outcomes.	Quality improvement documentation 　Problem-solving techniques 　Tracking and trending: selection of population source data 　Development of monitoring tool 　Analysis of data 　Evaluation and follow-up

and what the federal government calls acceptable. The case manager must understand the reimbursement system completely and must be fluent with the terms related to it. Guest lecturers who have expertise in this area or others should be invited to speak whenever possible.

Following this discussion should be one on managed care reimbursement systems. Case managers need to understand the finer points as they relate to case management in a managed care environment. Much of this discussion will relate back to the utilization management discussion.

Cover the role functions and responsibilities of the case manager, with a review of the case manager job description. Emphasis should be placed on the collaborative relationship between the case manager and all other disciplines. The specific responsibilities of the case manager can be covered during this time. These responsibilities include education, discharge planning, and facilitation of the patient's progress through the system.

The case management plan can be reviewed for form, content, and purpose. Possible topics to be covered in a discussion of case management plans include design, documentation, relationship to length of stay, use as a collaborative tool, and quality-of-care monitoring. Review case management plans in detail, as they are one of the more visible and tangible changes in case management. It is also important to review methods for writing the case management plan, especially how a case management plan can be used to track variances in care and quality data. Tracking and trending for selected patient problems or entire disease entities can be followed concurrently or retrospectively through the case management format.

Day Three

On the third day (see Table 25-4) offer a review of the roles and functions of the case manager. A "train the trainer" approach is useful during this portion of the curriculum. If someone already in the role of case manager is available, it is much more worthwhile for the new case manager to hear exactly how the role is carried out from someone who is already functioning in it. Provide a thorough review of how the case manager should collect data on patients. These data provide a framework from which the case manager can track the patients both while in the hospital and after discharge. Although each case manager will individualize the data collection process, some standard methods can be reviewed. In addition, walking the case manager through the day is also helpful.

Review the roles of the case management team. If at all possible, representatives from each discipline should lecture on their role and on how their role relates to case management and to other members of the case management team. Include the social work, utilization management, discharge planning, and home care disciplines. This overview should be followed by in-depth discussions on discharge planning, utilization review and management, social work, and planning for home care.

A workshop dedicated to managed care plan writing is a must for the third day. Each case manager should be given the opportunity to write a managed care plan from beginning to end. Going through the process step by step helps identify areas of confusion or uncertainty.

Variance analysis is a unique opportunity provided by the case management model. A retrospective analysis of what did or did not happen and looking for patterns as well as causes of the variances can be used to justify changes in care (Cesta, Tahan, & Fink, 1998). The case manager should be well versed in this process. In addition to providing the rationale for changes in care plans, variance analysis allows for future upgrading of the quality of care. It is much easier to track clinical outcomes with the variance analysis format. Include methods for identifying and monitoring outcomes. Outcomes can be identified as clinical and nonclinical, diagnosis specific, and generic. Also discuss continuous quality improvement (CQI) in relation to case management and case management plans.

Table 25-4	CASE MANAGER EDUCATION DAY 3 CONTENT OUTLINE

OBJECTIVES	CONTENT

Identify role of case manager.	Role functions
	    Planning and facilitation
	    Patient/family education
	    Discharge planning
	    Utilization management

Review the roles of the case management team.	Team members
	    Social work
	    Utilization
	    Discharge planning
	    Home care

Understand the in-depth roles of the case management team.	In-depth reviews
	    Discharge planning
	    Utilization management
	    Social work
	    Home care

Review case management assessment and documentation.	Assessment
	    On admission
	    Daily
	    Documentation
	    In-take assessment
	    On-going

Complete the case management plan.
Discuss variance analysis or outcomes.
	Review plans, practice writing
	Variances
	    Definition
	    Types
	    Monitoring
	Outcomes
	    Definition
	    Monitoring

Understand continuous quality improvement.	Continuous quality improvement
	    Definition
	    Relationship to case management

Discuss differentiated practice. Role play.	Relate differentiated practice to case management Relate to other disciplines in case manager role

Many case management programs use differentiated practice methods. Differentiated practice calls for the assignment of personnel based on employee level of education, experience, and expertise (American Hospital Association, 1990). An effective case management program should include a differentiated practice system so that optimal use can be made of the nurse's experience and education. One part of case management training should cover the levels of education for nurses, including a discussion of the strengths and weaknesses associated with each level.

Devote one part of the curriculum to role playing. This helps case managers by walking them through some of the situations they will encounter. One of the hardest areas for some new case managers is explaining to patients, physicians, and others exactly what the case manager role encompasses.

Giving out business cards to patients is equally difficult because case managers are not familiar with such formalities. Practice with the card can address and solve these problems. This may seem rudimentary, but it is crucial that the case manager feel at ease with these tasks.

Role playing can also be used to practice how to confront and resolve conflicts that arise during the change process.

Time Allotments

An allotment of 3 days to this curriculum represents the absolute minimal amount needed. A highly desirable approach to take would be to expand the detail of the 3-day program and spend more time on each topic. In this way, the program might be 6 to 9 days long. The longer the time devoted to the program, the higher is the likelihood that the case managers will receive the complex didactic materials needed to function in this complex role.

In addition to this didactic portion, the case manager should be given the opportunity to precept with an experienced case manager and to apply the strategies and theories learned in the classroom.

References

American Association of Colleges of Nursing (1997). *A vision of baccalaureate and graduate education: The next decade,* Washington, DC: The Association.

American Hospital Association (1990). *Current issues and perspective on differentiated practice.* Chicago: American Organization of Nurse Executives.

Bennis, W., & Nanus, B. (1985). *Leaders.* New York: Harper & Row.

Cesta, T.G., Tahan, H.A. , & Fink, L.F. (1998). *The case manager's survival guide: Winning strategies for clinical practice,* St. Louis: Mosby.

Doyle, R.L., & Schibanoff, J.M. (1997). *Healthcare management guidelines, Vol. 1,* Milliman & Roberston, Inc.

Fineman, L. (1996). Developing a formal education program for case managers. *Journal of Case Management,* 5(4), 158-161.

Holle, M.L., & Blatchley, M.E. (1987). *Introduction to leadership and management in nursing.* Boston: Jones & Bartlett.

Kahn, R.L., Wolfe, D.M., Quinn, R.P., Snoek, J.D., & Rosenthal, R.A. (1964). *Organizational stress: Studies in role conflict and ambiguity.* New York: Wiley.

O'Malley, J. (1988). Nursing care management, part II: Dimensions of the nurse case manager role. *Aspen's Advisor for Nurse Executives,* 3(7), 8-9.

Tahan, H.A. (1998, Nov.). *The case manager's excellence: Skills, traits and competencies.* Presented at the Medical Case Management Conference, Philadelphia.

Toran, M. (1998). Academic case management. *The Case Manager,* (1) 43-46.

The Competency Outcomes and Performance Assessment Model Applied to Nursing Case Management Systems

Carrie B. Lenburg

CHAPTER OVERVIEW

The assessment of competence at all levels of nursing personnel, as well as other applied disciplines, historically has been fraught with many concerns, problems, and uncertainties about its development, implementation, and evaluation. As healthcare delivery systems experience continuing seismic change, the need for, and confidence in, assessment of competence has become even more problematic and essential. Which competencies must be assessed, who should do it, when to do it, and how to do it in a objective, fair, and consistent manner are persistent and challenging questions. Those responsible for assessing the expected performance abilities of others typically experience concern about how to organize the evaluation of multiple, complex aspects of practice. They worry about how much, or how little, detail to include and the consequences of the evaluation outcomes, including potential personal, legal, and professional fallout. Moreover, the increasing interest in documented competence by regulators, employers, those in management and leadership positions, and consumers creates a new urgency for a different perspective of content and process. The evaluation of employee competence influences an agency's accreditation and quality standing and, therefore, its public image and reputation, recruitment of qualified employees, and financial viability. The use of competency outcomes and performance assessment methods, therefore, is crucial in today's healthcare and education systems (Lenburg, 1999a; Bargagliotti, 1999).

Case managers, regardless of the particular model or type of agency, frequently are engaged in assessing the competence of others, so they are challenged by these same questions and concerns. They also are subject to being evaluated themselves, which is a powerful stimulus for improving competency assessment methods throughout the agency. The ideas presented in this chapter are intended to help case managers develop and use a different conceptual framework for assessing competence—their own and that of other team members. As the role of case manager is redesigned by circumstances and creative professional determination, the model described allows for both flexibility and specificity in the ongoing evaluation of self and others. It is a guide for rethinking which competencies define practice and, therefore, must be documented through relevant and effective assessment methods.

Among the many problems to be considered is the historical practice of focusing on a multiplicity of specific but unorganized tasks, using a different approach and checklist for each level of employee and each different setting. The list of specific tasks, however, keeps changing, sometimes more rapidly than forms can be revised and staff can be oriented to use them. This situation becomes more complex with each institutional merger and the resulting changes in rules and procedures. In addition, anxiety associated with job security with each staffing correction influences the assessment process overall. Other related problems include the ever-decreasing time and personnel available to develop and administer relevant performance assessment methods that meet regulatory and professional standards, and avoid legal pitfalls. Ironically, institutional accreditation depends more on assessment of competence than ever before, at a time when it is more complex and difficult to implement with certainty.

THE COMPETENCY OUTCOMES AND PERFORMANCE ASSESSMENT (COPA) MODEL

The Competency Outcomes and Performance Assessment (COPA) model, developed by Lenburg over the past decade, offers a different perspective and approach to evaluating performance abilities of various levels of employees. While primarily developed for students in various types of educational programs, the model also is applicable to case managers in diverse practice settings and with various levels of personnel. The COPA model provides a comprehensive framework for re-visioning and organizing performance expectations in actual practice and thus it influences related learning and assessment of abilities in the context of those expectations (Lenburg & Mitchell, 1991). This chapter focuses on the essential core practice competencies identified in the model and illustrates how they apply to case management systems of care delivery. The following concise description of the model is included to help readers understand some of its primary components as a context for determining the usefulness of this approach in different clinical environments.

The elegance of the COPA model is its simultaneous universality and specificity. Four essential questions are used to guide the process of development and implementation of performance-based assessment:

1. What competencies outcomes are essential for practice? This question requires the identification of performance-based competencies considered mandatory for a given area of practice; once fully developed they collectively define practice.
2. What skills and related actions or behaviors provide sufficient evidence to substantiate individual competence? This question focuses on specific practice skills and the actions or inactions that must be observed to verify designated abilities. These statements define what competence looks like in actuality.
3. What are the most effective ways to learn these competencies (to upgrade, improve, achieve them)? This third question requires the integration of actual practice expectations and the use of effective learning strategies consistent with the characteristics of the learners (employees, orientees, students) and job classification.
4. What are the most effective methods to assess achievement of designated competencies? This question requires determination of associated assessment methods, logistics, policies, and related resources.

Briefly, the COPA model requires that the preferred outcomes, or results, be specified, clarified, and justified before determining how they can be achieved and subsequently assessed. In this model, the end is the beginning. Unlike traditional objectives that typically focus on directions, activities, and process, outcomes are the practice-oriented and performance-based expected results of those activities and processes. The outcomes approach is focused on the preferred end product; once that is clear, the map can be drawn to get there. Learning and practice strategies are customized to promote the most effective and efficient course to achieve those outcomes. Thereafter, specific methods of assessment are invented to document the achievement of actual performance of those outcomes. Thus, it is essential to begin with the competency outcomes, including some that are usually considered too ambiguous to assess, like ethical practice or cultural competence. An example of specifying preferred outcomes for cultural competence is described in Lenburg et al. (1995).

The assessment component of the COPA model is effective and supportable because it is based on the integration of 10 psychometrically based concepts developed by Lenburg (1979). These concepts include examination (as different from traditional evaluation), specified skills or dimensions of practice to be assessed, critical elements that define competence for each skill, level of acceptability, sampling, objectivity, comparability, consistency, flexibility, and systematized conditions. This constellation of concepts creates the framework for developing and implementing practice-based performance assessments; all of them are required, sometimes simultaneously, like transparencies that overlay each other to create the "whole picture." Lenburg and Mitchell (1991) describe and illustrate these concepts for actual and simulation performance assessments (performance examinations).

THE EIGHT CORE PRACTICE COMPETENCIES

The practice competencies in the COPA model are derived from many years of analyzing the kinds of skills nurses are required to perform effectively in the context of diverse and multiple client needs in contemporary health care delivery. Over time, the categories have been revised, refined, and tested for applicability and comprehensiveness in diverse situations. All of the resulting eight core practice competencies are required in practice, albeit to a different extent depending on various position descriptions, legal and regulatory requirements, and setting characteristics. The model makes it possible to use the same organizing framework to develop assessment instruments, which tends to promote consistency and objectivity across levels of employees (or learners) (Lenburg, 1999b). Ultimately, after the initial components are developed, this model requires less time to develop additional skills (instruments) or to revise existing ones and implement various required processes. Typically, when employees are subjected to similar expectations and believe the process is fair, they are more willing to do their best and they feel more satisfied with the content and process of competency performance examinations (CPEs), which are described later. Through such assessments they also become more competent and efficient employees.

The model provides structure for developing specific subskills under each category to correspond with different levels of staff and specialized work environments. More traditional approaches begin with a long list of specific skills that often seem unorganized and may or may not include all of the competencies required for the designated position. In contrast, the core practice competencies approach organizes essential skills into a more cohesive and useful manner and provides more assurance that all dimensions of practice are included, with emphasis on the most relevant skills for designated staff positions.

It is crucial to understand the meaning, relevance, and distinctions of the eight core competencies to appreciate their central place in the COPA model. The brief descriptions listed here provide an initial step in this direction. Taken in their broadest and most generic meaning, each competency (sometimes thought of as a category or dimension of practice) is applicable to some extent to individual employees from the most subordinate to the most senior position. Figure 26-1 lists an array of examples under each competency category to illustrate the continuum from the simpler to the more complex skills expected for diverse positions and circumstances:

1. Assessment and Intervention Skills: This competency includes all forms of assessment, data gathering, monitoring, and technical or therapeutic intervention skills.

2. Communication Skills: This competency includes oral, written, and computer communication skills used to exchange information and to transmit messages with or about clients and others.
3. Critical Thinking Skills: This competency includes a broad array of skills along a continuum from simple problem solving to scientific inquiry and reflective judgment.
4. Humanistic Caring Relationship Skills: This competency includes skills related to client-focused interests and concerns, interpersonal behaviors that demonstrate care for and with clients and significant others, sensitivity to individual cultures and preferences, client advocacy, and social justice concerns.
5. Teaching Skills: This competency includes the transmission of information intended to instruct clients and related others about topics essential to health care and well-being, from the simple telling and showing to the more advanced skills of formalized teaching episodes.
6. Management Skills: This competency pertains to such skills as managing time and resources, implementing activities to promote cooperation among staff and others, creating and implementing budgets, planning, delegating and supervising responsibilities of others, collaboration across disciplines, and similar activities.
7. Leadership Skills: This competency includes activities to promote staff morale and cooperation, assertiveness and risk-taking, creative planning for change and innovations, creating new policies or other protocols, and professional development.
8. Knowledge Integration Skills: This competency stretches along the practice continuum from using factual information, prior learning, basic principles, and procedures while fulfilling responsibilities, to supporting decisions and actions with relevant evidence, and applying knowledge from nursing and other health-related disciplines, humanities, arts, and sciences.

In this model, specific skills (subskills) are listed under each competency category, consistent with the expectations for the particular level of practitioner. The targeted content and process for performance-based learning and evaluation are based on the specific subskills listed under each competency category and the corresponding critical elements. Critical elements are defined as the single, discrete, and observable behaviors mandatory for that skill and for that level of staff. They specify the baseline of acceptable performance and define "how good is good enough." The critical elements for any given skill, therefore, guide the content and processes for learning and evaluation. Lenburg (1979), Lenburg and Mitchell (1991), and Luttrell, Lenburg, Scherubel, Jacob, and Koch (1999) offer further descriptions and examples.

APPLICATION TO CASE MANAGEMENT SYSTEMS

Writings related to nursing case management often describe the variety of complex roles and abilities required for nurses in various settings. Tahan (1997) describes the three role dimensions for the nurse case manager as the clinical role, the managerial role, and the financial/business role. While his overall categories differ from the COPA model, the competencies (skills) are essentially the same. These competencies are elaborated further by Cohen and Cesta (1997). Taylor (1997) makes a valuable contribution in describing the competencies of nurse case managers regarding ethical issues. Lenburg (Lenburg et al., 1995) chaired an Expert Panel of the American Academy of Nursing charged to explore cultural competence. Their work resulted in the monograph, *Promoting Cultural Competence in Nursing Education,* which contains multiple recommendations related to expected outcomes and competencies.

The predominant skills cited for nurse case managers include collaboration, negotiation, decision making, delegation, assessment, monitoring, planning, creating alternatives, applying specific interventions, teaching, supervision, and evaluating others. In the COPA model these and other essential skills expected of the case manager are clustered under the eight core practice competency categories. Using this approach, it becomes easier to determine whether or not all general and specific competencies are included and which are emphasized, overemphasized, or inadequately represented. This kind of competency analysis is fundamental for planning, revising, and evaluating orientation, instructional, or evaluation programs; it makes inconsistency and redundancy evident and identifies where corrective revisions need to be focused.

Box 26-1 illustrates the eight core competency categories with several examples for each of how and where to cluster subskills that may be required in case management practice. This is a cryptic overview of essential competencies and subskills; some of them already may be emphasized and others may be deficient and need to be targeted for quality improvement. These categorical examples are intended to stimulate discussion that ultimately could result in a revised draft with more specific skills for case managers in a particular health care institution or system. The list is not all-inclusive, and some subskills potentially could be shifted to other competency categories, depending on preferences and practice circumstances. Clearly, case managers engage in many competencies simultaneously, and to some extent their judgment and agency protocols in the particular system will determine where specific skills should be listed. This probably will vary for different levels of care providers in the system.

Figure 26-1 is a blank form that could be used as a worksheet on which case managers can list particular skills under each of the core competencies as they apply to the several primary roles of the position. The specific subskills vary by staff levels, practice settings, and types of case management system. For example:

What *specific assessment and intervention skills* are performed by the nurse case manager?
What specific forms of written, oral, and computer *communication skills* are required from them?
What different forms of *critical thinking* apply to various levels of staff on the case management team?

Name of Staff member:_____ **Position:**_____ **Date:**_____

List specific subskills for each competency category required for three – four primary roles for each particular position

Core Competencies	Role 1	Role 2	Role 3	Role 4
Assessment and intervention				
Communications				
Critical thinking				
Humanistic caring relationships				
Teaching				
Management				
Leadership				
Knowledge integration				

FIGURE **26-1**   Individual skills identification worksheet.

Box 26-1	**LENBURG'S CONSTELLATION OF CORE PRACTICE COMPETENCIES WITH APPLICATION TO CASE MANAGEMENT**

1. Assessment and intervention skills
   a. Promoting safety and protection: clients, families, personnel
   b. Assessing and monitoring: clients, personnel, practice protocols, audits, systems
   c. Managing therapeutic treatments and procedures: conventional, adaptive, innovative
   d. Promoting human-technology interaction and effectiveness
2. Communication skills
   a. Oral skills
      (1) Interacting, listening, processing, reflective feedback
      (2) Interviewing, history taking, data collection
      (3) Group discussion: interacting, leading, persuading
      (4) Giving directions, verifying, conflict resolution
      (5) Reporting, presenting
   b. Writing skills
      (1) Clinical reports, histories, clinical pathways, Multidisciplinary action plans (MAPs), Nursing care plans (NCPs), documentation
      (2) Agency documents: reports, forms, memos, letters
      (3) Manuscripts for publication, manuals, proposals
   c. Computing skills
      (1) Documentation related to/for clients, employers, authorities
      (2) Information search, investigation, discovery, synthesis, dissemination
3. Critical thinking skills
   a. Integrating, synthesizing pertinent data from multiple sources
   b. Problem solving, diagnostic reasoning, clinical decision making
   c. Outcomes and variance analysis, reflective judgment, ethical reasoning, prioritizing
   d. Scientific inquiry, investigation, research, evidence-based perspective
   e. Adaptation, creativity and innovation, quality improvements
4. Humanistic caring and relationship skills
   a. Moral, ethical, legal responsiveness and implementation for clients and others
   b. Cultural and individual respect, supportive interpersonal relationships
   c. Advocacy, sensitivity and compassion, social justice
5. Teaching skills
   a. Individuals and groups: clients, intradisciplinary and interdisciplinary staff development, others
   b. Health promotion, restoration, and maintenance, quality improvements
6. Management skills
   a. Administration and organization responsibilities; coordinate care and delivery systems
   b. Planning, delegation, supervision of others; maintain standards
   c. Interdisciplinary and intradisciplinary coordination, care conferences, discharge planning
   d. Human and material resource utilization, budgets, personnel, supplies, equipment
   e. Accountability and responsibility, performance appraisals, quality improvement
7. Leadership skills
   a. Intradisciplinary and interdisciplinary collaboration and negotiation, team building
   b. Creative vision to formulate alternatives, practice protocols, implement change
   c. Supportable assertiveness, persuasion, risk-taking, persistence, flexibility
   d. Anticipatory planning, policy making, stimulating evidence-based decisions
   e. Ensure professional standards, adapt as needed, represent the profession to community leaders
   f. Continued professional development.
8. Knowledge integration skills
   a. Use current knowledge pertaining to nursing and health-related disciplines and practice
   b. Incorporate humanities, arts, and sciences as well as business, economics, and politics into practice

The competency outcome categories facilitate the development of a comprehensive but specific framework to ensure that the learning, implementation, evaluation, and quality improvement processes are customized to the mission, environment, staffing patterns, and assigned staff roles of the agency or institution.

After the particular subskills are listed under each of the eight core practice competencies required for the designated positions and setting, specific critical elements can be identified. Collectively, critical elements define practice expectations related to that skill, whether that is assessment, critical thinking, communication, or management. The process of identifying the precise behaviors expected in practice is crucial to promoting competent practice and decreasing avoidable errors. The resulting document that includes the specific skills for each core competency with required critical elements provides the blueprint for instruction, orientation, and assessment; it also becomes one of the components for quality improvement planning. These components pertain to two of the four essential questions already described and provide the basis for the remaining questions. Specifying the core practice competencies with their related subskills and critical elements provides clear direction for further development of both product and process to improve quality of care delivery.

Box 26-2 outlines a draft of a few potential examples of subskills under several core competencies with related potential critical elements. The examples cited here pertain to the case manager and are general in nature to allow flexibility in development; specific skills, their wording, and the critical elements depend on many factors, as already noted, and can be written several different ways or to different levels of expectation. Both skills and critical elements will be more relevant if developed by the staff

---

Box 26-2 ▷ **SUGGESTED EXAMPLES OF SKILLS FOR SEVERAL CORE COMPETENCIES TO ASSESS PERFORMANCE OF THE NURSE CASE MANAGER**

A. CORE PRACTICE COMPETENCE: ASSESSMENT AND INTERVENTION

Subskill:
1. Monitor effectiveness of clinical path protocols in achieving patient outcomes

Critical Elements: The Case Manager is Able to:
1. Obtain pertinent data to substantiate implementation of established protocols
2. Analyze obtained data in context of protocols to identify variances
3. Interpret findings to identify root cause factors associated with the variance
4. Recommend strategies to maximize implementation of protocols while promoting patient outcomes and satisfaction

B. CORE PRACTICE COMPETENCE: CRITICAL THINKING

Subskill:
1. Plan a study to investigate differences in variance for a designated protocol among patients with similar conditions or DRG classification

Critical Elements: The Case Manager is Able to:
1. Write the specific question to be explored, with related components
2. Write the justification for investigating the specified problem
3. Describe methods to be used, including subjects, time line, and methods of data collection and analysis
4. Develop a budget that is adequate and efficient for the purpose
5. Outline potential consequences of positive and negative findings

Continued

Box 26-2	**Suggested Examples of Skills for Several Core Competencies to Assess Performance of the Nurse Case Manager—cont'd**

C. Core Practice Competence: Teaching
Subskill:
1. Teach a group of staff to implement changes in performance evaluation methods

Critical Elements: The Case Manager is Able to:
1. Develop a plan for a staff workshop to include the following:
   a. Specific outcomes to be achieved
   b. Strategies to promote learning and support
   c. Methods to evaluate comprehension and agreement with new methods
2. Interact with the group to determine perceptions of new methods described in material previously distributed
3. Implement persuasive strategies to maximize comprehension and support of new methods
4. Engage all members in discussion to maximize input of diverse examples, applications, and concerns
5. Evaluate comprehension and support of methods

D. Core Practice Competence: Management:
Subskill:
1. Maintain practice standards by holding self and other providers accountable

Critical Elements: The Case Manager is Able to:
1. Ensure that each staff member has completed orientation or education programs pertaining to specific standards
2. Implement specific methods by which staff will be oriented and evaluated
3. Evaluate staff performance of specific skills during designated periods using the pre-established standards
4. Use evaluation findings to assess the need for change to promote quality improvement in staff performance
5. Implement procedures designed to promote compliance with practice standards
6. Communicate with relevant agency authorities to report findings and recommendations

E. Core Practice Competence: Leadership
Subskill:
1. Collaborate with multidisciplinary team members to develop cost-effective protocols to achieve patient outcomes and patient and staff satisfaction

Critical Elements: The Case Manager is Able to:
1. Collaborate with multidisciplinary team in ways that:
   a. Contribute to achievement of outcomes from a nursing perspective
   b. Show respect for differing perspectives and positions
   c. Promote evidence-based decisions
   d. Promote team-building and cooperation
   e. Promote accuracy, clarity, precision, and relevance of findings, outcomes, interventions
2. Seek leadership opportunities to coordinate activities that promote achievement of outcomes
3. Use creative strategies to promote effectiveness and efficiency of care delivery protocols

in the particular setting and system to comply with various position descriptions. These examples, therefore, are intended to be suggestive, to illustrate the concept; they are not complete, conclusive, or necessarily the most relevant. They are ideas to stimulate more precise development. Other examples are suggested in some of the references.

The competency performance examinations (CPEs) are developed from this beginning (see Box 26-3). Space in this chapter does not permit description of all the components of this aspect of the COPA model (Lenburg, 1999b; Lenburg & Mitchell, 1991; Luttrell, 1999). Suffice it to say that the specified competencies and related critical elements form the basis for the assessment of competence of each

---

Box 26-3   **EXAMPLES OF COMPETENCY PERFORMANCE EXAMINATIONS (CPEs)***

CPE 1: IMPLEMENT THE NURSE CASE MANAGER ROLE AS MANAGER OF CARE FOR A GROUP OF ASSIGNED PATIENTS
AT THE DESIGNATED TIME FOR ASSESSMENT, THE CASE MANAGER WILL BE ABLE TO:

MET	NOT MET	COMPETENCIES AND CRITICAL ELEMENTS
____	____	1. Manage care delivered to assigned patients consistent with assessment of their needs
____	____	2. Delegate specific aspects of patient care to relevant staff according to qualifications
____	____	3. Prioritize patient care activities
____	____	4. Monitor patient care provided by assisting personnel
____	____	5. Ensure accurate administration of all therapeutic interventions to assigned patients
____	____	6. Manage time and resources consistent with patient needs and agency protocols
		7. Incorporate universal competencies and related critical elements:*
____	____	a. Safety and protection
____	____	b. Standard precautions
____	____	c. Interpersonal communication
____	____	d. Critical thinking
____	____	e. Humanistic caring relationships
____	____	f. Professional responsibilities
____	____	g. Documentation
____	____	8. Integrate knowledge relevant to the roles of nurse manager

CPE 2: IMPLEMENT THE CASE MANAGER LEADERSHIP ROLE ON THE DESIGNATED UNIT(S)
AT THE DESIGNATED TIME FOR ASSESSMENT, THE CASE MANAGER WILL BE ABLE TO:

MET	NOT MET	COMPETENCIES AND CRITICAL ELEMENTS
		1. Coordinate care of a full caseload of patients with designated staff:
____	____	a. Assign staff to patients consistent with patient needs, staff qualification, and unit needs
____	____	b. Delegate tasks to staff consistent with their qualifications and needs of the unit
____	____	c. Prioritize patient care activities
____	____	d. Monitor care for all patient care provided by assisting personnel

*Based on listing of critical elements for specific skills under competency outcome categories.   *Continued*

Box 26-3	**EXAMPLES OF COMPETENCY PERFORMANCE** **EXAMINATIONS (CPEs)*–cont'd**	

MET	NOT MET	COMPETENCIES AND CRITICAL ELEMENTS
_____	_____	2. Manage time, human, and material resources consistent with patient needs and agency protocols
_____	_____	3. Communicate essential information during and at conclusion of shift to designated others
_____	_____	4. Collaborate with other health care providers to promote achievement of patient outcomes
_____	_____	5. Integrate knowledge relevant to the role of nurse manager
		6. Monitor staff to ensure universal competencies are implemented (using critical elements)*
_____	_____	a. Safety and protection
_____	_____	b. Standard precautions
_____	_____	c. Interpersonal communication
_____	_____	d. Critical thinking
_____	_____	e. Humanistic caring relationships
_____	_____	f. Professional responsibilities
_____	_____	g. Documentation

*Based on listing of critical elements for specific skills under competency outcome categories.

employee at each level. Other components require the integration of the 10 psychometric concepts, such as critical elements, sampling, objectivity, consistency, and comparability. Moreover, relevant policy statements and procedural directions must be developed, including, for example, exactly how the Competency Performance Examination will be administered, by whom, when, and with what consequences. Holding staff accountable for competent practice is essential, and the COPA model provides a different and comprehensive approach to this complex issue.

SUMMARY

The COPA model has the potential for increasing the efficiency and effectiveness of case management systems and quality improvements in the care delivery organization. Some key characteristics that make the model attractive include its clarity and specificity of expected performance, potential for a universal practice framework to guide both the learning and assessment of competence, flexibility, and adaptability to diverse staff levels and practice environmental settings. As designed, the eight core practice competency categories in the model are useful as a guide for developing or revising statements pertaining to mission, practice-based outcomes, orientation programs, content and processes related to staff performance evaluation, and quality improvement strategies.

The creativity and commitment of the staff in a given setting will influence how this model can be developed and implemented, in part or in whole. It evolves from a belief in the need for an integrative and organizing framework grounded in psychometric concepts and applied to complex practice environments. Once the fundamental concepts are understood, it can serve the needs of multiple purposes and situations. It presents a different approach or perspective. When implemented as suggested in this chapter, this model presents a significant paradigm shift in learning and assessing competence, and the focus of practice itself.

References

Bargagliotti, T., Luttrell, M, & Lenburg, C.B. (Sept, 1999). Reducing threats to the implementation of a competency-based performance assessment system. *Online Journal of Issues in Nursing.* Washington, D.C.: Amer. Nurs. Assoc.

Cohen, E.L., & Cesta, T.G. (Eds). (1997). *Nursing case management: From concept to evaluation* (pp. 153-160). (2nded). St Louis: Mosby.

Lenburg, C.B. (Sept, 1999a). Redesigning expectations for initial and continuing competence for contemporary nursing practice. *Online Journal of Issues in Nursing.* Washington, D.C.: Amer. Nurs. Assoc.

Lenburg, C.B. (Sept, 1999b). The framework, concepts and methods of the competency outcomes and performance assessment (COPA) Model. *Online Journal of Issues in Nursing.* Washington, D.C.: Amer. Nurs. Assoc.

Lenburg, C.B. (1991). Assessing the goals of nursing education: Issues and approaches to evaluation of outcomes. In M. Garbin (Ed.), *Assessing educational outcomes.* New York: NLN.

Lenburg, C.B. (1979). *The clinical performance examination: Development and implementation.* New York: Appleton-Century-Crofts.

Lenburg, C.B., Lipson, J., Demi, A., Blaney, D., Stern, P., Schultz, P., & Gage, L. (1995). *Promoting cultural competence in nursing education.* Washington DC: American Academy of Nursing.

Lenburg, C.B., & Mitchell, C.A. (1991). Assessment of outcomes: The design and use of real and simulation nursing performance examinations, *Nursing & Health Care, 12,* 68-74.

Luttrell, M., Lenburg, C.B., Scherubel, J.C., Jacob, S., & Koch, R. (1991). Competency outcome for learning and performance assessment: Redesigning a BSN curriculum. *Nursing and Health Care Perspectives, 20,* 134-141.

Tahan, H. (1997). The role of the nurse case manager. In E.L. Cohen & T.G. Cesta (Eds), *Nursing case management: From concept to evaluation* (pp. 197-209). (2nded). St Louis: Mosby.

Taylor, C. (1997). Ethical issues in case management. In E.L. Cohen & T.G. Cesta (Eds), *Nursing case management: From concept to evaluation* (pp 314-334). (2nded). St Louis: Mosby.

The Role of the Nurse Case Manager

Hussein A. Tahan

CHAPTER OVERVIEW

There is no standardization in the job description of the nurse case manager. Each institution implementing case management systems has established its own version of the role. This chapter, however, presents a thorough description of the roles, responsibilities, and functions of the case manager. It delineates the role's clinical, managerial, and financial aspects, and discusses why nurses are, among all health care professionals, best fit to become case managers. In addition, it describes the skills and selection criteria required for the role. A special section of this chapter is designated for the various functions assumed by case managers while delivering patient care. Among these functions are change agent, clinician, consultant, coordinator and facilitator of care, educator, negotiator, manager, patient and family advocate, quality improvement coordinator, researcher, and risk manager.

Nurses have played a crucial role in the success of case management as a patient care delivery system since its inception. This is evidenced through the drastic changes such delivery systems have undergone. In the early 1980s case management models were implemented by nursing executives as nursing efforts to meet the demands and challenges of the ever-changing health care system: cost containment and higher quality care. Today, however, these models are being implemented in a broader perspective as patient care delivery systems that are interdisciplinary, surpassing the boundaries of nursing care.

Despite the fact that for a decade and a half case management models have been successful in improving quality of patient care and containing the incurred costs, the literature regarding the nurse case manager's role description and functions is conflicting. Nurse case managers are introduced as integral members of interdisciplinary health care teams every time a health care institution implements a case management system for patient care delivery. The presence and achievements of case managers in such institutions are important for the success of the case management system. Regardless of the patient care setting in which these systems are implemented, the institutions rely heavily on the nurse case manager, who acts as the gatekeeper of the interdisciplinary health care team and as the coordinator, facilitator, and evaluater of care activities. The case manager in most institutions is a registered professional nurse who assumes an advanced practice nursing role.

There is no standardization in the role of the nurse case manager. The institutions that have implemented case management systems have created their own case manager's role in a way that correlates with their organizational chart and operations, policies and procedures, financial status, and the goals and aims of the case management system. Regardless of the type of health care institution, there is some common ground in the role of nurse case managers. A summary of these commonalties is based on the role dimensions defined by Tahan (1993) and revised in 1998 (Tahan, 1998a,b), which are related to clinical/patient care, managerial/leadership, financial/business, information management/communication, and professional development/advancement.

THE NURSE CASE MANAGER'S ROLE DIMENSIONS

Case management is a compilation of activities that a case manager performs within a particular care setting (i.e., acute care, home care, managed care organization), or provided by an independent practitioner such as the case in community nursing centers or private case management practices. Case management activities may also be provided to specific patient populations and communities such as the elderly, those with mental disorders, or residents of an underserved neighborhood (Goodwin, 1994).

Regardless of the care setting of the institution providing case management services, the following are some commonly used case management activities:

1. Patient outreach, identification, and intake
2. Assessment and problem identification
3. Development of the plan of care
4. Implementation of the plan
5. Care coordination, facilitation, expedition, and management
6. Transitional planning and referral to other health care providers (e.g., social worker) and brokerage of services (e.g., home care)
7. Ongoing assessment, reassessment, and follow-up
8. Patient/family education regarding health care needs and lifestyle changes.
9. Monitoring and evaluation of care activities, patient responses to treatments, and outcomes
10. Patient/family advocacy
11. Quality assurance and improvement
12. Conducting research and research utilization
13. Cost control activities such as eliminating duplication and fragmentation, and expediting care provision
14. Writing reports and providing feedback to key stakeholders/personnel
15. Staff mentoring, coaching, and education (continuing education sessions)
16. Variance identification, analysis, and management
17. Managed care reviews, authorizations, and certifications
18. Public speaking
19. Writing for publication
20. Public health policy and politics
21. Data entry, analysis, and management
22. Documentation
23. Committee participation
24. Development and evaluation of case management plans

In acute care settings, for example, the nurse case manager is responsible for coordinating the care delivered to a group of patients (case load/case mix) that begins at the time of admission and extends beyond discharge. This is carried out through applying the nursing process (assessment, diagnosis, planning, implementation, and evaluation) . . . The nurse case manager ensures the delivery of cost-effective, outcome-oriented quality care, . . . and access to health care . . . The nurse case manager is accountable for applying nursing case management successfully to the daily activities of patient care (Tahan, 1993, pp. 55-56).

Nurse case managers can make sound decisions that reflect what is best for the patient and family, the interdisciplinary team, and the health care organization by applying Tahan's five role dimensions. Clarifying the nurse case manager's role by applying these five dimensions provides a generic conceptual framework health care organizations can use as a guide to better design the case manager's job description, functions, and responsibilities (Table 27-1).

The Clinical/Patient Care Role Dimension

Nurse case managers are responsible for the assessment of patients and families every time a patient comes with a problem. They identify the existing or potential health problems by evaluating the pa-

---

Table 27-1 ▶ THE NURSE CASE MANAGER'S ROLE DIMENSIONS AND ACTIVITIES	
ROLE DIMENSION	**ACTIVITIES**
Clinical/patient care	Patient outreach, identification, and intake
	Assessment and problem identification
	Development of the plan of care
	Implementation of the plan of care
	Ongoing assessment, reassessment, and follow-up
	Patient and family education
Managerial/leadership	Care coordination, facilitation, expedition, and management
	Transitional planning an referrals
	Monitoring and evaluation of care activities and outcomes
	Patient and family advocacy
	Quality assurance and improvement
	Staff mentoring, education, and coaching
	Committees participation
	Development of case management plans/clinical pathways
Financial/business	Cost control/reduction activities
	Variance identification, analysis, and management
	Managed care review, authorizations and certifications
Information management/ communication	Data entry, analysis, and management
	Documentation
	Writing reports
	Providing feedback to key stakeholders/personnel
Professional development/ advancement	Conducting research and research utilization
	Public/health policy and politics
	Writing for publication
	Public speaking

tient's physical, functional, psychosocial, financial, cognitive, and spiritual condition. They then, in collaboration with other members of the interdisciplinary health care team, develop a plan of care that meets the patient's needs (Bower, 1989; Ethridge & Lamb, 1989; Giuliano & Poirier, 1991; Tahan, 1993, 1998a,b; Zander, 1988a). The plan of care lists the key tasks or events that must be accomplished in handling patient problems and meeting the care goals, the patient and family teaching activities based on the identified health care needs, and the transitional plan that assures a timely and appropriate patient discharge. The plan of care also includes prospectively determined/desired outcomes. The patient care activities and expected outcomes are presented with a specific time line that delineates when an activity should be completed, and a particular outcome is expected to be achieved, denoting the patient's progress toward expected goals. Nurse case managers may use prospectively developed protocols/case management plans if any are available that meet patients' needs, diagnosis, and problems. If protocols are used, they are usually reviewed and revised to meet the individual patient's needs. Case managers use these protocols to direct, monitor, and evaluate patient treatments and nursing interventions, and the outcomes or responses to treatments (Cohen & Cesta, 1993; Tahan, 1993; Tahan and Cesta, 1995; Thompson et al., 1991; Zander 1988a).

Nurse case managers, when caring for patients, follow a holistic approach to care and spend a considerable amount of time discussing preventive services. They may or may not provide direct patient care activities. They assess the patient's and family's coping abilities, social support systems, and financial/health insurance status, and intervene if a problem is identified. Case managers are also responsible for facilitating the patient's journey through the health care system, arranging for consultation with specialists or specialized services, and assuring that transfers to more appropriate level of care areas are made when needed (Brockopp, Porter, Kinnard, & Silberman, 1992; Henderson & Collard, 1988; Leclair, 1991; Zander, 1988b).

As to case management plans, case managers play an active role in their development, implementation, and evaluation. They participate in an interdisciplinary health care team for that purpose. When these plans are implemented to guide patient care, nurse case managers identify any variances from the standards and work with other team members to analyze and, when possible, resolve these variances (Cohen & Cesta, 1993; Ethridge & Lamb, 1989; O'Malley, 1988a; Tahan & Cesta, 1995).

The Managerial/Leadership Role Dimension

The managerial role dimension refers to the case manager's responsibility for facilitating, expediting, and coordinating the care of patients during the course of their illness (Cohen & Cesta, 1993; Ethridge & Lamb, 1989; Kruger, 1989; O'Malley, 1988a; Tahan, 1993, 1998a,b; Zander, 1988a). Some examples of these functions are scheduling of and follow-up on tests, procedures, and treatments; patient and family teaching; transitional planning; negotiating community resources; monitoring patient care outcomes; and obtaining certification and authorizations from managed care organization (Cesta, Tahan, & Fink, 1998). The nurse case managers manage care by planning the treatment modalities and interventions necessary for meeting the needs of patients and families and the goals of the health care team. They determine, in collaboration with the interdisciplinary team, the goals of treatment, the projected length of stay, and the necessary treatments and services. This provides a clear time frame for accomplishing the care activities needed (Cesta, Tahan, & Fink, 1998; O'Malley, 1988b; Tahan, 1993).

Case managers also guide the patient care activities, nursing treatments, and interventions to be carried out by nurses and other health care professionals. They continuously evaluate the quality of care provided and the outcomes of treatments and services to prevent duplication, fragmentation, or misuse of resources (Ethridge & Lamb, 1989; Kruger, 1989; Loveridge, Cummings, & O'Malley, 1988; O'Malley, 1988b; Tahan, 1993; Zander, 1988a). They also conduct retrospective and concurrent chart reviews to evaluate the efficacy and efficiency of care and to identify any quality improvement opportunities (Cohen & Cesta, 1993; Tahan, 1993).

Nurse case managers act as gatekeepers of the interdisciplinary care team. They facilitate communication among the various members and disciplines involved in the care of patients internally (e.g., medicine, nursing, rehabilitation, occupational therapy, social services, pharmacy, medical records, nutrition, and radiology) and externally (e.g., managed care organizations, home care agencies, nursing homes, and durable medical equipment companies). They are continuously involved, directly or indirectly, in the care of their patients. On one occasion, nurse case managers are busy ensuring the timely implementation of necessary care activities. On another occasion, they are seen communicating certain outcomes of care to key health care providers such as physicians, or reassessing patients' conditions and updating managed care organizations of the latest developments so that they maintain appropriate reimbursement requirements/standards.

One informal responsibility of case managers is that of teacher and mentor. The case manager assesses staff development needs, especially among less experienced practitioners, and makes referrals to the appropriate person or resource (Brockopp et al., 1992; Cronin & Maklebust, 1989; Kruger, 1989; Leclair, 1991; Tahan, 1993). It is not uncommon to see nurse case managers conduct educational sessions related to the practice of case management for other health care providers, including physicians, nurses, therapists, and others. They may also function as preceptors for novice case managers, providing training on becoming successful case managers.

The Financial/Business Role Dimension

In collaboration with physicians and other health care team members, case managers initiate case management plans to assure that patients do not receive inadequate care while trying to maintain appropriate resource allocation and length of stay and containing cost (Collard, Bergman, & Henderson, 1990; Tahan, 1993).

Case managers access information related to diagnosis-related groups (DRGs) and current procedural terminology (CPT), the allocated cost for each diagnosis/procedure, the predetermined length of stay, and the treatments and procedures generally used for each diagnosis. They use this information to review resources and evaluate the efficiency of services related to the diagnosis. They exert a great influence over the quality and cost of care by determining, in a timely manner, the most important treatment for the patient. Case managers also assess variances (i.e., delays and deviations from the norm) and act immediately to control these variances to contain costs and improve quality (Cohen & Cesta, 1993; Crawford, 1991; Tahan, 1993; Tahan & Cesta, 1995). They assure consistency, continuity, facilitation, integration, and coordination of care activities to control any duplication or fragmentation in health care delivery, resulting in better allocation and consumption of resources and further cost containment (Henderson & Collard, 1988; O'Malley, 1988a).

To be effective, nurse case managers must access information on case mix indexes, cost and consumption of resources, and practice patterns and must be familiar with the prospective payment systems, current third party reimbursement procedures, and the operations of managed care organizations in today's health care environment of managed competition (Ethridge & Lamb, 1989; Kruger, 1989; Loveridge, Cummings, & O'Malley, 1988; McKenzie, Trokelson, & Holt, 1989; O'Malley, 1988b).

Case managers may work closely with utilization review nurses or may assume utilization review responsibilities, particularly in institutions that dissolved utilization review departments, in identifying long-stay patients, and in planning to control and prevent inappropriate hospital stays (Cohen & Cesta, 1993; McKenzie et al., 1989; Tahan, 1993), and in ensuring the necessary care activities, treatments, and procedures are completed within acceptable and reimbursable time frames.

The Information Management/Communication Role Dimension

Information management and communication are integral functions of the nurse case manager. Without communication, information management, or feedback, nurse case managers cannot possibly succeed in their role. All their roles, responsibilities, and functions depend on information. No matter what type of activity they may be involved in, some form of information is usually managed, transformed, or transmitted. Aspects of the nurse case manager's role that rely heavily on information are communication, negotiation, reporting, explanation, teaching, discussion, reinforcement, clarification, collaboration, coordination, facilitation, evaluation, monitoring, case-conferencing, and feedback. Information included in these activities is always directed toward improving patient care processes, achieving clinical and organizational outcomes, or eliminating variances (i.e., delays, deviations, and omissions) of care.

Nurse case managers are involved in information management and communication in a variety of ways. The following are some examples:

1. Data collection, analysis, trending, and reporting (e.g., variances, data, quality assurance and improvement data, research data, or outcomes management data)
2. Report generation (e.g., logs of case managed patients, variances, cost analysis, cost-benefit analysis, cost-effectiveness analysis, denials and appeals, length of stay, admission and readmission rates, and outcomes management)
3. Communicating and disseminating information (e.g., educational sessions, reports, case conferencing, grand rounds, patient and family education, managed care utilization reviews, authorizations/certifications)
4. Presentations/public speaking, storyboards, posters, and publishing
5. Providing feedback to case management plan development teams
6. Developing or revising policies and procedures
7. Sharing patient-related information with members of the interdisciplinary teams
8. Documentation
9. Obtaining authorizations for services from managed care organizations and reporting findings of utilization review and management activities

The success of nurse case managers depends on how well they communicate with their patients and families, care providers, and payers. Special attention is paid to how influential they are with the customers and stakeholders of the health care organization and the case management system. Two types of stakeholders are highlighted here: internal (e.g., members of the interdisciplinary team) and external (e.g., managed care organizations). In some situations, success is also a factor of computer literacy. As information networks in the field of case management have become highly dependent on and better facilitated by information technology, computer literacy skills have gained increased attention in the role of the case manager.

The Professional Development/Advancement Role Dimension

Professional development and advancement are necessary for nurse case managers. Professional practice aids nurse case managers in gaining the respect and confidence of members of the interdisciplinary health care team. It is highly beneficial that nurse case managers maintain membership in related professional organizations, share their successes and innovations with others, and improve the conditions under which health care services are provided. Some of the advantages of maintaining memberships in related professional organizations such as the Case Management Society of America, the American Nurses Association, and other specialty organizations are as follows:

1. Networking with other case managers and case management societies
2. Exchanging information regarding the latest innovations in case management
3. Obtaining professional support from other case managers

4. Maintaining acceptable professional practice standards
5. Identifying common and national practice standards
6. Developing acceptable standards that promote ethics-based practice and help reduce ethical dilemmas or guide nurse case managers through the process of ethical decision making
7. Maintaining a political voice to advocate for the health of the population at large
8. Making the public policy agenda of case management practices known to other constituencies

There are two types of scholarly activities nurse case managers can involve themselves in to promote their professional development and advancement status: (1) activities that focus on improving the health care practice environment and (2) activities that focus on the nurse case manager's self-development. Examples of the activities that focus on improving the case management practice environment are the following:

- Conduction of research and utilization of research findings
- Promotion of evidence-based practice
- Outcomes management
- Patient and family advocacy
- Legislation and public policy
- Sharing of information at public forums (e.g., public speaking, poster presentation)
- Consulting and entrepreneurial activities

Examples of activities that focus on the nurse case manager's self-development are as follows:

- Pursuing higher education (e.g., graduate degrees in area of practice)
- Becoming certified in the area of specialty or in the practice of case management
- Writing for publication
- Training novice case managers
- Participating in continuing education forums
- Admitting to areas of deficit and seeking improvement in these areas
- Obtaining new skills that improve practice
- Remaining up-to-date with the latest health care practices and innovations

THE NURSE CASE MANAGER'S SKILLS

To be successful in their role, nurse case managers need to have certain skills that make them capable of carrying out their clinical, managerial, business, information management, and professional responsibilities. These skills and traits transcend the issues of where or by whom case managers are employed and are needed by case managers regardless of the care setting where they function. Table 27-2 presents a comprehensive list of the desired skills and personality traits of case managers. It is not mandatory that each case manager exhibits all of these skills and traits. The list may be used by administrators of case management systems or supervisors of case managers to evaluate potential candidates for the case manager role and the actual performance of case managers.

As to their clinical skills, case managers need to be clinically astute and competent in all related diagnostic and therapeutic practices, tests and procedures. They are considered role models and clinical experts for nursing and other staff. They should be skilled in coordinating patients' discharge and patient and family teaching and should be particularly knowledgeable in adult learning theory and the health belief model. Nurse case managers should also be able to function as mentors for less experienced staff.

Since they function as members of interdisciplinary health care teams, nurse case managers should be highly skilled in communication, negotiation, contracting, teamwork, delegation, and conducting meetings. They also should be able to make sound decisions and resolve conflicts. To do all of this suc-

Table 27-2	DESIRED SKILLS AND TRAITS FOR NURSE CASE MANAGERS

SKILLS	TRAITS
CLINICAL/PATIENT CARE	
Direct/indirect care provision	Caring attitude
Expertise in clinical area	Tolerance
Patient and family teaching	Helpfulness
Transitional planning	Sensitivity
Coordination, facilitation, and expedition of care activities/treatments	Respect
Patient and family advocacy	Knowledge
Holistic and pastoral care	Resourcefulness
Crisis intervention and counseling	
Development and implementation of case management plans	
MANAGERIAL/LEADERSHIP	
Problem-solving	Charisma
Conflict resolution	Emotional intelligence
Critical thinking and clinical judgement	Independence, autonomy
Project management	Vision
Conducting meetings	Confidence and self-esteem
Goal-setting	Flexibility and adaptability
Management of change	Self-direction and motivation
Management of ethical and legal issues	Stress tolerance
Time management	Innovation and creativity
Priority-setting	Commitment
Delegation	Advocacy
Negotiation	Cultural sensitivity
Cultural competence	
Consensus-building	
Integration	

cessfully, they should acquire critical thinking and problem solving skills. Because of their managerial responsibilities, case managers are required to write progress reports and quality improvement and length of stay reports, to speak publicly, and possibly to write for publication.

Looking at the business responsibilities embedded in the role of nurse case managers, one can see it is crucial that they have skills in financial analysis, contracting procedures of managed care organizations, financial reimbursement procedures, marketing, and customer relations. These skills are important, since nurse case managers are pressured to improve quality of care and reduce length of stay, hence containing cost.

Table 27-2	DESIRED SKILLS AND TRAITS FOR NURSE CASE MANAGERS—cont'd	

SKILLS	TRAITS
BUSINESS/FINANCIAL	
Resource allocation	Tolerance to numbers
Utilization review and management	Ability to compromise
Certification/authorization of care activities	Attention to details
Financial analysis	Open-mindedness
Cost-effectiveness analysis	Risk-taking
Financial reimbursement procedures	Team player
Quality improvement	
Outcomes management	
Gatekeeping	
Claims and denials	
Health benefits and entitlements	
Variance analysis and management	
INFORMATION MANAGEMENT/COMMUNICATION	
Customer relations	Presentation of self
Cultural sensitivity	Acceptance to criticism
Writing reports	Assertiveness
Information sharing	Motivated
Communication	Pleasant
Documentation	Practical
Brokerage	Teamwork
Dealing with challenging people	Diplomatic
Active listening	Realistic
Collaboration	
PROFESSIONAL DEVELOPMENT/ADVANCEMENT	
Membership in professional organizations	Success
Political and public policy issues	Excellence
Legislation	Willingness to learn
Specialty certification	Eager to gain new skills
Writing for publication	Admit to areas of deficit
Public speaking	Open to improvement
Research	
Advanced education	
Networking	
Consulting	

SELECTION OF NURSE CASE MANAGERS

Health care administrators and policy makers have always struggled and still struggle with deciding who is best qualified to become the case manager. The question focuses on the following:

1. Should the case manager be a nurse-clinician or a paraprofessional staff member?
2. Are nurses the ideal candidates or are other professionals such as social workers and utilization reviewers equally effective in this role?

3. What is the financial implication of such a decision? Can the institution absorb the incurred cost?
4. Who best fits the institutional policies, procedures, and systems?

To respond to these issues, it is necessary to evaluate the case management system to be implemented and the proposed scope of practice and extent of responsibilities of case managers. Schwartz, Goldman, and Churgin (1982) argue that case managers should be clinicians because case management activities require substantial clinical knowledge and decision making skills. Grau (1984) describes case management as a set of clinically based functions that require a clinician to obtain the optimum benefit for the client. This definition also stresses that the background of the case manager is important because it influences the kind of direct and indirect care activities to be provided and other aspects of care delivery and monitoring.

Cohen and Cesta (1993) and Mundinger (1984) support the argument that nurses are best for case management roles because they can provide most services that other professionals offer to clients. Professionals, other than nurses, are neither prepared for nor capable of providing the direct care activities nurses are responsible for, which makes it more difficult for them to assume case management roles. Bower (1992) recommends nurses for case management roles because of their clinical abilities and skills that prepare them for better coordination of services to meet the total needs and concerns presented by patients and their families. Bower also argues that "nurses have skills and knowledge that extend beyond the biophysical and pathological aspects of care, bringing a holistic perspective and knowledge base to the care of case-managed clients" (p. 15). This strengthens the argument that nurses are the best prepared professionals for this role.

According to Zander (1990a), nurses are born for the role of case managers because they are "the generalists; they are the detail people, and they excel in managing care. They are at the juncture of cost and quality, and they know the human implications of trade offs such as early discharge, patient education in groups, or the use of new technology" (p. 201). Case management responsibilities are an extension of the traditional role of nurses. These new functions advance the role, promote professionalism, and bring nursing to a higher level of professional standards among the other health care professions.

One might say that physicians are the case managers of their patients. This may not work well in case management systems, since physicians' care basically is centered on the medical management of the disease. The patients need professionals who can attend to all their other needs, however, not just the medical ones. Nurses can fill this need. They are prepared to address the total picture of patient care, the actual and potential problems (i.e., physical, psychological, social, spiritual) their patients may experience. Nurses in the case manager role act as facilitators and coordinators of care, a role that complements that of the physician. Because of their educational preparedness and clinical experience, nurses bring a wholeness approach to the total management of patient care. Such an approach complements the physician's role and the medical plan.

The literature is clear that nurses should be selected to assume the case manager role. But the question regarding the criteria that make the best nurse case manager remains to be answered. These criteria, as considered by most institutions implementing case management systems, are related to the educational preparation of nurses, communication skills, leadership skills, and clinical knowledge and experience. The personality traits of nurse case managers are important to their success as interdisciplinary team players, negotiators of care, and patient and family advocates.

Tahan, in 1993, examined the selection criteria for nurse case managers. In his study, 26 nursing administrators of case management systems were surveyed on their preferences and perceptions of the criteria that make a successful case manager. It was found that:

- 40% of the nursing administrators recommended a BSN as the minimum requirement for the role
- 48% recommended 4 to 6 years of nursing experience, and 38% recommended 2 to 4 years

- 38% did not approve of the clinical ladder as a requirement for the role
- 61.9% did not have any preference for generalized versus specialized nursing experience; 28.6% preferred specialized practice
- Communication skills and certification in area of practice or specialty were recommended as prerequisites for the role

Most institutions employ registered nurses in the role of case manager. Some of them require a BSN degree as the minimum educational level; however, others use a combination of BSN and associate degree-prepared nurses. Bower (1992), in her book *Case Management by Nurses,* recommends a BSN degree as an entry level for nurse case managers. Loveridge et al. (1988) suggest that nurses with a BSN degree can assume case management responsibilities on a professional level, that is, no direct care activities, and that those with associate degrees can act as case associates, that is, function on a technical level or be responsible for the provision of direct care activities.

Zander (1990b), on the other hand, suggests that other skills and experiences may be as important as the education level. These areas should be looked at when screening nurses for case management roles. Examples of such skills and experiences are (1) knowledge of the nursing process, (2) skills in collaborative practice and interdisciplinary teams, (3) managerial and leadership characteristics, and (4) communication skills.

Advanced educational degrees, graduate nursing degrees, or graduate degrees in a health care–related field are currently more commonly used as requirements for the nurse case manager's role, especially in academic medical centers. This shift has happened because administrators of case management programs view the case manager's role as an advanced practice role. Other reasons are the availability of more graduate degree programs in nursing case management today than ever existed during the past decade and the awareness of the complex and progressive skills a master's prepared case manager brings to the role. In a survey of acute care case managers regarding staff development activities and needs, baccalaureate prepared case managers identified clinical issues as most useful compared to master's prepared case managers who identified systems-related issues as more important. This may indicate that master's prepared case managers have acquired a comfortable degree of clinical experience within their graduate degree preparation, making clinical issues of lesser need. In addition, graduate education may also have played a role in helping case managers become more attentive to systems-related issues (Nolan et al, 1998). After all, case managers spend a great deal of their time and efforts managing the system and resolving the system-related problems.

CHARACTERISTICS OF THE ROLES OF NURSE CASE MANAGERS

Nurses who assume case management roles are given the opportunity to demonstrate effectiveness and efficiency in patient care. It is imperative that nurse case managers be able to assure that the benefits of providing case-managed care exceed the incurred costs while maintaining or improving quality. The wide scope of functions, characteristics, and activities provided by nurse case managers illustrate many of the opportunities, challenges, and threats faced by nurses who are a part of any case management system. As a result, when delivering care, they tend to activate more than one role function or characteristic simultaneously. The nurse case manager's role characteristics and functions are best described in the following general categories.

Change Agent

Successful implementation of any case management system relies heavily on the change agents in the institution. Nurse case managers are integral to this change process (Cohen & Cesta, 1993). They are important in selling the new patient care delivery system to others in the institution, such as physicians, staff nurses, social workers, and personnel in the ancillary departments who are affected by the change. Nurse case managers act as role models and experts when promoting this change. They play a crucial role in teaching all health care personnel about case management systems and answer their questions and concerns. Nurse case managers act to spearhead change by encouraging health care personnel in their efforts to adapt to a new way of delivering care and by encouraging patients in their attempts to quit smoking or to abstain from alcohol, or in other healthful lifestyle changes.

Implementation of case management systems is not an easy process. Some resistance (Cohen & Cesta, 1993; Tahan, 1993), mainly from those most affected by the change, may be encountered. Nurse case managers are prepared to meet this challenge before assuming their new role. They understand that resistance is one way some people might choose to deal with the change. But helping people go smoothly through the process is the case managers' number one challenge. They are well educated in how to conquer resistance and are empowered by administration to employ any approaches deemed appropriate for dealing with resistance and helping make the transition as easy and smooth as possible.

Clinician

Nurse case managers use their clinical expertise in assessing the patient's and family's current status and in identifying their actual and potential problems. They depend on their clinical knowledge and previous experiences when implementing the approaches to care that will help resolve these problems. Keeping abreast of the current advances in medical technology and the latest strategies in patient care is crucial to their meeting the client's needs across the health care continuum.

It is important for nurse case managers to be astute in the nursing process (Bower, 1992), that is, to have assessment skills that enable them to identify the patient's actual and potential health problems and to be able to implement the interventions required to successfully resolve these problems and to evaluate the outcomes of care and responses to treatments.

The clinical skills enable nurse case managers to assess their clients as biopsychosocial beings and to plan the treatments to meet the clients' needs as a whole system and not just the disease. These skills allow them to establish more effective treatment goals and deliver better coordinated and timely care that helps the case-managed patients recover in a timely fashion.

Nurse case managers are also popular for their role modeling and clinical expert function. Because of their extensive clinical background, they act as a resource for less experienced practitioners, some of whom may be from disciplines other than nursing.

Consultant

Nurse case managers guide the interdisciplinary team through the case management process of patient care. They act as consultants to physicians, house staff, fellow nurses, and other providers (Green & Malkemes, 1991; Meisler & Midyette, 1994). Because of their knowledge of institutional policies and procedures, operations, and systems, they provide the interdisciplinary team with a better understanding of the standards of care and practice and facilitate the coordination of tests and procedures, hence the provision of care. They play an important role in identifying the practices that best support efficient and effective care.

They also act as consultants on clinical and administrative issues regarding the delivery of care. Nurse case managers coordinate the needs for consultants, especially for those patients with multiple, complicated needs, and ensure that consultations are obtained in a timely fashion. They are involved, as consultants, in comparing and evaluating medical products that provide the best patient outcomes in the most cost-effective manner (Meisler & Midyette, 1994).

Some nurse case managers may provide consultation services for patients and families via the telephone. This is best accomplished if case managers function in ambulatory care settings such as the emergency department, outpatient clinic, or home care or in the managed care organization setting when a client contacts the case manager for guidance or authorization regarding care.

Coordinator and Facilitator of Care

As patient care coordinators, nurse case managers collaborate with the interdisciplinary team members to meet the patient's needs and the goals of treatments. They are held responsible for coordinating and facilitating the provision of care on a day-to-day basis, the transitional plan, and the patient and family teaching efforts. They also coordinate the required tests and procedures as specified in the case management plan to facilitate a timely delivery of care and patients' movement through the complex health care system, to reduce fragmentation or duplication of care activities, and to promote a collaborative practice atmosphere among the various care providers.

Nurse case managers consult and collaborate on an ongoing basis with other team members every time a problem regarding the provision of care arises or the patient's condition changes. This aspect of the role is important because it permits immediate intervention and change in the plan of care, timely communication with the appropriate personnel, and better decision making regarding patient care. As coordinator and facilitator, the nurse case manager also prevents any delays in patients' discharge and helps control length of stay and resources, and hence, costs. This role responsibility makes nurse case managers important in the institution because they acquire the reputation of being "able to get things done." Health care providers then seek them out every time a problem arises or a certain care activity is not getting done.

It is easier for nurse case managers to assume responsibility for patient care coordination and facilitation because of their understanding of the operations of the institution, the existing systems, and the policies and procedures but mainly because of the power implicit in their role as granted to them by the organization's administration.

Educator

Patient and family education and staff development are other aspects of the nurse case manager's role (Cohen & Cesta, 1993; Meisler & Midyette, 1994; Smith, Danforth, & Owens, 1994; Tahan, 1993). Nurse case managers assess the patient's and family's educational needs at admission to the hospital and ensure that a teaching plan to meet these needs is put together to guide the nursing staff in the process of patient/family teaching. They may or may not be directly involved in conducting the actual teaching sessions. Case managers are responsible for making sure that patient and family teaching is completed, however, as indicated by the assessed needs. They also may act as members of institutional patient teaching committees responsible for developing patient and family teaching materials and overseeing the patient teaching process. Nurse case managers in most institutions play a significant role in assuring compliance with the standards of regulatory and accreditation agencies associated with patient and family teaching and in promoting any institutional policies and procedures.

Regarding staff development, nurse case managers help the clinical staff in professional growth and development by enhancing and disseminating new knowledge and skills. They assess the teaching needs of the nursing and support staff and plan educational sessions to meet these needs or make referrals to the training and development or continuing education departments. They also act as mentors and preceptors for junior and less experienced staff. In reference to case management systems, nurse case managers assume a crucial role in disseminating knowledge regarding case management models, case management plans, and the role of case managers with all health care providers. This is done either formally through prescheduled classes or informally whenever the opportunities arise.

Manager

The manager aspect of the nurse case manager's role entails managing patient care and allocation of resources. As gatekeepers of care, nurse case managers assure the completion of patient care activities in a timely fashion and the use of resources as appropriate and based on the needs of patients. As managers of care, they ensure that the plan of care or the case management plan reflects the patient's needs. They also direct and supervise the provision of care and optimize positive financial outcomes.

Nurse case managers conduct a review of current and past medical records to evaluate the cost of resources and quality of care. This review is important because it provides data regarding inefficient use of resources, medically unnecessary services, and the incurred costs. It also provides administrators with feedback regarding organizational performance.

Negotiator

Nurse case managers assume a significant role in negotiating the plan of care of patients—the length of stay, the required services, and the time in which patient care activities should be completed—with members of the interdisciplinary team and, more importantly, with the patient and family. They are popular for their negotiation skills in getting tests and procedures scheduled with ancillary departments in a timely manner and even in expediting reporting of results. Nurse case managers also play the role of gatekeeper of the interdisciplinary team, a role that requires a tremendous amount of negotiation. Using these skills, they improve the productivity of the team and assure successful completion of its goals.

Nurse case managers are also responsible for working closely with managed care organizations and insurance companies. They negotiate the approval (certification/authorization) of patient care services before the patient's hospitalization and the length of stay as determined by the patient's condition. This task is done before and on a regular basis during hospitalization. They exchange information with the representatives of the managed care organizations regarding patient care and the continued need of patients for medical attention.

Nurse case managers also negotiate the need for community services or nursing home placement with the physician and the patient and family. They then negotiate the approval of such services with appropriate managed care organizations and community resource agencies.

Patient and Family Advocate

Patient and family advocacy is an integral component of the case manager's role. This role is important in case management systems because nurse case managers are responsible for assuring that the needs of patients and families are met. They always inform their clients of their treatment plans and of their progress and support them while they are struggling with decision making regarding the available options for care. Nurse case managers may act as spokespersons for their patients with other health care team members or managed care organizations.

Nurse case managers convey the care options to the patients, which may include the appropriate treatment plan, medications, tests and procedures, expected length of stay, and whether there is a need for any community services after discharge. They answer those questions raised by the patient or family that they can and seek answers to those they do not know. The role of nurse case managers as patient and family educators and facilitators of care are excellent examples of advocacy.

Quality Improvement Coordinator

Nurse case managers are responsible for assuring that quality of patient care is maintained or improved at all times. With the current increased pressure on the health care system for cost containment, case managers are given the authority to ensure that quality of care is not compromised at the expense of reducing length of stay and costs. They act as quality improvement coordinators through their assigned responsibility for collecting and analyzing patient care–related data.

Case managers usually evaluate the provision of care by monitoring delays in patient care and deviations (variances) from the preestablished case management plans. They are proactive in improving patient care quality through developing, in collaboration with an interdisciplinary team of care providers, case management plans that reflect the ideal or best practices and delineate patient care activities, including time frames for completion.

They also participate in continuous quality improvement teams as active members for monitoring patient care activities, system problems, care quality, patient satisfaction, length of stay reduction, and so forth. They provide feedback on improvement efforts to all those involved in patient care on a unit level as well as on an administrative/organizational level. By virtue of their roles as case managers, they are always sought by health care providers, physicians and nonphysicians, to resolve delays in care processes and to investigate any patient care problems that arise.

Nurse case managers generate monthly variance reports that summarize patient care delays, omissions, and changes from the established case management plans. Such reports are an analysis and trending of the data collected. On the basis of these reports, case managers usually make recommendations for improving the organization's way of operating. They also suggest to the interdisciplinary teams any necessary revisions to be made in the case management plans to improve patient care and reduce delays or variances.

Researcher

In most institutions, research is considered an integral component of the role of nurse case manager. Case managers are encouraged to write grant and research proposals for studying patient care. They are active members of committees researching development, dissemination, and utilization of nursing knowledge. They evaluate patient care through research and make recommendations for changes in care standards, policies, and procedures on the basis of research results. They help bridge the gap between theory and practice by applying research in the clinical setting.

Nurse case managers are the best supporters of research related to product-line quality, health care issues, accessibility to care, professional issues, cost, system problems, and effectiveness of case management plans. Such research is important in the evaluation of the effectiveness of case management systems as patient care delivery models. Since they are at the forefront of patient care, case managers are the best people for data collection in such research efforts.

Risk Manager

Risk management is scrutinized in all health care institutions. Nurse case managers play an important role in identifying patient care issues that present legal risk. As coordinators, facilitators, and managers of patient care, they pay close attention to patient care outcomes and ensure that these outcomes meet the preestablished patient care goals and that care is delivered in compliance with the following parameters:

- The institutional policies, procedures, and standards of care and practice
- The requirements and standards of managed care organizations
- Regulatory and accreditation agencies on the state and federal level

It is important that there be a complete description of the case management system to be implemented and a clear definition of the nurse case manager's role. Most institutions expect case managers to:

- Develop case management plans that presumably will improve quality of care
- Select the treatment that is best for the patient
- Manage the patient's total care to ensure optimum outcomes

It is through these role functions that case managers reduce the medical liabilities an institution may face. They work closely with the legal or risk management department to prevent any patient care problems from escalating into a medical liability. In their role as patient and family advocate and in their proactive approach to patient care, they are influential in preventing and reducing legal risk and potential law suits. Case managers may also minimize liability through the following:

- Immediate investigation and solving of patient care problems
- Constant review and revision of hospital policies and procedures and standards of care and practice
- Knowledge of managed care contracts and assuring that care is precertified and provided in compliance with these contracts
- Supervision of appropriate allocation and utilization of resources
- Dissemination of information in a timely manner to key players and decision-makers

With the constant and rapid changes of health care delivery models, the role of nurse case managers has become more important than ever before. The popularity and success of case management systems have made these changes desirable. Nurse case managers have been empowered to function in advanced roles and to prove that their presence in such roles is crucial whenever any efforts are made to improve patient care quality and reduce cost and to help institutions maintain their financial stability, survival, and marketability.

References

Bower, K.A. (1989). Managed care: Controlling costs, guaranteeing outcomes. *Definition: The Center for Case Management, 3*(4), 3.

Bower, K.A. (1992). Case management by nurses (pp. 13-15). (2nd ed.). Kansas City, Mo.: American Nurses Association.

Brockopp, D.Y., Porter, M., Kinnard, S., & Silberman, S. (1992). Fiscal and clinical evaluation of patient care: A case management model for the future. *Journal of Nursing Administration, 22*(9), 23-27.

Cesta, T., Tahan, H., & Fink, L. (1998). The case manager's survival guide: Winning strategies for clinical practice, St. Louis: Mosby, Inc.

Cohen, E.L., & Cesta. T.G. (1993). Nursing case management: From concept to evaluation. St. Louis: Mosby.

Collard, A.F., Bergman, A., & Henderson, M. (1990). Two approaches to measuring quality in medical case management programs. *Quality Review Bulletin, 16*(1), 3-8.

Crawford, J. (1991). Managed care consultation: The "house supervisor" alternative. *Nursing Management, 22*(5), 75-78.

Cronin, C..J., & Maklebust, J. (1989). Case-managed care: Capitalizing on the CNS. *Nursing Management, 20*(3), 38-47.

Ethridge, P., & Lamb, G. (1989). Professional nursing case management improves quality, access and costs. *Nursing Management, 20*(3), 30-35.

Goodwin, D. (1994). Nursing case management activities: How they differ between employment settings. *Journal of Nursing Administration, 24*(2), 29-34.

Grau, L. (1984). Case management and the nurse. *Geriatric Nursing, 5*(8), 372-375.

Green, S.L., & Malkemes, L.C. (1991). Concepts of designing new delivery models. *Journal of the Society for Health Systems, 2*(3), 14-24.

Giuliano, K.K., & Poirier, C.E. (1991). Nursing case management: Critical pathways to describe outcomes. *Nursing Management, 22*(3), 52-55.

Henderson, M.G., & Collard, A. (1988). Measuring quality in medical case management program. *Quality Review Bulletin, 14*(2), 33-39.

Kruger, N.R. (1989). Case management: Is it a delivery model system for my organization? *Aspen's Advisor for Nurse Executives, 4*(10), 4-6.

Leclair, C. (1991). Introducing and accounting for RN case management. *Nursing Management, 22*(3), 44-49.

Loveridge, C.E., Cummings, S.H., & O'Malley, J. (1988). Developing case management in a primary nursing system. *Journal of Nursing Administration, 18*(10), 36-39.

McKenzie, C.B., Trokelson, N.G., & Holt, M.A. (1989). Nursing case management improves both. *Nursing Management, 20*(10), 30-34.

Meisler, N., & Midyette, P. (1994). CNS to case manager: Broadening the scope. *Nursing Management, 25*(11), 44-46.

Mundinger, M. (1984). Community-based care: Who will be the case managers? *Nursing Outlook, 323*(6), 294-295.

Nolan, M., Harris, A., Kufta, A., Opfer, N., & Turner, H. (1998). Preparing nurses for the acute care case manager role: Education needs identified by existing case managers. *The Journal of Continuing Education in Nursing, 29*(3), 130-136.

O'Malley, J. (1988a). Nursing case management. 1: Why look at a different model of nursing care delivery. *Aspen's Advisor for Nurse Executives, 3*(5), 5-6.

O'Malley, J. (1988b). Nursing case management. 2: Dimensions of the nurse case manager role. *Aspen's Advisor for Nurse Executives, 3*(6), 7.

Schwartz, S., Goldman, H., & Churgin, S. (1982). Case management for the chronic mentally ill: Models and dimensions. *Hospitals and Community Psychiatry, 33*(12), 1006-1009.

Smith, G.B., Danforth, D.A., & Owens, P.J. (1994). Role restructuring: Nurse, case manager, and educator. *Nursing Administration Quarterly, 19*(1), 21-32.

Tahan, H. A.(1998a). *The case manager's core competencies: Implications for education, training, and evaluation.* Contemporary Forum-Case Management Along the Continuum Conference. Chicago, March 16-18, 1998

Tahan, H.A. (1998b). *Assuring success in the case manager's role: Skills, traits, and competencies.* Issues and Trends in Nursing Case Management Conference, Princeton, NJ: June 2, 1998.

Tahan, H.A. (1993). The nurse case manager in acute care settings: Job description and function. *Journal of Nursing Administration, 23*(10), 53-61.

Tahan, H.A., & Cesta, T.G. (1995). Evaluating the effectiveness of case management plans. *Journal of Nursing Administration, 25*(9), 58-63.

Thompson, K.S., Caddick, K., Mathie, J., Newlon, B., & Abrahams, T. (1991). Building a critical path for ventilator dependency. *American Journal of Nursing, 91*(7), 28-31.

Zander, K. (1988a). Nursing group practice: "The cadillac" in continuity. *Definition: The Center for Case Management, 3*(2), 1-3.

Zander, K. (1988b). Why managed care works. *Definition: The Center for Nursing Case Management, 3*(4), 3.

Zander, K. (1990a). Case management: A golden opportunity for whom? In J.C. McCloskey & H.K. Grace (Eds.), *Current issues in nursing* (p. 301). (3rd ed.). St. Louis: Mosby.

Zander, K. (1990b). Managed care and nursing case management. In G.G. Mayer, M.J. Madden, & E. Lawrenz (Eds.), *Patient care delivery models* (pp. 37-61). Rockville, Md.: Aspen Publishers.

Credentialing for Case Management

Licensure, Certification, Certificate Programs, and Accreditation

Jeanne Boling, Marlys Severson

CHAPTER OVERVIEW

Licensure, certification, and certificate programs all play key roles in the assurance of a level of competence and quality for case management services provided by individuals. Accreditation programs give the professional and public assurance of a level of competence and quality for case management organizations. This chapter describes the role of each type of credential and the benefits and concerns surrounding each. In addition, practical tips for evaluation are included to assist in navigating the expanding horizon of case management.

HISTORY OF CASE MANAGEMENT CREDENTIALING

In 1992 the National Case Management Task Force assembled representatives from 29 national stakeholder organizations in case management to discuss the need for standardization of case management services. The need was to protect the valuable services case management professionals were providing to patients and their families from inexperienced, uneducated, and wrongly motivated individuals calling themselves case managers. The result of this meeting was to appoint the Commission of Certification of Insurance Rehabilitation Specialists, now known as the Commission for Disability Management Specialists, to develop a certification for individual case managers using the criteria developed by the National Task Force. The resulting new credential became known as the Certified Case Manager (CCM). This credential was conceived as a multidisciplinary entry level credential for the advanced practice of case management. The estimated 25,000+ nationally certified case managers have demonstrated a basic professional licensure, a level of specific case management professional experience, and a knowledge level by obtaining a passing score on a research-based examination. The certification process, therefore, serves to distinguish a basic level of expertise to the vulnerable public.

Since the initial development of the CCM examination, the number of additional certifications for case managers has grown with the specific interests of case managers as the field has developed. Once case management was recognized as a successful strategy in the management of health care quality, efficiency and cost, it began to be practiced in every conceivable setting: hospitals, home care, subacute care, behavioral health care, all forms of managed care organizations, rehabilitation facilities, insurance and reinsurance carriers, independent case management organizations, elder care, long-term care, military, pediatric specialty, all clinical specialties, Medicare, Medicaid, Champus/Tricare, occupational health, and workers' compensation settings. It became obvious that individual case managers could be practicing at the highest level but could be severely impeded by the system in which they practiced. Thus came the need for evaluation of the system used by the organization supporting the individual case manager. This then called for the accreditation process. In the same manner that a valid certification process assures the public of a level of individual competence, an accreditation process assures purchasers of case management services (employers, health plans, insurers) of the competence of the case management organization's structure and system. Initiated in 1997 and 1998, both the Commission of Accreditation of Rehabilitation Facilities (CARF) and the American Accreditation of HealthCare Commission/URAC accreditation programs for case management organizations were scheduled to roll out in 1999.

What Questions Does Credentialing Answer?

Case management professionals provide a service to a medically less knowledgeable and vulnerable public. At the time of their greatest need and lowest ability to evaluate, they are asked to trust a case manager to assist them in making highly complex decisions and access necessary resources. How can they be assured that the case manager they are working with has the level of knowledge and expertise to guide them through this process? How do they know it is safe to trust the case manager with whom they are working? A hospital human resources department needs to hire for case management positions. How will they evaluate the skill level of the individuals interviewed? A manufacturer buys health care coverage for employees. Three health plans respond to an employer's request for proposal. All have case management. How can the company do a comparative analysis for the quality of the case management services marketed? The answers to these questions rest in the credentialing provided by state licensure, certification, and accreditation bodies charged with protecting the public. In this chapter, we will look at the messages sent to the public by licensure, certification, certificate programs, and accreditation in case management.

LICENSURE

Licensure by individual states assures the public that the individual health care professional has completed the basic education for the profession, passed a knowledge-based exam, and has not committed any criminal acts (Box 28-1). Licensure conveys to the public a minimal level of competency to practice. Each profession defines the parameters of the basic entry practice.

Box 28-1   LICENSURE

A license or permit to practice medicine or a health profession within a defined scope issued by any state of the United States.
Examples include RN, MD, LCSW, and RPT.

Case management, as outlined in the Case Management Society of America's (CMSA) *Standards of Practice*, is recognized as a multidisciplinary function and requires that:

The case manager will:

Maintain current professional licensure or national certification in a health and human services profession or both (Case Management Society of America, 1995).

Because case management is not yet recognized as an independent professional discipline, the licensure of case managers is critical to the evaluation of the practice of case management.

CERTIFICATION

When practice requires experience, expertise, or knowledge beyond the basic level of practice, disciplines have addressed advanced practice with additional requirements for education, demonstrated competency, or experience (Box 28-2).

The choice of which certification to obtain is a very individual decision based on the person's discipline, specialty, geographical location, and practice area.

INDIVIDUAL CONSIDERATIONS FOR SELECTION OF A CREDENTIAL

Additionally, consideration must be given to the following:

- Do you practice case management throughout the continuum of care, or is it limited to a part of that continuum?
- Does your case management practice encompass the entire process of case management as described in the Case Management Society of America *Standards of Practice for Case Management* (Box 28-3), or does your job entail completing a part of the process of case management?
- Does the state in which you practice mandate any particular certificate in the practice arena in which you function?

Box 28-2 ▶ **CERTIFICATION**

An adjunctive credential available to an individual who meets eligibility criteria of a particular examination and subsequently achieves a passing score on the examination. The certification can be granted by a national certifying body, signifying that an individual has met the qualifications for case management practice established by that certifying body.

Examples include CCM, CRRN, CDMS, A-CCC, COHN, CMC, C-MAC, and CPHQ.

Box 28-3 ▶ **CASE MANAGEMENT PROCESS**

Common to performance of case management functions is the process used, including assessment, problem identification, outcome identification, planning, monitoring, evaluating, and outcome reporting.

- How does the certification relate to your discipline?
- How will the certificate benefit you in your present position and fit into your career path?

Once all of these questions have been answered, a review of the available certifications must be made. Care must be taken to review the employment situation and to match it with the eligibility criteria of whatever certification is felt to be most appropriate. Without a match between eligibility criteria of the examination and the present job description of the individual, the process cannot continue.

Evaluating Certification Programs for Validity

The certification program must also be examined for validity. Questions to ask are as follows:

- Is it a not-for-profit agency with a program that is national in scope?
- Is it administratively and financially independent of the parent association and free from conflict of interest?
- Is the examination free of bias and nondiscriminatory with published demographic data?
- What is the program for periodic recertification to ensure continued competence?
- How are pass/fail cutoff scores established? Has anyone been granted the credential without achieving a passing score?
- Is there a formal disciplinary policy designed to protect the public?
- Is the certifying agency separate and independent from any associated educational body?
- Are the eligibility criteria logically appropriate to relevant job requirements?
- Does at least one public member serve as a member of the governing board?
- Are reliability statistics produced after each administration of the examination?
- Has the validity of the examination been established by conducting a national job analysis survey?
- Is the certification process research based?

This choice of a credential is a highly individual and personal choice that must be weighed carefully. As the practice of case management matures, there will continue to be more certifications available. It is not surprising that there is a great deal of confusion among the credentials. They may be related to particular disciplines, a particular practice arena, or particular disease entities. Carefully weigh the choices and choose the certification that is most appropriate. The various certifying bodies are able to forward eligibility criteria and information regarding the certification. Carefully review this information and contact them for clarification if necessary. Finding the best match is the priority. Table 28-1 illustrates a representative sample of the certifications available.

There are a number of perceived benefits of case management certification for the individual case manager, the case manager employer, the public client/patient and their families (Box 28-4).

Likewise, time and effort go into the offering and obtaining of any credential. This time is equivalent to value. Concerns about the relative value of the credential compared with the cost of obtaining it are the primary issues in case management as well as other professional disciplines (Box 28-5).

Box 28-4 ▶ **PERCEIVED BENEFITS OF A CASE MANAGEMENT CERTIFICATION**

- Provides a benchmark of knowledge and assurance to employers of case managers.
- Contributes to the ethical standards of the practice of case management.
- Most experts agree that having a certification indicates that a case manager is attempting to broaden his/her base of knowledge and stay current with trends in quality and patient care.[3]
- Provides assurance to the public that the case manager has attained a specific level of knowledge.

Table 28-1	CASE MANAGEMENT CERTIFICATIONS			
CERTIFICATION	**ACRONYM**	**PRIMARY FOCUS**	**ORGANIZATION PROVIDED BY**	**CONTACT INFORMATION**
American Board of Disability Analyst	ABDA	Rehabilitation medicine, case management	American Board of Disability Analysts	ABDA Central Office Park Plaza Medical Bldg. 345 24th Ave. N. Suite 200 Nashville, TN 37203-1520 Telephone 615-327-2984
American Board of Quality Assurance and Utilization Review Physicians	ABQAURP	Utilization management physicians and allied health physicians	American Board of Quality Assurance and Utilization Review Physicians	American Board of Quality Assurance and Utilization Review Physicians 2120 Range Rd. Clearwater, FL 33765 Telephone 800-998-6030
Advanced Certification Continuity of Care	A-CCC	Multidisciplinary discharge planners/case managers	National Board for Continuity of Care Certification	National Board for Continuity of Care Certification 638 Prospect Avenue Hartford, CT 06105-4250 Telephone 203-586-7525
Certified Case Manager	CCM	Multidisciplinary multiple practice setting case managers	Commission for Case Management Certification	Commission for Case Manager Certification 1835 Rohlwing Rd., Suite D Rolling Meadows, IL 60008 Telephone 847-818-0292
Certified Disability Management Specialist	CDMS	Disability managers, insurance-based rehabilitation specialists, vocational counselors	Certified Disability Management Specialist Commission	Certified Disability Management Specialist Commission 1835 Rohlwing Rd., Suite D Rolling Meadows, IL 60008 Telephone 847-818-0292
Case Management Administration Certified	CMAC	Case management administration	The Center for Case Management	The Center for Case Management 6 Pleasant St. South Natick, MA 01760 Telephone 508-651-2600
Care Manager Certified	CMC	Gerontology, counseling care management	National Academy of Certified Care Managers	National Academy of Certified Care Managers 3389 Sheridan St., Suite 170 Hollywood, FL 33021

Continued

This listing is not intended to represent that the certifications listed meet the National Organization for Competency Assurance standards.

Table 28-1	CASE MANAGEMENT CERTIFICATIONS—cont'd			
CERTIFICATION	**ACRONYM**	**PRIMARY FOCUS**	**ORGANIZATION PROVIDED BY**	**CONTACT INFORMATION**
Certified Managed Care Nurse	CMCN	Nurses in managed care	American Board of Managed Care Nursing	American Board of Managed Care Nursing 4435 Waterfront Dr., Suite 101 Glen Allen, Virginia 23060 Telephone 804-747-9698
Certified Occupational Health Nurse–Case Manager	COHN-CM	Occupational health case management	American Board of Occupational Health Nursing–Case Manager	American Board for Occupational Health Nurses 201 E. Ogden Ave., Suite 114 Hinsdale, IL 60521 Telephone 630-789-5799
Certified Professional Disability Management	CPDM	Disability managers	Insurance Educational Association	Insurance Educational Association 1201 Dove Street Newport Beach, CA 92660 Telephone 800-655-4432 ext. 1
Certified Professional in Healthcare Quality	CPHQ	Quality managers, utilization managers, risk managers	Healthcare Quality Certification Board of the National Association for Healthcare Quality	Healthcare Quality Certification Board of the National Association for Healthcare Quality P.O. Box 1880 San Gabriel, CA 91778 Telephone 818-286-8074
Certified Professional Utilization Review	CPUR	Utilization managers, case managers	InterQual	InterQual 44 Lafayette Road P.O. Box 988 North Hampton, NH 03862-0988 Telephone 800-582-1738
Certified Rehabilitation Registered Nurse Certified Rehabilitation Nurse–Advanced	CRRN CRRN-A	Rehabilitation nurses	Rehabilitation Nursing Certification Board	Rehabilitation Nursing Certification Board 4700 W. Lake Avenue Glenview, IL 60025-1485 Telephone 800-229-7530
Certified Nursing Case Manager	RN, CM	Nurse case manager	American Nurses Credentialing Center	American Nurses Credentialing Center 600 Maryland Ave. SW, Suite 100 West Washington, DC 20024 Telephone 800-284-2378

This listing is not intended to represent that the certifications listed meet the National Organization for Competency Assurance standards.

Certificate Programs

A growing number of programs provide continuing education certificates. Some certificate programs are based with for-profit continuing education entities, some are academically based, and some are based with not-for-profit organizations (see Box 28-6).

These programs may or may not screen applicants for experience or professional licensure. They may or may not test the individuals to demonstrate a knowledge level attained. They do offer an educational program for a fee at the conclusion of which is offered a certificate. Because there is considerable variation in the quality of these programs, care must be taken to evaluate the value of the certificate. Some certificate programs, although funded by a for-profit entity, offer not only the certificate but also grant the individual completing the class an acronym to use. This suggests to the untrained public, employer, or professional that the program is assuring the public of a level of expertise and therefore protection. However, such is not the case unless the program offers a research-based examination and generally follows the criteria set forth by the National Association for Certifying Agencies (NACA), a division of the National Organization for Competency Assurance (NOCA) based in Washington, D.C. It is important to distinguish a certificate program from a national research-based and recognized certification credential.

These certificate programs may be useful in obtaining an entry level of knowledge before entering the field of case management. Additionally, some certificate programs provide an overview of case management to prepare the participant for a case management certification examination.

Accreditation

Certification establishes a benchmark only for individual practice. However, with certification only, the health care industry still faces the problem of qualified individuals practicing within a system that may not understand or support the role of the case manager. Accreditation of case management organizations helps to shape the system and thereby assists individual case managers in reaching the full extent of their practice capability. Accreditation also serves as a measure of quality of a case management program to the public and to purchasers of case management services. Two organizations, the Commission

---

Box 28-5 ▶ **CONCERNS RELATED TO CASE MANAGEMENT CERTIFICATIONS**

- Some case managers feel pressured by an increasingly competitive job market to take advantage of the recent proliferation in case management credentials (Case Management Society of America, 1995).
- Some experts are critical of the trend toward raising the educational requirements for the top case management certifications. At issue is whether the bachelor of science in nursing should be regarded as a minimum standard for the practice of case management, since a baccalaureate degree is required in allied health professions (Case Management Society of America, 1995).
- Credentialed case managers command higher salaries. Some case management employers do not wish to pay more.

Box 28-6 ▶ **CERTIFICATE**

The award of a paper certifying completion of a given educational program.

on Accreditation for Rehabilitation Facilities (CARF) and the American Accreditation HealthCare Commission/URAC, offer accreditation standards for case management departments (Fig. 23-4). Both are scheduled to become available in 1999. The CARF standards are geared more toward acute rehabilitation care, while the Commission/URAC standards apply more to payer-based programs.

Sections that Commission for the Accreditation of Rehabilitation Facilities (CARF)

Several sections comprise the CARF Case Management Accreditation Standards.

LEADERSHIP. The leadership section addresses who is responsible for managing and directing medical rehabilitation case management. It also outlines who in leadership would be responsible for various areas of case management activity, such as fiscal management, ethics, strategy, health, safety, and transportation.

INFORMATION AND OUTCOMES MANAGEMENT. This section addresses how information is gathered at the level of the individual and the level of the program to determine the outcomes of interventions completed by case managers. It also discusses public disclosure of information gathered.

REHABILITATION PROCESS FOR PERSONS SERVED. The rehabilitation section addresses the rights of the client and how case managers interact with the client and the rehabilitation team, as follows:

- Full participation of the case manager in decision making related to the services, equipment, and supplies provided to the persons served, community resources used, and efficient movement of the client through the continuum of care
- The role of the case manager in the continuum of care and use of the continuum of care
- Coordination with all stakeholders
- Advocacy for clients

American Accreditation HealthCare Commission/URAC

The standards address the following areas:

STANDARDS FOR STRUCTURE AND ORGANIZATION
- Staff structure and qualifications
- Staff management and development
- Information systems
- Confidentiality
- Financial responsibility
- Oversight of delegated functions

STANDARDS FOR CASE MANAGEMENT PROCESS
- Accessibility
- Patient rights
- Appeals and grievances

Standards for Quality Improvement

- Quality improvement data
- Quality improvement program

Where do the URAC Standards Apply?

The standards apply to "case management organizations," which are defined as organizations and/or programs that provide telephone and/or on-site case management services in conjunction with a private or publicly funded benefits program. Such services may be provided by a stand-alone case management organization or by an organization that conducts case management in conjunction with a range of managed care services such as utilization management or disease management (AAHC/URAC, 1999).

Accreditation Process

Unlike licensure and certification, accreditation is not granted as the result of receiving a passing score on a content specific test. Rather, accreditation is the cumulative evaluation of the structure and processes that are in place within a case management organization. It not only reviews the documentation of policies and procedures, but looks at how well the organization implements the policies and procedures that exist.

The accrediting body develops a set of guidelines that become the basis of the evaluative process. These guidelines are usually established using experts in the field, may be based on the standards that exist for the industry being accredited, and, in most accrediting organizations, are opened for public comment.

The accreditation process is usually two-fold, including a review of documentation and on-site interviews. The review of documentation is an overview of policies, procedures, and processes of the organization. It is a cursory review to determine if the organization meets a basic level of compliance with the standards. For instance, does the organization have the necessary policies and procedures in place to meet the accreditation standards? During this review, the examiner may desire additional information from the organization or pose specific questions to be reviewed. This review may occur before or during the on-site assessment.

The accreditation process culminates in an on-site evaluation. During this phase of the process, reviewers engaged by the accrediting organization schedule an on-site assessment of the organization to evaluate if indeed the organization is functioning in a manner consistent with the guidelines established. The team usually conducts interviews of key staff members and may review additional internal documents for evidence of compliance (e.g., patient charts or minutes of meetings). If the organization displays a level of operation in keeping with the standards outlined, they are granted accreditation status for a specified period of time.

As you might imagine, any process that requires time and establishes a level of accountability is debated as to the relative value to society. Boxes 28-7 and 28-8 list the benefits and concerns of accreditation.

The following areas must be addressed by accrediting entities requiring outcomes data so criteria can be refined:

1. Case load size
2. Case management qualifications

Box 28-7 ▶ **BENEFITS OF ACCREDITATION**

- Encourages sufficient organizational support for case management
- Clarifies operational procedures and policies governing case management
- Encourages increasing organizational focus on quality management
- Promotes organizational accountability
- Ensures that case managers can practice in a manner consistent with the profession's standards (D'Andrea et al)
- Once the accreditation is established and recognized by state legislatures, it may substitute for organization licensure. This can save significant time and money for multistate organizations (Key to Quality Healthcare)

Box 28-8 ▶ **CONCERNS RELATED TO ACCREDITATION DEVELOPMENT**

- Some case management employers are concerned that the cost of preparation (American Health Consultants, 1998) for accreditation will add to the cost of case management and ultimately drive up the cost of health care.
- Small case management firms and individual case managers are concerned over the developmental costs of the accreditation and their continued survival in the marketplace.
- There is concern that state legislatures may require accreditation to conduct business within the state

---

3. Evaluation of quality in case management programs
4. Collection and analysis of data
   a. Cost
   b. Confidentiality
   c. Access
5. Outcomes studies

How Does Case Management Program Accreditation Impact Individual Case Managers?

Accreditation will help to standardize case management practices by measuring case management programs against consistent benchmarks. Hopefully, some of the results will be (1) increased organizational focus on quality, (2) clearer operational policies and procedures governing case management, and (3) sufficient organizational support for case management services. Accreditation can also make customers and clients more confident in the case management services they receive.

As the development of case management continues, the need for research-based continuing quality improvement will become critical. It is the hope of the industry that professional organizations can work jointly with certification and accrediting bodies to collect data, identify best practices, and advise practicing case managers concerning which case management strategies are most effective.

As you can see, licensure, certification, certificate programs, and accreditation all play a role in assuring the public and those purchasing case management services of a level of professional care (Box 28-9). The reader is strongly encouraged to evaluate and reach for the most appropriate credential.

Box 28-9	ACCREDITATION BODIES

American Accreditation HealthCare Commission/URAC
1275 K Street, NW Suite 1100
Washington, DC 20005
Telephone 202-216-9010
Fax 202-216-9006
www.urac.org

CARF. The Rehabilitation Accreditation Commission
4891 E. Grant Road
Tucson, AZ 85712
Telephone 520-325-1044
Fax 520-318-1129
www.Carf.org

References

Accreditation programs: Key to quality healthcare. http://www.urac.org/Key-to-quality.htm.

American Accreditation HealthCare Commission/URAC Case Management Accreditation Standards. 1999.

American Nurses Credentialing Center (1998). *Nursing Case Management Catalog.*

American Health Consultants (1998, Dec.). *Hospital case management.*

D'Andrea, G. & Hamill, C.T. (1999). Case management organization accreditation under way. *The Case Manager, 10*(1), 53-61.

Commission on Accreditation of Rehabilitation Facilities (1999). *1999 Medical rehabilitation standards manual, Medical Rehabilitation Case Management Program.*

Case Management Society of America. (1995). *Standards of practice for case management* (pp. 14-18).

Commission for Case Management Certification (1997). *CCM Certification Guide,* Certified Case Manager.

Mullahy, C.M. (1998). *The case manager's handbook* (pp 154-157, 435-441). (2nd ed). Aspen.

Powell, S.K. (1996). *Nursing case management.* Philadelphia: Lippincott—Raven.

Learning Partnerships

Online Case Management

Gayle Preheim

CHAPTER OVERVIEW

Today's competitive and chaotic managed care environment provides the impetus for acquiring or updating knowledge and skills to meet the demand for employment opportunities and expanded roles in case management. This chapter will describe the challenges and opportunities for developing case management competencies through innovative educational strategies and courses delivered via the Internet.

Current trends in education have redefined the who, what, where, and how of teaching and learning. The World Wide Web and interactive educational technology allow for the creation of virtual classrooms with increased relevancy and availability and without the rigid constraints of time, place, or pace. Best practices in education using interactive technology emphasize creating an active learning environment to promote discovery, critical thinking, and collaboration. Student and faculty roles are changed in a web-based environment, and the responsibilities for learning and teaching are shared. Experiences with online case management courses provide insights into the advantages and potential pitfalls. Innovative partnerships among case managers, employers, and educators have evolved to guide the design, delivery, and evaluation of web-based educational programs for competency development throughout professional nursing careers.

TRENDS IN EDUCATION

Roles and concepts of teaching and learning are being restructured (Sherry & Wilson, 1997). The rapidly expanding World Wide Web and emerging virtual communities provide professional nurses with previously unimagined access to multiple databases and a rich national and international community for collaborative practice. A recent focus of education is to rapidly respond to the learning needs of dynamic communities of health care professionals by designing and delivering quality and accessible educational programs. Innovative strategies integrate educational technology into teaching and learning to provide case managers with additional tools to achieve goals of personal growth and professional advancement.

Relationship of Case Management and Online Learning

The study and practice of case management are well suited to online learning and resources. Case managers recognize the need and benefit of updated skills. Current knowledge is needed to be able to impact the coordination of care and influence the organization for improved cost and quality outcomes in the delivery of health care. Self-directedness, flexibility, collaboration, effective communication skills, and commitment to inquiry and discovery for problem solving and decision making are skills necessary for both effective case management practice and successful web-based learning.

Proficiency in using technology is a commonly required competency in the workforce today (Twigg & Oblinger, 1996). The amount and type of information professionals must process and communicate are changing. As the use of computer technology and information increases, individuals who have not developed basic computer skills will be at a disadvantage. Case managers must be skilled and knowledgeable in the use of computers to access, manage, and communicate information (Robin, 1998). They must be able to access and use the rapidly changing and increasing volume of database resources, consumer information, clinical guideline and practice standards, and accrediting and regulatory information available on the Web.

"In a world of accelerated change, learning must be a lifelong process." (Knowles, 1980, p.19). Professionals are expected to build new skills on past knowledge, apply theory in practice, and become increasingly self-directed problem solvers and decision makers (Mast & Van Atta, 1986). Knowledge doubles every 7 years. The shelf life of a technical degree today has been estimated to be less than 5 years. Reskilling is becoming a requirement for employees. The American Society for Training and Development predicts that by the year 2000, 75% of the current workforce will need to be retrained due to rapidly changing skill sets (Verville, 1995). In reengineered organizations, employees have more complex roles and expanded work responsibilities (Foreman, 1995).

Nurses whose educational program integrates the essential competencies of case management with skill building in network telecommunications have greater potential to do the following:

- Be knowledgeable about health care issues and changes occurring locally, and nationally through the Internet and World Wide Web.
- Be knowledgeable about economic trends, local needs and resources, and alternative problem-solving and decision-making strategies through health care information systems.
- Develop skills in using clinical information systems for the practice of nursing case management and the delivery of nursing care.
- Develop skills to evaluate and manage programs and projects through the use of clinical knowledge, knowledge of health policy, knowledge of clinical and cost data management, and manipulation, analysis, and interpretation of data.
- Develop skills in using computerized information systems in health care to support clinical and administrative decision making.
- Develop information management skills to functionally collect, aggregate, organize, move, and present information in effective and economical ways useful to others.
- Improve communication, understanding, and management of information for care delivery and coordination.
- Maximize the accuracy, timeliness, and usefulness of information for improved health care planning, delivery, and monitoring.
- Transform data or information from one form to another to increase meaningfulness and usefulness.
- Provide insight into structures of information for processing and using appropriate transformations, including algorithms and rules of thumb useful in the practice of nursing case management.
- Work together across boundaries of time, multiple roles and responsibilities, and urban and rural geographies.
- Discover a vision of the future that includes technology and information systems in health care.

Shifts in Expectations and Approaches in Education

Four elements of teaching and learning, relevant to the professional development of case managers, are shifting (Boettcher, 1998) and will be outlined here.

WHO IS LEARNING?

Today's view of education is nontraditional. As pragmatists who face the realities of the workplace daily, case managers view education for its use-value rather than enrichment. Nurses are returning to school for retooling, an additional degree, or certification for professional advancement. Learner demographics show shifts from full time to part time, from younger to more mature, from inexperienced with computer technology to skilled in the use of computers and the Internet. Online teaching and learning strategies are appropriate for case managers who may be distant from campus, hold positions of employment, or have workloads that require the readily available course materials and opportunities for faculty and peer interaction at a flexible pace and convenient place. According to Fulkerth (1998), education is evaluated according to the expectations of a consumer-oriented culture: what do I get, how much will it cost, how convenient is it, how will it be delivered, and what's the warranty?

WHO IS TEACHING?

A collaborative movement between the teacher and student is shifting the teacher's role from controlling the course content and delivery to creating an environment for learning. The teacher as teller with the sole authority and single answer is drifting as an appreciation for the complexity of real world problems and diversity of possible responses is growing (Sherry & Wilson, 1997). As a facilitator, guide, and mentor, the teacher creates the learning environment with learning tools. Students are accountable for their own learning and share the responsibility for teaching each other (Fulkerth, 1998). In an innovatively designed web-based environment, interaction, and collaboration are promoted by providing access to unlimited numbers of case management experts in the field, clinical and educational resources, and knowledge bases.

WHAT IS IMPORTANT TO LEARN?

Expectations are changing about what students need to learn, as well as the delivery mechanism and technology available to serve the need. A shift is occurring from teaching content to enabling students to develop lifelong learning skills. Clinical practice disciplines are becoming more complex and more interdisciplinary. In addition to mastering the nursing discipline's knowledge base, case managers must know how to access, analyze, and use rapidly changing information such as clinical guidelines, health policy, and accrediting and regulatory criteria (Collins, 1996; Fulkerth, 1998). The focus is on the learner and authentic problems (Sherry & Wilson, 1997). The capacity for learning how to learn is essential. Facts are less important than processes, relationships, and interactions. Essential competencies in preparation for a successful career and a useful life are the ability to think critically, communicate effectively, and collaborate with others (Twigg, 1994).

WHERE IS LEARNING OCCURRING?

Accessibility to innovatively designed educational programs using technology is increasing to meet the case manager's changing learning needs and expectations. Online courses are leading the development of new learning environments (Campbell, 1997). The World Wide Web represents a new way of looking at teaching and learning. Used in combination with Internet communication tools such as email, the web can be used for material delivery or as an environment for interactive learning. Distributed learning allows faculty, case managers, and educational materials to be placed at independent locations so that teaching and learning can occur at any time, in any place, and at any pace (Boettcher, 1998).

The Impact of Educational Technology

Web-based or supported courses using new technological resources can be designed to address different learning styles, illuminate difficult concepts, accelerate knowledge acquisition, and prepare students for a lifetime of learning (Andriole, 1995). According to Sherry and Wilson (1997), educational technology impacts learning in the following ways:

- Enhancing the quality of education through active learning and teaching strategies.
- Guiding educational redesign from instructing to facilitating learning.
- Creating relevant and accessible learning environments for learners with differing learning styles and constraints of time and location.
- Promoting shared responsibility between the faculty and the learner for the quality of the learning process.
- Advancing active learning strategies that motivate and satisfy learners because of the improved quality of learning.

INNOVATIVE ONLINE TEACHING AND LEARNING STRATEGIES

A web-based learning environment can be attractive to both traditional and nontraditional nursing students who seek a rigorous learning experience yet require flexibility. Communications technology allows asynchronous learning experiences, providing continuous access to the course. Increasingly, learners use networks to interact with peers, their instructors, professional experts, and other information resources available on the World Wide Web (Twigg & Oblinger, 1996).

Assessing Readiness for Online Learning

A self-assessment of learning readiness and goals is necessary before investing time and energy in online learning. Consider motivations, ability to be self-directed and self-disciplined, the degree of direction and structure preferred, and skills for working in a virtual environment, including willingness to use a computer as a medium for interacting with people. The following questions will help determine if an online course is the learning alternative of choice:

- Why do I want or need to take this course?
- What are my available options, who else offers them, at what cost, with what schedule, and for what benefit?
- Is this the right time for me to take the course, given my workload, organizational support, family support, financial capability, availability of tuition reimbursement, and motivation?
- How will this course meet my needs in terms of content, schedule, outcomes, application, technical support, mentoring, and collegiality with other learners?
- Do the educational technology and delivery methods suit my learning style, and do I have access to the appropriate hardware, software, and computer skills?
- What skills do I have to contribute to promoting a community on line? (Billings, 1996)

Recommendations for Selecting an Online Offering

An online course should have comprehensive requisites to support learning, including a resource team for assuring quality in design, delivery, and technical support. Essential factors to consider include the following:

- Evidence of design team (expert content faculty, web developer, instructional designer/graphic designer, technical assistance) collaboration and commitment to excellence in the use of educational technology with a valued place in the school.

- Evidence of a well-organized educational offering that includes planning, course materials, specific computer hardware and software requirements, access instructions, timelines, computer literacy expectations for students, enrollment procedures, and a plan for obtaining necessary help/support.
- Faculty reputation as skilled facilitator, group mediator, communicator, and proven demonstrations of attentiveness, empathy, patience, flexibility, humor, and ability to establish trust in the faculty-learner relationship.
- Evidence of student involvement and feedback integrated in the course offering, and reflection of student evaluation data from previous offering integrated into the current offering.
- User-friendly enrollment procedures, advising, and access to text, course materials, and library resources that assure careful and prompt attention to student needs, including those of distant learners.
- Availability of technical assistance at the educational institution and clear protocol for accessing as needed.
- Appropriate opportunities for orientation to the technology before the course begins and socialization to the roles of the learner (self-directed learning, independent learning, collaborative learning) and faculty and as a member of an online learning community.
- Availability of help for students to learn how to learn online via learning guides, presentation handouts, or introductory training modules.
- Peer support; success of online learning depends on shared commitment and enthusiasm of learners.
- Opportunities for formative and summative evaluation by the students of the course/delivery so recommendations for improvements can be integrated in an ongoing manner.
- Access to information systems support at the workplace if Internet access is expected during work hours.
- Administrative or employer support for your enrollment, including opportunities to integrate course learning activities with workplace issues or initiatives (Billings, 1996).

Innovative Strategies to Promote Learning Outcomes

The Internet as a delivery method has potential advantages relevant to access, convenience, and flexibility. However, the teaching and learning strategies used to facilitate the mastery of higher order learning are more important than the delivery method (Campbell, 1997). The course design, whether unstructured or highly structured, should increase the learner's competency through purposeful interaction. Instruction includes the elements of motivating the learner, explaining what is to be learned, linking new information with previous knowledge, providing instructional material, and testing comprehension (Ritchie & Hoffman, 1998). Online strategies may include a wide variety of tools and techniques, such as distributed lectures and instructional materials, interactive media textbooks, one-to-one communication using email, access to library resources, asynchronous group communications for posting messages and submitting assignments, synchronous group discussions or chat areas for same-time, different-place meetings, simulation exercises, and online assessment and evaluation (Billings, 1996).

Instruction, however, is not learning. Learning requires initiative, interest, interaction, innovation, and involvement. In 1987 the American Association of Higher Education recognized that networked communication systems and information technologies were becoming major resources for teaching and learning. The "Seven Principles of Best Practice in Education" (Chickering & Ehrmann, 1987) describe appropriate ways to maximize the use of educational technology, as follows:

1. Encourage contacts between students and faculty. Interacting encourages students to think about their own experiences and learning goals and is a most important factor in student motivation.
2. Develop reciprocity and cooperation among students. Learning is a social process. Thinking is improved and understanding is deepened when student-student interaction and collaboration are promoted.
3. Use active learning techniques. Learning involves thinking, speaking or writing reflectively, relating to experience, and applying to daily lives.

4. Give prompt feedback. Knowing what you know and what you don't know focuses learning. Frequent opportunities to perform and receive feedback on performance should be provided. Students can learn to self-assess their learning needs.
5. Emphasize time on task. Allocating realistic amounts of time and energy promotes learning.
6. Communicate high expectations. Expecting the student to perform well becomes a self-fulfilling prophecy. Peer evaluation and learning teams can encourage investment in learning.
7. Respect diverse talents and ways of learning. Different students bring different strengths and styles of learning. Self-direction, self-discovery, and self-discipline are worthwhile learning tasks.

A "constructivist" learning environment to promote active learning outcomes is appropriate for the World Wide Web. This environment creates opportunity for involvement and the generation of self-directed learning. Generative learning is based on the ability to reflect on existing knowledge and integrate alternative points of view. "Students must work with information, manipulate it, change it, relate it to existing knowledge structures, and use it to support problem solving. Students learn how to use or apply information they learn. Generative learning activities require students to take static information and generate fluid, flexible, usable knowledge" (Kommers, Grabinger, & Dunlap, 1996, p. 273).

A learning environment should be created that includes activities such as collaboration, autonomy in learning, critical reflection, and authentic interactions with real-world problems. Students should participate in activities that promote high-level thinking processes, including problem solving, experimentation, original creating, and discussion and examination of topics from multiple perspectives (Bostock, 1997). However, to become capable problem solvers, students must know how to learn and be willing and able to take responsibility for identifying learning deficits, setting learning goals, managing the learning process, and monitoring the learning strategies they use (Grabinger & Dunlap, 1996).

Role Expectations and Shared Responsibilities

In a web-based environment, teaching and learning come together as a partnership. Faculty provide the framework and manage the learning process. The learner actively participates and collaborates with other learners and resources to enhance comprehension, understanding, and knowledge (Doherty, 1998). Students become investigators and problem solvers. Teachers become facilitators and coaches rather than presenters of knowledge (Knowles, 1980).

The goals of online learning are consistent with the principles of adult and active learning, whereby nurses tend to be self-directed and accept responsibility for their own learning. Adult learners have developed individualized learning styles, depending on what works best for them. Some learn most effectively through action, interaction, or participation; others through reading and reflection. A web-based environment blends these approaches. Online learning provides the opportunity and expectation that individuals will select learning materials that they perceive have immediate applicability to life tasks. The focus of learning is on problem solving and generating products of value. It emphasizes self-determination, self-assessment, and the involvement of the whole person in the learning process (Kinzie & Sullivan, 1989; Lawless & Brown, 1997). Learner control is enhanced in online learning because the case manager can direct his or her own learning experiences, including the path and pace. Depending on learning style and needs, the depth of study, range of content and type of media, and time spent are tailored by the individual. The learner's perceptions of competence, self-determination, and intrinsic interest may increase (Lawless & Brown, 1997).

The faculty role in online learning has often been described as the "guide on the side" rather than the "sage on the stage." As facilitators, faculty should be resources for self-directed learners rather than imparters of a body of knowledge. Designing a framework for constructive discourse and negotiation of meaning among students is a primary responsibility. Learning guides and content resources may be provided. Learners' participation and activities are monitored, and social support for the learning community is provided through encouragement, feedback, and mentoring.

As important as the concepts of self-directed learning and active involvement are for the student, and facilitation and guidance are for the faculty, the critical element for successful online learning is the development of a community of learners. Through the dynamic community, peers and experts in the field develop and share toolkits with useful application for professional development and personal growth. The new model for education is a learning network: a community of learners who work together in an on-line environment. The American Association for Higher Education (1998) outlined Learning Principles and Collaborative Action, as follows:

1. Learning is fundamentally about making and maintaining connections.
2. Learning is enhanced by taking place in the context of compelling situations.
3. Learning is an active search for meaning by the learner, constructing knowledge rather than receiving it, and shaping it as well as being shaped by experiences.
4. Learning is a developmental and cumulative process.
5. Learning is by individuals who are intrinsically tied to others as social beings.
6. Learning is strongly affected by the educational climate.
7. Learning requires frequent feedback if it is to be sustained.
8. Learning takes place informally and incidentally.
9. Learning is grounded in particular contexts and individual experiences.
10. Learning involves the ability of individuals to monitor their own learning.

"Network learning enables anyone, anywhere, at anytime to be a learner or a teacher. It enhances the link between theory and practice, and the classroom and the real world" (Kersley, p. 70, 1993). A community of learners has come together when learners gather to provide mutual support and scaffolding for learning and performance. Indicators of an effective learner support environment are as follows:

- Learners solve their own problems and share solutions.
- Effective learning resources are located or developed and made available to the entire learning community.
- Learners are encouraged and rewarded for taking initiative.
- Learners' areas of expertise are valued.
- Technical support and guidance are made available to each other through online resources and a buddy system.
- The informal culture encourages risk-taking and innovation (Sherry & Wilson, 1997).

EVALUATION OF AN ONLINE LEARNING EXPERIENCE

The Web is effective in providing quality and accessible educational opportunities, promoting interaction among learners across geographical boundaries, and guiding application to practice. However, offerings must be carefully designed and strategies cautiously implemented to achieve the desired outcomes of content mastery and competency development. What engages, motivates, and reinforces student learning? What student/faculty preparation is needed and how can barriers be managed? Which methods are most useful for redesigning roles, structuring learning experiences, assessing competencies, and facilitating learners' ability to perform in the practice setting?

Many models, instruments, and methodologies exist to evaluate the use of educational technology and the value of the virtual classroom. The Flashlight Evaluation Project (Ehrmann & Zungia, 1997) uses a conceptual model for evaluating the impact of informational technology on teaching and learning. Changes in learning outcomes, access, and cost are measured. Examples of key learner-focused educational issues include active and collaborative learning strategies, using time productively, high expectations for all students regardless of learning style, rich and rapid feedback, engagement in learning, faculty and student interaction, cognitive and creative outcomes, accessibility, respect for diversity, and application to work (Ehrmann & Zungia, 1997).

Courses designed to provide opportunities for collaboration, problem- or project-based experiences, and focus on high-level activities, such as integration and critique, are most effective in promoting learning (Billings, 1996).

Learners' Perceptions of the Benefits of Online Learning

Satisfaction is directly related to the availability of learner support for using the technology and changes in approaches to teaching and learning. In comparisons of online courses with real-time courses offered on campus, students' responses to online courses were positive (Andriole, 1996; Billings, 1996; Forsyth, 1996; Saltzberg & Poyson, 1996; Twigg & Oblinger, 1996). Themes related to online learning included the benefits of accessibility, convenience, and flexibility. Students believed they spent more time with the course material because learning was more meaningful to them. They generally felt connected, interacted more with faculty and peers, learned to use classmates as resources, and reflected more on their interactions with the course content (Carlton, Ryan, & Siktberg, 1998). The ability to share examples, discuss works in progress, and critique each other's work was valuable. The need to take more responsibility for their learning was acknowledged, as was the high technology learning curve. The consensus was that course and personal learning goals were accomplished.

Lessons Learned by Exploring, Experimenting, and Evaluating

In 1997 an existing didactic case management course offered at the University of Colorado School of Nursing was redesigned for Internet delivery. Ongoing modification has occurred with each of its subsequent offerings. A design team consisting of content experts, instructional designer, and webmaster developed and operationalized the course using WebCT (1999), an authoring software program. The conceptual framework for the content includes the Case Management Society of America Standards of Practice and the Commission for Case Manager Certification Essential Activities and Core Areas of Case Management. The course features six content modules with competency outcomes, interactive learning activities and resources, a conference center for asynchronous discussion, and individual and group assignments with critical elements for competency evaluation. A teaching and learning environment emphasizes a caring educative pedagogy and reinforces the "Seven Principles of Best Practices in Education" (Chickering & Gamson, 1987).

The process of transforming a course for internet delivery includes *exploring* a variety of traditional and innovative strategies for consistency with the goals of competency-based education within an educative caring pedagogy; *experimenting* with multiple learning strategies to determine usefulness and effectiveness in content mastery and competency development, including problem-based learning projects, presentations, peer review, quizzes, reflection papers, group work, and research using Internet resources; and *evaluating* the efficacy of methods from student and faculty viewpoints. Formative and summative evaluation methods are used to assess the impact of learning strategies and competency assessment methodologies. Consistent themes include agreement that the course design supported learning, confidence in ability to learn difficult and complex material was enhanced, meaningful communication was encouraged, and application of learning to the real world was emphasized. Students agreed they would enroll in another Internet course and recommend the course to others. Responses were used in an ongoing manner to improve content, teaching strategies, and level of presentation. Recommendations for design and evaluation strategies have guided subsequent web-based offerings and facilitated the evaluation of curriculum concepts and organizing frameworks.

INNOVATIVE PARTNERSHIPS FOR TEACHING AND LEARNING

Design-Develop-Deliver-Decide Model

Partnerships among case managers, employers, and educators are evolving for the purpose of achieving shared goals. Nursing case managers play critical roles in satisfying the need for quality health services in a cost-effective environment and require updated knowledge and skills. Nursing administrators recognize the immediate need for quality educational programs and professional development to support the evolving role of nursing case manager and to positively impact clinical and cost outcomes. Nursing educators are committed to promote the fusion of learning and work and to design and deliver educational programs using interactive learning strategies and technology to increase accessibility and relevance. The result was the faculty-developed **"Design-Develop-Deliver-Decide"** model to create, market, implement, and evaluate a case management web-based course offered by the University of Colorado, School of Nursing. Health care professionals from a variety of tertiary care and health maintenance organizations have successfully completed the course for credit toward degrees or for professional development.

In **Design,** the educational setting, strategies, and players are redefined. The employing organization demonstrates to its members a commitment to learning, the expectation and support for competency development, and continuous improvement. The educator-employer partnership is established to assist in achieving the goals. A needs analysis identifies the employer's performance expectations of the practicing nurse. Competency outcomes are determined collaboratively. The return on investment must be determined: will the educational program result in increased knowledge, evidenced by improvement in the performance of essential skills at a reasonable cost?

Collaborative planning in the **Develop** phase assures course structure and process to enhance competency development. A design operationalizes the course, which features interactive strategies selected to promote self-directed learning, content mastery, and application to practice. Responsibility is shared among the employer and the course development team to assure a learner-centered Web environment.

In traditional educational settings the student-teacher relationship starts and ends with the **Delivery** or offering of the course. In a collaborative partnership the relationship with the employer has preceded the learner-facilitator relationship and may be extended beyond the duration of the current course offering. After expectations are mutually clarified, protocols are established for participant identification, tuition reimbursement, assessment of basic computer skills and Internet access, and time frames. Recognition, encouragement, and reward by the employer are important, as the responsibility for the quality of the process is shared among educator, employer, and learner.

Throughout the course, learners, employers, and educators must **Decide** whether the anticipated outcomes are achieved. Evaluation data provide a quantitative and qualitative picture of the strengths and areas of improvement. Recommendations from formative data collected at the end of each module are incorporated to continually shape the educational experience to meet learning needs and expectations. Key learning, continued learning needs, and one-word journals clarify students' perspective of competency achievement. Summative course evaluation data provide a comprehensive review of the web-based learning environment and evidence of learning. Finally, evidence of learning relevant to practice, including functional, interpersonal, and critical thinking competencies, are summarized and presented in educator-employer conferences. Employer feedback is solicited, providing an opportunity to assess their perspective of the success of the project, strategize about future possibilities, and forge partnerships that enhance both service and education.

Implications for Building Learning Partnerships

Partnerships among case managers, nursing administrators, and educators promote professional development and achievement of shared goals to improve care coordination, quality, and cost outcomes. When innovative teaching and learning strategies are planned by employer and educator partners and operationalized in a web-based environment, learners have an opportunity to demonstrate initiative in self-directed learning to achieve cognitive, attitude, and skill outcomes. As the learner is guided by the structured modular activities and resources, continuing learning needs are identified and new learning is reinforced by online interaction. Involvement is maximized as convenience and accessibility are increased by altering time and space constraints through networked educational technologies. Professional working relationships, networking, and mentoring among nurses, administrators, and faculty are enhanced when nontraditional learners are provided educational options that are supported by nursing leaders in their workplace.

Learning as a part of life and work is reinforced as the educational experiences integrate current practice roles and responsibilities with education throughout professional nursing careers. Employer and educator models for competency development that align goals, strategies, and resources are key to advance professional nursing practice and to demonstrate the valuing of professional development and the role of the nursing case manager. "Higher education is transitioning from asynchronous learning—anytime, anyplace, for anyone—to a pervasive learning environment—every time, every place, and for everybody." (Duderstadt, 1997, p.10).

References

American Association for Higher Education, American College Personnel Association, National Association of Student Personnel Administrators: Joint Task Force on Student Learning Final Report, "Powerful partnerships: A shared responsibility for learning", *June, 1998.* http://www.aahe.org/assessment/joint.htm

Andriole SJ: Asynchronous education and training networks: Lessons learned well and in progress, *October 9, 1995.* http://www.sloan.org/education/aln95.htm

Billings D: Distance education in nursing: adapting courses for distance education, *Computers in Nursing 14*(5):262-263,266, 1996.

Boettcher JV: The turtle is moving. *Syllabus Magazine, 12*(2), *September, 1998.* http://www.syllabus.com/sep98_magfea.html

Bostock S: Designing web-based instruction for active learning. In B.H. Kahn (Ed.), *Web-based instruction,* Englewood Cliffs, NJ, 1997, Educational Technology Publications. http://www.keele.ac.uk/depts/cs/Stephen_Bostock/wbi.html

Campbell J: Evaluating ALN: What works, who's learning? *ALN Magazine 1*(2), August, 1997. http://www.aln.org/alnweb/magazine/issue2/campbel_alntalk.htm

Carlton K, Ryan M, & Siktberg L: Designing courses for the internet: A conceptual approach, *Nurse Educator 23*(3), 45-50, 1998.

Collins B: *Tele-learning in a digital world,* London, 1996, Thomson Computer Press.

Chickering A, Ehrmann S: Implementing the seven principles: Technology as lever, AAHE http://www.aahe.org/technology/ehrmann.htm

Chickering, A.W. & Gamson, Z.F. Seven principles for good practice in undergraduate education. *American Higher Education Bulletin, March, 1987.*

Doherty, P.B. Learner control in asynchronous learning environments, ALN Magazine, 2(2), October, 1998. http://www.aln.org/alnweb/magazine/vol2_issue2/doherty.htm

Duderstadt, J.J. The future of the university in an age of knowledge, ALN Magazine, 1(2), August, 1997. http://www.aln.org/alnweb/journal/issue2/duderstadt.htm

Ehrmann, S., Zungia R. *The flashlight evaluation handbook,* Washington, DC, 1997, Teaching, Learning and Technology Group, AAHE.

Foreman, D. The use of multimedia technology for training in business and industry, *Multimedia Monitor* 13(7):22-27, 1995.

Forsyth, I. *Teaching and learning materials and the internet,* London, 1996, Kogan Page.

Fulkerth, B. A bridge for distance education: planning for the information-age student. Syllabus Magazine, Vol. 12, No. 4, November-December 1998. http://www.syllabus.com/nov98_magfea.html

Grabinger, S., Dunlap, J. *Make learning meaningful.* In Kommers P, Grabinger S, Dunlap J, *Hypermedia and multimedia learning environment: instructional design and integration,* Mahwah, NJ, 1996, Erlbaum Association.

Kersley, G. Speaking personal with Linda Harasim. *The American Journal of Distance Education, 7*(3):70-73, 1993.

Kinzie, M.B., Sullivan, H.J. Continuing motivation, learner control and CAI. *Educational Technology Research and Development, 37*(2):5-14, 1989.

Knowles, M. *The modern practice of adult education,* Chicago, 1980, Follet Publishing.

Kommers, P., Grabinger, S., Dunlap J. *Hypermedia and multimedia learning environment: instructional design and integration,* Mahwah, NJ, 1996, Erlbaum Association.

Lawless, K.A., Brown, S.W. Multimedia learning environments: Issues of learner control and navigation, *Instructional Science,* 25, March, 1997.

Mast, M., Van Atta, J. Applying adult learning principles in instructional module design, *Nurse Educator 11*(1), 35-39, 1986.

Ritchie, D., Hoffman, B. Instructional design principles in the world wide web, NAU/Web.com, Flagstaff, Arizona, May, 1998.

Robin, M. Models of online courses, *ALN Magazine, 2*(2), October, 1998. http://www.aln.org/alnweb/magazine/vol2_issue2/Masonfinal.htm Paper from conference proceedings, *Networked lifelong learning: innovative approaches to education and training through the internet* edited by L. Banks, C. Graebner, and D. McConnell, University of Sheffield, 1998.

Saltzberg, Polyson, S. Distributed learning on the world wide web. *Using the Web to Redefine Distance Learning, 1996.* http://www.umuc.edu/iuc/cmc96/papers/poly-p.html

Sherry, L., Wilson, B. Transformative communication as a stimulus to web innovations. In B.H. Kahn (Ed.), *Web based instruction,* Englewood Cliffs, NJ, 1997, Educational Technology Publications.

Twigg, C. The need for a national learning infrastructure, *Educom Review 29*(4,5,6,), 1994. http://www.educause.edu/nlii/keydocs/mongraph.html

Twigg, C. Notes for the June 4-5, 1997 NLII-ITPS Symposium on creating and delivering collegiate learning materials in a distributed (networked) learning environment: a business model for university-corporate collaboration. http://www.educause.edu/nlii/nliitpnotes.html

Twigg, C., Oblinger, D. *The virtual university: a report from a Joint Educom/IBM Roundtable,* Washington, D.C., November 5-6, 1996. http://www.educause.edu/nlii/VU.html

Verville, A.L. What business needs from higher education, *Educational Research, 76*(4):46-50, 1995.

WebCT. *World wide web course tools, software tools for creation of Web-based educational environments,* February, 1999. http://homebrew1.cs.ubc.ca/webct/

VII

IMPLEMENTATION
Taking a Systems
Process Approach

Building on Unit VI, Unit VII takes the reader on a journey through all the key steps in the implementation process. Of particular interest is the application of the case management design to a variety of clinical settings. In addition, an understanding of today's case management planning tools, including MAPS, and case management documentation tools are included in this section. Today's case managers deal with a myriad of ethical issues, which are explored here. A discussion of the information technology arena, and compliance and regulatory issues completes this very eclectic section.

The Cast of Characters

CHAPTER OVERVIEW

Primary nursing models no longer meet the changing needs of either the health care environment or the patients. In this chapter the multidisciplinary approach is discussed in terms of its relative value to the case management model. Both this approach and case management in general are presented in response to an increasingly complex health care environment. How to form teams and how to gain the support and trust of colleagues are two of the topics discussed.

GETTING OUT OF THE PARALLEL PLAY SYNDROME

Those who began their nursing careers in the 1970s were trained and educated to function as independent professional nurses. With the advent of the primary nursing model, *professional* meant doing everything oneself (Bakke, 1974). The team spirit and sense of esprit de corps were lost in the fight to prove nursing a worthy profession. In the attempt to show just how important nursing was to the patient, other disciplines, which also provided unique and necessary services, were neglected.

Perhaps nursing had to go through this process. Perhaps it was necessary as part of the profession's evolutionary growth. Because nurses were so used to nursing's being viewed as a second-class profession, they were riding high on the conviction that they could do it all and do it all well.

Out of this generation of parallel play came terms such as *burnout, fatigue syndrome,* and *fragmented care.* Under the primary nursing model, it was expected that the nurse would meet all the patient's needs, from the bed bath to the discharge plan. With the nursing shortage that began in 1985 and the prospective payment system that resulted in shortened lengths of stay, nurses found it almost impossible to function under the primary nursing system.

Increased complexity and technology required that registered nurses become experts in a narrower range of tasks, which meant that other tasks had to be relinquished or returned to the other disciplines. Nursing care had to become more specialized as it responded to changing patient needs both in the hospital and after discharge.

Because the hospital stay was shortened in response to the prospective payment system, the phrase "discharge them quicker, but sicker" was being quoted by both health care practitioners and patients. Members of the public were losing confidence in the health care system because they felt rushed through the process by the insurers as well as the health care providers, who now had to keep the hospital stay as short as possible.

Flexible time (flex-time) measures, which were designed to attract more people to the profession and to retain those already in the workforce, contributed to fragmented nursing care. Fragmentation was chiefly an outcome of these measures, which resulted in the advent of 10- and 12-hour shifts. Flex-time was very attractive to employees because it allowed them to have long blocks of time off to spend with their families and to continue their education. Unfortunately, these long blocks of time created a tremendous gap in patient care. Trying to be all things to the patient for 12 hours and then not being present for 3 days was meeting the worker's needs at the patient's expense. The accelerated hospital stay compounded the situation. It was conceivable that patients might see a different nurse during each day of an average 4-day hospital stay. Patients complained that no one knew them or their needs, and they were unable to develop professional relationships with any of their nurses. These patients felt that no one practitioner was responsible for their care. Nursing appeared to have failed because accountability for patient care had been lost.

Although nursing departments across the country tried to keep functioning in primary nursing systems, the new environment made it impossible to do so. Primary nursing had been founded on the notion that the registered professional nurse would be responsible for all aspects of the patient's care from admission to discharge. This became unattainable with the introduction of the flex-time system. Although theoretically nurses were responsible, extended absences from the unit prevented a true continuation of their relationship with the patient or the other members of the health care team.

In addition, patient assignments continued, in many instances, to remain geographic, with each nurse on the shift assigned a particular geographic part of the nursing unit. If the patient was moved to some other area of the unit, it was likely that the primary nurse would no longer be caring for that patient. Such changes meant care had become extremely fragmented.

At the same time, the role of the head nurse or nurse manager was moving away from the bedside. More and more administrative responsibility was given to these middle managers as upper management positions were eliminated. In the past the nurse manager had been able to clinically monitor all the patients on the floor and still carry out managerial responsibilities. As the administrative duties increased, this became more difficult to accomplish. In addition, the average length of stay was dramatically shortened, so that patients were admitted and discharged from the unit faster than they could be followed up by a busy manager with other responsibilities.

THE EFFECTS OF A CHANGING ENVIRONMENT

During the 1970s nurses and other health care providers first began to complain of stress-related problems such as chronic fatigue and burnout. In 1974 a psychologist named Freudenberger coined the clinical term *burnout*. Burnout was described as the degeneration of a once highly productive individual into a negative, exhausted one. It was seen as a direct response to work stress when the worker no longer had the resources available to deal with other people's emotional, psychological, and physical problems.

Burnout follows a particular pattern that generally begins with feelings of emotional exhaustion. Such exhaustion results from being emotionally overextended and exhausted by one's work with others (Maslach, 1976, 1978, 1982). This exhaustion is followed by feelings of depersonalization, which have been described as negative, unfeeling, and impersonal responses toward the recipients of one's care. As the syndrome becomes more severe, the worker may describe feelings of reduced personal accomplishment. Personal accomplishment is characterized by feelings of competence and successful achievement in one's work with people (Maslach, 1976, 1978, 1982). By placing registered nurses in a position that required them to be all things to the patient, the nurses experienced an incredible amount of on-the-job stress.

Role overload was yet another outcome of work stress that was identified in some nurses (Cesta, 1989). Role overload is characterized by the worker's subjective feelings of being unable to complete the work because of inadequate personal or environmental resources (French & Caplan, 1972; Hardy, 1976; Ritzer, 1977). These feelings have been reported to be particularly high in nurses who are in their first 2 years of employment (Cesta, 1989; Das, 1981; Maslach, 1982).

When role overload combined with feelings of burnout, the nurse's ability to deal with work began to change and gradually diminished (Cesta, 1989).

Nurses began to adjust the primary nursing system in an attempt to address changes in the health care arena. This new system eventually became known as *modified primary* and retained the theory that the nurse was accountable for all aspects of care. This did not mean, however, that the nurse retained responsibility for the patient from admission to discharge. Primary nursing responsibilities were applicable only to the day the nurse worked.

Once these modifications were made in the primary model, the stage was set for the development of a more appropriate model that addressed all the foregoing issues (Loveridge, Cummings, & O'Malley, 1988). The alternative model combined elements of team and primary nursing (Zander, 1985). There was really nothing new or revolutionary about the case management model for nursing care delivery. The basic premise of the model was a team or collaborative approach that allowed the case manager to function as the evaluator and coordinator of care or facilitator of the team. This new role was similar to that of the primary nurse, except that the case manager was now removed from direct patient care responsibility.

With the addition of this role, nursing moved away from attempting to be all things to the patient. Members of the profession began to admit that they could not do all things equally well and that other members of the team were needed to provide their particular areas of expertise. Nursing was finally getting out of the parallel play syndrome and was moving toward a more dynamic and interactive modality.

FORMATION OF THE COLLABORATIVE PRACTICE GROUPS

It is perhaps easier now for nurses to reintroduce themselves to the team approach. Although social workers and physicians had functioned that way for years, nurses had been struggling to achieve independence and autonomy. Nurses now feel more confident and ready to join the team after gaining prestige among other health care providers (Farley & Stoner, 1989).

Institutions implementing case management models for the first time must explain to team members why nurses are returning to the team approach. At first, this reintroduction of the team approach may be observed with some suspicion and doubt. Without making the intentions of the team clear, it will be impossible to institute collaborative practice groups.

Physicians and other health care providers may have preconceived ideas about case management, some of which stem from their familiarity with the managed care systems introduced in health maintenance organizations (HMOs). Generally, many health care providers see these managed care systems as negative or as one more way for their practices to be regulated and controlled and their services to be rationed (Knight, 1998; Schwartz & Mendelson, 1992).

Collaborative practice groups cannot be formed until all members adopt the model as their own and see its benefit for both themselves and the patient. It should be emphasized that case management is not just a nursing care model but a way for all the disciplines to form plans of care that avoid duplication of effort, unnecessary tests and procedures, or misuse of resources.

Each discipline involved in patient care activities develops a plan that meets the objectives for that discipline as they relate to the patient. Case management provides, for the first time, the opportunity for all the disciplines to come together in an effort to use each other's expertise for maximum benefit to the patient.

Cast of Characters

Who then comprises the cast of characters, and how do they come together as a group? Formation of these interdisciplinary groups is one of the first steps for implementation, and it must take place before any real clinical changes can occur.

In a unit-based case management approach, who is in the group depends on the types of case management plans being developed. At the least, each group should consist of members from the following disciplines: nursing, medicine, social work, discharge planning, and nutrition. People from these areas make up the core of any group, and each one provides input related to the clinical objectives of that member's discipline. Of course, the central figures in any such team are the patient and family.

Other members are added as they relate to the particular diagnosis or procedure planned. Other disciplines that might be included are physical therapy, occupational therapy, respiratory therapy, and nutrition.

In some cases the groups may have already been formed as part of the implementation of a non-unit-based case management approach. In this approach, groups are formed around a particular diagnosis, and all members of the team are experts in that clinical area. For example, a team might be formed to manage diabetic patients throughout the hospital. A diabetes case management team is often headed by a diabetologist and a nurse case manager who together provide the leadership to direct the other members of the team. A cardiac case management team might be headed by a cardiologist and a cardiac nurse case manager. The members of a case management team follow the patients' cases regardless of where they might be within the hospital. Therefore the team remains constant while the patients and their locations change.

Because the case management team is developed before the arrival of the patient, these groups have already determined protocols and care methods for their specific types of patients. It is not necessary for the case manager to identify the members of the team at the time of the patient's admission to the hospital because the team is already in place. In the unit-based case management model, however, the members of the team are determined by the patient problem. These teams are fluid and constantly changing.

After the patient's admission the attending physician, case manager, social worker, nutritionist, and others are identified and the specific plan of care for the patient is formalized. The use of internal techniques and relationships should not be underestimated in the formation of the multidisciplinary groups. If a nonthreatening, informal relationship has been developed first, it will be much easier to obtain the cooperation of some professionals. Inviting key players to lunch, meeting in the library, or just chatting on the unit can do much to gain trust and respect.

There may be occasions when a member of another discipline who is in a position of authority may be needed to intervene on the part of the case manager to obtain concurrence for collaborative practice. For example, some physicians admit large numbers of patients to the hospital every year and are therefore considered to have a great deal of power and independence in their everyday practice within the hospital. These individuals may not immediately see the advantage of joining a multidisciplinary team effort because it may not appear to benefit them, or they may view the effort to form teams as an attempt to control their practices. In a case like this, it may be necessary to have a physician administrator intervene on the behalf of the case management team. Usually, once the benefits are presented to the physicians, they give their support. Also, they may need to get their superiors' consent to participate.

Another technique to gain the support of some of the more resistant professionals is to begin working first with those who have already agreed to the model. It is sometimes more effective to begin with these individuals than to try to convert the resisters right away. Perhaps when success is proved with those who have been immediately receptive, the others will give their support. Once again, support may depend on people's perceptions of what the model can do for them. There will always be a certain percentage of players who will sit on the fence, waiting to see if implementation succeeds or fails. Once success is evident, they will cross over to the case manager's side.

In both the unit- and non-unit-based case management approach the team becomes the focal point for care delivery, with each member lending information from a specific area of expertise. Most institutions rely on the case manager to be responsible for smooth operation and communication among team members. In some instances, however, social workers or physicians have been used to coordinate communication. Nurses function well in this role because they are educated to take a holistic approach to care delivery and because they are the ones who become involved in all aspects of the patient's care.

For example, it is less likely that a social worker will have the clinical skills that a registered nurse has, but most registered nurses have the basic skills required to provide discharge planning and referral services to patients after discharge. Case managers should be able to identify patients at high risk and to refer such patients to the appropriate discipline. Patients with high-risk discharge planning needs can be referred to the discharge planner or social worker, as appropriate to the organization. At the very least, the case manager should be able to work the system to the patient's advantage, knowing the appropriate members to call as needs arise. An advanced understanding of the patient's medical and nursing needs helps to make this assessment complete. The case manager can then refer the problem to the appropriate practitioner.

In the unit-based approach, it may be difficult or impossible for the complete team to meet at one time. Once again, case managers fill this gap. They provide the thread that holds all the members together. In this sense the case managers must have excellent communication skills. The information they translate between team members and to patients and families must be accurate and concise or the thread is broken and the team falls apart.

The team should be assembled as a group whenever possible. Dialogue and opinion can thus be shared face-to-face. It is often during meetings of this type that difficult patient problems are resolved.

The case manager may spend a good deal of time during the beginning of implementation trying to ensure that the team becomes a reality and remains on target to provide the best possible care for the patient.

The case manager role consists of the following three dimensions (Tahan, 1993; chapter 17). The first dimension is the clinical role, which requires collaboration with the interdisciplinary team and involves the development of protocols that list the key tasks or events that must be accomplished for handling patient problems. Case managers use these protocols to direct, monitor, and evaluate patient treatment and the outcomes or responses to treatment (Thompson et al., 1991; Zander, 1988). Case managers identify variances from the standard protocols and work with other health care team members to analyze and deal with these variances of care (Cesta, Tahan, & Fink, 1998; Ethridge & Lamb, 1989; O'Malley, 1988b).

The second dimension is that of the managerial role, which refers to the case manager's responsibility for coordinating the care of patients during the course of hospitalization (Ethridge & Lamb,

1989; Kruger, 1989; O'Malley, 1988a; Zander, 1988). The case manager manages care by planning the nursing treatment modalities and interventions necessary for meeting the needs of the patient and the family. Goals of treatment are set at admission, and length of stay is determined as it relates to the diagnosis-related group (DRG). The discharge plan is formed as early in the hospital stay as possible (O'Malley, 1988b).

Case managers also guide the activities, nursing treatments, and interventions of other nursing staff members (Ethridge & Lamb, 1989; Kruger, 1989). They continuously evaluate the quality of care provided and outcomes of treatments and services to prevent misuse of resources (O'Malley, 1988a).

One of the informal responsibilities of the case manager is that of teacher and mentor (Cronin & Maklebust, 1989; Kruger, 1989). The case manager assesses staff development needs, especially among the less experienced practitioners, and refers them to the appropriate person or resource (Leclair, 1991). As part of the teaching responsibilities of the role, case managers conduct patient and family teaching sessions during the hospitalization period (Cronin & Maklebust, 1989; Zander, 1988).

The third dimension of the case manager role involves financial aspects. In collaboration with the physician and other health care members, case managers activate a caregiving process for each patient and use a case management plan, which is a generic tool for managing care and keeping it consistent with the predetermined financial outcomes for a defined case type (Adams & Biggerstaff, 1995; O'Malley, 1988b; Zander, 1988). The use of such clinical treatment standards helps ensure that patients do not receive inadequate care because of cost containment measures (Collard, Bergman, & Henderson, 1990; Mass & Johnson, 1998).

Case managers access information related to DRGs and case types, the cost of each diagnosis, the allocated length of stay, and the treatments and procedures generally used for each diagnosis. They use this information to review resources and evaluate the efficiency of care related to the diagnosis (Cronin & Maklebust, 1989). The case manager has a great influence on the quality and price of care by helping to determine in a timely manner the most pertinent treatment for the patient (Henderson & Collard, 1988). Case managers also assess variances for each case type and act immediately to control these variances to contain costs (Cesta, Tahan, & Fink, 1998; Crawford, 1991). They assure consistency, continuity, and coordination of care to control for duplication and fragmentation in health care delivery, which results in better resource allocation and further cost containment (Henderson & Collard, 1988; O'Malley, 1988a).

To be effective, case managers must access information on case mix index, cost of resources, and consumption and must be familiar with the prospective payment system and current third-party reimbursement procedures, including managed care and capitation (Ethridge & Lamb, 1989; O'Malley, 1988b).

Case managers work closely with the utilization review department in identifying long-stay patients and planning with that department to control and prevent inappropriate hospital stays (Cronin & Maklebust, 1989). In other cases the case manager assumes the functions of utilization review/management. These functions generally include reviewing cases for medical necessity and resource utilization and providing this information to third party payers, particularly managed care organizations (MCO). When these functions are integrated into the role of the case manager, work with third party payers becomes less fragmented and better coordinated. Communication and cooperation with the MCO is enhanced.

References

Adams, C.E., & Biggerstaff, N. (1995). Reduced resource utilization through standardized outcomes-focused care plans. *Journal of Nursing Administration, 25*(10), 43-49.

Bakke, K. (1974). Primary nursing: Perceptions of a staff nurse. *American Journal of Nursing, 74*(8), 1432-1434.

Cesta, T.G. (1989). The relationship of role overload and burnout to coping process in registered professional staff nurses newly employed in a hospital setting. Doctoral dissertation. University Microfilms, Inc., Publication Number: 9016399.

Cesta, T.G., Tahan, H.A., & Fink, L.F. (1998). *The case manager's survival guide: Winning strategies for clinical practice.* St. Louis: Mosby.

Collard, A.F., Bergman, A., & Henderson, M. (1990). Two approaches to measuring quality in medical case management programs. *Quality Review Bulletin,* 3-8.

Crawford, J. (1991). Managed care consultant: The "house supervisor" alternative. *Nursing Management, 22*(5), 75-78.

Cronin, C.J., & Maklebust, J. (1989). Case-managed care: Capitalizing on the CNS. *Nursing Management, 20*(3), 38-47.

Das, E.B.L. (1981). Contributing factors to burnout in the nursing environment. Doctoral dissertation, Texas Woman's University. *Dissertation Abstracts International, 42,* 04B.

Ethridge, P., & Lamb, G. (1989). Professional nursing case management improves quality, access and costs. *Nursing Management, 20*(3), 30-35.

Farley, M.J., & Stoner, M.H. (1989). The nurse executive and interdisciplinary team building. *Nursing Administration Quarterly,* 24-29.

French, J.R.P., & Caplan, R.D. (1972). Organizational stress and individual strain. In A.J. Morrow (Ed.), *The failure of success* (pp. 30-66). New York: AMACOM.

Freudenberger, H.J. (1974). Staff burn-out. *Journal of Social Issues, 30,* 159-165.

Hardy, M.E. (1976, Aug.). Role problems, role strain, job satisfaction, and nursing care. Paper presented at the annual meeting of the American Sociological Association, New York.

Henderson, M.G., & Collard, A. (1988). Measuring quality in medical case management programs. *Quality Review Bulletin,* 33-39.

Knight, W. (1998). *Managed care: What it is and how it works.* Gaithersburg, Maryland: Aspen.

Kruger, N.R. (1989). Case management: Is it a delivery system for my organization? *Aspen's Advisor for Nurse Executives, 4*(10), 4-6.

Leclair, C. (1991). Introducing and accounting for RN case management. *Nursing Management, 22*(3), 44-49.

Loveridge, C.E., Cummings, S.H., & O'Malley, J. (1988). Developing case management in a primary nursing system. *Journal of Nursing Administration, 18*(10), 36-39.

Maslach, C. (1976). Burned-out. *Human Behavior, 5,* 17-21.

Maslach, C. (1978). Job burn-out: How people cope. *Public Welfare, 36,* 56-58.

Maslach, C. (1982). *Burnout. The cost of caring.* Englewood Cliffs, N.J.: Prentice-Hall.

Mass, S., & Johnson, B. (1998, Nov.). Case management and clinical guidelines. *The Journal of Care Management.* Special Edition.

O'Malley, J. (1988a). Nursing case management. I: Why look at a different model for nursing care delivery? *Aspen's Advisor for Nurse Executives, 3*(5), 5-6.

O'Malley, J. (1988b). Nursing case management, part II: Dimensions of the nurse case manager role. *Aspen's Advisor for Nurse Executives, 3*(6), 7.

Ritzer, G. (1977). *Working.* Englewood Cliffs, N.J.: Prentice-Hall.

Schwartz, W., & Mendelson, D. (1992 Summer). Why managed care cannot contain hospital cost without. *Health Affairs* 100-107.

Tahan, H.T. (1993). The nurse case manager in acute care settings: Job description and function. *Journal of Nursing Administration, 23*(10), 53-61.

Thompson, K.S., Caddick, K., Mathie, J., Newlon, B., & Abraham, T. (1991). Building a critical path for ventilator dependency. *American Journal of Nursing,* 28-31.

Zander, K. (1992 Fall). Quantifying, managing, and improving quality: III. Using variance concurrently. *The New Definition, 7*(4), 1-4.

Zander, K. (1985). Second generation primary nursing: A new agenda. *Journal of Nursing Administration, 15*(3), 18-24.

Zander, K. (1988). Managed care within acute care settings: Design and implementation via nursing case management. *Health Care Supervisor, 6*(2), 27-43.

Variations Within Clinical Settings

CHAPTER OVERVIEW

Case management models provide an opportunity for health care institutions to provide quality, cost-effective services regardless of the type of setting or financial resources. The model is flexible and can be adapted to meet the needs of both clinical and institutional settings.

This chapter describes how the case management model can be adapted to a variety of clinical settings, including medicine, surgery, critical care, nursing homes, clinics, and other ambulatory care settings. The way a case management model is used depends on the goals of the organization using it. The chapter also discusses the challenge facing case management in linking the inpatient and outpatient settings.

FLEXIBILITY OF CASE MANAGEMENT

One thing that makes case management models particularly appealing is that the structure is extremely flexible. A case management design can be modified to fit the needs and budgets of any clinical setting. Because the primary goals of case management are to reduce costs while maintaining quality, the model can, in many circumstances, be implemented for a minimal cost (Ethridge & Lamb, 1989).

There are probably as many variations on the case management theme as there are nursing units in the United States. There is no right or wrong way to design a case management system. The design is not as important as the roles and functions of the system's members. Each person's functions are what make the model unique, not the number of workers involved. Today's health care environment calls for flexibility and creativity, and the institutions that display these features will probably be the most successful ones over the next 10 years (Armstrong & Stetler, 1991).

For an institution implementing case management for the first time, the exact design structure for the units will be based on an array of factors. Choosing the first units to participate is an important decision. If the first units are successful, the institution will be more likely to support continued implementation. On the other hand, if the first units are less than successful, the leaders of the organization may not be willing to allow the implementation process to continue. Therefore the first units should be chosen carefully.

The units selected for initial implementation should have the following characteristics:

Homogeneous patient population
High-volume case types
Potential for improvement in length of stay
A committed nurse manager
A receptive physician group
An interested nursing staff
An open full-time equivalent (FTE) position (if possible)

Of course, it may not be possible to obtain each of these elements on every nursing unit. Finding a unit with as many of these factors as possible will help ensure a positive transition to a case management model.

A homogeneous patient population is beneficial because it may mean a smaller number of professionals involved in patient care on the unit. A homogeneous population also reduces the number of case management plans that need to be written. Most units that specialize in certain diseases or surgical procedures will have a smaller physician group with which to interact. A smaller group will allow for a more rapid transition to the model and will be more helpful in formulating the case management plans because the group will probably be more likely to agree on plans of care.

A large percentage of high-volume case types will also help when generating case management plans that will cover a wider number of patients on the unit. In general, if a unit admits more than 50% of its patients to five or fewer diagnosis-related (DRG) categories, the unit may be a good candidate for conversion to case management.

However, it is important to analyze these high-volume case types for their potential in reducing length of stay. High volume does not necessarily mean a reduction in length of stay. For example, some patient problems are on protocols that are already as brief as possible. Chemotherapy is one example. Reductions might not be attainable around the diagnosis, but other elements of hospitalization, such as preadmission blood work or prehydration therapy, may allow for reductions.

The transition to a case management system will require total commitment from those on the unit. One of the most important people in the change process is the nurse manager. The nurse manager has 24-hour responsibility and accountability and has the primary administrative responsibility for the smooth functioning of the unit. Most of the other professionals enter and exit the unit because their responsibilities take them to other areas of the hospital. The nurse manager's sole responsibility is the nursing unit. It is vital that nurse managers have a working knowledge of case management so that they can function both formally and informally as advocates for change. Nurse managers can be instrumental in obtaining the cooperation of physicians with whom they have long-standing relationships.

Most of the activities on a nursing unit revolve around nurse managers who have administrative authority for their units. Their responsibilities may include staffing, budgeting, maintaining supplies, and caring for patients. No changes in these responsibilities should be made without the nurse managers' input and support.

When selecting units for conversion to case management, at least a majority of physicians affiliated with the unit should support the change. This, of course, may not always be possible. Obtaining the support of some physicians can be enough for making a positive transition.

It is important that the chief medical officer be supportive of the conversion to case management. Chairpersons of individual clinical areas should also be engaged in the change process as early as possible and should be supportive of case management.

When a case management model is implemented, it is helpful but not crucial to begin with a nursing staff that volunteered to be among the first units in the institution to convert. Often such enthusiasm came from the unit's nurse manager and filtered down to the other nurses on the unit. Again, this may be a factor that is not immediately obtainable.

Most institutions converting to a unit-based model try to do so at minimal cost to the organization. This may mean using an already existing FTE position or a budgeted position that has never been filled. It is not wise to eliminate an employee to make room for a case manager. The open FTE position should be acquired through attrition whenever possible because elimination of an employee can cause ill will, resentment, and insecurity among other staff nurses on the unit.

Some organizations have had to use other creative approaches to obtaining case management positions. Some have converted existing departments or positions, such as utilization managers, discharge planners, social workers, or nurse managers. No position should be eliminated unless others in the organization are able to absorb the workload of the eliminated position(s). During this time, job descriptions should be reviewed and, if necessary, role functions reallocated. Examples might include the development of discharge planning criteria for patients that slot them into either high- or low-risk categories. Lower risk patients might remain the responsibility of the staff nurse or case manager, whereas high-risk patients are referred to the discharge planner or social worker. Retaining these additional FTE positions raises the cost of the overall design of the model. As organizational resources continue to dwindle, these types of designs will become less and less possible. During the initial design phase, it is always preferable for the organization to look for opportunities to integrate these functions under the role of the case manager. This provides for the most efficient, least expensive design.

It is often possible to create additional positions once some success has been shown. For these reasons it is again imperative that the initial units selected indicate a great potential for successful transition.

MEDICAL UNIT

Medical units may be among those with the most case management patient needs. Medical patients are often elderly and have more complex discharge plans. These patients are often the least likely to be advocates for themselves and can fall through the cracks during an extended and complicated hospital stay. They are among the most costly to hospitals and are often resource intensive.

Medical patients are also among the most difficult to plan for because their hospital course can be unpredictable. Ironically, these are also reasons that a case manager can be a great asset to a medical unit. The medical patient whose hospital course changes daily needs someone to ensure that everything is happening as planned and that nothing is missed.

There are usually more case managers on a medical unit than on any other type of unit in the hospital. Because of the increased complexity and severity of the cases, the organization should aim to have every medical patient under the authority of a case manager. The number of case managers should be based on an average case load of about 15 to 20 patients. If every patient on the medical unit cannot be followed by the case manager, then criteria must be developed for selecting those patients who will benefit the most by being followed. In general, the case load of the case manager on the medical unit must be somewhat smaller than what would be seen on either a specialty unit or a surgical unit because these patients tend to need more resources and the number of interventions per patient will probably be greater.

Criteria for selecting patients on a general medical floor must be individually determined through a retrospective audit of those patients who seem to represent patterns of increased resource use. However, this is not the only factor to be evaluated. Other patients who might benefit from a case manager include those with the following characteristics:

Advanced age (older than 70 years)
Noncompliance with treatment
Potential for falls
Potential for skin breakdown
Discharge placement problems/complicated plan
Complicated medical plan
Home care needs
Complicated teaching needs

SURGICAL UNIT

Surgical cases can be as complicated as medical cases. Generally, though, the hospital course of a surgical patient is somewhat more predictable and amenable to a predetermined plan. Many surgeons practice with protocols, which manage the patient's postoperative course in the same way that the case management plan does. Although there are exceptions to every rule, the expected course can be planned around an anticipated length of stay. Surgical patients are often elective admissions, which means that there may be less potential for in-hospital complications.

For these reasons, a surgical case manager may be able to carry a larger patient case load than a case manager on a medical unit. A case load of about 25 patients is probably manageable on most surgical units. One complication to this equation is the extremely short lengths of stay on surgical units that will translate to rapid turnover for the surgical case manager. While the patients may be less complex clinically, this accelerated turnover may mean a workload for the surgical case manager that is comparable to that of the medical case manager. The rapidity of turnover should be factored in when determining an appropriate case load for the surgical case manager.

It may not be necessary to have every surgical patient under the direction of a case manager. Criteria for selecting patients should include patient need and complexity or severity of condition. Patients who are admitted for emergency surgery and who require medical clearance before surgery also might need the attention of the case manager. Patients who develop postoperative complications, which may result in a prolonged length of stay, should also be considered.

CRITICAL CARE UNIT

The critical care unit may be the last area of the hospital to convert to case management. Because this area has a lower nurse-patient ratio and a more responsive health care team, these patients are already receiving a form of case management.

Critical care can be viewed as one episode in the course of hospitalization. Case management in critical care can help with clinical management issues such as admission and discharge criteria. These criteria can support patient throughput.

The case manager and case management plans may be the only elements missing from these areas. Most intensive care units have a 2:1 or a 1:1 nurse/patient ratio. In these situations, it may be possible to use the nurses, in their current positions, to function in a case management role. Thus all registered nurses working in the unit would be case managers and would carry out the functions and responsibilities of the case manager as well as provide direct patient care.

Case management plans can be developed around particular clinical problems, such as ventilator weaning, which would support and assist the staff nurses acting as case managers. Protocols for withdrawing patients from care as they improve could be incorporated into critical care case management plans.

There are problems with this system, but solutions do exist. The first problem is that continuity of care is still an issue if the unit is on flextime. Also, it may be difficult for nurses working with critically ill patients to take on the added responsibilities associated with the case manager role. They may not have the time needed to create managed care plans or to be involved in team formation. They may simply be absent from the unit too much to care for patients and function as case managers.

One option for staffing critical care areas with case managers is to cohort the acute unit with the critical care unit. For example, the surgical case manager would also be responsible for patients transitioning in or out of the surgical intensive care unit. The cardiology case manager might also be responsible for the critical care unit, and so on. This type of design provides continuity for the patients and does not require a case manager dedicated to those areas.

The emergency department lends itself to the development of case management plans. Plans can be developed for the efficient treatment of specific disease entities such as asthma or for the clinical management of patient treatments such as conscious sedation. Case management plans can also be developed for beginning the "ruling-out" process, as in the treatment of abdominal pain, and the identification of tuberculosis or human immunodeficiency virus (HIV) infection. Emergency department case managers can perform a number of important functions including the following:

- Management of treat-and-release patients, including standardization of the treatment processes.
- Referrals of "soft admissions," who might be discharges from the emergency department instead of admitted. Referrals to primary care physicians, clinics, home care, or subacute care are possible referral options.
- Expeditious treatment and admission of patients admitted to the hospital, including beginning the appropriate treatment (e.g., antibiotics) in the emergency department.

NURSING SKILLED NURSING FACILITY

The skilled nursing facility (SNF) is an example of a non-acute-care facility that can financially benefit from a case management system. A case management model can ensure a higher quality of patient care with fewer resources. As the population ages and life expectancy increases, the needs of extended-care facilities will rise proportionally. As do most other health care institutions, nursing homes struggle with increased regulations and decreased resources (Smith, 1991).

In the nursing home setting a case manager can ensure patient outcomes. This can reduce the use of registered nurses and increase the use of ancillary personnel.

Skilled nursing facilities are required to provide plans of care and goals for their patients. Generally, personnel other than registered nurses can carry out these plans. Regulation requires that a registered nurse be present in most instances, but this nurse could be better used as a facilitator, educator, or coordinator of services to the patient. This approach can enhance quality of life and slow deterioration of functional ability.

SUBACUTE CARE FACILITY

Another area of consideration for case management are subacute units. Subacute care is defined as follows:

- A level of care that blends acute and long-term care skills and philosophies
- Care that bridges long-term and acute care
- One of the fastest growing segments on the continuum of health care

Subacute care is less invasive than acute care and less diagnostically oriented. Patient care is more intense but of shorter duration than that given in a skilled nursing facility. Care usually occurs immediately following hospitalization, but in some cases it may be used instead of hospitalization. For appropriate case management in a subacute setting, patients must be in stable condition, but well enough to go home. Subacute program models include the following:

- Short-term medically complex
- Short-term rehabilitative
- Long-term or chronic (20% of all subacute cases)

Short-term medically complex patients are usually postsurgical patients or those with complex medical conditions who are medically stable but still require intensive medical/nursing management and/or ancillary services. Examples include the following:

Wound care
Respiratory management
Total parenteral nutrition
Dialysis
IV therapy
Postsurgical recovery
Oncology
Acquired immunodeficiency syndrome (AIDS) care
Complications due to prematurity
Terminal care

Short-term rehabilitative patients are those who have a potential for functional improvement who also have significant medical and nursing needs and are too ill or unable to tolerate the intensity of acute rehabilitation. Short-term rehabilitative therapies include physical, occupational, and speech therapy. Typical diagnoses would include stroke, amputation, total hip or knee replacement, and brain injury.

Long-term or chronic care patients have an extended acute care stay (e.g., longer than 25 days), but can be discharged earlier to a subacute setting if an appropriate one is available. They may be medically stable, but have high nursing/ancillary care needs.

Long-term patients may include those requiring preventative maintenance, needing maintenance of functional level, those in a coma, patients who are ventilator dependent, and those with head injuries.

Subacute case managers may function in free-standing skilled nursing facilities, in hospital-based skilled nursing facilities, in acute care hospital rehabilitation units, in long-term care hospitals, or in specialty hospitals or units.

A team approach with the nurse manager as a case manager can be cost effective and ensure improved quality of care. Many institutions have attempted to use the nurse manager in this facilitator role. As in the acute care setting, this dual role has become increasingly difficult in the nursing home setting. By using a case manager in addition to a nurse manager, greater quality and more efficient clinical outcomes can be achieved.

AMBULATORY/OUTPATIENT SETTING

Case management crosses all boundaries of the health care spectrum. The patient's quality of life may depend on the kind of clinical management this person receives in the primary care setting. The approach used in most ambulatory settings is a form of case management. Continuity of caregivers is often attempted for a patient's return visits. For many patients without a private family physician, these clinic visits provide their only links to the health care system. Using the team approach to manage patients enhances quality of care. To this end the American Academy of Ambulatory Care Nursing (AAACN) included case management skills in their competencies for professional practice (AAACN, 1997).

The future challenge for case management models will be to link the inpatient and outpatient settings in a way that promotes a smooth transition for the patient and ensures continuity of care once the patient returns to the community.

Development of case management plans can be based on expected outcomes for each patient visit. Such an approach can control the resources applied and the goals of care for each visit. This approach can also be used for home care visits or for clinic visits. If care is guided by the expected outcomes, progress can be tracked and monitored and appropriate interventions made in response to the patient's reaction to treatment.

Documentation of the patient's level of compliance after discharge from the hospital can provide valuable data as to the effect hospitalization had on the patient's quality of life. Additionally, a case manager's unique relationship with the patient, as well as follow-up visits and phone calls, can ensure patient compliance with postdischarge health care follow-up.

References

AAACN (1997). *Nursing in ambulatory care: The future is here.* Monograph. Washington, DC: American Nurses Publishing.

Armstrong, D.M., & Stetler, C.B. (1991). Strategic considerations in developing a delivery model. *Nursing Economics, 9*(2), 112-115.

Ethridge, P., & Lamb, G. (1989). Professional nursing case management improves quality, access, and costs. *Nursing Management, 20*(3), 30-35.

Smith, J. (1991). Changing traditional nursing home roles to nursing case management. *Journal of Gerontological Nursing, 17*(5), 32-39.

Brainstorming

Development of the Multidisciplinary Action Plan (MAP)

CHAPTER OVERVIEW

The case management plan is the documentation that drives the case management system. Institutions implementing case management models need to determine the content of the documentation format they wish to adopt.

This chapter reviews the evolution of case management plans and the step-by-step process of development. This chapter also discusses the links between the prospective payment system, diagnosis-related groups (DRGs), and the case management plan.

Health care organizations must go beyond what the DRG suggests when designing these plans. The principal procedure or diagnosis should be used with the DRG as the underlying guide for determining the extent of the plan.

EVOLUTION OF THE CASE MANAGEMENT PLAN

Just as there are many ways to adapt case management models to fit the needs of a particular organization, there are multiple ways to develop a case management documentation system. Since case management's inception, most hospitals have been using the *critical path* label on their case management plans. When introduced in 1985 by the New England Medical Center in Boston, the critical path was the first system that attempted to incorporate expected outcomes within specified time frames. The term *critical path* means that the plan defines the critical or key events expected to happen each day of a patient's hospitalization (Giuliano & Poirier, 1991; Zander, 1991, 1992).

Since 1985 critical paths have been adapted to meet the needs of organizations implementing case management models. The paths remain an extremely flexible method of planning and documenting. In addition to *critical path* and *clinical pathway*, other labels, such as *multidisciplinary plan, multidisciplinary action plan (MAP)*, and *action plan*, have been attached to these case management plans. All these terms are the same in theory. Each of the plans attempts to outline the expected outcomes of care for each discipline during each day of hospitalization. Some of these care plans place greater emphasis on the nursing plan, while some emphasize the medical plan of care. Some others, such as the MAP discussed here, incorporate all disciplines.

Some case management organizations use case management plans as one-page guides. Essentially these one-page plans are multidisciplinary protocols for the problem or diagnosis. The detail of the plan depends on the goals of the organization in which the plan is being used. In some cases, nursing documentation can be recorded directly onto the form. This format is also easily adapted to a hospital computer system. Computerization of the plan allows the case manager the flexibility of changing the plan as the patient's needs change. For those organizations without a computer system, the case management plan is still an easy, flexible tool to use.

The case management plan can also be used in place of the traditional nursing care plan. Nursing care plans have been criticized by some as useless exercises in writing. The plans are written to meet the needs of regulatory agencies but are often not used by nurses to guide or plan their day-to-day care. Once written, the plans are often never looked at again. These plans are not even written to provide a plan of care that correlates with the expected length of stay. For this reason these plans are not the preferred form for planning care in case management models.

It is no accident that the critical path or MAP format came into existence. These MAPs are the driving force behind case management models because they help determine the plan of care and arrange that plan around the expected length of stay. Unlike the nursing care plan, MAPs are multidisciplinary and take into account the unique contributions of each discipline. MAPs also link case management with the prospective payment system by using the DRG for determining the appropriate length for the plan. The most current reimbursements are consulted when any plan is started.

When developing the MAP, keep in mind that the state reimbursable length of stay may be longer or shorter than the federal length of stay. Also, it would be impractical to develop standard plans for patients with varying types of insurance coverage. Instead, these variations in reimbursable length of stay can be averaged. Another technique is to determine the length of stay the physician expects and measure it against the reimbursable length of stay. It may turn out that the stay the physician hoped for is shorter than the reimbursable length of stay. In a case like this, the physician's preference would determine the length of stay outlined in the MAP.

National guidelines such as Milliman and Robertson (1997) should also be used as a benchmark reference. Guidelines such as these provide not only length of stay expectations, but also alternative settings and options for managing the length of stay. They are used by many managed care organizations during the review process for determining reimbursable hospital days.

If the length of stay the physician expects is longer than the reimbursable length of stay, a compromise must be reached. The federal and state rates should be reviewed with the physician in relation to the physician's plan. Areas for reduction should be discussed to reduce the length of stay so that it matches or comes below the reimbursable length of stay. A general guideline is to design the plan so that it is shorter than the reimbursable length of stay. This allows for some margin of error in case the patient requires an additional day of hospitalization.

The case manager can control the length of stay by overseeing the movement of the patient through the system. It is difficult to implement MAPs that will be effective without the position of case manager in place. Instituting plans without a professional to drive the process is not a likely way to achieve the desired results. The staff nurse and the case manager are responsible for ensuring that the expected outcomes, as outlined on the MAP, are carried out. If the expected outcomes cannot be achieved, the case manager analyzes the patient's situation and documents the outcome that cannot be accomplished. This outcome is then documented as a variance, which is anything that does not happen when it is supposed to happen.

The DRG must be used as a guide for projecting the length of stay indicated on the MAP. Because the DRG categories are designed for determining hospital reimbursement rates, they are too heterogeneous to assess the effectiveness of the clinical plan at the bedside. For example, if a MAP is written to plan the care of a lumbar laminectomy patient, the discharge diagnosis of lumbar laminectomy might fall under a wide variety of DRGs, such as "medical back procedure" or "spinal procedure." Therefore, if someone wanted to look at the length of stay of all laminectomy patients within a case management system in the hospital, then asking for length of stay records for one DRG would not include the majority of laminectomy patients, who might have been classified under other DRG categories.

Other DRGs are heterogeneous in another way. For example, the DRG for chemotherapy, DRG 410, includes any and all chemotherapy protocols, whether they are for 1 day or for 5 days. The Health Care Finance Administration (HCFA) reimbursement rate for chemotherapy is 2.6 days, regardless of the type of chemotherapy being given. Once again, the DRG system will not be a suitable tool for analyzing whether the MAP decreases the length of stay, reduces resource use, or provides the most effective quality care for that problem.

If an organization wants to determine the true effectiveness of case management plans used among a specific patient group, the DRG cannot be used. Clinicians must dig deeper, using a microanalysis approach. Patients' reviews should be based on their principal procedure or diagnosis at the time of discharge. This way the plan's effectiveness can be determined. After all, there is no MAP called "medical back problem," and there cannot be one called "chemotherapy" because these would be too general. It follows, therefore, that analysis must be as specific as the level of the diagnosis. Once again, it should be emphasized that other data sets, such as the Milliman and Robertson guidelines, should be referenced when making care planning decisions.

The case management plan for chemotherapy would be specific to the type of chemotherapy being administered and the specific protocol being followed. In the interest of cost-effectiveness, several chemotherapy protocols can be combined on one MAP. At the time of admission the patient's specific protocol is identified from a menu of several possible choices on the MAP. All these plans would fall under the same DRG, even though they would be different.

The process for developing the case management plan must be based on several specific elements. The organization must first decide on the form that the plans will take. Factors that affect the form include degree of complexity, extent to which the plan will include other disciplines, and whether the form will include nursing documentation. These factors help determine the plan's design and content. Each factor must be decided before the content is developed.

Once the format has been decided and approved, the organization must decide which diagnoses or procedures are to be planned first. It is obvious that every plan cannot be developed simultaneously. Some general guidelines can be useful in making these decisions. If the model being implemented is a case management, diagnosis-specific approach, then these decisions have probably already been made. Many organizations begin with a few specific diagnoses that are easily planned. Some examples of commonly used diagnoses include "fractured hip," "open heart surgery," and "transurethral prostatectomy" (TURP). These are easily written and followed because these types of procedures are already the subjects of many protocols. It is generally easier to get the cooperation of surgeons who are managing these cases because they are already managing their patients in a protocol-oriented way. It is also easier to reduce length of stay because the chance of complication or comorbidity is slightly lower in these patient populations than in some others.

If the organization is adopting a unit-based case management model, then deciding which diagnosis to begin with is slightly more complicated, although technically it is the same as for the non-unit-based approach. One of the first factors to consider is the number of patients to include in the implementation of one plan. This involves examining the high-volume case types for the organization. Once this is done, an attempt should be made to match these high-volume case types to the units being converted to a case management model. These two factors point to the types of patient problems that should be considered first. After these determinations a match is then made to physicians who work with these patients and who are willing to help develop and adopt case management plans.

Only after all these steps have been taken can the actual process of writing begin. There will be several parts to each plan. Generally the longest of these are the nursing and medical plans. Plans for medical problems are developed from chart review, consultation with experts in the field, and literature review, all to create the "best possible plan" or ideal plan for that patient problem. To make the most of each person's time, individual brainstorming sessions between the case manager and a representative from each discipline are most effective. The case manager can make some preparation to begin the shell of the plan before meeting with anyone. The case manager can determine the approximate length of the plan, based on state and federal reimbursements, and then can begin to plan out the nursing portion of the plan, indicating the expected nursing outcomes for each day of hospitalization.

Once these pieces are complete, the case manager then arranges to meet with members of the other disciplines. The most logical person to begin with is the physician. Plans need to be physician specific, but this means that several physicians agree as a group to the same plan. Under no circumstances should a completed plan be presented to a physician until it is first made clear that the individual preferences and practice patterns of that practitioner will be taken into consideration. Plans should be individualized as much as possible.

Another technique to use is a team approach in which the members of the team physically meet as a group at specific, assigned times. The team can begin the process by developing a tool to review patient records. The tool should include demographic and clinically specific information. Clinical issues that "appear" to be affecting length of stay should be highlighted. Examples of these include progressive ambulation, timing of removal of tubes or drains, switches from intravenous to oral medications, and response time for consults. The clinical issue being studied will drive this list. Once the tool is developed, the team can begin reviewing charts. A representative number of charts should be selected randomly. For most diagnoses at least 30 charts should be reviewed. Validating the issues that "appear" to be affecting length of stay will help drive the clinical content of the plan (Adler, Bryk, Cesta, & McEachen, 1995).

Most physicians have a clear sense of their expectations or of what they would routinely order for the average patient with a particular problem. Of course, not every patient can or will fit into this projected plan exactly. Each plan must be tailored to the patient after admission. The physician should remember that the projected plan is designed for the average patient with a particular problem. This plan could be considered an aggregate of all patients the physician has treated, discounting unusual or aberrant conditions or circumstances.

On average the plan-development process can be completed in less than an hour. This hour is a small contribution compared with the amount of time it would take for the physician to individually inform all the health care providers of the care plan. Development of a MAP not only saves the physician time but also eliminates the second guessing that sometimes occurs.

One approach for developing a MAP is to simply ask the physician what would routinely be ordered for each day of hospitalization. Systematically running through each day ensures that nothing is neglected. Once all disciplines have completed this process, each should be afforded the opportunity to review the plan one last time. If a group of physicians is involved, each physician should have the chance to provide input. This content should be checked against the data collected on chart review.

The decision as to which disciplines will be represented in the plan depends on the diagnosis or procedure being planned. For some, physical therapy will be important. For others, respiratory therapy may be necessary. In most institutions, social work is a separate component but an integral part of the patient's plan, so this department should be given its own section on every plan. In other institutions some specialties such as skin care nurse may always be included. The disciplines involved will vary from institution to institution, but in general, nursing, medicine, and social work should be on every plan (Tahan, 1998).

Once each representative has participated in the plan-development process, it would be beneficial to have as many of these people as possible sit down together to review the plan. This form of brainstorming may expose redundant treatments or procedures. This is another way of significantly reducing resource utilization while providing the best quality of care possible.

MAP TIMELINES

MAPs can be time lined in hours, days, weeks, or months, depending on the clinical area. Emergency room treatment might be mapped out in terms of hours or parts of an hour. Typical diagnoses, including common medical problems or surgeries, usually fall within a day's time frame. Weeks might be used for those diagnoses that have a longer length of stay, such as those that might be found in a neonatal intensive care unit where the length of stay is 3 or 4 months. Month time frames might be relevant in long-term care facilities, such as those for patients with chronic mental disorders, where clinical progress is extremely slow and lengths of stay are measured in years. Nursing home patients provide another example of patient goals that might be evaluated in terms of months.

Once these time frames are determined, variance time frames must be decided. In other words, when does something become a variance? In what time period should every outcome listed for a particular day be achieved? A variance is anything that does not happen when it is supposed to happen. The hospital must decide what kind of leeway will be allowed for achieving these outcomes. Day 1 will seldom begin at 6 AM on the day of admission because most patients are admitted later in the day. For example, emergency admissions may arrive on the unit in the late afternoon or night shift. It is clear that the beginning and end of any one day in the hospital is a loose concept. Institutions should be generous when deciding on variance time frames. If not, it is possible to set up a situation where almost everything becomes a variance. A plan lasting at least 5 days might not place something into the variance category unless it is not completed within 24 hours. The expected time frame should drive the time frames for variances. For example, if the plan is developed around 15-minute intervals, anything beyond that time period becomes a variance.

Documentation of Variances

An area designated for documenting variances should be on the plan. Each variance can be identified and categorized, if desirable. Typical variance categories include the following:

Operational
Health care provider
Patient
Unmet clinical indicators

An example of operational variances is the breakdown of a piece of equipment, which prevents the completion of a test. Another example is the inability to discharge a patient because no long-term care facilities in the area have an available bed. These are examples of operational variances that go beyond the confines of the hospital. More examples are presented in the Boxes 32-1 and 32-2.

Health care provider variances include any situations in which a health care provider is the cause of the delay in achieving an expected outcome. Discretion must be used when documenting these variances because some may involve a risk management issue. For example, if the resident is paged several

---

> ### Box 32-1 ▶ OPERATIONAL VARIANCE EXAMPLES

Broken equipment
Lost requisition slips causing delays
Departmental delays due to staffing or other causes
Interdepartmental delays
Larger system delays affecting discharge, such as home care services, equipment, or insurance availability

---

> ### Box 32-2 ▶ HEALTH CARE PROVIDER VARIANCE EXAMPLES

Deviation from plan because of physician's varying the practice pattern
Change related to health care provider's practice patterns, level of expertise, or experience

---

times during the night because a patient has pulled out the nasogastric tube and the resident does not respond for several hours, the patient misses several doses of medication. Other variances in this category may be associated with the physician's alteration or adjustment of the traditional plan of care.

Patient variances include any patient-related delays (see Box 32-3). The patient delay may be caused by complications of the patient's medical condition, which require a delay in completion of a test or procedure. For example, the patient may have spiked a fever and may be unable to leave the floor for magnetic resonance imaging (MRI). In other circumstances the delay may be because the patient refused to allow the test or procedure. Noncompliance frequently causes patient delays. When a patient refuses a test or procedure, the absolute need for the test or procedure should be questioned and evaluated. This sort of stringent review and follow-up is an example of how a checks-and-balances system in case management can help reduce unnecessary resource use. Tests and procedures cost the institution money not only in terms of the expense of the supplies and equipment but also in terms of the human resources needed to administer the test and evaluate the results. More timely completion of appropriate tests means a reduction in the length of stay for all patients.

Another type of patient variance is called *patient variance on admission*. This variance type is also known as a preexisting condition or comorbidity. Case management plans are simple guidelines or expected plans for particular diagnoses or procedures. Regulatory agencies require individualization of any predetermined plans of care during patient admission. This process should be a routine part of putting any patient on a case management plan. The patient's case should be reviewed in relation to the prewritten plan. Anything different or unusual about the patient's case should yield a change in the plan to make it specific to the patient. One plan is not going to be appropriate for every patient. This process ensures that the plan meets the needs of the patient in question. For example, if the plan calls for a specific medication and the patient is allergic to that medication, the plan should be altered to adjust to that particular patient's clinical condition.

The fourth type of variance is unmet clinical quality indicators (see Box 32-4). Clinical quality indicators are developed in conjunction with the MAP. They are created by the physicians to benchmark clinical outcomes that reflect quality of care rendered. These clinical outcomes can be either intermediate or discharge patient outcomes (Morrison & Beckworth, 1998). The box contains examples of clinical quality indicators that would be developed for asthma team patients.

Box 32-3	**PATIENT VARIANCE EXAMPLES**

Refusal
Change in status
Emotionally or physically unable

Box 32-4	**UNMET CLINICAL QUALITY INDICATORS**

ASTHMA
Intermediate Outcomes
Patient is off IV Solu-Medrol when peak flow >200

Discharge Outcomes
Peak flow measurement >250 L/s
Patient is out of bed without shortness of breath
Patient is able to return demonstration of the use of metered dose inhaler (MDI) with spacer

---

Variance data are abstracted from the patient's medical record and MAP. The analysis of these data is invaluable in determining why an expected patient outcome or clinical quality indicator has not been met. In addition, these data allow for trending of patient outcomes, length of stay, and evaluation of the quality of patient care.

Appendix 7-1 at end of Chapter 7 is an example of a MAP developed and used at the St. Vincents Catholic Medical Centers of New York. This MAP is clinically specific, not DRG specific. The format illustrated is a preprinted, bound booklet that outlines the expected outcomes for care for each day of hospitalization for each discipline involved. Medicine, nursing, social work, and discharge planning are automatically included on every plan. Other departments are included as needed. Each department is given a standard place on the form, and content is filled in by members of the discipline during formation of the plan.

The length of the booklet is guided by the reimbursement for the DRGs usually associated with the diagnosis or problem. This information is correlated with what the physician expects the length of stay to be. Generally the physician will adapt to the reimbursement length of stay if this information is supplied in a positive way. If more than one DRG is involved, which is usually the case, then some judgment must be used in determining the shortest possible plan that takes into account the possibly varying reimbursable lengths of stay. In other words, it may be necessary to look at the most commonly used DRGs and follow an average or usual length of stay. Clearly, these expected lengths are "guesstimates" and will not be completely accurate every time. Each plan may be lengthened or shortened, depending on patient-related variations, but some professional judgment must be used. If a plan is 7 days in length and the patient is ready to go home on the sixth day, an earlier discharge would be completed, and the documentation would be written to reflect the reasons why. A delayed discharge must be documented in the same way with variances that caused the delay being documented and explained.

During the early phases of DRG use in case management systems, the finer points of the DRG were not always synchronous with the system itself. As the system evolved into more of a financial one, clinical applications of the system needed to remain flexible, and the limitations of such uses needed to be clarified for those clinicians using the system.

Space for nursing documentation has been incorporated into the form of some MAPs. In this space the registered nurse documents whether expected outcomes for the day were achieved and any appropriate responses of the patient. Progress notes are included only when a more elaborate or detailed form of documentation is needed, and narrative nurse's notes are eliminated unless an exception arises. This detailed list of outcomes provides the nurse with an action plan that is specific for that day and keeps the patient on track toward discharge.

For the novice nurse who is less able to project patient needs because of a lack of experience, the MAP provides a plan that is outcome-oriented and guides the new nurse through that particular day of hospitalization. Rather than correcting problems after they have happened, the MAP provides an advanced, detailed plan with tasks that can be carried out in a timely fashion.

The case manager is the driving force behind the success of the managed care plan. It is generally the case manager who checks on variances related to both cause and remedy and who is accountable for the patient's continued success in moving through the system. Using the plan as a guide, the case manager directs all other health care providers toward achieving the expected daily outcome of care.

Another responsibility of the case manager is to provide patient teaching when necessary and to find out why a test or procedure has not been done. The case manager also reviews the care plan with the physician and ensures timely outcomes. Finally, the case manager coordinates with the social worker, discharge planner, family, and patient to ensure that the best possible discharge plan has been made and that it is ready when the patient goes home. This entire process is communicated to other members of the team through the MAP format and through the case manager's documentation. All in all, the case manager views the whole picture and ensures proper and accurate progress of the patient through the hospital system.

Staff nurses work in collaboration with the case manager and other members of the health care team to ensure that the outcomes of care are achieved within the time frames specified on the MAP. The patient's outcomes are documented by the staff nurse and relate the clinical story of the patient's progress during hospitalization. Appendix 32-1 contains a sample critical path that has been adapted to the needs of a particular institution; Appendix 7-1, at the end of Chapter 7 provides an additional example.

PATIENT PATHWAYS

The case management plan can be adapted for use by patients and families. The existing plans rewritten in language understandable to patients and their families can be an effective tool. It is not necessary for these adapted plans to contain as much in-depth information as the case management plans used by the health care providers. Rather, only specific information relevant to the patient's needs can be summarized from the more detailed plan.

An issue to consider in the selection of the content is the inclusion of a discussion in patient-friendly language of the general course of events patients can expect during their hospital stay. Care should be taken not to be too specific clinically because as changes are made to the medical plan, patients may become concerned that there is something wrong or that their clinical progression toward discharge is not going as planned.

Benchmarks should be outlined in the patient's version of the case management plan. These benchmarks should include milestones during the course of the hospital stay as well as discharge indicators. For example, asthmatic patients might be told that their intravenous medication will be stopped when their peak flow reading is 200 L/s. In this way the patient will clearly understand the goal of care as well as why their IV medication was switched to an oral medication. Other benchmarks should relate to the patient's clinical condition and should reflect the benchmarks or indicators outlined in the clinician's case management plan.

Another useful technique is to give the patient and family a patient version of the critical pathway. Such a document presents the discharge indicators or the factors that indicate when a particular case type is safe and ready for discharge. Again, these pathways should be written in language that is understandable to lay people and given to the patient soon after admission to the hospital. In this way the patient once again knows the indications for safe discharge and can work with the health care team toward these goals. In addition, the patient also sees that a decision to discharge is based on predetermined criteria and is not arbitrary in any way.

References

Adler, S.L., Bryk, E., Cesta, T.G. & McEachen, I. (1995). Collaboration: The solution to multidisciplinary care planning. *Orthopaedic Nursing, 14*(2), 21-29.

Doyle, R.L. & Schibanoff, J.M. (1997). *Healthcare management guidelines*, vol. 1, Milliman & Roberston, Inc.

Giuliano, K.K., & Poirier, C.E. (1991). Nursing case management: Critical pathways to desirable outcomes. *Nursing Management, 22*(3), 52-55.

Morrison, R.S., & Beckworth, V. (1998). Outcomes for patients with congestive heart failure in a nursing case management model. *Nursing Case Management, 3*(3), 108-114.

Tahan, H.A. (1998). The multidisciplinary mandate of clinical pathways enhancement. *Nursing Case Management, 3*(1), 46-51.

Zander, K. (1991). Care MAPs: The core of cost/quality care. *The New Definition, 6*(3), 1-3.

Zander, K. (1992). Physicians, care MAPs, and collaboration. *The New Definition, 7*(1), 1-4.

APPENDIX 32-1

ST. MICHAEL HOSPITAL MILWAUKEE, WISCONSIN
Uncomplicated MI Critical Path

DRG: _____

HCFA LOS: _____ EXP. LOS: _____

PHYSICIAN: _____

DATE REVIEWED BY PHYSICIAN/RN: _____

DAY/DATE	DAY 1 ED	DAY 1 CCU	DAY 2	DAY 3 TRANSFER TO MCU	DAY 4
FLOOR:					
Consults:			Cardiac Rehab PT and OT – – – – Dietitian	– – – – →	
Tests:	CBC ECG Electrolytes Glucose BUN Creatinine CXR Cardiac enzymes	CCU Standing Orders – – – → ECG – – – → Assess Need: CPK Isoenzymes × 3 (total) per protocol Chem profile & electrolytes	ECG – – – –	ECG – – – – – Stress test/cath ordered Day 7 or 8	ECG
Activity:	Bed rest – – –	– – – →	Bed rest with commode PRN	Up in chair & progress – – – – → Progression of self-care ADL – – – – – →	
Treatments:	IV D₅W Ko – – – → Cardiovascular Assessment & VS q 10-15 min & PRN – – – → Monitor – – –	Daily weights I & O VS q 4° & PRN – – –	Heplock VI – – –	VS q 8° & PRN – – –	– – – – → – – – – → – – – – – – – – – – – –
Medications:	Nitrates – – – – O₂ 2-4 PNC – – – – Analgesics – – – – Lidocaine	– – → – – – – – – – – → Stool softener Beta blockers Calcium channel blockers	O₂ PRN – – – →		

Diet:		Low cholesterol			
Discharge planning:	Complete ED data base	Complete data base. Assessment of home situation	Mutual goal setting — — — → *Multidisciplinary Staffing (T or F) Assessment of IP & OP plans of care. (*Inpatient Cardiac Rehab only)		Assess D/C needs & date Contact SW/HC PRN
Key nursing diagnosis/interventions:	Orientation to ED, staff & equipment. *Assess & monitor:* -Heat-to-toe assessment ×1 -Hemodynamic & cardiovascular stability (4) *Instruct:* -Pain scale 1-10 (1) -Preparation for admission to CCU(2) [ ] brochure given [ ] family/sig. other notified -Offer emotional support	-Orientation to CCU routine, equipment, CCTV, & care delivery system. -Assess pain q 30′ until under control (1) -Reinforce use of pain scale (1) -Position for comfort q 2 ° or prn (1) *Assess & Monitor:* -Head-to-toe assessment q 4° or prn -Activity restriction (3) -Hemodynamic & cardiovascular stability (4) -Arrhythmatic disturbances (4)	Position for comfort q 2° or prn (1) -Patient booklet given(2) -Orient to CCTV, channels 3 & 11 (2) Review basic medication instruction with administration of routine doses (2) *Instruct:* -ID risk factors specific with patient (2) -Diet modification (2) -Gradual progression of activity (3) — —	Assess patient readiness to learn, observe verbal/nonverbal cues, patient's condition (2) *Instruct:* Stress Reduction (2) -Stress management relaxation techniques — — — -Time management -ID support systems & resources — — — — — — → — — — → — — — →	— — — ↑ — — — ↑ — — — ↑ — — — ↑ — — — ↑ — — — ↑ — — — ↑

continued

ST. MICHAEL HOSPITAL MILWAUKEE, WISCONSIN—CONT'D
Uncomplicated MI Critical Path

Key patient activities/ outcomes:				
-Patient &/or significant other verbalizes fears & anxiety -Patient rates pain & intensity on 1-10 scale (1) —→ -Patient &/or significant other verbalizes reason for hospitalization (2)	-Patient demonstrates use of call light —→ - - - - - → - - - - - → Patient's behavior indicates pain reduction or elimination (1) Patient verbalizes that pain is decreased, alleviated, or under control (1)	-Patient verbalizes understanding of diagnosis (2) -Patient voices specific concerns related to coping with illness (2) -Patient watches CCTV (2)	-Patient behavior shows progress toward acceptance of illness (2) - - - - - -Patient able to identify own learning needs (2) - - - - - -Patient demonstrates readiness to learn (2) - - - - - -Patient verbalizes own risk factors (2) -Patient demonstrates gradual progression of energy using energy-conservation techniques (3&4)	- - - - - → - - - - - → - - - - - → Behavior shows signs of: -Stress management (2) -Relaxation techniques (2) -Patient verbalizes time management skills (2&4) -Patient verbalizes support system & resources (2)

Day/Date	DAY 5 Transfer to 2N with telemetry	DAY 6	DAY 7-8
Floor:			
Consults:		Assess need OP cardiac rehab	
Tests:			Stress test/Cath
Activity:	Ambulate bid	Up ad lib	
Treatments:	CS q 8° & PRN I&O	VS bid or q shift D/C I&O	D/C Heplock
Medications:			
Diet:	Low cholesterol →		
Discharge planning:		D/C orders D/C meds Follow-up MD appointment	

Key nursing diagnosis/interventions:	Review previous learning (2)	Review home program (2)
		-Post-MI status
		-Diet
		-Meds
		  a) Schedule
		  b) Indications/side effects
		  c) Med sheet given
		-Follow-up with MD
		-Program given by patient
			OP cardiac rehab
			Post list
				Possible nursing diagnoses
				1. Pain
				2. Knowledge deficit (learning needs with diagnosis of MI)
				3. Activity intolerance
				4. Decreased cardiac output
				*Nursing care guide available

Key patient activities/outcomes:	Patient verbalizes understanding of cardiac disease and/or MI (2)	Patient plans activity progression and after D/C (home, work, sexuality, social) using energy conservation/work simplification techniques (2,3,4)	Patient describes home med schedule with indications/side effects (reference med sheet) (2)
			Patient verbalizes follow-up MD, early warning signs, and emergency plan (2)
				WIPRO Criteria →
				All Met and Documented before Discharge
				72 hours before D/C
				  No evidence of ECG changes.
				48 Hours before D/C
				  No change in type/dosage of antiarrhythmic drug(s).
				  Chest pain controlled with anti-anginal drugs.
				  Vital signs WNL for patient
				24 Hours before D/C
				  Lab values WNL for patient (electrolytes, BUN, enzymes)
				  Oral temp <99° without antipyretic.
				  Invasive monitoring devices removed.
				  Activity/mobility/ambulation documented as improved/stabilized.
				  Improved clinical status (e.g., chest clear, rales & wheezing, absence of friction rub & S, gallop).
				  If DC'd to self-care, document completion of patient education.
				  D/C plan documented.
				If hospital stay < 3 days for rule out MI, no evidence of ECG changes or enzyme rise.

DEFINITIONS

Decreased cardiac output: A state in which the blood pumped by the individual's heart is sufficiently reduced that it is inadequate to meet the needs of the body's tissues.

Pain: A state in which an individual experiences and reports the presence of severe discomfort or an uncomfortable sensation.

Activity intolerance: A state in which an individual has insufficient physiological or psychological energy to endure or complete required or desired daily activities

©St. Michael Hospital, Milwaukee, Wisconsin.

Standardizing Documentation

The Next Generation in Pathway Development

Vivienne Smith, Kathleen Smith

CHAPTER OVERVIEW

Documentation systems have the potential to integrate clinical pathways and clinical charting. Standardized nomenclatures are necessary to clearly describe, examine, and evaluate the work of health care providers. Clinical information systems can provide a framework for organizing and planning care, as well as support data collection that can be used to determine the best practices for desired patient outcomes. All three elements are necessary to develop an automated, comprehensive, multidisciplinary record of patient care. This chapter will review the different elements necessary to accomplish this goal.

INTRODUCTION

Of all the activities performed by professional nurses, possibly the least popular, and the one with the least *perceived* value, is documentation (charting). Despite this, nurses spend an extraordinary amount of time documenting patient care. They may spend more than 15% of their time involved in activities directly related to charting (Miller & Pastorino, 1990). One study cites 27% of an 8.5-hour shift (Short, 1997)! Many institutions still use paper systems for nurse charting, and information is recorded on everything from official forms and flowsheets to hastily scribbled, handwritten notes (information intended for transfer later into the patient's legal record). Duplication of effort is not unusual, as the documentation tools that exist in many institutions lend themselves to redundancy and fragmentation. Review of documentation confirms that nurse charting often shows scattered attention to care issues such as discharge planning, teaching, and continuity of care. Tasks seem unrelated to individual patient problems, and specific care plans are not always evident. In most cases nurses are *providing* appropriate, high-quality care, but documentation systems rarely support or reflect this.

The problems associated with this method of documentation are obvious. When regarded in combination, they lead to a series of undesirable events and lost opportunities. Nurses become exhausted trying to keep up with a series of cumbersome and problematic documentation requirements. They re-sent time taken from direct patient care and perceive the documentation system as something that, far from facilitating care planning, actually *distracts* from it. However, there is enormous potential for documentation to become more than a mere chronological record of events.

Designing and implementing a documentation system that facilitates planning, enhances interdisciplinary communication, records and reports patient response to interventions, and still saves valuable nursing time at first seems impossible. The challenges are overwhelming. However, today's health care market demands that all professionals document their contribution to patient outcomes, which may prove to be the trigger that forces nurses to finally document their worth. Ultimately, data collection systems must be in place to measure and report the contribution of all disciplines, including nursing, to patient outcomes.

INTEGRATING CLINICAL PATHWAYS, CARE PLANNING, AND DOCUMENTATION

Since the early 1980s, health care environments have increasingly developed clinical paths for planning care and monitoring expected outcomes. They can be thought of as "a visualization of the patient care process" (Coffey et al., 1992). However, one downfall is that they often remain in the domain of the case manager and the physician. Other direct caregivers, including bedside nurses, frequently plan their care independent of the pathway because it is not always visible to the entire team. In some cases, pathways are regarded as a financial tool with little clinical significance. One unfortunate result is that nursing's contribution to patient advancement on the path is often overlooked.

Nursing care plans have been around in one form or another since the 1930s. However, their use is frequently limited to the academic setting, a useful exercise for students learning the nursing process. Use of written care plans by seasoned nurses is rare, with knowledge and experience acquired "on the job" driving day-to-day care planning. Consequently, care planning is not necessarily linked to predetermined outcomes (goals), and the level of critical thinking applied to clinical situations by nurses is not always evident. It has become clear that the traditional nursing care plan must somehow be merged with the clinical path so that the elements of the path, including expected outcomes, become the core of the nursing care plan. At the same time there must be enough flexibility to allow nurses to identify additional problems and appropriate interventions for individual patients. In this way the unique contribution of the nursing assessment can be incorporated into the main, multidisciplinary plan of care.

One of the first challenges for integrating clinical pathways and documentation is overcoming the reality that a large number of staff nurses really do not understand the nature or purpose of the clinical path. A first step toward integrating nursing practice is to develop a paper system that requires shift by shift registered nurse (RN) review of the pathway. Nurses should learn to recognize and understand the concept of "phase of care" and be able to relate this to appropriate, expected outcomes. Pathway format must be standardized to eliminate the confusion associated with pathways that "look" different. Case managers and staff nurses from both specialties can be instrumental in reformatting the pathways, leaving space for RNs to indicate shift review of the path. Charting by exception might be considered as an efficient documentation method to use as it removes the burden of requiring a written response to every pathway element.

Pathways can be broken into 24-hour segments, capturing a 24-hour "snapshot" of the patient's status, so that all members of the care team can see at a glance the patient's location on the path in relation to expected outcomes. Staff nurses must be required to note variances or unmet outcomes and follow up with a written note to ensure the item is incorporated into future planning. Since case managers often feel the greatest "ownership" of the paths, they should plan to work very closely with the nurses to monitor and evaluate the project, enlisting the help of other clinicians wherever possible.

The nursing Kardex is the tool most often used to plan nursing care. However, all too often it appears as little more than a place to transcribe medical orders. One possibility is that as long as the Kardex remains available, nurses will continue to rely on it for shift reports and care planning, ignoring the path. This proved to be the experience of one institution (Newell, 1996). Replacing the Kardex with the clinical path hopefully encourages the type of critical thinking that links daily planning to expected outcomes and facilitates communication between caregivers.

STANDARDIZED LANGUAGES

As nurses begin to use clinical pathways as a framework for planning and documenting their care, it is important that standardized languages be used when describing that care. Structured vocabularies are necessary to clearly describe, examine, and evaluate the work of nursing. Because nurses may use multiple terms to describe the same phenomena, it becomes impossible to collect the data necessary for comparing similarities or differences in the care and outcomes of particular patient populations (McCloskey & Bulechek, 2000). Classification systems of nursing care elements have been developed to address these problems. The benefits of incorporating standardized nursing languages into clinical documentation are that they enable us to explicitly describe the nursing process, thereby increasing the visibility of the contributions of nursing. They also improve communication between caregivers and continuity of care for patients. Additionally, computerization of clinical documentation, if it is to provide useful outcome data, is only possible through the use of standard, codified language systems.

Background

Werley and Lang (1988) first recognized the need for nursing to develop a standard set of data elements that could be collected by nursing to measures outcomes. This data set, called the Nursing Minimum Data Set (NMDS), is defined as a minimum set of items of information with uniform definitions and categories concerning the specific dimension of professional nursing that meets the information needs of multiple data users in the health care system (Werley & Lang, 1988). The elements of the NMDS are divided into three categories (Table 33-1). Elements in the first two categories are collected by existing standardized data sets, for example, the Uniform Hospital Discharge Data Set. The nursing care elements of diagnoses, interventions, outcomes, and intensity of nursing care are not collected. Medicine has developed several classification systems to describe medical care, such as the International Classi-

Table 33-1	NURSING MINIMUM DATA SET		
DEMOGRAPHIC ELEMENTS	**SERVICE ELEMENTS**	**NURSING CARE ELEMENTS**
Personal identification	Facility or service agency number	Nursing diagnosis
Date of birth	Health record number of client	Nursing intervention
Sex	Number of principal registered nurse	Nursing outcomes
Race and ethnicity	Provider	Intensity of nursing care
Residence	Episode admission or encounter date	
	Discharge or termination date	
	Disposition of client	
	Expected payer of bill	

fication of Diseases (ICD), Current Procedural Terminology (CPT), and Diagnostic Related Groups (DRG). Major work has been undertaken and is ongoing to develop standard language and classification systems for nursing elements. Interestingly, the nursing components from the nursing minimum data set can already be found within the body of any care plan/clinical pathway.

Languages Approved by the American Nurses Association

The Steering Committee on Databases to Support Clinical Nursing Practice was established by the American Nurses Association (ANA) to oversee the development of nursing languages within the framework of the NMDS (Bowles & Naylor, 1996). Terms from these classification systems have been incorporated into the National Library of Medicine's Unified Medical Language System (UMLS), which is a resource and cross-link for assisting health professionals to retrieve and integrate vocabularies of medical information (McCormick & Jones, 1998). ANA-approved nursing languages also provide the foundation for a Unified Nursing Language System (UNLS). Currently the ANA recognizes several standardized nursing languages: North American Nursing Diagnosis Association (NANDA) taxonomy, Nursing Interventions Classification, Nursing Outcomes Classification, Omaha System, Georgetown University Home Health Care Classification, Ozbolt Patient Care Data Set, and the Perioperative Nursing Data Set. Table 33-2 is a comparison of the various classification systems.

NANDA's Nursing Diagnosis Taxonomy

Nursing diagnosis was originally introduced in the early 1970s (Gebbie & Lavin, 1975). Since then, NANDA has been formed to further the work of classifying nursing diagnoses. A nursing diagnosis is defined as a "clinical judgment about individual, family, or community responses to actual or potential health problems/life processes" (NANDA, 1990, p. 5). The definition contains a label with defining characteristics and related or etiologic factors. The NANDA taxonomy contains 150 approved diagnoses classified into nine domains. It is important that these diagnoses be clearly identified in the documentation of care in order to provide the links to interventions and outcomes. The diagnoses are continually being updated, and presently members of a project called the Nursing Diagnosis Extension and Classification (NDEC) is working to refine and extend the nursing diagnosis classification system (Utz, 1998).

   Unfortunately, over the years, nurses have not embraced the concept of nursing diagnosis, even though the diagnosis may accurately describe real problems experienced by patients. However, it remains quite evident that the way nurses treat these problems greatly influences the patient outcomes for which nurses should be held accountable. Although many nurses are not comfortable with the language in the NANDA taxonomy, computerization may help by providing structure and clarification.

Omaha System

The Visiting Nurse Association of Omaha, Nebraska developed the Omaha system over a 20-year period (Martin & Scheet, 1992). It is widely used in community health settings, including home care, school health, public health, and other outpatient care. It includes problem classification and intervention elements, as well as a problem-rating scheme for outcome evaluation. The Problem Classification Scheme of the system comprises four domains into which all identified problems are distributed: physiological, health related behavior, psychosocial, and environmental. The interventions are organized in four categories: health teaching, guidance, and counseling; treatments and procedures; case management; and surveillance. The taxonomy includes 63 targets that are the object of the nursing interven-

Table 33-2 NURSING CLASSIFICATION SYSTEMS

LANGUAGE SYSTEM	NANDA	OMAHA SYSTEM	GEORGETOWN HOME HEALTH	NIC	PATIENT CARE DATA SET	PERIOPERATIVE DATE ELEMENT SET	NOC
Elements	Nursing diagnosis	Problem, intervention, outcome	Diagnosis, intervention, outcomes	Interventions	Problem, goals, orders	Diagnosis, outcomes, interventions	Outcomes
Setting	All	Community	Home health	All	Acute care	Perioperative	All
Structure	**Diagnosis** • 9 domains • 150 diagnoses with a definition, defining characteristics and related or etiologic factors	**Diagnosis** • 4 domains • 44 problems with modifiers and signs and symptoms **Intervention** • 4 categories • 63 targets with 3rd level client information **Outcome** • Problem rating scale (1-5) in area of knowledge, behavior and status	**Diagnosis** • 20 home health care components • 50 major diagnostic categories • 95 subcategories • 3 outcome modifiers **Intervention** • 20 home health care components • 60 categories • 100 subcategories • 4 type action modifiers **Outcome** • Included with diagnostic code and rated improved, stabilized, or deteriorated	**Interventions** • 7 domains • 30 classes • 486 interventions with a definition and cluster of activities	**Problem** • 22 components • 363 terms • 10 atomic level elements **Goals** • 22 components • 311 terms • 7 atomic level elements **Orders** • 22 components • 1357 terms • 6 atomic level elements	**Outcomes** • 4 domains • 29 outcomes statements **Diagnosis** • 4 domains • 64 diagnoses **Intervention** • 4 domains • 127 interventions	**Outcomes** • 7 domains • 29 classes • 260 outcomes with a list of indicators measured by one of 17 different 5-point Likert scales

tions. Outcomes of patient problems are measured on a five-point scale evaluating a patient's progress in terms of knowledge, behaviors, and status at scheduled intervals.

Georgetown Home Healthcare Classification (HHC)

The HHC was created from a study funded by the Health Care Financing Administration (Saba, 1992). The purpose was to develop a method to predict resource needs and measure outcomes of home health Medicare patients. The diagnoses and intervention are organized under a classification and coding framework of 20 home health nursing components. The diagnosis element uses an expanded version of the NANDA taxonomy to include new home health diagnoses for classifying patient problems and contains 50 major diagnostic categories and 95 subcategories. The coding for expected outcome/goal (improved, stabilized, or deteriorated) is included in the diagnostic code as a fifth digit modifier. The intervention classification contains 60 major nursing intervention categories, 100 nursing intervention subcategories, and a modifier for one of four types of intervention: assessment, direct care, teaching, and management. Thus each nursing diagnosis/expected outcome and nursing intervention is represented by a five-digit alphanumeric code.

Nursing Interventions Classification (NIC)

The NIC is a comprehensive taxonomy of 486 interventions that describe treatments nurses perform (McCloskey & Bulechek, 2000). NIC was developed by a large team of researchers at the University of Iowa funded by a grant from the National Center for Nursing Research. An intervention is the label given to a set of specific activities that nurses perform to assist patients as they move toward an outcome. Interventions can be both nurse-initiated and physician-initiated. The interventions are organized into a three-level taxonomy with 7 domains and 30 classes. The domains include physiological (basic), physiological (complex), behavioral, safety, family, health system, and community. The interventions are listed under classes such as activity and exercise management, elimination management, electrolyte and acid-base management, and drug management. Each intervention has a label name with a definition that is coded. The suggested activities for each intervention are not coded and can be modified to individualize the care of the patient. The taxonomy is quite comprehensive and contains both basic and complex interventions that can be used for all types of patients in all settings. NIC can also be used by other disciplines such as physical therapy, dietitians, and respiratory therapists to describe their care.

Patient Care Data Set (PCDS)

The PCDS was developed to provide a comprehensive set of standard terms to represent and capture clinical data for use in patient care information systems in the acute care setting (Ozbolt, 1996). In collaboration with the University Health System Consortium the terms were derived from patient care planning and documentation materials from nine hospitals and tested for reliability and validity in six of the hospitals. The data set contains a data dictionary and sets of terms and codes representing 363 patient problems, 311 patient care goals, and 1357 patient care orders. The terms are organized into 22 components. Within each component are three axes: problems, goals, and orders. Each axis contains a set of defined atomic-level elements. For example, under the component "activity" on the axis of patient care orders the values of each of the following atomic-level elements are coded: subject, object, action, indicators, method, and risk factors. The PCDS captures a more detailed level of care than the other classification systems.

Perioperative Nursing Data Set (PNDS)

The PNDS provides the data elements that define and describe professional nursing practice in the perioperative setting. Language development efforts were led by a committee of clinical experts from the Association of Perioperative Registered Nurses. The elements of nursing diagnosis, interventions, and outcomes were derived from literature review and validated by an expert panel review and by surveying the membership of the organization. The PNDS consists of three patient domains—safety, physiology, and behavior responses, individual and family—and one structural domain of health system. Each domain includes relevant nursing diagnoses (NANDA-approved), outcomes, and interventions. The intervention contains a label, intervention definition, and a list of activities and is linked to one or more outcome statements and nursing diagnoses (Kleinbeck, 1999).

Nursing Outcomes Classification (NOC)

The NOC provides the language for the evaluation step of the nursing process and outcome element of the NMDS (Johnson, Maas, and Morehead, 2000). Researchers at the University of Iowa also developed this classification. It includes a set of 260 outcome labels sensitive to nursing care. A nursing-sensitive outcome is defined as a "variable concept representing a patient or family care giver state, behavior, or perception that is measurable along a continuum and responsive to a nursing interventions" (Johnson, 1998). The taxonomy is organized into 7 domains and 29 classes. Each domain contains classes or groups of related outcomes. The outcomes each have a definition, label name, and list of indicators with a five-point scale for use in rating the status of the outcome. For example, in the domain of "Functional Health" under the class "Mobility" is the outcome, "Mobility Level." It contains a list of indicators such as "ambulation: walking" that is evaluated on a scale from 1 to 5 and ranges from dependent to completely independent. The classification contains 17 different five-point Likert scales. The outcome is coded by a 10-digit alphanumeric code, which designates domain, class, outcome, indicator, what scale was used, and the 1-to-5 evaluation score. The development of a standard language for outcomes enables the examination of links between diagnoses, interventions, and outcomes. It allows the measurement of patient status at different points along the clinical path. Without the inclusion of nurse-sensitive outcome measures in pathways, the contributions and quality of nursing care cannot be recognized or measured.

Worldwide Implications

Development of standard nursing language systems has implications worldwide. In 1988 the ANA submitted the approved diagnostic labels of the NANDA Taxonomy to the World Health Organization (WHO) for inclusion in the International Statistical Classification of Diseases and Related Health Problems (ICD-10). Because the classification had not been approved by all member countries of the WHO, it was withdrawn and referred to the International Council of Nursing (ICN). Subsequently, the ICN has established an international task force to develop an International Classification of Nursing Practice (ICNP), which would include a standardized vocabulary and classification of nursing phenomena (nursing diagnosis), nursing interventions, and nursing outcomes. An Alpha Version was published in 1996, and a Beta Version is to be published in 1999 for further testing.

The ICNP three-fold purpose is to provide a vocabulary, a new classification system for nursing, and a framework into which existing vocabularies and classifications can be cross-mapped to enable comparison of nursing data collected using other nursing vocabularies and classifications (Clark, 1998). It has been recognized that no single language and classification system can meet the needs of nurses in a variety of settings in all countries, therefore ICNP may be able to provide the unifying framework for all nursing language systems throughout the world.

USING STANDARD NOMENCLATURES IN CLINICAL PATHWAYS

By incorporating standardized languages into clinical pathway/care plans, documentation becomes more consistent and efficient. Information about nursing care can be retrieved and aggregated, and the effectiveness of specific interventions can be determined. Additionally, other disciplines can document their care using the same standardized language. Knowledge gained through the analysis of this information can be used to demonstrate the contribution of nursing to patient outcomes. Pathways can continually be improved, reflecting the most effective and efficient interventions for a given population.

Table 33-3 illustrates an example of the languages of NANDA, NIC, and NOC being used to describe nursing care and evaluate outcomes for patients on a renal transplant clinical path. The example is not intended to provide a comprehensive plan for a patient having a renal transplant (tests, medications, and other features were omitted to simplify for publication). The intent is to demonstrate the incorporation of standard languages and the links between diagnosis, interventions, and outcomes.

AUTOMATING THE PROCESS

Clinical information systems (CIS) are an essential part of any plan to develop a documentation system that seeks to describe and standardize nursing care. They can provide the framework for organizing patient care. Most systems already provide features that support input, display, and reporting of patient information. However, not all systems have kept pace with the rapidly changing needs of the industry. It is essential that in addition to a framework for nurses to use at the bedside, the CIS have the ability to codify data that can later be retrieved and analyzed. The system should support data collection that can be used to determine best practices for desired outcomes, variability in practice, and the most effective utilization of resources.

In 1998 the ANA created the Nursing Information and Data Set Evaluation Center (NIDSEC). The purpose of NIDSEC is to ensure that information systems are equipped to recognize and report the contribution of nursing to patient outcomes. Carol Bickford, a senior policy fellow in the ANA's Department of Nursing Practice, states ". . . a patient's response to treatment or a nursing intervention can help or hinder an outcome. But such variables aren't routinely captured, because there is no standard framework to convert nurses' observations and actions into retrievable sets of data" (Morrissey, 1999). So far, McKesson/HBOC's Pathways 2000 Care Manager Clinical Charting software has been certified as meeting ANA standards. Others are expected to follow suit because the market is demanding better nursing data.

At this time, one of the greatest challenges is in trying to find ways to make current CIS support the vision of a problem-oriented, multidisciplinary care plan. Such plans represent major practice changes for nurses, so the CIS must facilitate and support this. Merely replicating what exists today on paper will not accomplish the goal of linking documentation to care plans. In other words, the nursing process should drive the documentation system, not vice versa. Basically, each time a charting entry is made, it should be clearly linked to a patient problem. Reports should display this correlation, and data must be retrievable for later analysis.

When entering into discussions about technical feasibility with software vendors, it is imperative to bring this clinical perspective to the table, shifting the paradigm away from traditional charting systems.

	PHASE: ONE DAY: ADM-PRETX-OR day	PHASE: TWO DAY: POST-OP DAY 0/1	PHASE: TWO DAY: POST-OP DAY 2
	NANDA	NANDA	
Nursing diagnosis/ Patient problems	**Knowledge deficit related to procedures**	**Risk for fluid volume deficit** **Risk for infection** **Pain** **Risk for altered nutrition** **Impaired physical mobility** **Knowledge deficit: medications** **Knowledge deficit: disease process**	
Nursing treatments/ intervention	NIC–ADMISSION CARE: Pre-op nursing admit history assessment per standards	NIC–FLUID MANAGEMENT: VS q2hr until stable Daily wt I&O q hr CVP q4hr × 24hr Monitor lab values Monitor skin turgor Monitor for edema Monitor breath and heart sounds	NIC–FLUID MANAGEMENT: VS q4hr Daily wt I&O CVP q8hr × 24hr Monitor lab values Monitor skin turgor Monitor for edema Monitor breath and heart sounds
		NIC–IV THERAPY: IV fluids D5 1/2NS—@50ml/hr + urine replacement IV site checks Site care, central line Instruct patient IV therapy	NIC–IV THERAPY: IV fluids D5 1/2NS—@50ml/hr DC urine replacement IV site checks Site care, central line Instruct patient IV therapy
		NIC–TUBE CARE: URINARY Foley to gravity Irrigate with 20-30 ml NS prn Follow Foley care protocol Instruct patient Foley care	NIC–TUBE CARE: URINARY Foley to gravity: Irrigate with 20-30 ml NS prn Follow Foley care protocols Instruct patient Foley care
		NIC–INCISION SITE CARE: Monitor healing process of incision site Remove operative dressing and leave open to air Instruct patient incision site care	NIC–INCISION SITE CARE: Monitor healing process of incision site Instruct patient incision site care
		NIC–PAIN MANAGEMENT: Assess pain using pain assessment protocols PCA protocols Implement pain control measures Evaluate effectiveness of pain control measures Instruct patient pain management	NIC–PAIN MANAGEMENT: Assess pain using pain management protocols DC PCA pumps Administer oral analgesics Evaluate effectiveness of pain control measures Instruct patient pain management
Diet	NIC–DIET STAGING: NPO except meds with sip of H2O	NIC–DIET STAGING: NPO except sips water/chips for meds × 8hr, then clear liquids. Advance to regular diet as tolerated.	NIC–DIET STAGING: Progress to regular

Continued

	PHASE: ONE DAY: ADM-PRETX-OR DAY	PHASE: TWO DAY: POST-OP DAY 0/1	PHASE: TWO DAY: POST-OP DAY 2
Activity	Ad lib pre-op	NIC–EXERCISE THERAPY: AMBULATION OOB with assist at least TID	NIC–EXERCISE THERAPY: AMBULATION Ambulate with assist qid
Teaching	NIC–TEACHING: PREOPERATIVE: Instruct patient/family using renal pre-op teaching standards.	NIC–TEACHING: PRESCRIBED MEDS Instruct patient/family medications using renal teaching standards.	NIC–TEACHING: DISEASE PROCESS Instruct patient/family teaching based on renal transplant teaching standards
Consults			NIC–TEACHING: PRESCRIBED DIET Transplant dietician
Discharge planning	NIC–DISCHARGE PLANNING: Collaborate with health team in planning for continuity of health care Identify patient teaching needs for post-discharge care Develop discharge plan	NIC–DISCHARGE PLANNING: Review discharge plan in daily ward rounds	NIC–DISCHARGE PLANNING: Review discharge plan in daily ward rounds
Outcomes	NOC KNOWLEDGE: TREATMENT PROCEDURE Description of procedure: 1 2 3 4 5 Performance of IS treatment: 1 2 3 4 5		NOC FLUID BALANCE BP in expected range 1 2 3 4 5 Body weight stable 1 2 3 4 5 24 hr I&O balanced 1 2 3 4 5 CVP in expected range 1 2 3 4 5 Serum electrolytes in expected range 1 2 3 4 5 INFECTION Fever 1 2 3 4 5 WOUND HEALING: PRIMARY INTENTION: Skin approximation 1 2 3 4 5 RESOLUTION OF DRAINAGE 1 2 3 4 5 PAIN Reported pain 1 2 3 4 5 NUTRITION Food and fluid intake 1 2 3 4 5 MOBILITY LEVEL Ambulation: walking 1 2 3 4 5 KNOWLEDGE: TREATMENT REGIMEN Description of prescribed medication 1 2 3 4 5 Description of prescribed diet 1 2 3 4 5 Description of self-care responsibilities for ongoing treatment 1 2 3 4 5 Description of expected effects of treatment 1 2 3 4 5

Table 33-3	**EXAMPLE OF STANDARDIZED LANGUAGES IN CLINICAL PATHWAY** **Diagnosis: Renal Transplant—cont'd**		
	PHASE: THREE **DAY: POST-OP DAY 3**	**PHASE: THREE** **DAY: POST-OP DAY 4**	**PHASE: THREE** **DAY: POST-OP DAY** **5/DISCHARGE DAY**
Nursing diagnosis/ Patient problems	NANDA **Risk for fluid volume deficit** **Potential for urinary retention** **Risk for infection** **Pain** **Risk for altered nutrition** **Impaired physical mobility** **Knowledge deficit: medications** **Knowledge deficit: disease process**		
Nursing treatments/ interventions	NIC–FLUID MANAGEMENT VS q4hr Daily wt I&O Monitor lab values Monitor skin turgor Monitor for edema Monitor breath and heart sounds NIC–IV THERAPY Buff cap IV IV site care NIC–TUBE CARE: URINARY Foley to gravity: Irrigate with 20-30 ml NS prn Foley care protocol NIC–INCISION SITE CARE: Monitor healing process of incision site NIC–PAIN MANAGEMENT: Assess pain using pain management protocols Administer oral analgesics Evaluate effectiveness of pain control measures Instruct patient pain management	NIC–FLUID MANAGEMENT VS q4hr Daily wt I&O Monitor lab values Monitor skin turgor Monitor for edema Monitor breath and heart sounds NIC–IV THERAPY IV site care NIC–URINARY ELIMINATION MANAGEMENT: D/C Foley Monitor for urinary elimination and retention Instruct patient s/s urinary retention NIC–INCISION SITE CARE: Monitor healing process of incision site NIC–PAIN MANAGEMENT: Assess pain using pain management protocols Administer oral analgesics Evaluate effectiveness of pain control measures Instruct patient pain management	NIC–FLUID MANAGEMENT VS q4hr Daily wt I/O Monitor lab values Monitor skin turgor Monitor for edema Monitor breath and heart sounds NIC–URINARY ELIMINATION MANAGEMENT: Monitor for urinary elimination and retention NIC–INCISION SITE CARE: Monitor healing process of incision site NIC–PAIN MANAGEMENT: Assess pain using pain management protocols Administer oral analgesics Evaluate effectiveness of pain control measures Instruct patient pain management
Diet	Regular	Regular	Regular
Activity	NIC–EXERCISE THERAPY: AMBULATION Ambulate with assistance qid Shower	NIC–EXERCISE THERAPY: AMBULATION Ambulate Shower	NIC–EXERCISE THERAPY: AMBULATION Ambulate Shower

Continued

Table 33-3	EXAMPLE OF STANDARDIZED LANGUAGES IN CLINICAL PATHWAY Diagnosis: Renal Transplant—cont'd		
	PHASE: THREE DAY: POST-OP DAY 3	**PHASE: THREE DAY: POST-OP DAY 4**	**PHASE: THREE DAY: POST-OP DAY 5/DISCHARGE DAY**
Teaching	NIC–TEACHING, INDIVIDUAL Patient and family teaching based on renal transplant teaching standards	NIC–TEACHING, INDIVIDUAL Patient/family teaching based on renal transplant teaching standards	NIC–TEACHING, INDIVIDUAL Patient/family teaching based on renal transplant teaching standards
Consults			
Discharge planning	NIC–DISCHARGE PLANNING: Review discharge plan in daily ward rounds	NIC–DISCHARGE PLANNING: Review discharge plan in daily ward rounds	NIC–DISCHARGE PLANNING Review discharge plan and prepare discharge sheet
Outcomes		FLUID BALANCE BP in expected range 1 2 3 4 5 Body weight stable 1 2 3 4 5 24 hr I&O balanced 1 2 3 4 5 Serum electrolytes 1 2 3 4 5 INFECTION Fever 1 2 3 4 5 WOUND HEALING: PRIMARY INTENTION: Skin approximation 1 2 3 4 5 Resolution of serosanguineous drainage 1 2 3 4 5 PAIN Reported pain 1 2 3 4 5 NUTRITION Food and fluid intake 1 2 3 4 5 MOBILITY LEVEL Ambulation: walking 1 2 3 4 5 KNOWLEDGE: TREATMENT REGIMEN Description of prescribed medication 1 2 3 4 5 Description of prescribed diet 1 2 3 4 5 Description of self-care responsibilities for ongoing treatment 1 2 3 4 5 Description of expected effects of treatment 1 2 3 4 5 URINARY ELIMINATION Elimination pattern in expected range 1 2 3 4 5	

The current version of an existing product may support the concept to some extent, but frequently not all needed functionality is available. One feature to consider would be integrating the documentation system with orders so that orders and clinical charting are connected. When phases are initiated, orders (which should reflect nursing interventions) are activated, and completion of these orders will link to appropriate documentation screens, keeping the pathway current and also allowing the nurse to continually link activities to the plan. Programming changes take time, however, so in the meantime it is wise to explore creative ways to use existing products while continuing to communicate needs to vendors. The CIS are an essential tool as we seek to optimize the use of clinical paths.

SUMMARY

Clinical charting has been a burdensome task for nurses because of the inefficient documentation systems that exist in most hospitals. Consequently, when reviewing the medical record it is difficult to obtain a clear and cohesive picture of the patient's care. The merging of the clinical pathway and the nursing care plan is one step toward providing a structured framework for documentation. This also would increase the visibility of the contribution of nursing to the care and outcomes of patients on a pathway. Standardized languages also should be used in that documentation to enable the collection and aggregation of data related to nursing that affects patient outcomes. Automated clinical documentation systems must be designed to demonstrate a multidisciplinary plan, implementation of that plan, and evaluation of outcomes for patients.

References

Bowles, K.H., & Naylor, M.D. (1996). Nursing intervention classification systems. *IMAGE: Journal of Nursing Scholarship, 28*(4), 303-308.

Clark, J. (1998, Sept 30). The international classification for nursing practice project. *Online Journal of Issues in Nursing.*

Coffey, R.J., et al. (1992). An introduction to critical paths. *Quality Management in Health Care, 1*(1), 45-54.

Gebbie, K.M., & Lavin, M.A. (Eds.) (1975). *Classification of nursing diagnosis: Proceedings of the first national conference.* St. Louis: Mosby.

Johnson, M., Maas, M. & Moorhead, S. (Eds.) (2000). *Iowa outcomes project. Nursing outcomes classification (NOC).* (2nd ed.) St. Louis: Mosby.

Johnson, M. (1998). Overview of the nursing outcomes classification (NOC). *On Line Journal of Nursing Informatics, 2*(2).

Kleinbeck, S. (1999, in press). The development of a specialty nomenclature: The perioperative nursing data set. *AORN Journal.*

Martin, K., & Scheet, N. (1992). *The Omaha System: Applications for community health nursing.* Philadelphia: W.B. Saunders.

McCloskey, J.C., & Bulechek, G.M. (Eds.) (2000). Iowa Intervention Project. In *Nursing intervention classification (NIC)* (3rd ed.). St. Louis: Mosby.

McCormick, K., & Jones, C. (1998, Sept. 30). Is one taxonomy needed for health care vocabularies and classifications? *Online Journal of Issues in Nursing.*

Miller, P., & Pastorino C. (1990). Daily nursing documentation can be quick and thorough! *Nursing Management, 21*(11), 47-49.

Morrissey, J. (1999). Quantifying nursing's impact—slowly. *Modern Healthcare, 28*(1), 40.

Newell, B.A. (1996). We killed the kardex so the care path could live. *Nursing Management, 27*(12), 51.

North American Nursing Diagnosis Association. (1990). Taxonomy I, revised 1990. St. Louis: NANDA.

Ozbolt, J.G. (1996). From minimum data to maximum impact: Using clinical data to strengthen patient care. *Advanced Practice Nursing Quarterly, 1*(4), 62-69.

Saba, V.K. (1992). A classification of home health care nursing diagnosis and interventions. *Caring, 11*(3), 50-57.

Short, M.S. (1997). Charting by exception on a clinical pathway. *Nursing Management, 28*(8), 45-46.

Utz, S.W. (1998). Computerized documentation of case management: From diagnosis to outcomes. *Nursing Case Management. 3*(6), 247-254.

Werley, H., & Lang, N. (Eds.) (1988). *Identification of the Nursing Minimum Data Set.* New York: Springer.

Ethical Issues in Case Management

Sister Carol Taylor

CHAPTER OVERVIEW

This chapter explores the ethical issues related to case management. The essential elements of ethical competence are described, and strategies for developing and evaluating ethical competence are offered. The nurse case manager's potential for influencing the well-being of patients is highlighted with a discussion of advocacy. The principle- and care-based theoretical and practical approaches to clinical ethics are presented with a discussion of the nurse case manager's role in clinical ethics. The chapter concludes with a discussion of moral integrity and with an examination of the six recurrent issues confronting nurse case managers.

Nurse case managers literally hold human well-being in their hands. Repetitious execution of the multiple administrative and clinical tasks that make up the workday of each nurse case manager often blinds us to the truth of this statement. Renewed attention to what we do and reflection on *why* we do what we do will quickly remind us that the "cases" we "manage" are actually people with unique life histories and needs. Moreover, we will readily see the links between who we are and how we conduct ourselves professionally and the well-being of those society entrusts to our professional care. This concluding chapter examines why ethical competence is essential for nurse case managers, explores the role of the nurse case manager in clinical ethics, and examines specific challenges to the professional and personal integrity of nurse case managers.

ETHICAL COMPETENCE AND THE NURSE CASE MANAGER

Ethical Competence as a Core Competence

Is ethical competence a core or an elective competence? Is it like knowing the general principles of asepsis or like knowing how to run a neonatal intensive care unit? Although some nurses continue to think about ethical competence as a specialized expertise that nurses can choose to develop, the American Nurses Association (ANA) in 1991 published standards of professional performance that hold all nurses accountable for ethical practice. Boxes 34-1 and 34-2 present the ANA Code of Ethics and Standards of Professional Performance. Today nurses are legally liable if their practice is ethically deficient.

| Box 34-1 | **The American Nurses Association's Code of Ethics** |

The nurse provides services with respect for human dignity and the uniqueness of the client, unrestricted by considerations of social or economic status, personal attributes, or the nature of health problems.

The nurse safeguards the client's right to privacy by judiciously protecting information of a confidential nature.

The nurse acts to safeguard the client and the public when health care and safety are affected by the incompetent, unethical, or illegal practice of any person.

The nurse assumes responsibility and accountability for individual nursing judgments and actions.

The nurse maintains competence in nursing.

The nurse exercises informed judgment and uses individual competence and qualifications as criteria in seeking consultation, accepting responsibilities, and delegating nursing activities to others.

The nurse participates in activities that contribute to the ongoing development of the profession's body of knowledge.

The nurse participates in the profession's efforts to implement and improve standards of nursing.

The nurse participates in the profession's efforts to establish and maintain conditions of employment conducive to high quality nursing care.

The nurse participates in the profession's effort to protect the public from misinformation and misrepresentation and to maintain the integrity of nursing.

The nurse collaborates with members of the health professions and other citizens in promoting community and national efforts to meet the health needs of the public.

From American Nurses Association. (1985). *Code for nurses with interpretive statements.* Washington, DC: The Association. (EDMNA, Appendix C, p. 266).

Elements of Ethical Competence

Part of the difficulty in holding ourselves and one another accountable for ethical competence lies in the failure to define exactly what it is that constitutes ethical competence. When hiring a new nurse case manager, we generally have a clear idea of the intellectual, clinical, and administrative competencies essential to the successful execution of the role. Rarely, however, are the requisite ethical competencies clear in our mind, and we thus fail to evaluate candidates in this arena. Listed below are some basic characteristics of the ethically competent nurse case manager. Following the list are reasons why these characteristics are important and ways they can be evaluated in a prospective employee interview. Ethically competent nurse case managers are able to:

Be trusted to act in ways that advance the best interests of the patients entrusted to their care

Hold themselves and their colleagues accountable for their practice

Act as effective patient advocates

Mediate ethical conflict among the patient, significant others, the health care team, and other interested parties

Recognize the ethical dimensions of practice and identify and respond to ethical problems

Critique new health care technologies and changes in the way we define, administer, deliver, and finance health care in light of their potential to influence human well-being

Commitment to Patient Well-Being

Commitment to patient well-being as an element of ethical competence would seem to be self-evident, since all those in helping professions in general and in health care professions in particular have as their reason for being commitment to human well-being. Unfortunately the health care system is changing

Box 34-2	THE AMERICAN NURSES ASSOCIATION'S STANDARDS OF PROFESSIONAL PERFORMANCE

STANDARD V. ETHICS: THE NURSE'S DECISIONS AND ACTIONS ON BEHALF OF CLIENTS ARE DETERMINED IN AN ETHICAL MANNER

Measurement Criteria

The nurse's practice is guided by the *Code for Nurses*

The nurse maintains client confidentiality within legal and regulatory parameters

The nurse acts as a client advocate and assists patient in developing skills so that they can advocate for themselves

The nurse delivers care in a nonjudgmental and nondiscriminatory manner that is sensitive to client diversity

The nurse delivers care in a manner that preserves/protects client autonomy, dignity, and rights

The nurse seeks available resources to help formulating ethical decisions

From American Nurses Association. (1998). *Standards of clinical nursing practice,* ed 2 Washington, D.C.: The Association.

in ways that make it increasingly difficult to assume this orientation. The nurse case manager's first challenge and core responsibility is to keep the entire system of care and the caregiving team focused on meeting the needs of the patients it purports to serve. One nurse case manager voiced frustration when she was unable to find a bed on the unit a patient with acquired immunodeficiency syndrome (AIDS) requested when he was being readmitted for new complications. She was told that worrying about which unit had a bed was not "her job." She quickly responded to her colleague that if this was important to the patient, then it was important to her because she didn't know who else was going to worry about it.

EXAMPLE. Nurses working in an oncology unit are discovering that patients enrolled in certain managed care companies have had their access to mental health services severely restricted. Their options are to accept the restricted services as a given or to begin to gather the data that will demonstrate that these restrictions are dramatically influencing the health and well-being of the patients being served. If commitment to the health and well-being of patients is their primary commitment, they will not allow this change in the system to go unchallenged.

RESPONSIBILITY AND ACCOUNTABILITY

As systems for delivering health care continue to fragment, it is not unusual for patient health problems to go undiagnosed or, when diagnosed, to be ignored or inadequately addressed. The diffusion of power and authority in complex caregiving teams makes it easy to assume that "someone else" is responsibly monitoring the problem. By virtue of the coordinating role they play in the caregiving team, nurse case managers are well positioned to monitor the effectiveness of the plan of care and to call to accountability those whose efforts remain uncommitted: *If I hold myself accountable for the well-being of those committed to my care, I need more than a task orientation to each day's work. It isn't enough for me to be "busy" doing professional activities. These activities must be contributing to the well-being of those I serve. My workday is complete when I am confident that everything necessary is being done for those entrusted to my care.* This critical distinction is often overlooked in practice today.

EXAMPLE. Nurses on your unit are pleased that the newly implemented critical pathway for women undergoing a modified radical mastectomy seems to be streamlining care and ensuring a better quality of care for all. Each staff nurse has been encouraged to keep women "on the path" postoperatively so that discharge outcomes can be met within specified time intervals. One nurse voices a concern that one patient seems to need more time and that she is afraid that nurses are impatient with her lack of outcome achievement. The nurse case manager who assumes responsibility for patient well-being is able to counsel staff nurses about the importance of respecting individual patient needs and about their need to assume responsibility for advocating that patients receive the time they need to meet critical outcomes. At issue is our ability to remember that we are first accountable to the patient and then to a new system of care.

Example.   Although everyone in your hospital knows something about advance directives and some are even enthusiastic about their potential for eliminating or reducing conflict over end-of-life decision making, the hospital has not identified who is responsible for actually helping patients to specify their preferences in a meaningful way. Each patient receives literature on advance directives in the admitting office but after that is at the mercy of any health care professional who elects to pursue this conversation. More often than not no one pursues this concern. You can elect to raise this issue and attempt to change the system to ensure that this need is being addressed or you can accept the status quo.

ABILITY TO ACT AS AN EFFECTIVE ADVOCATE

Most of us have heard stories from friends or acquaintances about someone's terrifying hospitalization. "I don't know how people in hospitals survive without a family member in constant attendance to make sure the patient gets the ordered care and to prevent mix-ups!" Although numerous variables influence the amount and type of advocacy required by different patients, it is generally true that someone must act as advocate for the patient on multiple levels and in particular for the patient whose self-advocacy is impaired. Again the nurse case manager is in the ideal position to "work the system" both within and outside the hospital to ensure that the patient's needs are met. In the current climate of financial "bottom-line" decision making the need for strong patient advocacy is even more pronounced.

Example.   A managed care company decides to reimburse hospitals for only the first 12 to 24 hours after delivery, and nurses begin to find women who need a longer hospital stay after delivering to realize valued maternal-infant outcomes. The nurse case manager must choose whether to advocate for these women. A nurse case manager can decide to accept that some outcomes simply cannot be realized in this short time frame or can work to change the system to ensure that these needs are met either in the hospital or at home. An effective advocate will work with individual patients on a case by case basis as well as try to marshal forces to change the system.

ABILITY TO MEDIATE ETHICAL CONFLICT

Ethical conflict is inherent in health care practice today. Among the forces contributing to this conflict are the following:

The multiple therapeutic options available for most health problems and the lack of consensus about their medical effectiveness, benefit, and burdens

The raging debate about who should get how much of our scarce health care resources and the increasing tendency to dismiss certain patients as "poor investment risks" or as simply "unworthy" of indicated medical care

The condition of moral pluralism; the fact that we seem to grow more heterogeneous daily in our religious and cultural beliefs and values

Ethically competent nurse case managers need to be skilled in identifying patients, families, and caregiving teams that are at risk for ethical conflict and in addressing the factors contributing to this conflict. When nurse case managers can effectively mediate problematic situations or invite ethics consult teams to perform this service, the conflict does not escalate and the alienation that sometimes results between patient and families and caregiving individuals, team, or institution can be avoided. A chief objective is to identify the sources of common problems and to change the system to prevent their recurrence.

EXAMPLE.   The wife of one of the patients on your unit comes to you and tells you that a gastrointestinal consultant has just informed her that they need to take her husband back to surgery because he has developed a mesenteric infarct. She tearfully tells you that she knows her husband would refuse this surgery if he were able to speak but that no one seems to be listening to her. He did not do well after surgery to remove a recurrent meningioma. She said that he only reluctantly consented to repeat surgery after much pleading from his adult children. You can side with the medical team who seems to be of the mind that this is a reversible problem that must be addressed or you can try to find out more about the wife's reluctance to consent and get the caregiving team to sit down with the wife and family to decide what actually is in the patient's best interests. The nurse case manager must choose whether to ignore the conflict (or hope that someone else assumes responsibility for its resolution) or to intervene to mediate the conflict.

ABILITY TO RECOGNIZE ETHICAL DIMENSIONS OF PRACTICE

The ethical dimensions of practice range from sensitivity to threats to human dignity in the caregiving environment to concerns about limited access to basic health care services. The nurse case manager who recognizes the ethical dimensions of practice and who knows how and when to intervene can provide effective leadership in this domain.

EXAMPLE.   Nurses in a medical intensive care unit are voicing frustration with the unevenness with which ethical dimensions of care are addressed in the unit, depending on which attending physician is leading the resident team that month. Two of the four attending physicians who make rounds with the residents are supportive of and encourage discussion of ethical questions, whereas the other two seem to believe that these discussions distract attention from the "critical," that is, medical, aspects of the case. At issue is how comfortable the nurses and medical residents are in addressing the topic of do-not-resuscitate (DNR) orders and in initiating advance planning for critical end-of-life decisions. While one case manager allows the attending physician to determine what can be discussed in morning rounds, another invites all four attending physicians to a meeting in which nurses present a plan to make ethical concerns a priority item in the discussion of each patient during rounds. The time gained with patients for whom there are no current ethical questions will allow for a timely discussion of issues when they do come up.

ABILITY TO CRITIQUE POTENTIAL TO INFLUENCE HUMAN WELL-BEING

A final critical element of ethical competence for the nurse case manager is the ability to critique new health care technologies and changes in the way we define, administer, deliver, and finance health care in light of their potential to influence human well-being. The nurse skilled in this ability remains sufficiently distant from and critical of all aspects of caregiving to evaluate them in terms of their human consequences. Examples of successful intervention in this regard occur in both beginning and end-of-life care. In the not so distant past physicians always interjected the latest medical technology into the processes of childbearing and dying. Although this type of care continues to meet the needs of some high-risk patients, we fortunately now have the options of natural childbirth and hospice care for patients who elect to go a different route. These alternative types of care were made available after reflective health care professionals challenged the need for the latest medical treatment for all beginning and end-of-life care.

EXAMPLE.   A critical care nurse comments there is almost no need to spend time in the patient's room any more because sophisticated monitoring equipment allows everyone at the nurses' station to know more than they ever wanted to know about each patient at any moment in time. A nurse case manager listening to this comment begins to wonder how beneficial this equipment is, in its totality, to the patient. How much of it is merely a convenience to the nurses and doctors? What benefits are gained for the patient and at what cost in terms of burden and discomfort? He decides to study this concern and involves other interested nurses. As a result of the data they collect and especially because of what they learn from patient interviews, one type of monitor is "retired" and another is used only for patients with special monitoring needs. When they share their findings with the company who manufactures many of the products they use they discover that the company is interested in the topic of humanizing technology and seeks their collaboration in a research project.

Evaluating Ethical Competence

To evaluate ethical competence in prospective nurse case managers it is helpful to present case scenarios common to the practice setting and elicit their response (Box 34-3). Responses should demonstrate their ease and competence in recognizing and addressing ethical concerns. Box 34-3 offers sample scenarios for evaluating ethical competence and highlights the specific competencies they test. These scenarios could also be used in an informal or formal staff meeting to spark conversation about ethical competence and to encourage reasoning about how case managers identify and meet ethical obligations to individual patients and to society. After several hypothetical scenarios are explored, staff can be invited to present situations they have experienced so that the team can talk together about different ways of responding. When these discussions are regularly scheduled, they communicate the expectation that ethical competence is critical to the performance of the nurse case manager's roles and that it needs to be consciously developed and updated in the same way that clinical and administrative competencies are approached.

Theoretical and Practical Approaches to Clinical Ethics

Ethics broadly defined concerns itself with right and wrong moral conduct, with how we ought to live (and die) and why. Clinical ethics, a relatively new branch of ethics, addresses ethical issues and problems that arise in the context of caring for actual patients in varied clinical settings, in the hospital, residential facility, clinic, and home. The ethically competent nurse case manager will be familiar with at least two common approaches to clinical ethics: the principle-based approach and the care-based approach. Brief descriptions of these follow, and references are cited for those wishing to learn more about these methods.

PRINCIPLE-BASED APPROACH

One of the leading theories of bioethics and clinical ethics has been termed the four-principle approach. Popularized by Beauchamp and Childress (1994), this approach identifies four ethical principles derived from common moral beliefs and uses them to identify, discuss, and analyze the moral features of particular situations. The four principles include autonomy (self-determination), beneficence (benefiting or helping), nonmaleficence (avoiding harm), and justice (treating fairly). Other theorists list as key principles veracity (truth telling), confidentiality (respecting privileged information), fidelity (keeping promises), and avoiding killing. All of these are held to obligate health care professionals in a prima facie manner; that is, all things being equal, I am obligated to respect patients, benefit them, cause them no harm, treat all fairly, be truthful, and so on. A moral dilemma results when I am unable to simultaneously execute two prima facie obligations. For example, a woman with AIDS begs you not to inform her sexual partner and the father of her child that she has AIDS because she is afraid that he will leave her. While you have an obligation to respect her privacy and to keep privileged information confidential, you also have an obligation to prevent harm to identifiable third parties. Seemingly you can-

> Box 34-3 **EVALUATING ETHICAL COMPETENCE**

SAMPLE CASE SCENARIOS FOR INTERVIEWING PROSPECTIVE EMPLOYEES
INTERVIEWER: "Among the competencies we find to be essential for our nurse case managers is ethical competence. I'd like to get a sense of your competence and confidence in responding to some hypothetical situations. I'll describe a situation and invite you to tell me how you would respond if you were the responsible case manager."

SCENARIO 1
The wife of a patient with end-stage cancer seeks you out and tells you that she is afraid that her husband is "losing hope" and "giving up." She tells you that she has just learned that one of the patients on the unit was evaluated for inclusion in a clinical trial that offers some promise of arresting the disease if the patient receives the experimental drug. She wants you to get her husband in this trial and to do whatever you can to ensure that he receives the experimental drug. You are not familiar with the criteria for inclusion in this trial and think that it would probably be futile for her husband given his condition. You have to be at an administrative meeting in 20 minutes. What do you say to her?

Evaluate Response for:
Commitment to patient well-being
Sense of responsibility and accountability
Ability to be an effective patient advocate

SCENARIO 2
One of the staff nurses on your unit complains that the medical staff is treating patients differently and that it is making a lot of the nurses "mad." The unit has both wealthy, well-insured patients and a large number of minority, Medicaid, and Medicare patients. She reports that a number of the attending physicians seem to bend over backward to ensure that the preferences of the wealthy patients are known and met while doing the bare minimum for other patients. You suspect that she is probably right but also know that this system is well entrenched.

Evaluate Response for:
Commitment to patient well-being
Sense of responsibility and accountability
Ability to be an effective patient advocate
Ability to recognize ethical dimensions of practice

SCENARIO 3
A woman who has just delivered her first baby and who appears utterly fatigued after a lengthy labor and overwhelmed by the new demands of parenting confides to you that she needs to stay in the hospital for a couple of days until she feels comfortable caring for her newborn. You are concerned about her level of stress but also know that her health maintenance organization will only fund the first 24 hours of care after delivery and that this couple has limited financial resources.

Evaluate Response for:
Commitment to patient well-being
Sense of responsibility and accountability
Ability to be an effective patient advocate
Ability to critique system's potential to influence human well-being

Continued

Box 34-3 ▶ EVALUATING ETHICAL COMPETENCE—CONT'D

SCENARIO 4

Marita, a 16-year-old high school junior with congenital heart defects and a long history of hospitalizations, surgical and pharmacological interventions, and chronic illness, now needs a heart transplant or she will die. She adamantly refuses the transplant and says she prefers death to the ordeal of the transplant. Her mother cannot accept this decision and refuses to even discuss this with her daughter. The staff is split as to whether to side with the patient or her mother and differ in their assessments of the probability of the transplant's ultimately benefiting her. You sense the team's growing frustration and know that if the transplant option is pursued, the sooner it is done the better the prognosis.

Evaluate Response for:
Commitment to patient well-being
Ability to be an effective patient advocate
Ability to mediate ethical conflict

SCENARIO 5

While making rounds you encounter an 82-year-old patient who was admitted from the local prison with complications secondary to his emphysema. You recognize him from previous admissions and in talking with him listen to his descriptions of how horrible the conditions are in the prison for the aging convicts like himself. Listening to his story you recall other elderly prisoners who have been on your unit during the last 3 or 4 years who have shown some signs of neglect. He tells you that he will do anything to get admitted to the hospital and that most of the other elderly prisoners would too. "Not even a dog should have to live the way we do." You sense that he is probably being honest and that he does not seem to be manipulative or playing on your sympathies.

Evaluate Response for:
Commitment to patient well-being
Sense of responsibility and accountability

SCENARIO 6

An 11-year-old Native American boy in the pediatric oncology unit tells you to make sure that "Ellen never takes care of me again." When you question him, he tells you how "mean" she is and that she never treats him nicely like the other nurses do. You respect Ellen's clinical competence and know that this patient has a reputation for being a problem.

Evaluate Response for:
Commitment to patient well-being
Sense of responsibility and accountability
Ability to be an effective patient advocate

not do both. Unfortunately there is no agreed on hierarchy of principles that specifies which principles may supersede others. Clouser and Gert (1994) offer a strong critique of this method, which they term *principlism.* Many nurses have been critical of this methodology because popularized versions seem to promote a type of quandary ethics of the to-pull-the-plug-or-not variety, which has not been sensitive to the everyday ethical concerns of practicing nurses.

CARE-BASED APPROACH

Dissatisfaction with the principle-based approach to nursing ethics combined with attentiveness to Gilligan's (1982) ground-breaking work in moral development led some nurse theorists to begin to articulate an ethic of care (Benner & Wrubel, 1989; Fry, 1989; Watson, 1985). Central to this perspective is the nature of the nurse-patient relationship and attention to the particulars of individual patients viewed within the context of their lives. Operating within this methodology, nurses pay attention to the human needs and interests that underlie ethical conflict with the intent of restoring and strengthening bonds between professionals, patients, and families. Characteristics of the care perspective include the following:

Centrality of the caring relationship
Promotion of the dignity of and respect for patients as people
Acceptance of particular patients and health care professional variables (beliefs, values, relationships) as
    morally relevant factors in ethical decision making
Norms of responsiveness and responsibility
Redefinition of fundamental moral skills (Taylor, 1993)

ETHICALLY RELEVANT CONSIDERATIONS

Whichever ethical approach the nurse case manager uses, the following list of ethically relevant considerations is helpful in the analysis of ethically problematic cases and in the discussion of these cases with others. Fletcher, Miller, and Spencer (1995) suggest that the following eight considerations offer a bridge between ethical principles, an ethics of caring, and the clinical situation:

1. Balancing benefits and harms in the care of patients
2. Disclosure, informed consent, and shared decision making
3. The norms of family life
4. The relationships between clinicians and patients
5. The professional integrity of clinicians
6. Cost-effectiveness and allocation
7. Issues of cultural and religious variation
8. Considerations of power (pp. 11-13)

Ethical Resources for the Nurse Case Manager

Since clinical ethicists in general and nurse ethicists more specifically are still something of a rarity and infrequently are employed by health care agencies and institutions, nurse case managers who are interested in developing ethical competence may need to look outside their institutions for resources. Many professional nursing organizations such as the American (and states') Nurses Association and the Association of Critical Care Nurses have task forces and committees that deal exclusively with ethical matters. These organizations and others frequently host conferences and seminars that address ethical issues and can refer nurses to the educational resources most likely to address their needs. Box 34-4 highlights some of the better known ethics resources. Some geographical areas are served by regional networks of ethics centers or by university-based ethics centers.

Advocacy and the Nurse Case Manager

Nurse ethicist Sally Gadow defines advocacy as the moral commitment to enhance patients' autonomy. "Among all of the professionals surrounding a patient, nurses often are the most capable of fostering patient self-determination. The practice of advocacy in nursing thus involves development of the nurse-patient relationship as the medium for expression of patients' values" (1989, p. 535). To function effectively as a patient advocate, nurse case managers must understand the basic dynamics in health care decision making.

Box 34-4 ▶ **ETHICAL RESOURCES**

American Nurses Association Center for Ethics and Human Rights
600 Maryland Avenue, SW
Suite 100 West
Washington, DC 20024-2571
(202)651-7055
   Publishes the *Ethics and Human Rights Communiqué,* which provides an ongoing vehicle of communication for nurses facing ethical and human rights dilemmas in practice. *Communiqué* informs readers about important upcoming events and resources of interest such as bibliographies, surveys, grants, ANA conferences, ethical continuing education offerings, and new ANA publications.
   National Reference Center for Bioethics Literature
   Kennedy Institute of Ethics
   Georgetown University
   Washington, DC 20057
   800-MED-ETHX
   A specialized collection of library resources concerned with contemporary biomedical issues in the fields of ethics, philosophy, medicine, nursing, science, law, religion, and the social sciences. Call for bioethics information, BIOETHICSLINE searches (computerized data base), search strategies, reference help, and publication orders.
   The Hastings Center
   255 Elm Road
   Briarcliff Manor, NY 10510
   914-762-8500
   A nonprofit, nonpartisan organization that carries out educational and research programs on ethical issues in medicine, the life sciences, and the professions. Publishes *The Hastings Center Report.*

   Basically there are three models of health care decision making that are "alive and well" in most clinical settings (Table 34-1). In paternalism or maternalism the clinician is "boss" and makes decisions to benefit patients, who are viewed as generally lacking sufficient knowledge to make right decisions. When this model works well, patients are spared the anguish of making tough decisions, and competent and compassionate clinicians make good decisions in the patient's best interests. When this model does not work well, patients receive unwanted care and live with the consequences long after the clinician exits the scene. The patient sovereignty model evolved to correct the problem of patients receiving unwanted care. Championing the patient as "boss" and the principle of autonomy, this model claims that no one knows what is best for the patient better than the patient himself or herself. In this model, patients receive the care they desire or demand, and the chief drawback is that there is often no one to protect patients from their poor or ill-advised choices.

   In the early 1980s the President's Commission for the Study of Ethical Problems in Medicine and Biomedical and Behavioral Research rejected both these models and recommended a model of shared decision making. This model is also based on autonomy but respects the fact that both the patient and clinicians bring something of importance to the process of decision making and calls for both to participate in the decision. The objective in this model is not simply that patients choose but that patients make the choice that is right for them, that is, a choice consistent with their values, moral identity, and decisional history. In this model clinicians are obligated to provide the support patients need to make good decisions. It is in this respect that the decision-making model differs from the patient sovereignty model, which is a model of noninterference.

Table 34-1	MODELS OF HEALTH CARE DECISION MAKING			
MODEL	**DESCRIPTION**	**PRINCIPLE**	**JUSTIFICATION**	**DANGERS**
Paternalism	Physician is the boss.	Beneficence	Patients often do not understand enough about medicine to make the "right" decision.	Patients may receive care they do not want and must live with the consequences.
Patient sovereignty	Patient is the boss.	Autonomy (self-determination)	No one knows better than the patient what is in his or her overall "best interests"; right to be self-determining ought always to take precedence.	No one protects patients from a "poor" or "ill-advised" choice; "easy-out" for health care practitioners.
Shared decision making	Patient and health care team work together.	Authentic autonomy	Patient may need support in being authentically autonomous.	Can easily slide into paternalism.

Even this brief introduction of models will make clear why the advocacy role of the nurse is problematic. Although most ethicists agree with the President's Commission and recommend a model of shared decision making, clinicians may be found who subscribe to each of the three models. Not surprisingly these clinicians differ in their estimate of whether patients and families need advocates and in their acceptance of the differing responsibilities of advocates.

CLINICAL ETHICS AND THE NURSE CASE MANAGER

Promoting Autonomy

Among our most prized human abilities is the freedom to make choices in light of what we value or deem good. Individuals are autonomous to the extent that they are self-determining. Much of the bioethics debate in the United States has focused on how we can safeguard the right of patients to be autonomous. Nurse case managers by virtue of their position and authority in the health care system can play a critical role in safeguarding patient autonomy.

Individuals with an intact decision-making capacity have the right to consent to and to refuse all medically indicated therapy. Since judgments about decision-making capacity ideally are made by those who know patients best, nurse case managers ought to participate in efforts to determine and document capacity. Criteria for decision-making capacity include the following:

1. The ability to comprehend information relevant to the decision at hand
2. The ability to deliberate in accord with a relatively consistent set of values and goals
3. The ability to communicate preferences

Nurse case managers who are effective advocates will help patients with decision-making capacity to anticipate the types of health care decisions they may need to make in the future and to explore their treatment options. It is important that patient preferences be documented and that nurses be familiar with state law about advance directives. Nurse case managers can play a leading role in making sure that the agency or institution they are affiliated with has a policy that identifies the parties responsible for obtaining and documenting patient preferences.

It is important that case managers working with patients with complex needs support authentically autonomous decision making, that is, ensure that decisions reflect the identity, decisional history, and moral norms of the patient. This frequently will mean walking patients through the various treatment options to see what each will mean for this patient in terms of real-life benefits and burdens. When institutional, caregiver, or family interests interfere with the autonomy of the patient, nurse advocates will support the patient and ensure that his or her interests are protected.

Lack of decision-making capacity does not of itself negate the right to be self-determining. Known preferences of the incapacitated individual are to be respected. Advance directives—a living will or durable power of attorney for health care—legally protect an individual's preferences concerning health care. Case managers advocate for incapacitated patients by supporting their surrogate decision makers. The role of the surrogate decision maker is to be a voice for a patient who can no longer speak for himself or herself. Surrogates should be instructed to use their knowledge of the patient and the patient's values to make the choice the patient himself or herself would make if he or she were able to do so.

Valid moral surrogates have intact decision-making capacity, understand the information pertinent to the decision at hand, know the patient's preferences to the extent that this is possible, have no undue conflict of interest, and are not experiencing severe emotional problems. Relatives who are legally valid surrogates but who are financially or emotionally dependent on a patient may make treatment decisions based on their own needs rather than on the interests of the patient. Nurse advocates can teach such surrogates that their charge is to be a voice for a now incapacitated patient and that they should decide as the patient would decide. If surrogates persist in making decisions that run counter to the patient's previously expressed wishes, health care professionals may need to explore legal means to challenge the surrogate's decision-making authority.

Promoting Patient Well-Being

The first task of the nurse advocate is to work with the patient, family, and health care team to clarify and communicate the appropriate goal of therapy: cure and restoration, stabilization of functioning, or preparation for a comfortable, dignified death. Although this would seem to be a given, often confusion makes it difficult to ensure that all interventions are consistent with the goal. Obviously, treatment goals may need revision when a patient makes unexpected progress or fails to progress. In one tertiary medical center a decision was made to terminate aggressive treatment for a man with an advanced stage IV glioblastoma. He was transferred out of the neurology step-down unit to a general floor. Unfortunately the transfer was made on a weekend evening when communication was poor, so when the patient spiked high temperatures, an aggressive workup was done and therapy for sepsis was initiated. If the intent of the therapy was comfort and the therapy was consistent with preparing him for a dignified death, the intervention was appropriate. If, on the other hand, it was merely a knee-jerk response to a life-threatening complication and was aimed at restoration and cure, it was inappropriate for this patient. The families of incapacitated, frail, debilitated patients may need great support in determining what is in the best interests of the patient and in deciding when to treat a condition aggressively and when to let nature take its course. Unfortunately there is no clear line to be drawn between promoting life and needlessly prolonging dying.

Pellegrino (1989) recommends analysis of therapy along two lines: effectiveness and benefit/burden ratio. A treatment is effective to the degree that it reverses or ameliorates the natural progression of the disease. Surgical repair has a high probability of being effective treatment for a mesenteric infarct. This is an objective medical determination—to the degree that medicine as a science can be objective. Whether the benefits of that surgery would advance the overall best interests of the patient described earlier who had had a recurrent meningioma and outweigh the burdens of the surgery is, however, a subjective determination that can be made only by the patient or by those who know the patient best. Nurses may need to remind physicians that more is at stake in treatment decisions than whether the proposed therapy is "medically indicated." Nurses' knowledge is also critical in the determination of the probability that a particular intervention will contribute to or compromise a goal such as comfort.

Nurses advocating for the patient's interests will also ensure that the patient's priority needs are addressed (biologic, psychosocial, and spiritual needs). As health care reform increasingly fragments services, the likelihood that patients will be cared for by health care professionals, including nurses, who know them well is decreasing. Nurse managers must critique nursing systems of care in which no one nurse is responsible for the overall plan of care and the identification and resolution of concerns of high priority to patients and families. All too frequently the only patient problems receiving attention today are physical problems. It is nursing's charge to ensure that holistic, individualized, prioritized care is a reality, especially for today's elders.

Preventing and Resolving Ethical Conflict

Nurse case managers who wish to prevent ethical conflict will work in care settings where it is established that preventing and resolving ethical conflict fall within the authority of each health care professional engaged in patient care. This conviction will facilitate early recognition of problematic situations and timely communication among all those involved in decision making. When communication among the patient, family, and caregiving team fails to resolve the problem, an ethics consult or meeting of the institutional ethics committee may be indicated. Sensitivity to and the ability to communicate about the factors contributing to ethical conflict are essential to successful mediation of these conflicts. When mediation is not attempted, conflicts tend to escalate, and it is not unusual for patients and families to develop hostile adversarial relationships that all too frequently end in litigation or at the very least in alienation and a distrust of health care professionals that colors future interactions with caregivers. Nurse case managers should be aware of the ethics resources available in their institutions and professional community and use them when needed (review Box 34-4). Mastery of a process of ethical decision making to simplify conflict resolution is also important, as shown in Box 34-5. Box 34-6 summarizes critical elements of the advocacy role of the nurse case manager.

MORAL INTEGRITY AND THE NURSE CASE MANAGER

Mark Siegler (1984), a physician ethicist, describes three stages in the evolution of medicine and notes how medicine's focus has changed from one stage to the next. In the first stage, the age of paternalism, physicians focused on the good of the patient as defined by the physician. In the second stage, the age of autonomy, the focus remained the good of the patient but as defined by the patient himself or herself. In the third stage of medicine, which Siegler termed *the age of bureaucratic parsimony,* the good of the patient is weighed against the good of society. Today we can add a fourth stage of medicine to Siegler's list, which might be termed *the age of for-profit medicine,* in which health care professionals (or other decision makers) weigh the good of the patient against the good of stockholders. These are profound paradigmatic changes that have the potential to dramatically influence the practice of profes-

| Box 34-5 | **A PROCESS OF ETHICAL DECISION MAKING** |

ASSESSMENT

Gather and document pertinent medical and nonmedical facts:

- *Who:* persons who have the authority for decision making and the responsibility for its consequences and the effect on them personally of the decision needing to be made
- *What:* patient's medical condition, prognosis, and therapeutic options and probable consequences of treatment and nontreatment; patient's beliefs, values, interests; related family, caregiver, and institution beliefs, values, and interests; pertinent legal and administrative considerations
- *When:* time parameters
- *Where:* setting
- *Why:* variables creating or fueling conflict

DIAGNOSIS

Identify the ethical issue(s) as clearly as possible. Distinguish ethical problems from communication or general patient care management problems.

PLANNING

1. Identify the objective of doing the ethics workup.
2. List and explore courses of action likely to achieve this goal. Think through the short- and long-term consequences of each.
3. Think of the ethical justification for each course of action and defend it against competing options:
   a. Compatibility with aims of nursing and demands of nurse-patient relationship
   b. Approaches to ethical inquiry: ethical principles, care perspective, virtue theory, communitarianism
   c. Grounding and source of ethics: philosophical (based in reason), theological (based in religion), sociocultural (based in custom)
4. Clearly identify what you believe to be the moral obligations of the nurse.
5. Select the course of action you are best able to defend against counter arguments.
6. Seek assistance if unable to work through the above steps independently.

IMPLEMENTATION

Implement the selected course of action and assess consequences.

EVALUATION

Critique your decision, incorporating feedback from involved participants if possible. Decide how you would respond to a similar case in the future. Determine whether you need to do something now to optimize future responses. Interventions may be personal (e.g., learn more about advance directives) or institutional (e.g., clarify the hospital's DNR policy and reeducate caregivers about the policy).

From Taylor, C. (1997). Ethical perspectives. In M.M. Burke & M.B. Walsh (Eds.), *Gerontologic nursing: Care of the elderly* (2nd ed.). St. Louis: Mosby.

sional nursing. Nurse case managers who wish to preserve their moral integrity in today's changing health care milieu face multiple challenges. Six of these challenges are explored on the following pages.

Challenge 1: Fidelity to the Unique Needs of Individual Patients

When asked to list descriptors of quality care many nurses use words like *holistic, individualized, prioritized,* and *continuous.* It is interesting to reflect on the reality that underlies these descriptors and to ask if we are still able to practice nursing in a way that makes this type of care anything more than in-

Box 34-6   **ADVOCACY COMPETENCIES**

SUPPORTING AUTONOMY
1. Determining and documenting the patient's decision-making capacity; ensuring that agency or institution policies specify how this is to be done, and identify responsible parties
2. Protecting the right of patients with decision-making capacity to be self-determining
   a. Facilitate communication and documentation of the patient's preferences
   b. Anticipate the types of treatment decisions that likely will need to be made
   c. Assist in the preparation of advance directives
3. Promoting authentic autonomy; authentic decisions reflect the individual's identity, decisional history, and moral norms
4. Identifying the morally as well as legally valid surrogate decision maker for patients who lack decision-making capacity
5. Supporting the surrogate decision maker, clarifying the surrogate decision maker's role
6. Identifying limits to patient or surrogate autonomy and limits to caregiver autonomy
7. Developing agency or institution policies that identify the caregivers responsible for and the procedures to be used to identify and support the appropriate decision makers

PROMOTING PATIENT WELL-BEING
Clarifying the goal of therapy: cure and restoration, stabilization of functioning, preparation for a comfortable, dignified death
1. Determining the medical effectiveness of therapy
2. Weighing the benefits and burdens of therapy
3. Ensuring that all interventions are consistent with the overall goal of therapy
4. Ensuring that the patient's priority needs are addressed (biologic, psychosocial, and spiritual needs)
5. Ensuring continuity of care as patient is transferred among services and within and without the institution
6. Weighing the moral relevance of third-party interests (family, caregiver, institution, society)
7. Identifying and addressing forces within society and the health care system that compromise patient well-being

PREVENTING AND RESOLVING ETHICAL CONFLICT
1. Establishing that preventing and resolving ethical conflict falls within the authority of all health care professionals engaged in the care of a patient
2. Developing awareness of and sensitivity to the conscious and unconscious sources of conflict
3. Facilitating timely communication among those involved in decision making: one-on-one meetings and periodic meetings of the patient, family, and interdisciplinary team to clarify goals and plan of care
4. Documenting pertinent information on the patient record
5. Referring unresolved ethical issues to the ethics consult team or the institutional ethics committee
6. Identifying and addressing system variables that contribute to recurrent ethical problems

From Taylor, C. (1997). Ethical perspectives. In M.M. Burke & M.B. Walsh (Eds.), *Gerontologic nursing: Care of the elderly* (2nd ed.). St. Louis: Mosby.

teresting rhetoric. Are the type of nurse-patient relationships that make holistic, individualized, and prioritized care possible a reality today or are they mere relics of a bygone past when nurses had the time to really get to know their patients? For example, nurses in a medical center were discussing the care received by a patient who had recently died from end-stage breast cancer. Apparently she was concerned about seeing her two children, ages 17 and 20 years, who had stopped coming to visit because they were overwhelmed by the degree of her illness, especially since their father had died of a brain tumor 2 years earlier. What the staff realized after she died was that no one had picked up on her requests to see her children and had not arranged a visit, so the patient died without ever seeing her children again. Horrified that this had been allowed to happen, the nurses realized that not one of them had seen this request as his or her responsibility in their attempts to provide highly technical rescue medicine that was responsive to each medical complication and crisis. One nurse caught herself saying, "I am familiar with 'the case' but didn't really know this woman."

Clinical practice guidelines based on aggregate data, critical pathways, and algorithms all seem to draw attention away from individual patients to population aggregates. Each of these standardizing methodologies has the potential to improve patient outcomes by keeping achievable target outcomes consciously before patients and the caregiving team. Whether these methodologies are used to improve care for individual patients or to force individuals to jump through predetermined hoops that may or may not contribute to their well-being may in large part be determined by the stance adopted by nurse case managers. Never before have patients been so in need of nurse advocates who know the system well enough to ensure that it is responsive to the unique needs of individual patients and their families. In the past our lack of skill in "working the system" limited our power to effectively serve as advocates for patients. Today the nurse case manager has the authority to pull together and to coordinate the services each individual patient needs and to modify systems that are unresponsive to patient need. How this authority will be used remains to be seen.

Challenge 2: Competing Loyalties

The nurse case manager's ability to modify the system to meet individual patient needs depends on his or her loyalties. When asked to whom are you accountable, nurse case managers may reply, "to the patient," "to the hospital," "to my boss," "to myself," "to the caregiving team." If I see myself as primarily accountable to an employing institution who pays my salary and who is driven by a financial bottom line, I may be reluctant to advocate for a patient who needs additional time to achieve target outcomes before discharge. It is helpful to consciously reflect on one's loyalties and to identify potential conflicts. Once again, the rhetoric of nursing reminds us that our primary concern is the patient. Unfortunately, today it is not uncommon for nursing practice to reflect concern for anything but this reality.

Challenge 3: Resolving Role Conflict

Among other things, the nurse case manager is a service coordinator, an advocate, a counselor, and a gatekeeper. Obviously, where one works, the needs of the patients served, and the mix of professionals on the caregiving team will all influence the roles played by the nurse case manager and the amount of time spent in each role. It can be helpful to use a pie chart to record the portion of time you spend in each role, on average, on any given day and to compare your chart with those of others in comparable positions. Reflection and discussion should yield greater insight into whether your personal mix of roles is adequately serving your patients and your employing institution. An important question to ask is, "What determines which of your roles takes precedence when role conflict exists?"

> The needs of your employer: "Utilization review says she has to be out of here by noon tomorrow at the latest."
>
> The needs of your patient: "We just have to get her pain under better control before she goes home, and this might take another day or two; they just changed her medicine this evening."
>
> Your unique talents: "I don't know how utilization review does it. . . . I could never talk with an already overburdened family about the need to take their mom or dad home before they think they are ready."

Our moral integrity makes it imperative for us never to allow our priorities to be dictated solely by our employing agency or institution. As the health care system changes, we need to reflect more carefully on what may be termed the "nonnegotiables" of our practice. What are those elements of professional nursing care that we cannot surrender without ceasing to be nurses?

Challenge 4: Owning Responsibilities to Underserved Populations

Nurses have both individual and corporate responsibilities to underserved populations. Nurse case managers are uniquely situated to gather the type of data that can be used to demonstrate to policy makers that the needs of select groups of patients are not being adequately addressed. Recurrent admissions of patients whose problems could have been more successfully addressed had the patients been seen earlier should be a signal that health needs are not being adequately met. Whether the patients be homeless men and women; a large population of abused children, spouses, or the elderly; incarcerated individuals; those with psychiatric or mental health problems; or simply those with inadequate insurance, nurse case managers can, if they choose, lead caregiving teams in gathering the type of data that will convince policy makers of the need for system reform.

Challenge 5: Identifying Personal Biases

In the interests of providing care that is just and oriented to giving each person his or her due, it is essential that nurse case managers attempt to identify personal sources of bias or discrimination. Reflection usually reveals the presence of some factors that positively or negatively predispose us to patients. An air of helplessness in a patient may elicit one nurse's mothering instinct and disgust in another. Similarly, age, gender, body size, occupation, skin color, nationality, culture, religion, financial status, and lifestyle factors can all influence the way we perceive and relate to patients. One nurse case manager who had worked in an AIDS unit for several years confided that she slowly realized after reflecting on her work that she treated patients differently on the basis of how they had acquired AIDS. "I'm much more patient and giving of myself to those who acquired it through sexual transmission rather than by sharing needles." This brief vignette illustrates the importance of identifying our personal biases. We need to be as conscious as we can of what inclines (or disinclines) us to "go to bat" for a patient whose needs are not being met.

Challenge 6: Balancing Care for Others With Appropriate Self-Care

A final word of caution. The tremendous potential nurse case managers have for influencing the delivery of health care in the United States may result in some nurses literally sacrificing themselves on the altar of quality care for those entrusted to their practice. While responsibility and accountability are essential elements of ethical competence, in excess they can fan the flames of burnout and quickly reduce a competent, caring professional to a lifeless mannequin. When deficient, nurses poorly serve their patients and colleagues, who quickly learn not to trust nurses who consistently place their needs and well-being over and above the needs of those they work for and with. The ethically competent nurse knows how to balance competing responsibilities to self, family, and work and is able to skillfully meet both professional and personal obligations. This dimension of moral integrity merits ongoing reflection and may be aided by discussion with colleagues. Because no two nurse case managers will view their responsibilities to patients, the caregiving team, and themselves in exactly the same way, discussions about what constitutes acceptable boundaries of responsibility and accountability can be helpful.

• • •

These are exciting times. More individuals than ever before are claiming as an achievable goal quality affordable care for all. Unfortunately, some of the means being used to achieve this goal are already suspect. Nurse case managers are on the front lines of the revolution in health care. Never before have the everyday choices of practicing nurses had greater potential to set standards of excellence that will serve us all. Ethical competence is not an option for nurse case managers. The health and well-being of all those we serve literally depend on their ethical competence.

References

American Hospital Association. (1991). *Put it in writing: A guide to promoting advance directives.* Chicago: The Association.

American Nurses Association. (1998). *Standards of clinical nursing practice.* (2nd ed.) Washington, DC: The Association.

American Nurses Association. (1985). *Code for nurses with interpretive statements.* Washington, DC: The Association.

Beauchamp, T.L., & Childress, J.F. (1994). *Principles of biomedical ethics,* (4th ed.). New York: Oxford University Press.

Benner, P., & Wrubel, J. (1989). *The primacy of caring. Menlo Park,* Calif: Addison-Wesley Publishing Co.

Clouser, K.D., & Gert, B. (1994). Morality vs. principlism. In R. Gillon, (Ed.), *Principles of health care ethics.* New York: John Wiley & Sons.

Concern for Dying. (1991). *Advance directive protocols and the patient self-determination act: A resource manual for the development of institutional protocols.* New York: Concern for Dying.

Fletcher, J.C., Miller, F.G., & Spencer, E.M. (1995). Clinical ethics: History, content and resources. In J.C. Fletcher, C.A. Hite, P.A. Lombardo, & M.F. Marshall (Eds.), *Introduction to clinical ethics* (pp. 3-17). Frederick, Md.: University Publishing Group.

Fry, S. (1989). The role of caring in a theory of nursing ethics. *Hypatia, 4,* 88-103.

Gadow, S. (1989). Clinical subjectivity: Advocacy with silent patients. *Nursing Clinics of North America, 24*(2), 535-541.

Gadow, S. (1980). Existential advocacy: Philosophical foundations of nursing. In S.F. Spicker & S. Gadow (Eds.), *Nursing: Images and ideals: Opening dialogue with the humanities* (pp. 79-101). New York: Springer.

Gilligan, C. (1982). *In a different voice: Psychological theory and women's development.* Cambridge, Mass.: Harvard University Press.

The Hastings Center. (1987). *Guidelines on the termination of life-sustaining treatment and the care of the dying.* Bloomington and Indianapolis: Indiana University Press.

Jameton, A. (1993). Dilemmas of moral distress: Moral responsibility and nursing practice. *AWHONN's Clinical Issues in Perinatal and Women's Health Nursing, 4*(4), 542-551.

Patient Self-Determination Act of 1990, In OBRA 1990 (P.L.101-508, H.R.5835). Pellegrino, E.D. (1989). Withholding and withdrawing treatments: Ethics at the bedside. *Clinical Neurosurgery, 35,* 164-184.

Pellegrino, E.D. (1989). Withholding and withdrawing of treatments: Ethics at the bedside. *Clinical Neurosurgery, 35,* 164-184.

President's Commission for the Study of Ethical Problems in Medicine and Biomedical and Behavioral Research. (1982). *Making health care decisions* (Vols. 1-3). Washington, DC: U.S. Government Printing Office.

President's Commission for the Study of Ethical Problems in Medicine and Biomedical and Behavioral Research. (1983). *Deciding to forego life-sustaining treatment: Ethical, medical, and legal issues in treatment decisions.* Washington, DC: U.S. Government Printing Office.

Siegler, M. (1984). Should age be a criterion in health care? *Hastings Center Report,* 14(5), 24-27.

Taylor, C. (1993). Nursing ethics: The role of caring. *AWHONN'S Clinical Issues in Perinatal and Women's Health Nursing, 4*(4), 552-560.

Taylor, C. (1995). Rethinking nursing's basic competencies. *Journal of Nursing Care Quality, 9*(4), 1-13.

Watson, J. (1985). *Nursing: The philosophy and science of caring.* Boulder, Co.: Colorado Associated University Press. Content adapted from Taylor, C. (1997). *The morality internal to the practice of nursing.* Unpublished doctoral dissertation, Georgetown University, Washington, D.C.

Clinical Career Ladders

CHAPTER OVERVIEW

Nursing career ladders can be linked intrinsically to a case management model. The case manager position can be integrated as the third or fourth rung of a clinical career ladder. In this way, greater experience and education are rewarded in a bedside position that recognizes and rewards experience. Traditional clinical career ladders often do not accommodate educational and experiential qualifications of the advanced practitioner. The autonomous case manager role is attractive to nurses with experience who wish to remain in bedside nursing but who are looking for a position of increased responsibility and independent practice.

When considering clinical career ladders, institutions must assess the cost of maintaining a ladder and evaluate the positive effects such a ladder has on recruitment and retention.

GOALS AND OBJECTIVES OF A CLINICAL CAREER LADDER

The nursing case management model can provide the framework for the integration of a true clinical ladder. Traditionally, clinical ladders have not provided a system for promotion at the bedside that included true changes in job title and responsibility.

Most promotions at the bedside have provided the staff nurse with an elevated title, such as staff nurse level II or senior staff nurse. This change in title may also have included a financial reward and an altered job description. However, analysis of such positions reveals that the actual day-to-day responsibilities remained the same.

Each organization implementing a career ladder will have different goals and objectives for an addition of this kind. Generally the integration of a career ladder will cost the organization money. The long-term savings that come because of decreased turnover or lowered vacancy rates are difficult to measure. Even more difficult is showing a cause-and-effect relationship between the career ladder and the decreased turnover and vacancy rates (Vestal, 1984).

Nevertheless, there are some generic goals and objectives that most organizations will hope to achieve by implementing a career ladder. Whether the achievement of these goals offsets the cost of the increased salaries that accompany the ladder will be a determination each organization must make for itself (Del Bueno, 1982).

An effective clinical career ladder has some inherent benefits, as follows:

Provides the opportunity for professional advancement in a direct patient care position
Promotes individual professional growth and development
Attracts nurses to the organization and helps retain them
Rewards individual expertise
Provides a framework for the development of performance evaluation tools
Increases job satisfaction
Positively affects patient care

Most clinical career ladders reflect what the name suggests. The ladders are designed to promote clinical advancement, usually at the bedside. Therefore the emphasis is on the direct care provider, generally the staff nurse. Other ladders may be designed for career or professional advancement, such as administration or education, or they may be a combination of clinical, administration, and educational roles.

Each step or level must be defined by specific behaviors and levels of performance that are identifiable and measurable. They should also be realistic and achievable (AORN, 1983).

Advancement in the clinical ladder is initiated by the nurse through a request. It is the nurse's responsibility to produce documents supporting a claim for advancement to the next level. Evaluation will then take place through a review of the documents. The documents should include the nurse's periodic evaluations and any other evidence of professional education, certification, and the like.

The documents are weighed against the performance expectations of the level to which the nurse is striving. Theoretically any nurse who has met the criteria should be eligible for advancement. In a true career ladder situation there should be no quota of positions per level, and any qualified nurse should be eligible for advancement.

All nurses within the career ladder should be evaluated periodically. These evaluations result in advancement, retention in the current position, or demotion (AORN, 1983).

Incentives for promotion include advanced title, salary benefits, and heightened status. Each promotional level should move the nurse toward a higher level of empowerment and self-actualization.

Just as there are benefits to the implementation of a ladder, there also are some problems (McKay, 1986). As already mentioned, the cost/benefit ratio may not be suitable for the organization. There is always the potential for a ladder to have a negative effect because it implies a hierarchical organizational structure.

For the ladder to produce a truly supportive environment and improve the quality of care, staffing patterns for each day and for each shift should incorporate representatives from each level. This may not always be feasible or realistic, particularly on the evening or night shift when staffing levels are low.

Monetary awards are often greater for those advancing within an administrative career ladder than for those advancing within a clinical ladder.

Other difficulties arise if the nursing department is represented by a union. The goals of the department and the goals of the clinical ladder must meld with those of the union. Each aspect of the ladder must be negotiated for integration into the bargaining union contract. Nursing departments represented in this way should include union representatives in the negotiations from the very beginning. In most cases the institution of a clinical career ladder will be best implemented at the beginning of a new contract.

The number of levels of any ladder will depend on the philosophy, goals, and budget of the organization. The following are qualifications a nurse from a particular level should have:

Level I
Entry level capabilities
A license or temporary permit to practice professional nursing
An understanding of the hospital policies and procedures
A basic familiarity with patient care
General skills needed to function at a beginning level of nursing practice

Level II
A more holistic understanding of patient care delivery
A career orientation with goals and direction
An ability to prioritize needs of patients and families and to delegate responsibilities to other members of the nursing staff as appropriate
An ability to act as a resource for other nursing staff members
An understanding of the relationship between career goals and personal growth

Level III
Ability to act as a resource for the health care team
Self-directed in most aspects of learning
Involvement in professional committees or organizations
An understanding of the health care team as a whole that comes together to meet mutual patient goals
A change agent for the institution within the department of nursing
An active seeker of additional professional responsibility
Commitment to nursing as a career
Ability to plan patient care based on current and future patient care needs
Ability to plan for appropriate discharge
Financial awareness incorporated into daily practice, including resource use, length of stay, and discharge planning needs

The level I registered nurse is expected to apply basic nursing theory to practice. Nursing care is delivered to the nurse's assigned group of patients based on actual needs, physician orders, and nursing diagnoses. The registered nurse at level I is able to complete all required treatments for a particular shift in accordance with the policies and procedures of the organization. This nurse may begin to learn the skills necessary to assess patient and family learning needs and begin meeting those needs (Barr & Desnoyer, 1988).

The level II practitioner begins to shift from actual patient problems to identifying potential problems and applying interventions that will prevent those problems from occurring. At this level the nurse's organizational skills begin to develop. Focus becomes more global as the nurse develops an awareness not only of the nurse's own patients but also of those throughout the unit. Patient problems are seen on a health care continuum that extends beyond hospitalization (Barr & Desnoyer, 1988).

The level III practitioner sees the health care team as a whole and seeks to begin to bring the team together to meet patient needs and to provide the best possible care. At this level the nurse begins to take a more active leadership role on the unit, serving as preceptor and informal leader. The registered nurse at this level is involved in seeking advanced education in some specialty or certification category. The nurse applies this knowledge and skill in practice and becomes an expert in the chosen area. This knowledge is used by the expert nurse to create an environment for positive change both on the unit and in the department (Barr & Desnoyer, 1988).

Differentiated practice is a personnel deployment model designed to better use the skills and education of the experienced nurse. An educational requirement within a clinical performance framework is incorporated into the differentiated practice model. By using a differentiated practice modality, the design of the clinical ladder can clearly delineate the evolving knowledge base and expanded level of functioning of the experienced nurse. Some institutions may want to include criteria for educational level and mandate that those at the third or fourth level have a master's degree. Using this model within a clinical career ladder bases employees' roles on both educational preparation and clinical performance.

In other models the fourth or fifth level is that of the clinical nurse specialist. If this role is seen as a bedside clinical position and not as a management or educator position, it belongs in a clinical career ladder. Once again, this depends on the perception of the role within the department (Metcalf, 1984).

THE CASE MANAGER POSITION WITHIN THE CLINICAL LADDER

The case manager position provides the opportunity for the development of a true career ladder, one that integrates a title change and financial incentive with significant changes in job description and job responsibilities.

The staff nurse position incorporates all the direct nursing tasks associated with providing nursing care. Included among these are the physical assessment, vital signs, medication administration, blood drawing, wound care, skin care, ambulation, and patient feedings.

The generic nurse case manager role removes the staff nurse from direct nursing functions. Her role becomes one concerned with the indirect nursing tasks provided to patients. Among these are patient and family teaching, care planning, coordination and facilitation of patient care and services, and discharge planning.

Shifting the focus to these functions also involves a substantial increase in the number of patients who can be taken care of on a daily basis. A case manager's focus is much broader than just the tasks at hand. The case manager must constantly focus on the plan of care for the days ahead by coordinating and facilitating services whether for discharge planning or patient teaching.

For the first time, this group of nurses has been given responsibility for controlling costs and length of stay. In this position, nursing holds the purse strings of health care.

Furthermore, this is the first time a registered nurse who wishes to remain at the bedside can do so while accepting promotion and change in job status. This position can be attractive to nurses who are not interested in positions within administration or education but who are looking for a change that still involves bedside nursing. In other cases the position might be attractive to a nurse who has been in the field for 1 or 2 years but who does not yet have the skills or education needed to advance to administrative or educational roles.

The case manager position is usually found at the third or fourth level of a clinical career ladder. The position empowers the staff nurse to create an environment for change in the organization, and it has the potential to generate a tremendous amount of job satisfaction. Research shows that longevity and job satisfaction are related (Malik, 1992). The career ladder, therefore, provides an incentive for the more experienced nurse to remain in a clinical position. Increased job satisfaction may have a trickle-down effect on the other staff nurses on the unit.

The autonomous case manager role may be the best argument thus far for creating clinical career ladders. Malik (1992) reports that clinical career ladders may not provide a position that affords the experienced staff nurse the opportunity to use her advanced skills and knowledge. The case manager role, which requires a higher level of functioning and skills, may serve to fill this gap.

References

AORN. (1983). Guidelines for developing clinical ladders. *AORN Journal,* 37(6), 1209-1224.

Barr, N.J., & Desnoyer, J.M. (1988). Career development for the professional nurse: A working model. *The Journal of Continuing Education in Nursing, 19*(2), 68-72.

Del Bueno, D. (1982, Sept.). A clinical ladder? Maybe! *Journal of Nursing Administration,* 19-22.

Malik, D.M. (1992). Job satisfaction related to use of career ladder. *Journal of Nursing Administration, 22*(3), 7.

McKay, J.I. (1986). Career ladders in nursing: An overview. *Journal of Emergency Nursing, 12*(5), 272-278.

Metcalf, J. (1984, Fall). The clinical nurse specialist in a clinical career ladder. *Nursing Administration Quarterly,* 8-19.

Vestal, K.W. (1984, Fall). Financial considerations for career ladder programs. *Nursing Administration Quarterly,* 1-8.

Case Management and Information Technology

Roy L. Simpson

CHAPTER OVERVIEW

Information technology will be pivotal to the future success of case management because of its potential to help professional nurse case managers perform their jobs more effectively and efficiently. This is especially true for those who are involved in beyond-the-walls case management, which still depends heavily on paper-based processes. Because of its pervasiveness, information technology's greatest opportunity for case managed care lies in the development of a national information network that links nursing information systems with patients in their own homes via computers. Such a network would allow nursing professionals to satisfy the patient's need for confidentiality and 24-hour access to information support while meeting nursing's need to reach ever-growing patient populations.

Among innovative efforts already under way that successfully offer case-managed care via computer networks to patients with diseases such as acquired immunodeficiency syndrome (AIDS) and Alzheimers is ComputerLink, a special computer network designed to help nurses support home-based care. The computer's capacity to offer daily follow-up contact, to serve as a medium for asking and answering questions, to provide voice reminders or alarms to signal anything from medications to checkups, and to contain costs are characteristics that will contribute to the success of networks that both case management professional and patient alike can access. The acceptance of a universal nursing minimum data set to codify nursing knowledge will also be crucial to this process.

Despite advances in information technology, case management in the mid-1990s continues to be a largely manual, labor-intensive process. Yet information technology, like no other tool available to professional nurse case managers, promises to make case management more viable, effective, and powerful. To be sure, technologically sophisticated hospitals using within-the-walls case management protocols likely are already benefiting greatly from existing clinical information systems and patient tracking systems. In these institutions, automation primarily is used for documentation assistance and managing patient follow-up schedules.

When it comes to beyond-the-walls case management, however, few institutions have the information technology tools needed to liberate professional nurse case managers from intensive paper-based processes. Yet it is precisely in this area—in case management beyond the walls of the institution—that information technology holds the greatest promise.

The real opportunity for case-managed care lies in the direction in which technology is currently and rapidly moving—toward the advent of *pervasive* technology or *pervasive* health care information networks or infrastructures.

A pervasive technology is one that is more noticeable by its absence than its presence, in the same way that automobiles, televisions, and telephones are today. In other words, a hotel room—or even a hospital room—today without a phone or television would be an unpleasant surprise. Yet it is likely that within 10 years, a hotel room or a hospital room without a *computer as well* will also be an oddity. The wild excitement over the Internet and the World Wide Web is only a hint at how powerfully the information superhighway is beginning to permeate the consciousness of American society.

This is particularly true of younger generations who are as comfortable with computers as toddlers of previous generations were with telephones. With this in mind it is important to remember that only people born before a technology becomes pervasive think of it as "technology"; all others think of it as part of the environment. Thus today's schoolchildren do not think of television and telephones as technology; they simply cannot imagine life without them. They are part of the landscape of modern existence. Tomorrow's children—and tomorrow's nurses—will feel the same way about computers.

In this march toward pervasiveness, technology historically passes through the following four predictable stages:

1. Development as experimental curiosities as individuals try to solve a particular problem in laboratories or—in the case of computers—in their garages or basements
2. Usage by a small number of specialists to solve a specific problem
3. Mass development as it becomes easily manufactured and commonplace (although still used primarily by a small fraction of the population who have specialized training)
4. Total pervasiveness and accessibility by the average citizen, as exemplified by telephones, televisions, and radios.

Although health care technology will never move beyond the third stage (after all, it will always require individuals with specialized training to operate), the *network* in which information is shared will indeed become pervasive. One need only look at the explosion of current interest in the Internet and the World Wide Web to get a glimpse of how information networks will pervade American society. Indeed the technology to deliver multimedia services over telephone wires via the television has existed since the early 1990s. Cable television companies and telephone operating companies are fighting it out to determine who will "own" the ability to deliver information technology services to the home. In other words, this convergence of technology means that the television—the current focus of entertainment in most American homes—will also be the focus for computer interaction (i.e., the television will also *be* the computer—it will be possible to go from watching a TV show to attaching a keyboard to the set and to instantly begin "surfing" information networks or communicating with caregivers via bulletin boards).

The development of a pervasive national information network has tremendous ramifications for the nurse case manager. A national network will link nursing information systems and, as a result, nurse case managers, to patients in their own homes via computers (or multimedia centers—the TV as computer or vice versa). It is even imaginable that within 10 years all homes will come equipped with a TV, just as they come equipped with ovens. Prognosticators also predict that there will be a computer company or information company, similar to the phone company, that individuals will call to get their computer turned on and linked into the network (just as one calls the power company to get the power turned on). Taken to its logical conclusion, this prediction sees an information utility company just like the telephone or electrical utility. This information utility will likely be run like any other utility, with some sort of public service commission in charge and with hefty governmental laws that regulate distribution of services.

NETWORK LINKAGE AND HOME CARE

With network linkage connecting patients with each other and with nurses through a computer network, the nursing professional can satisfy the patient's need for confidentiality and 24-hour access to informational support. Network linkage also supports nursing's need to reach out to an ever-expanding patient population. Today nurses are already experimenting with case-managed care via computer networks for such diseases as AIDS and Alzheimer's with immensely positive results.

Consider the work of Patricia Brennan, associate professor of nursing and systems engineering at the Frances Payne Bolton School of Nursing at Case Western Reserve University, who used computer networks to link AIDS and Alzheimer's disease patients' family caregivers to nurses and with each respective subgroup. Participants in the study were provided with terminals and modems and given access to ComputerLink—a special computer network designed to help nurses support home-based care. Users were free to access the network any time of the day or night at no cost. Each participant was provided with 1.5 hours of free training and ongoing assistance in using the system.

The ComputerLink network offered the following three primary modules:

1. A communications module, which included a bulletin board area for "conversing" with others in the same predicament and a question-and-answer section for anonymous postings to nurses
2. A decision support model, which helped participants make self-care choices using a structured decision analysis method
3. An information module, a database filled with encyclopedic data about the disease.

A project nurse was assigned as chief moderator, responsible for reading all public "conversations" and notations (and therefore for assessing information gaps in the participating populations), maintaining the currency of the electronic encyclopedia, troubleshooting for all participants, and acting as clinical expert in all capabilities.

The results were positive. The typical user got on the system 125 times, or an average of four to five times a week. According to Brennan, "testimonial evidence of perceived support abounded in both groups of participants. Postings on the public forum contained messages of encouragement, ideas for self-care and for managing with the formal health system, and counsel to peers" (Simpson, 1994).

There were also many nursing benefits. Case managers were able to disseminate information to patients more easily and quickly. Nurses could also control misinformation by ensuring that outdated information was not accessible to users. Privacy over the network ensured that all users could learn from an interaction, not just one patient at one time.

Brennan's research project proved that "continuity of care in home care can be achieved through both traditional and non-traditional means,—sending nurses out to the homes or through novel use of existing technology such as computer terminals" (Simpson, 1994).

NETWORK LINKAGE AND CASE MANAGEMENT

Having a network that can be accessed by case management professionals and patients alike will be key to the success of case management in the future. If computers do indeed become as ubiquitous as phones and televisions in people's homes, case management beyond the walls becomes a viable reality. Without ever leaving the hospital, nurses could have daily contact with patients for follow-ups, questions about medications, patient follow-through, and so on.

With voice or sound computer-generated reminders or alarms, nurses could remind patients or family members about everything from taking insulin shots, to changing their dressings, to coming in for a check-up. Via the same network, patients could report to the caregiver unusual symptoms or concerns about their care. Although such communications could never replace the personal contact and personal care that is so important to the professional practice of nursing, they would certainly alleviate the strain on nurses who must manage the details involved in community-based health care delivery.

In addition, using networked computers would support the institution's desire to contain costs. If day-to-day communications and educational issues are addressed via computer, resources could be allocated more cost effectively, ensuring that nursing professionals spend their face-to-face time with more critical situations.

Once a nationwide network of health care information is in place, it can be surmised that "back-office" linkage will be an important part of the network. And it will likely be expected that the case manager will manage the various critical pathways and treatment protocols outlined by different payers. In this way the case manager truly becomes an advocate for the patient and an intermediary for the institution—ensuring not only that the patient receives the best care but also that the institution follows prescribed protocols to obtain reimbursement.

Insurance companies and third-party payers are already playing a big part in the development of the health care information network so that benefit and financial information can be managed quickly and efficiently on the patient's behalf. Payers and institutions alike will likely be the focus for collecting all the data related to patient care, performing variance analyses and indicating benchmark outcomes in an ongoing attempt to determine the best protocols while containing costs. The debate as to who will set critical pathways and treatment protocols continues to rage (i.e., the payers or the providers?). To have a strong voice in this process, nursing must be able to identify and codify nursing services and outline its contributions to the patient's outcomes.

The result of establishing benchmarks and of being held to standards of care will be profound. For example, if 3 patients out of 10 with a cholecystectomy develop a nonsocomial infection after surgery and the benchmark is 1 out of 10, the competence of the nursing care will be closely scrutinized. Nurse managers and case managers must be prepared for this eventuality.

Clearly a pervasive network of this kind will empower nurses, particularly case managers, at the same time that it makes them more accountable for their actions. The case manager of the future needs to be an expert not only in clinical care but also in critical analysis of enormous amounts of data on which decisions will be based.

PREPARING FOR THE FUTURE

A common health care network would not, and could not, replace nursing contact. However, it would serve as a powerful support tool in the evolution of case management. It may be 10 years or more before a pervasive network is in place whereby nursing would have both the informational infrastructure and the ability to contact and communicate with patients electronically. The advent or acceptance of a universally accepted nursing minimum data set is critical to this process. Nursing must be able to codify its knowledge in order to be able to properly use computer networks and share nursing information and outcomes with other medical and nonmedical caregivers.

Nursing has always been able to adapt to technological advances. Fifty years ago there was no such thing as an intensive care unit (ICU). Today, nurses are critical to the success of ICUs. In the same way we must prepare for a future that will be dramatically different—a future of vast computer connections that can link patients with caregivers, caregivers with each other, and more. The promise of case management will be achieved by using information technology to share information and communicate with patients and caregivers beyond the walls of the institution. It is up to nurses *today* to prepare themselves for such a future.

REFERENCE

Simpson, R.L. (1994, Winter). Computer networks show great promise in supporting AIDS patients. *Nursing Administration Quarterly, 18*(2), 92-95.

Compliance and Regulation

Rebecca F. Cady

CHAPTER OVERVIEW

Because of developments over the last 10 years in state and federal law and law enforcement, case management has become inextricably intertwined with the legal issues of compliance and regulation. Nursing case managers must be aware of the key issues in compliance and regulation as they pertain to the nursing case manager's professional activities to avoid both personal and corporate liability.

INTRODUCTION

Compliance and regulation have become, in recent years, issues about which all health care providers must be aware. Unfortunately for most of us, the laws and the regulations developed to enforce the laws are among the most confusing ever created. Entire volumes have been devoted to explaining the intricacies of these two issues. To understand these issues as they relate to case management, it is necessary to first review the applicable government health care programs and the laws that govern them.

Overview of Governmental Health Care Programs

Case managers deal with many patients who are insured by Medicare and Medicaid. Medicare, enacted in 1965, is a federally funded health insurance program contained in Title 18 of the Social Security Act (42 USC Sections 1395 et. seq.). In general, it is designed to provide health insurance benefits to Social Security recipients over age 65 years and to those who are permanently disabled as defined under the Social Security Act. Medicare is entirely a federal program and pays only for services that are "reasonable and necessary for the diagnosis or treatment of illness or injury or to improve the functioning of a malformed body member" (42 U.S.C. Section 1395y(a)(1)(A)). Participating providers are required to ensure that any services rendered to Medicare recipients are supported by sufficient evidence of medical necessity (42 U.S.C. Section 1320c-5(a)(1)). Under the statutes that govern Medicare, the Secretary of

Health and Human Services regulates the administration of the program via the Health Care Financing Administration (HCFA) with regulations totaling over 1600 pages. Medicaid, also enacted in 1965, is jointly financed by the federal and state governments and is administered by the states. Medicaid provisions are contained in Title 19 of the Social Security Act (42 U.S.C. Sections 1396 et. seq.). Medicaid authorizes federal grants to states for medical assistance to low-income persons who are age 65 years or over, blind, disabled, or members of families with dependent children or qualified pregnant women or children (42 C.F.R. Section 430.0).

The Secretary of Health and Human Services is primarily responsible for the administration of the government's various health care programs established under the Social Security Act. In 1978 the Office of the Inspector General (OIG) was created by Congress to detect and prevent fraud and abuse in the Medicare and Medicaid programs (5 U.S.C. App. Section 2(2)). State Medicaid Fraud Control Units are authorized by the Medicare-Medicaid Anti-fraud and Abuse Amendments to the Social Security Act. The purpose of these state units is to conduct a statewide program for the investigation and prosecution of violations of all applicable state laws regarding all aspects of fraud in connection with any aspect of the provision of medical assistance and the activities of providers of such assistance under the federal Medicaid program (42 U.S.C. Section 1396b(q)(3)). To obtain Medicaid funding, a state must have a plan for medical assistance, which must contain procedures relating to payment for services sufficient to ensure that payments are consistent with quality of care (42 U.S.C. Section 1396 a(a)(30)(A)). Each state must have a fraud detection program, and the state plan must provide for exclusion of persons who have committed fraud or abuse. The federal statute defines abuse as "provider practices that are inconsistent with sound fiscal, business, or medical practices, and result in an unnecessary cost to the Medicaid program, or in reimbursement for services that are not medically necessary or that fail to meet professionally recognized standards for health care" (42 C.F.R. 455.2).

CHAMPUS is the federal health insurance program for Department of Defense employees. Like Medicare, CHAMPUS pays only for medically necessary services and supplies (32 C.F.R. Section 199.4(a)(1)(i)).

Nursing Case Management

To understand how nursing case management activities are affected by laws regarding compliance and regulations, the role and duties of the nursing case manager must be reviewed. Nursing case management is noted to be a model of care delivery that focuses on achieving optimal patient outcomes in expected time frames while containing costs, which meets the standards of regulatory agencies and is in line with health care reform activities at the federal level (Elizondo, 1994). The goals of nursing case management are (1) achieve expected patient outcomes within specific time frames; (2) improve quality of care; (3) deliver multidisciplinary care throughout hospitalization; (4) contain costs; (5) ensure appropriate length of stay; and (6) improve patient, family, and caregiver satisfaction (Elizondo, 1994). Bower (1995, p.166) defines case management as follows:

> A clinical system that focuses on the accountability of an identified individual or group for coordinating a patient's care (or group of patients), across an episode or continuum of care; negotiating, procuring, and co-ordinating services and resources needed by patients/families with complex issues; insuring and facilitating the achievement of quality, clinical, and cost outcomes; intervening at key points for individual patients; addressing and resolving patterns of issues that have a negative quality-cost impact; and, creating opportunities and systems to enhance outcomes.

Nursing case management activities must meet compliance requirements as well as conform to many federal and state regulations. This chapter will identify the critical issues that nursing case managers must be aware of, outline rules to follow, and illustrate the consequences of not following these rules by discussing the penalties and punishments that may ensue.

Historical Background: Compliance and Regulation

In May 1995 the Department of Health and Human Services (HHS) began a 2-year demonstration project entitled Operation Restore Trust (ORT). The purpose of this project was to test several new approaches to fighting fraud and abuse in the Medicare and Medicaid programs. This program initially targeted five states: California, Florida, Illinois, New York, and Texas. These states were chosen because collectively, these states' residents included more than one third of all Medicare and Medicaid beneficiaries. The goal of ORT was to increase enforcement in health care programs where the government believed that fraud and abuse were prevalent. The project also focused on high-growth program areas, which included home health agencies, nursing homes, hospice care, and durable medical equipment suppliers.

In 1996 the Office of the Inspector General's (OIG's) fiscal year medical and audit review indicated that 30% of all claims reviewed did not comply with Medicare laws and regulations. This report estimated that the dollar value of improper Medicare benefit payments made during fiscal year 1996 was $23.2 billion, or approximately 14% of the $168.6 billion in processed fee-for-service payments reported by the HCFA. This report also estimated that improper home care claims accounted for $3.6 billion, or 15.74% of the improper payments (Gibbs-Brown, 1997). This report identified the four leading causes of improper Medicare payments as (1) insufficient or no documentation (46%); (2) lack of medical necessity (36.78%); (3) incorrect coding (8.53%); and (4) noncovered or unallowable services (5.26%).

The OIG's fiscal year 1997 medical and audit review revealed that only 11% of the total Medicare outlays constituted payment of improper claims, a 3% reduction from the previous years' statistics (Schorr, 1998). This suggested to the OIG that overall claims accuracy was improving. It was also found that claims submitted without documentation had decreased as well, from more than $3 billion in erroneous payments during fiscal year 1996 to only $850 million in fiscal year 1997 (Schorr, 1998). As a result of the initial success of this program, HHS has decided to expand it over the next 3 years to include all 50 states.

THE REAL COST OF HEALTH CARE FRAUD

Experts estimate conservatively that 3% of the $1 trillion health care costs ($30 billion) was lost to fraud in 1997 (White, 1998). A 1998 report by the OIG estimated that losses to fraud and abuse may exceed 10% of annual health care spending, or $100 billion per year (OIG, 1998). In 1997 the Department of Justice expected to recover more than $1 billion in fines and settlements just from fraud against government health care programs (White, 1998). Criminal convictions for health care fraud in 1997 increased threefold over the 1992 total (U.S. Department of Justice, 1997) The crimes included submitting false claims to Medicare, Medicaid, and other insurance plans; home health care fraud; fake billing by foreign doctors; and needless prescriptions for durable medical equipment by physicians in exchange for a kickback from manufacturers (DOJ, 1997). Fraud is also a problem in the private sector. A survey done by the Health Insurance Association of America revealed that nine out of 10 private insurers has launched antifraud programs since 1995. The savings from these private insurers' antifraud programs totaled a staggering $260 million, an average $2.3 million per insurer, which constituted a savings of $7.50 for each dollar spent on fraud detection (White, 1998). According to Greg Anderson, director of corporate finance investigations for Blue Cross-Blue Shield of Michigan, billing for services not rendered and upcoding fraud*[1] constitute 100% of the provider fraud in fee-for-service plans (White, 1998, p. 32).

In 1998 a review by the Department of Health and Human Services' Office of the Inspector General (OIG) found that portable chest x-rays performed in long-term care facilities cost up to nine times more than nonportable chest x-rays. The OIG also found, after reviewing medical records in California, New York, Florida, Texas, and Illinois, that there was "no indication in more than 50% of the beneficiaries' medical records that they would be unable to be transported outside of the nursing home for medical services." As a result, the OIG recommended that the HCFA enforce the Medicare requirement that a physician must justify the need for portable services. According to HCFA, the result of such enforcement would be a savings of as much as $63.7 million per year and $371.9 million over 5 years (Schwartz, 1998). In 1998 Cambridge Information Services, a Massachusetts-based health care information research company, used data obtained from HCFA to determine that U.S. hospitals may have overbilled Medicare for as much as $482 million for laboratory tests performed between 1990 and 1997. As a result, they estimated that the Department of Justice could potentially recover at least $750 million in overbillings and penalties (Medicare Report, 1998).

Ultimately, the cost of this fraud is passed on to consumers and their health care providers in the form of lower payments for services rendered, higher copays, and higher costs of health insurance.

FALSE CLAIMS

The False Claims Act

The Federal False Claims Act (31 U.S.C. Section 3729) prohibits presenting any false claim for reimbursement to the United States if the provider knows the claim is false or where there is deliberate ignorance or reckless disregard of the claim's falsity. This law also prohibits submitting or causing to submit a false claim, conspiring to obtain a false claim, and making or using false records to obtain a payment. This means that employers may be liable for the acts of employees as well as contractors who submit claims that are false. In the health care setting the False Claims Act can be used to prosecute the institution, entity, or individual provider for a variety of actions, including the following (Kleiman, 1999):

1. Billing for goods and services not provided
2. Billing for unnecessary goods and services
3. Submitting false cost reports
4. Billing for substandard care
5. Acceptance or giving of kickbacks
6. Unbundling of services or supplies that should be grouped together

It is important for clinicians to realize that the False Claims Act allows for actions against individual clinicians. Therefore false claims are not merely a problem for the health care corporation. Nursing case managers must exercise caution when billing for their services to avoid the submission of potentially false claims.

---

*Upcoding is a term used to describe the practice in which a different billing code is used to maximize reimbursement for a service or procedure done instead of using the specific code designated for that service or procedure.

Whistleblowers

The False Claims Act also authorizes the filing of a lawsuit by a "whistleblower" when institutions or organizations violate federal prohibitions on fraud and abuse. Kleiman (1999) reminds us that fraud in any program depending on federal funding* may be prosecuted under this act. The whistleblower can be a current or former employee, a patient, a competitor, or any other individual who obtains knowledge of fraudulent and or abusive behavior. Generally, the knowledge must be firsthand, that is, it cannot come from a public source. If the federal government decides to join the whistleblower as a plaintiff in the lawsuit, the whistleblower may collect up to 25% of the government's ultimate recovery in the case (31 U.S.C. Section 3730(d)(1)). Given the stiff penalties that apply in fraud and abuse cases, the whistleblower can receive a great deal of money if the government prevails in such a case. As a result, the number of these lawsuits, known as "Qui Tam" cases, has increased dramatically since 1993, with 131 cases filed in 1993 and 530 cases filed in 1997 (DOJ, 1997). According to figures from the Department of Justice, over 50% of the Qui Tam cases filed in 1997 were home health care related (DOJ, 1997). Recoveries in Qui Tam cases as of October 1997 were $625 million (DOJ 1997).

Under the False Claims Act, an employee who is fired, demoted, or otherwise discriminated against for furthering an investigation into false claims is entitled to double back pay with interest, litigation costs, attorney's fees, general damages, and reinstatement (31 U.S.C. Section 3730(h)). This reflects the fact that whistleblowers are protected by law against retaliatory actions for investigating or reporting fraud. Both federal and state laws protect whistleblowing employees. In addition, the U.S. Supreme Court has recently ruled that federal civil rights law protects employees who are fired to deter them from testifying in a federal trial against their employers (*Haddle v. Garrison, 1998*). Kleiman (1999) notes that since all False Claim Act suits must be filed under seal, the defendant may not know about the suit for months or even years, with the result that the whistleblower may remain anonymous and may continue working in the industry during most of the time the suit is in process.

DEALING WITH WHISTLEBLOWERS

When the case manager must deal with a subordinate employee who is a whistleblower, great caution must be exercised. The case of *Neal v. Honeywell, 826 F. Supp 266 (7ᵗʰ Cir. 1994)* is instructive in how not to deal with a whistleblower. In this case a human resources department psychologist reported fraud to the company hotline. She immediately experienced retaliation, despite promises of anonymity. After she was forced to quit, she sued her employer under the False Claims Act for the retaliation. In this case, the plant manager, who had been involved with the fraud, was promoted with a salary increase. The whistleblower, Dr. Neal, was given a 1-month paid leave when she was subjected to death threats and was denied a routine promotion. Dr. Neal was eventually awarded $294,000. Her employer was also required to pay nearly $1 million of Dr. Neals' attorney's fees. Even though she did not file a false claims case, this whistleblower was able to use the False Claims Act to receive compensation for the retaliatory actions of her employer.

Kleiman (1999) notes that retaliation does not always mean firing the employee. Courts may also consider actions such as breaking promises of confidentiality, reducing the responsibilities of employees who come forward with problems, or subtly punishing them in other ways to be retaliation. This means that when faced with the need to take action regarding an employee who has reported fraud and or

---

*This includes Medicare, Medicaid, the Veterans Administration, Tricare, CHAMPUS and private health insurance purchased for federal employees, as well as federal support for medical or nursing education or biomedical research.

abuse, it would be prudent to discuss the matter with your institution's risk manager or in-house attorney before acting.

QUI TAM CASE STUDIES

Kleiman (1999) reports the results of three different whistleblower cases. He notes that three whistleblowers will be splitting $52.5 million as their share of the recovery for the SmithKline laboratory case. The claims clerk who reported that Illinois Blue Cross/Blue Shield was shredding claims has recovered more than $29 million (20.8% of the government's $140 million recovery). A whistleblower at the University of Texas' San Antonio Health Center filed a Qui Tam case resulting in a $17 million fine, of which the whistleblower received $4.2 million. In the University of Texas case the medical center had to agree to an extremely rigorous Corporate Integrity Agreement, which amounts to a court-supervised compliance plan.

CORPORATE COMPLIANCE: MANAGING THE RISK

The nursing case manager must be aware of the requirements regarding compliance plans for several reasons. First, if the nursing case manager is involved in developing or administering the compliance program, it is imperative to be familiar with the standards against which the program will be judged. Second, each nursing case manager must be familiar with his or her own employer's compliance plan and program, and being aware of the standards will provide a background of understanding why the plan was developed as it was.

The Compliance Program and Plan

If an agency or institution finds itself in question of having violated legal prohibitions against fraud and abuse, one of the most beneficial defenses it will have is a well-developed corporate compliance program. The Federal Sentencing Guidelines (1991) provide for decreased monetary fines and other penalties if the defendant entity had in place at the time of the alleged fraud and abuse a corporate compliance program that was developed and carried out in accordance with these guidelines. Stahl (1998) notes that while adopting and implementing a compliance program is voluntary, the OIG believes that such programs prevent fraud, abuse, and waste and at the same time further providers' fundamental mission to provide quality care.

There are two aspects to corporate compliance described by Cantone (1999): the corporate compliance program, which is the total of a corporation's efforts to comply with the various laws and regulations, and the corporate compliance plan, which is a detailed document specifically addressing those areas identified as presenting the corporation with significant liability.

Cantone (1999) identifies several benefits to a corporate compliance plan for healthcare organizations, including the following:

1. Potential reduction of civil or criminal wrongdoing
2. Potential reduction of administrative or civil penalties if a violation occurs
3. Provision of a more accurate view of employees' behaviors
4. Identification and elimination of criminal and unethical conduct
5. Provision of a means for efficient dissemination of information relating to changes in government requirements
6. Establishment of a structure that encourages employees to deal with concerns internally, which reduces the potential for Qui Tam actions and governmental investigations

Stahl (1998) identifies additional benefits of a compliance program, cited by the OIG in its guidelines for compliance, which were released on February 11, 1998:

1. Ensures that accurate claims will be submitted to government and private payers
2. Enables the hospital/facility to fulfill its caregiving mission
3. Assists hospital/facility in identifying any weaknesses in internal systems and management
4. Demonstrates a strong commitment to honest, responsible provider and corporate conduct
5. Improves quality of care
6. Develops a procedure that allows for prompt, thorough investigation of alleged misconduct by corporate officers, managers, employees, independent contractors, physicians, other health care professionals, and consultants
7. Initiates immediate and appropriate corrective action
8. Minimizes the loss to the government from false claims, and thereby reduces the hospital's/facility's exposure to civil damages and penalties, criminal sanctions, and administrative remedies

Developing a Compliance Plan

When developing a corporate compliance plan, the Federal Sentencing Guidelines must be referred to carefully. To meet the Federal Sentencing Guidelines, a compliance plan must include the following (Federal Sentencing Guidelines, 1991; Cantone, 1999):

1. Compliance standards and procedures
2. Overall compliance program oversight by high-level personnel
3. Due care delegating authority
4. Employee education and training
5. Monitoring, auditing, and reporting systems
6. Consistent enforcement and discipline
7. Response and corrective action

In developing a compliance plan, the first step is to perform a baseline risk assessment to determine responsibilities and existing processes for compliance, focusing on the most common types of compliance problems (Cantone, 1999). Part of this risk assessment should include auditing clinical charts, financial operations, policies and procedures, contracts, and billing processes to search for miscoding, double billing, and credit balances (Cantone, 1999). Common areas of risk can include the following:

Billing for services not provided
Plan of care documents not signed by the physician
Falsification of physician signatures
Backdating physician signatures
Physician consultation and administrative fees
Kickbacks
Cost report fraud

The second step is to establish a code of conduct, which will apply across the board in the organization. A code of conduct should include the following:

Ethical principles
Explanation of laws
Schedule for amending the code
A vehicle to report potential compliance issues
A nonretaliation policy for whistleblowers
Description of disciplinary measures

Third, oversight for the compliance program must be assigned to a high-level person in the organization. In some institutions a corporate compliance officer (CCO) is solely responsible for compliance. In others the functions of the CCO are assigned to a high-level corporate officer such as the chief financial officer or the executive director. Some organizations also appoint a compliance committee that provides oversight to all compliance activities.

It is crucial to remember that to meet federal guidelines the compliance plan must be more than just artfully written documents. The plan must truly function in accordance with the guidelines provided by the Federal Sentencing Guidelines, as follows:

1. The organization must have established compliance standards and procedures to be followed by its employees and other agents that are reasonably capable of reducing the prospect of criminal conduct.
2. Specific individuals within high-level personnel of the organization must have been assigned overall responsibility to oversee compliance with the standards and procedures.
3. The organization must have used due care not to delegate substantial discretionary authority to individuals whom the organization knew, or should have known through the exercise of due diligence, had a propensity to engage in illegal activities.
4. The organization must have taken steps to communicate effectively its standards and procedures to all employees and agents.
5. The organization must have taken reasonable steps to achieve compliance with its standards.
6. The standards must have been consistently enforced through appropriate disciplinary mechanisms, including as appropriate, discipline of individuals for failure to detect an offense. Adequate discipline of individuals responsible for an offense is a necessary component of enforcement; however, the form of discipline that will be appropriate will be case specific.
7. After an offense has been detected, the organization must have taken all reasonable steps to respond appropriately to the offense and to prevent further similar offenses, including any necessary modifications to its program to prevent and detect violations of law.

(Federal Sentencing Guidelines, 1991).

Documentation

Good documentation can be an important way to defend against charges of fraud and abuse. Stahl (1998) suggests that policies and procedures related to the processing and submitting of claims should do the following:

1. Provide for proper and timely documentation of all physician and other health care professional services that substantiate billed services.
2. Specify the documentation requirements in the patient's medical records, which, at a minimum should include the length of time spent in providing the service, who provided the service, why the service was provided, and the clinical outcomes. This documentation is essential to justify reasonableness and medical necessity.

It is imperative, however, that documentation never be falsified. The Federal False Entry Statute provides:

> . . . [W]hoever, in any matter within the jurisdiction of the executive, legislative, or judicial branch of the Government of the United States knowingly and willfully:
> 1. falsifies, conceals, or covers up by any trick, scheme, or device a material fact;
> 2. makes any materially false, fictitious, or fraudulent statement or representation; or
> 3. makes or uses any false writing or document knowing the same to contain any materially false, fictitious or fraudulent statement or entry;
> shall be fined under this title or imprisoned not more than five years, or both.
> (18 U.S.C. Section 1001).

Providers have an obligation to ensure that their Medicare-funded services are "supported by evidence of medical necessity . . . as may reasonably be required by a reviewing peer review organization. ." (42 U.S.C. Section 1320c-5(a)(3)).

Duty to Report

If an institution receives an overpayment from Medicare, whether this arises from simple negligence or from the presentation of false claims, it must report this overpayment to the HCFA. Stahl (1998) notes that when violations of the compliance program are identified, the matter must be reported to the appropriate governmental authority within a reasonable time frame, but no later than 60 days after the violation is identified. If administrators are aware of overpayments and fail to report them, they could be liable for concealment of a felony. U.S. Code Title 18, Section 4 states: "Whoever, having knowledge of the actual commission of a felony cognizable by a court of the United States, conceals and does not as soon as possible make known the same to some judge or other person in civil or military authority under the United States, shall be fined under this title or imprisoned not more than three years, or both." To date, no health care professionals have been prosecuted under this law; however, personnel who fail to report knowledge of false claims do so at risk of their entire professional and personal lives.

POTENTIAL PENALTIES FOR LACK OF COMPLIANCE

Penalties for fraud and abuse can literally ruin a health care provider's personal and professional life. Cantone (1999) notes that the potential consequences for failing to comply include the following:

1. Probation and a court imposed, government designed program.
2. Fines set at an amount sufficient to divest the organization of all of its net assets.
3. Exclusion from the Medicare and Medicaid programs.
4. Management liability.
5. Stockholder lawsuits.
6. Qui Tam lawsuits.

Exclusion

Section 1320a-7 of Title 42 provides that individuals can be excluded from participation in Medicare and state health care programs under certain circumstances, including (1) conviction relating to fraud, (2) conviction relating to obstruction of an investigation of Medicare fraud, (3) claims for fraud or excess charges, and (4) furnishing patient services of a quality that fails to meet professionally recognized standards of health care (42 U.S.C. 1320a-7(b)). A minimum 5-year exclusion from participation in Medicare and/or any state health care program is mandatory for any individual or entity that (1) has been convicted for Medicare-related crimes, (2) has been convicted of a criminal offense relating to neglect or abuse of patients, or (3) has been convicted of a criminal offense related to the delivery of an item or service under Medicare, Medicaid, or any state health care program (42 U.S.C. Section 1320a-7(a) and 1320a-7(c)(3)(B)). Generally, when a provider is going to be excluded, that provider is provided with a notice indicating that within 60 days of the notice, they can request a hearing before an administrative law judge to challenge whether they were in fact convicted, whether their convictions were related to the delivery of an item or service, and the length of their exclusion from the program.

Suspension of Payments

A state Medicaid agency is also allowed to suspend provider payments "upon receipt of reliable evidence that the circumstances giving rise to the need for a withholding of payments involve fraud or willful misrepresentation under the Medicaid program" (42 C.F.R. Section 455.23 (a)). The regulation provides that payments may be suspended "without first notifying the provider," but requires that notice be given within 5 days of taking such action and specifies that the provider may request and must be granted administrative review where state law so requires (42 C.F.R. Section 455.23(a)).

Financial Penalties

The False Claims Act allows potentially enormous financial penalties for individuals or facilities found liable under the act, including treble damages and straight fines of up to $10,000 for *each* false claim submitted.

License Revocation

The individual state in which a practitioner convicted of fraud against a government program is licensed can also take action against that practitioner, including revocation of professional licenses and imposition of fines in addition to those imposed by the federal government. For example, in Louisiana the statutory maximum penalty for Medicaid fraud is 5 years with or without hard labor and/or a fine of not more than $10,000 (Louisiana Statutes Annotated –R.S. 14:70.1). Many states have adopted the Federal Sentencing Guidelines as mandatory in dealing with Medicaid fraud cases on a state basis. In the New York case of *Bhatt v. DeBuono (1997),* the New York appeals court upheld the decision of the State Board for Professional Medical Conduct to revoke the medical license of a physician who was convicted upon his plea of guilty to a felony charge of insurance fraud.

FALSE CLAIMS ISSUES RELATED TO NURSING CASE MANAGEMENT

False Claims Resulting From Substandard Care

The most potentially devastating type of false claims case to a case manager is a case involving false claims as a result of substandard care. There have been several important recent cases alleging fraud in substandard care. The first case occurred in the Eastern District of Pennsylvania in February of 1996. At this time, the U.S. Attorney's office filed a civil complaint against the owner and former manager of Tucker House, a 180-bed nursing facility located in Philadelphia. This lawsuit alleged that three former residents had been subjected to substandard care, in that inadequate nutrition was maintained, as evidenced by the development of multiple Stage III and IV pressure ulcers, secondary infections in the ulcers, precipitous and severe weight loss, and other symptoms of malnutrition, as well as improper wound care. The government also found that the staff failed to recognize the malnutrition or intervene early enough to prevent further decline of the patients' health.

The suit was based on both the False Claims Act and the Nursing Home Reform Act (NHRA, 42 U.S.C.A. Section 1396r et. seq.). The government's contention was that the defendants had violated the False Claims Act by submitting claims for services provided to these residents when the residents had not been provided with adequate care. The government's argument was that noncompliance with quality of care standards applicable to nursing facilities under both federal and state law was the same as intentional noncompliance with the required Medicare and Medicaid provider certification agreement between the government and the facility. This is because, under the certification agreement, all providers are charged with knowing all federal and state laws that apply to them and to the services they provide; the government has interpreted the knowledge requirement to be a compliance requirement as well. Because submitting claims for services to the government is a certification that all such services were provided in compliance with all quality of care laws and regulations, submitting such claims while not complying with the quality of care standards was false certification actionable under the False Claims Act.

The NHRA requires nursing facilities participating in Medicare and Medicaid to ensure that their residents are cared for adequately and appropriately. The regulations under the NHRA specifically require that facilities identify when a resident's nutritional status falls below what is considered acceptable for that patient's age and health status and must correct, if possible, whatever is causing the nutritional problem (42 C.F.R. Section 483.25(i)). This act also requires comprehensive assessment and treatment of pressure ulcers (42 C.F.R. Section 483.25(c)). In this case, state laws in Pennsylvania also required that facilities meet daily nutritional requirements of patients (28 PA Code Section 211.6a), and that the director of nursing services ensure that all prescribed health services for patients are properly implemented (28 PA Code Section 211.12e).

One of the important facts of this case was that the medical records of these patients indicated that the facility's staff had or should have had some knowledge that the nutritional intake of the residents was not sufficient. Even worse, the nursing staff's treatment notes were not entirely consistent with the severe problems obviously present in these patients. The fact that the facility failed to determine what the patients' true conditions were before submitting the claims constituted, in the government's eye, reckless disregard for the truth. The case was settled for $500,000 and consent orders imposing rigorous quality of care standards on the facility (Kleiman, 1999; Kurlander, 1997).

Two years later, in January 1998, the same U.S. attorney filed a similar action against three additional nursing homes. This case also settled for $500,000 and an agreement to implement the same kinds of quality of care standards as in the Tucker House case (Kleiman, 1999). Finally, in August of 1998, the U.S. attorney's office in Baltimore filed suit against Greenbelt Nursing and Rehabilitation Center. The suit was settled only 1 month after it was filed. In a detailed court order agreed to by both parties, Greenbelt's owner agreed to strict standards for staffing, staff training, quality assurance, medical and nursing care, nutritional needs, psychiatric services, wound care, and resident safety. Greenbelt was also required to hire a monitor and an interim manager to be approved by the government. Most importantly, Greenbelt agreed that the United States government could interview its staff outside the presence of supervisors and without company lawyers present (Kleiman, 1999).

The Problem of the Dually Eligible Client

Compliance presents a potentially very complicated problem for all health care providers, but most especially for nursing case managers. Often the case manager is forced to juggle the regulations and rules of both Medicare and Medicaid simultaneously when dealing with a single patient. Mitchell (1997) notes that Medicare and Medicaid overlap significantly, especially where persons with chronic conditions are concerned. Saucier (1995) noted that nearly all elderly Medicaid beneficiaries and up to a third of Medicaid beneficiaries with disabilities also qualify for Medicare. When patients are dually eligible, the federal government (through Medicare) is responsible for primary, acute, and a growing amount of chronic care and the state (through Medicaid) is responsible for long-term care and wraparound coverage (Mitchell, 1997). Although the two funding sources complement each other in that Medicaid covers gaps in Medicare coverage for the dually eligible, the existence of two payers does not, by itself, ensure coordination of care. Mitchell (1997) suggests that this is due to the fact that the systems remain bifurcated, which potentially undercuts the benefits of managed care for those dually eligible patients, as the current system creates obstacles to providing good and cost-effective care. What this means for the nursing case manager is that extra care must be taken when dealing with dually eligible clients to avoid potential compliance issues.

Management and Evaluation of Medicare Patients

Under the Medicare management and evaluation regulations, which were published in 1989, nurses can provide reimbursable case management services for home health patients with chronic problems to prevent rehospitalization of those patients. This regulation was significant because it was the first time Medicare rules did the following:

1. Recognized and reimbursed nurses as case managers in the home
2. Reimbursed for prevention and health promotion in the home
3. Acknowledged and reimbursed chronic rather than exclusively acute care (Allen, 1994; Knollmeuller, 1993; National Association for Home Care, 1992).

Management and Evaluation (MAE) is defined as providing case management for patients with chronic illnesses and multiple skilled or nonskilled disciplines involved, where rehospitalization or non-adherence to the care plan is likely (Allen 1994; HCFA, 1989). Allen (1994) notes that the regulation provides for the continued care of persons at high risk for rehospitalization who can benefit from a registered nurse assuring that the care plan developed with the patient and family is maintained.

The rules regarding MAE resulted from a lawsuit brought in 1987, which asserted that fiscal intermediaries of HCFA had randomly and without permission narrowed the definition of eligible Medicare home services and denied reimbursement of home care agencies, and that HCFA had failed in its oversight of these intermediaries. The suit also challenged HCFA's 1986 modification of the definition of eligible care regarding part-time/intermittent care, as well as its narrow definition of "medically necessary" and arbitrary reimbursement decisions based on the semantics of the claim rather than on medical need (Allen, 1994). The courts agreed with the claimants and ordered HCFA to rewrite the eligibility rules and broaden the definition of allowable Medicare-reimbursed services provided in the home. As a part of these rule changes, MAE of the patient's care plan was introduced as a reimbursable skilled service under Medicare (Allen, 1994). MAE services have the following three goals:

1. To allow registered nurses to monitor the delivery of skilled and unskilled care provided in the patient's home.
2. To coordinate services with an appreciation for the interrelationship of the caregiving services given the potential for adverse consequences.
3. To provide a reimbursement avenue to respond to care plan complications.

(Allen, 1994).

Allen (1994) notes that MAE is a skilled service and thus may be provided as a stand-alone service to Medicare recipients. Criteria for identifying patients who could benefit from MAE services include various physical, environmental, psychosocial, and health-related behaviors and conditions. The physical criteria include potential for deterioration and complex, multiple care needs. Environmental criteria include an unhealthy or unsafe environment and actual or potential safety issues. Psychosocial criteria include unorganized or fragmented informal caregivers, lack of or inconsistent support system, and limited financial, mental, or intellectual resources. Health-related behavior criteria include multiple health care providers and/or community services, unstable or inconsistent self-care, need for coordination and teaching of formal or informal unskilled care, and high turnover of caregivers, with a need for continuity and instruction of unskilled providers (Allen, 1994). To avoid potential trouble with false claims arising from MAE services, the case manager must document the criteria in nursing notes, must evaluate the criteria at regular intervals to assure that they are current problems, and must document interventions (Allen, 1994). Documentation is critical in this area because although the regulations do not limit the visit frequency or duration, the documentation must reflect that the patient continues to need the skilled service.

Allen (1994) notes that there are three potential problems with use of MAE. First, MAE cannot be used only to continue a home health aide, as MAE is not meant to provide long-term homemaker or activities of daily living assistance only. Second, MAE is not appropriate for continued management of an unstable situation. Third, MAE requires an updated working care plan that reflects the skilled and unskilled care that is being provided. Nursing case managers performing MAE must be careful to avoid these problems and to document thoroughly.

OTHER RELEVANT FEDERAL AND STATE LAWS PERTAINING TO COMPLIANCE AND REGULATION OF NURSING CASE MANAGEMENT

In addition to charges under the False Claims Act, providers may be charged with mail fraud in violation of 18 U.S.C. Section 1341 if they have used the U.S. mails in furtherance of their fraudulent behavior, and may be charged with wire fraud in violation of 18 U.S.C. Section 1343 if they have engaged in telephone conversations or used wire transmissions in furtherance of their fraudulent behavior.

The Medicare anti-kickback statute (42 U.S.C. Sections 1320a-7b(b)) represents a cumulation of several years of congressional effort to combat fraud and abuse in the Medicare and Medicaid programs. Congress first enacted these laws in 1972. The law made it a misdemeanor to solicit, offer, or receive any "kickback or bribe in connection with" furnishing covered services or referring a patient to a provider of those services (Social Security Amendments, 1972).

In 1977 Congress expanded on the 1972 statute, making violations of the statute a felony and additionally proscribing the solicitation or receipt of any "remuneration," including any kickback, bribe, or rebate, in return for referring a patient to a provider of covered services, regardless of whether the prohibited act was done "directly or indirectly, overtly or covertly, or in cash or in kind" (Medicare–Medicaid Anti-Fraud and Abuse Amendments, 1977). The statute was revised again in 1980, because there was uneasiness regarding the application of the statute, to include what is known as a "scienter" requirement, which means that the person accused must have knowingly and willingly engaged in the prohibited conduct to be subject to criminal sanctions. This does not mean that the accused had to know that the conduct was illegal.

In 1987 Congress streamlined this statute into a single statutory scheme, 42 U.S.C. Section 1320a-7b(b). The current version of the statute provides in part:

1. Whoever knowingly and willfully solicits or receives any remuneration (including any kickback, bribe, or rebate) directly or indirectly, overtly or covertly, in cash or in kind—
   (A) in return for referring an individual to a person for the furnishing or arranging for the furnishing of any item or service for which payment may be made in whole or in part under a Federal health care program, or
   (B) in return for purchasing, leasing, ordering or arranging for or recommending purchasing, leasing, or ordering any good, facility, service, or item for which payment may be made in whole or in part under a Federal health care program, shall be guilty of a felony and upon conviction thereof shall be fined not more than $25,000 or imprisoned for not more than five years, or both.

Providers can also be punished under state laws for accepting kickbacks.

Safe harbor regulations were issued by the DHHS in 1991 (42 C.F.R. Section 1001.952 (a)-(m), 1992). DHHS explained that "[I]f a person participates in an arrangement that fully complies with a given [safe harbor] provision, he or she will be assured of not being prosecuted criminally or civilly for the arrangement that is the subject of that provision" (Background to Safe Harbor Provisions, 56 Fed. Register 35952, 35958, July 29, 1991). The safe harbor provision allowing for payments pursuant to personal services and management contracts provides as follows:

> The following payment practices shall not be treated as a criminal offense under section 1128B of the Act and shall not serve as the basis for an exclusion:
>
> (d) Personal services and management contracts. As used in section 1128B of the Act, "remuneration" does not include any payment made by a principal to an agent as compensation for the services of the agent, as long as all of the following six standards are met—
>
> (1) The agency agreement is set out in writing and signed by the parties.
> (2) The agency agreement specifies the services to be provided by the agent.
> (3) If the agency agreement is intended to provide for the services of the agent on a periodic, sporadic, or part-time basis, rather than on a full-time basis for the term of the agreement, the agreement specifies exactly the schedule of such intervals, their precise length, and the exact charge for such intervals.
> (4) The term of the agreement is for not less than one year.
> (5) The aggregate compensation paid to the agent over the term of the agreement is set in advance, is consistent with fair market value in arms-length transactions and is not determined in a manner that takes into account the volume or value of any referrals or business otherwise generated between the parties for which payment may be made in whole or in part under Medicare or a State health care program.
> (6) The services performed under the agreements do not involve the counseling or promotion of a business arrangement or other activity that violates any State or Federal law.
>
> For purposes of paragraph (d) of this section, an agent of a principal is any person, other than a bona fide employee of the principal, who has an agreement to perform services for, or on behalf of, the principal. (42 C.F.R. Section 1001.952(d), 1992).

Kickbacks can be a major issue for nursing case managers because of the nature of their practice, which involves making referrals and procuring goods and services for clients. It is imperative to refuse to accept any type of gift or payment that depends on your making referrals of federally insured patients. If such gifts or payments are offered to you, your facility's risk manager or in-house attorney should be contacted at once.

References

Allen, S. (1994). Medicare Case Management. *Home Healthcare Nurse 12*(3) 21-27.

Bhatt v. DeBuono, 661 N.Y.S.2d 66 (1997).

Bower, K. (1995). Collaborative care: two effective strategies for positive outcomes. In K. Zander (Ed.), *Managing outcomes through collaborative care: The application of caremapping and case management* (pp.1-38). Chicago: American Hospital Publishing.

Cantone, L. (1999). Corporate compliance: Critical to organizational success. *Nursing Economics 17*(1) 15-19.

Department of Justice (1997, Oct.). Qui Tam cases filed and Recoveries. Available at http://www.taf.org/taf/docs/pub.html.

Elizondo, A. (1994, Dec.). Nursing case management in the neonatal intensive care unit part 1: Pioneering new territory. *Neonatal Network 13*(8), 9-12.

Federal Sentencing Guidelines, 1991.

Gibbs-Brown, J. (1997). Results of operation restore trust audit of medicare home health services in California, Illinois, New York and Texas (A-04-96-02121) (pp.4-22) (Report sent to HCFA from OIG). Washington, DC: U.S. Government Printing Office.

Health Care Financing Administration (1998). Financial report for fiscal year 1997. Washington, DC: US Department of Health and Human Services, Health Care Financing Administration.

Health Care Financing Administration (1989). Health Insurance Manual-11 (HIM-11). Revision 222. Washington DC: HCFA.

Kleiman, M. (1999, June). The False Claims Act. *JONA's Healthcare Law, Ethics, and Regulation 1*(2), 17-22.

Knollmeuller, R. (1993). The role of prevention in home health care nursing practice. *Home Healthcare Nurse 11*, 21-23.

Kurlander, S. (1997). Liability under the false claims act for inadequate care of nursing facility residents. *Advances in Wound Care, 10*(5), 47-49.

Medicare-Medicaid Anti-fraud and Abuse Amendments, Pub.L. No. 95-142, 91 Stat. 1179, 1181 (1977).

Medicare Report, The Bureau of National Affairs, Inc. Washington, DC, 1998, 9:9:220.

Mitchell, E. (1997, Spring). Medicaid, Medicare, and managed care: Case management for dually eligible clients. *Journal of Case Management 6*(1), 8-12.

National Association for Home Care. (1992). Home care management and evaluation: Understanding and documenting. Washington, DC: The Association.

Saucier, P. (1995). Federal barriers to managed care for dually eligible persons. Portland, Me.: National Academy for State Health Policy.

Schorr, B. (1998). OIG knocks DME claims for documentation & HHA claims for lack of necessity. *Home Health Line 23*(18), 9.

Schwartz, R. (1998, Feb.) OIG targets nursing homes—again. *Nursing Homes,* pp. 10-11.

Social Security Amendments Act, Pub.L. No. 92-603, Sections 242 (b) and (c), 86 Stat. 1419, 1972.

Stahl, D. (1998). Consolidated Billing and Compliance Program Part 2. *Nursing Management 29*(6), 12-15.

31 USC Section 3279 (False Claims Act).

42 U.S.C. Section 1320 (Medical Necessity of Medicare services).

42 USC Sections 1320 a-7 (Federal Provisions regarding exclusion from Medicare and Medicaid).

42 U.S.C. Sections 1395 et seq. (Medicare Law).

42 USC Sections 1396 et seq (Medicaid Law).

U.S. Department of Justice (1997). 1997 Annual report, Washington, D.C.: U.S. Department of Justice, p. 27.

White, J. (1998, March). How provider fraud flattens corporate profits. *Business & Health,* p. 28.

UNIT

VIII

EVALUATION, OUTCOMES MEASUREMENT, AND RESEARCH

Important Components of Decision Making

One of the most commonly overlooked areas in the process of designing and implementing case management is the evaluation component. While often neglected, it is by far among the most critical elements. Today's organizations are data driven, and case management evaluation and research data is among the most robust data available in health care delivery settings. What makes the data unique and beneficial is its focus on the combination of clinical, financial and quality issues. Unlike much of the data collected prior to case management, it does not compartmentalize the information, but places it in a context which makes it of use to practitioners, administrators and regulatory bodies. Finally, outcomes data seeks to answer many of the questions being raised in health care today in terms of efficacy and cost of care. Unit VIII provides a unique look into this complex and growing area for case management.

Key Functions and Direct Outcomes of Case Management

Sherry L. Aliotta

CHAPTER OVERVIEW

This chapter describes the four key functions of case management and how they can be used to identify and measure the direct outcomes of case management. The chapter presents the "Spectrum of Accountability" model developed by the Council for Case Management Accountability and how that model will be used to link case management outcomes to the end outcomes of the health care system. The implications of this model on the practice of case management are presented.

FOUR KEY FUNCTIONS OF CASE MANAGEMENT

The "Standards of Practice for Case Managers" list four key functions of a case manager. These functions are the assessor, planner, facilitator, and advocate.

Assessor

Without a thorough assessment, the probability of accurately identifying issues that can benefit from case management intervention is drastically diminished. Assessment by a case manager forms the database of information for the patient. The case manager should complete a comprehensive review of the key aspects of the patient and the situation. The case manager must be skilled in interviewing and gathering data. The manager must also be able to identify sources of information to obtain a detailed picture of the problems, issues, and barriers that may be present. In addition, the case manager must identify the strengths and resources that the patient possesses. The actual gathering of the information is just the first step of the process. The case manager must synthesize the information obtained to anticipate the problems, issues, or barriers, and how these will impact the patient's progress toward the achievement of their goals. The case manager must also recognize where the patient's strengths, talents, and abilities can be used, and where support, education, or further

417

intervention is required. This requires critical thinking and analytical skills on the part of the case manager.

Planner

The information gained and the analysis performed during the assessment phase forms the foundation for the planning phase. The case manager collaborates with the patient, the patient's family, significant others, and all treating professionals to develop a case management plan. The plan contains the long-term and short-term goals, the problems to be addressed, the pieces of the plan that are already in place, and the interventions necessary to achieve the established goals. The interventions in the plan should address the problems, issues, and barriers identified as a part of the comprehensive assessment and those revealed through joint planning with the patient. The plan should reflect where the patient is in relationship to the desired goals and anticipate the pitfalls and milestones in order to evaluate the success of the plan.

Facilitator

The case manager implements or ensures implementation and coordination of the care plan. The case manager maintains communication with all the parties. She looks for opportunities to prevent duplication, delays, and miscommunications in the care of the patient and intervenes when possible. The case manager is the "trouble-shooter" to resolve conflicts and expedite care. Case managers often accomplish the extraordinary on a routine basis.

Advocate

The case manager advises the patient of the available options and ensures that the patient's interests are identified and supported. Where possible, the case manager provides the patient with the information needed for the patient to be an effective advocate of his or her own requirements. The advocacy role of the case manager includes ensuring that the patient and significant others are the key architects of their own life and lifestyle choices. Often case managers decide what the patient's problems are, what the patient is going to do to solve them, and which problem the patient will tackle first. The fact that the patient later agrees to the case manager's plan does not mean the patient was a participant in the care planning. Such practices, although commonly used, do not fulfill the potential of the case manager as an advocate.

THE KEY FUNCTIONS OF CASE MANAGEMENT AND OUTCOME MEASUREMENT

Outcome measures for case management need to demonstrate two things:

1. Case managers are effective in performing the four key functions.
2. Effective performance of the four key functions has a positive impact on overall outcomes.

Much of the research published to date (Wagner et al., 1999) regarding the outcomes of case management have focused on indicators such as reduction in inpatient days, improved health status, and decreased in costs. These items and other related outcomes are more accurately described as "end outcomes." The challenge for case managers lies in quantifying exactly how its key functions impact the end outcomes.

END OUTCOMES OF THE HEALTH CARE SYSTEM

The major end outcomes reported by the health care system include the following:

- High quality care—This is often measured using proximate measures such as patient satisfaction, readmission rates, complications, morbidity and mortality, or adherence to recognized treatment standards. As with the key functions of case management, these proximate measures are based on assumptions. Sometimes the assumptions are supported by research evidence, and sometimes they are not. For example, in their landmark article on a nurse-led multidisciplinary intervention, Rich et al. used an instrument that was found to be responsive in measuring quality of life in patients with congestive heart failure (Rich et al, 1995). This measure is supported by research evidence.
- Decreased or appropriate costs—Measurements for costs include reductions in hospital admissions, emergency room visits, and overall "per case" costs. For example, researchers in Australia used their hospital's inpatient and outpatient costing systems to compare the costs of the study interventions as compared to costs of usual care (Stewart et al, 1998). Some measurements are obtained using "pre-post" comparisons where costs are measured before the case management intervention and then after the case management intervention. The before and after measurements are compared and the cost reductions calculated. Using measurements of appropriate costs is more difficult. It is often difficult to state what the cost of care *should* be. When these types of measurements are done, they are usually based on comparison with recognized standards or actuarial data and are often correlated with quality or health status measures.
- Improved health status—Often measured via use of questionnaires or surveys that examine the patient's perception of the impact their health has on their quality of life. Other indicators could include the absence of symptoms, resumption of employment, or other aspects of the patient's chosen lifestyle. As with quality of care, there are numerous proximate measure that are used as verification of improvement in health status.

If case management is to be able to conclusively establish a correlation between what the case manager does and the desired end outcomes of the health care experience, they must achieve clear definitions. Case management must define both the interventions and the impact of those interventions.

DIRECT IMPACT OF CASE MANAGEMENT

The first question that had to be answered was, "What are the direct outcomes of case management?" This question was proposed to case management leaders and to customers, recipients, purchasers, and colleagues of case management by the Council for Case Management Accountability. The three leading answers were as follows:

- Improved adherence
- Improved coordination of care
- Enhancement of patient empowerment and involvement

The Spectrum of Accountability from the Council for Case Management Accountability (Figure 38-1) describes and illustrates the relationship between the key functions of case management, the direct outcomes of case management, and the end outcomes of the health care system.

The Spectrum of Accountability is the model that the Council for Case Management Accountability developed to guide their approach to the development of outcome measures for case management. The model illustrates the functions of case management (assessment, planning, facilitation, and advocacy) resulting in the direct outcomes of patient knowledge, involvement and empowerment, increased adherence, and coordination of care. The final piece of the model depicts the direct outcomes of case management as contributing to the end outcomes of case management.

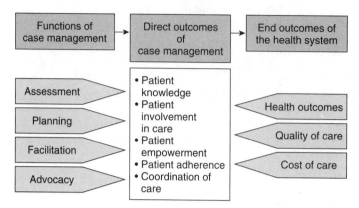

FIGURE **38-1**   Spectrum of accountability.
(Courtesy Case Management Society of America Council for Case Management Accountability, Little Rock, Arkansas © 1997. Used with permission.)

IMPROVED ADHERENCE

Improving adherence has long been a key focus for case management. In many case management models, nonadherence is a "trigger" to initiate an assessment by a case manager. All of the key functions of case management are applied to the problem of nonadherence. In the assessment the case manager specifically seeks information that will offer cues as to the cause of the nonadherence. As a planner, the case manager identifies the problem and collaborates with the patient to establish goals relating to better adherence and interventions to help the patient achieve the goal. In the role of facilitator the case manager helps to eliminate or minimize barriers to adherence. Finally, as an advocate the case manager offers solid, factual information on the impact of the nonadherence and supports the patient in the decision-making process. Which of these actions is most likely to enhance adherence? Which strategy is the one that all case managers should implement? Which of these examples is not as effective as the others? All of these questions remain unanswered without effective outcome measurements.

In adherence, as with the other "top three" case management outcomes, there is already a significant amount of information in the literature. Glenys A. Hamilton, authored a paper for The Case Management Society of America and the Council for Case Management Accountability titled, "Patient Adherence Outcome Indicators and Measurement in Case Management and Health Care." The paper details the results of Dr. Hamilton's comprehensive review of several hundred articles on adherence. The paper substantiates several concepts key to the development of case management outcomes. First, there are factors and interventions that enhance adherence. The presence of evidence in the literature documenting the ability to improve adherence is crucial for case management outcomes because it proves that adherence is a "modifiable" problem, issue, or barrier. If it was discovered that adherence could not be improved, then it would not be possible for case management to address nonadherence effectively. The second concept the Hamilton paper confirms is that there are barriers to adherence. This is important because it supports the idea that there are interventions that can minimize or eliminate the barriers to adherence. The final assumption validated in the Hamilton paper is that adherence can be measured. The impact of these three concepts:

- Adherence can be enhanced
- There are barriers to adherence
- Adherence can be measured

provides the evidentiary backing needed to establish the linkages between case management functions and the direct outcomes (impact) of case management. The final linkage to the end outcomes of cost savings, quality of care, and improved health status are also established.

IMPLICATIONS FOR PRACTICE

Using adherence as a model, case management can begin to develop the initial body of research that conclusively links case management actions with outcomes that impact the overall cost, quality, and health status of the individual. How might this work in clinical practice? First, valid and reliable measurements of adherence would be developed and tested. Once these measures are determined to be accurate, the case manager would include these measurements in the initial assessment of the patient. A specific set of interventions would be culled from the literature. The case manager would include these interventions in the care plan. As the plan was executed, the case manager would record the results of each intervention. At the conclusion of the case management episode, the case manager would administer the measures of adherence again. The improvement in the scores, or lack there of, would help to determine the effectiveness of the interventions and the case manager. Finally, overall end outcomes would be measured to demonstrate the impact of improved adherence on end outcomes. Once the link is firmly established, case managers could simply measure their own direct outcomes. Although the state of the science papers on empowerment and involvement and coordination of care have not been completed, similar findings are expected.

IMPLICATIONS FOR CASE MANAGEMENT

Case managers will need to develop a "measurement orientation." The days of "good faith" belief are rapidly coming to an end. A standard line in most any educational program for a health care professional is the phrase, "if it isn't documented, it wasn't done." The new mantra for case managers will be "if we didn't measure it, it didn't make a difference." Of course, we all know things were done even if they were not written down, and we all know that we are making an impact even if we do not measure the impact. The key element in both of these expressions is the ability to prove the action was taken or the impact was observed. Case managers will need to incorporate measurement into all key aspects of their practice.

The second key implication for practice lies in the ability to link interventions and outcomes. Case managers frequently initiate various interventions to help resolve or improve an identified problem. Anecdotal reports indicate that in most circumstances the case manager can impact the problem positively. What is often missing is the knowledge of which intervention or combination of interventions resulted in the positive outcome. In the quest to measure and demonstrate outcomes, we cannot forget process. It is obligatory to clearly delineate the processes employed to reach the outcome. Recently, a friend was having a computer problem that would result in having to redo a large and complicated spreadsheet. We both tried everything we could think of to resolve the problem. After I made one desperate move, the problem went away. My friend exclaimed, "How did you do that?" I had no idea what I had done, or why it worked. The immediate problem was resolved, but I had no way of reproducing the result because I did not define my intervention. Furthermore, I had no understanding of why it worked. Case management has a history of being apparently successful without clearly understanding why. Our future depends on reversing that trend.

Once we can measure our results and describe our interventions and rationale, standardizing of practice can be accomplished. Case managers can begin to base practice on proven interventions. Imagine the power of being able to measure a patient's level of nonadherence and identify this patient's barriers to adherence. Now imagine implementing a series of interventions proven to be effective in improving adherence where these particular barriers exist. Think of the savings in time when trial and error methods are eliminated and envision obtaining authorization for needed services and equipment when the outcome achieved by using that service is well documented. These are just two examples of what could be accomplished with solid outcome measurements. An additional benefit of standardized practice is the ability to perform comparisons and benchmarking.

Another barrier to outcome measurement for case management has been the numerous variations of interventions, outcome measurement, evaluation methodologies, and terminology. This variation has prevented across-the-board comparisons. Without the ability to compare, it is difficult to identify best practices and innovation. When there is marked variation, differences in outcomes may result from the methodology used to calculate the outcomes, the intervention, or any number of other factors. This often drives people or organizations assigned to evaluate the value of programs to force comparisons. This can result in conclusions based on incomplete or inaccurate comparisons.

With all of this uncertainty, the industry is reluctant to endorse standards of care for case management problems. However, the ability to benchmark and compare data would allow for the identification of best practices and the establishment of standards of care. This process resembles what happened when the Standards of Practice for Case Managers began to forge the requirements for the practice of case management and for what constitutes case management. Standards of care may serve to quell the debate over who is a case manager. Once the controversies over who case managers are, what they do, and what their qualifications should be are resolved, the efforts of case management can focus on shaping and improving practice.

The Council for Case Management Accountability (CCMA) was formed by the Case Management Society of America in 1995. The objectives are to establish a framework for accountability and define consistent mechanisms for reporting and comparing performance measurements industry-wide and to disperse those measurements to key stakeholders. They are looking to identify existing measures and indicators that can be linked to those currently available and used, and to identify where there are gaps and no measurements exist.

References

Council for Case Management Accountability. Informational Brochure Case Management Society of America, Little Rock, AR 1998.

Council for Case Management Accountability, Case Management Society of America. Little Rock, AR. "A Framework for Case Management Accountability" 1997.

Hamilton, Glenys A. Case Management Society of America-Council for Case Management Accountability State of the Science Paper. "Patient Adherence Outcome Indicators and Measurement in Case Management and Health Care, 1999.

Rich, Michael W, Beckman, Valerie, et al. "A Multidisciplinary Intervention to Prevent the Readmission of Elderly Patients with Congestive Heart Failure." *The New England Journal of Medicine.* November 2, 1995 Vol. 333 No. 18 pp. 1190-1195.

Standards of Practice for Case Managers. Case Management Society of America. Little Rock, AR 1995.

Stewart, Simon, Pearson, Sue, and et. al. "Effects of Home-Based Interventions on Unplanned Readmissions an Out-of-Hospital Deaths. *Journal of the American Geriatric Society.* 46:174-180, 1998.

Wagner, Edward H., Davis, Connie, and et. al. "A Survey of Leading Chronic Disease Management Programs: Are They Consistent with the Literature" *Managed Care Quarterly.* 1999 7(3):56-66.

The Data-Driven Health Care Environment

Methods of Gathering and Presenting Relevant Data About Health Care Systems

Amy J. Barton, Diane J. Skiba

CHAPTER OVERVIEW

Being information poor and data rich is a common phenomenon in health care. Health care professionals collect volumes of data but are unable to extract valuable information from these data. Clinical data represent an underutilized resource, yet they have the potential to make the greatest impact on the delivery of health care. According to Zielstorff, Hudgings, & Grobe (1993), the underutilization of data results from the current inability to manage large volumes of data and to determine patterns that will be useful in predictions. Rose (1999) uses the term *informaciation* to represent the phenomenon of having inadequate patient information and evidence to make patient decisions and guide choices for quality, cost-effective care. He believes that data toxicity, an overload of redundant, inaccurate, uninformative, or confusing facts, led to poor decision making.

How do we interpret data and how do we prepare data so we can transform it into meaningful information? These key questions need to be addressed by all case managers. Generally, data alone do not provide adequate information for decision making. Data are facts that must be summarized and displayed in meaningful ways for interpretation.

This chapter provides a foundation for data-driven decision making. In the world of best practices, evidence-based practice (EBP), and benchmarking, it is imperative that data-driven decision making is part of the case manager's role. In this chapter we view data-driven decisions from three interrelated lenses. The first view of data is through a traditional statistical lens, the second view of data is through an informatics lens, and the final view is through a continuous quality improvement lens. This chapter consists of three major sections. The first section defines data and highlights the issues related to data necessary for decision making, the second section focuses on data collection methods, and the final section highlights techniques for analysis and presentation of data.

WHAT ARE DATA?

First, what are data? According to Bauer (1996), "Data are the recorded and reported measures of real-world phenomena—the values of variables, which are the possible numeric measures of an event or experiment (p. 42)." This definition represents a statistical or research frame of reference. Data by themselves are not considered useful and must be viewed within a quantification framework. There are several frameworks proposed to view the quantification process that leads to data-driven decisions. One such model (Cleveland, 1985) conceptualized quantification as a five-step interactive process:

Thought (initial stage characterized by conjecture, hypothesis, and curiosity)
Data (undigested observations or unvarnished facts)
Information (numbers put into useful form, organized data)
Knowledge (organized, internalized information)
Wisdom (integrated knowledge that can be used to make decisions) (pp. 22-23)

In this model, according to Bauer (1996), descriptive statistics are the tools used for organizing data and creating information. Accordingly, inferential statistics are necessary for translating information into useful knowledge. Bauer (1996) considers wisdom as the art of being a good decision maker. Statistics provide the knowledge, but it is the wise human who makes the decisions.

In the world of statistics there are two types of data related to four levels of measurement (Table 39-1). Statisticians classify data as either parametric or nonparametric, and these distinctions are related to the levels of measurement. Parametric data are observations on variables that are consistent in their measure of distance between points on a scale. In other words, parametric data have consistent units of measure and have a uniform distribution of values. Interval and ratio levels of measurement are related to parametric data. On the other hand, nominal and ordinal data are related to nonparametric data. These data are not consistent, are arbitrarily measured, and are considered distribution free. Consequently, there is no uniform distance between units of measure, and the magnitude of the scale varies across and within groups. Definitions of the levels of measurement help to clarify the two types of data.

Each level of measurement corresponds to specific descriptive and inferential tools to translate data to information and information to knowledge.

Table 39-1 ▶ LEVELS OF MEASUREMENT

LEVEL OF MEASUREMENT	DEFINITION	DATA TYPE	EXAMPLE
Nominal	Numerical naming; numbers do not represent quantity or degree	Nonparametric	Gender (male/female)
Ordinal	Rank-ordered numbers	Nonparametric	Patient acuity rating
Interval	Equal differences between numbers represent equal differences in the variable	Parametric	Length of stay
Ratio	Numbers represent equal amounts to form an absolute zero	Parametric	Kelvin temperature scale

Another model from the informatics field presents a comparable quantification continuum. Graves and Corcoran (1989) view data as the initial stage of the continuum that eventually leads to discoveries and decisions. They use Blum's (1986) definitions as a basis for their continuum:

Data (discrete entities that are described objectively without interpretation)
Information (data that are interpreted, organized, or structured)
Knowledge (information that is synthesized, so relationships are identified and formalized)

Accordingly, datum is a fact about a variable that has both the attributes of value and type. Value is an attribute because datum represents a discrete entity in the real world. The attribute of type refers to this representation in terms of a restricted set of values and a restricted set of operations to manipulate or alter its values. Data types include numbers (integer or real), character strings (text), or media (sound, photo, etc.). Depending on the data type, certain mathematical operations are possible. For example, it is not possible to perform addition and subtraction on text, but you can do so on numeric data.

Data, information, and knowledge are considered three states of the phenomena generically termed information (Graves & Corcoran, 1989). To understand how data are viewed in the continuum, it is important to first define nursing informatics:

Combination of computer science, information science and nursing science designed to assist in the management and processing of nursing data, information, and knowledge to support the practice of nursing and delivery of nursing care (Graves & Corcoran, 1989, p. 227).

Given this definition, the management component is the ability to collect, aggregate, organize, move, and represent information, whereas the processing is viewed as the transformation of one state (data) to a more complex state (information). The progression of information to knowledge leads to the final transformation of knowledge into decisions or discoveries.

Let's take this view of data on the quantification continuum and apply it to health care. Stead (1991) defines five categories of health care data: historical data (about a particular patient or device), encounter patient data, subgroup data of a specified population or set of events, work-flow management data, and knowledge databases for use in decision making. Three primary users (administrator, support personnel, and direct care providers) retrieve these five categories of health data. In nursing, patient care data are of central concern and thus become the basic information unit. Atomic-level data, as defined by Zielstorff et al. (1993), are the elemental, precise data captured at the source in the course of clinical practice. These discrete, uninterpreted data are then available for processing. The processing of this atomic-level data allows it to be analyzed, combined, aggregated, and summarized with the end result of being transformed into information and knowledge. Transforming data from one state to a more complex state adds meaning and value to the data. In the following figure (Zielstorff et al., 1993), one can see how atomic-level data can be abstracted, aggregated, and summarized for use by other health care professionals. For example, outcome measures at the patient level can be aggregated and summarized by diagnosis for presentation to quality managers (Figure 39-1).

From an informatics point of view, the goal of moving along the continuum from data to knowledge is considered the process of informatting. This term, coined by Zubof (1991), describes a key consequence of information technologies on organizations. According to Zubof (1991), to informate means to translate or make visible as explicit information. In health care there has been limited success in making the data elements of nursing visible.

Data from a continuous quality improvement lens builds on the atomic level and moves up the pyramid to present cross-sectional data over time and across populations. Quality managers incorporate not only patient-level data but also financial and population-based data to make decisions. When

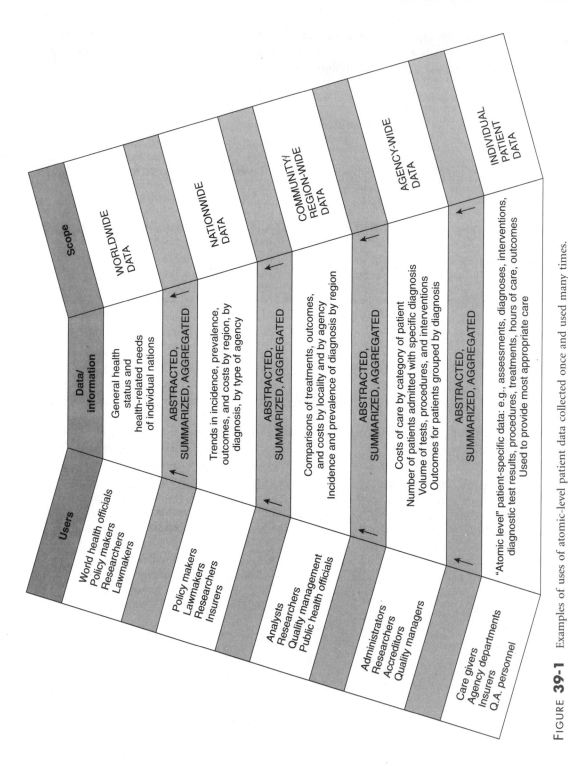

FIGURE **39-1**   Examples of uses of atomic-level patient data collected once and used many times.
(Reprinted with permission from Rita D. Zielstoff, Carole I. Hudgings, Susan J. Grobe and The National Council Implementation Project Task Force on Nursing Information, © 1993 American Nursing Publishing. American Nurses Foundation/American Nurses Association, Washington, DC.)

applied to case management, the case management plan serves as a foundation for data collection and analysis according to Cohen and Cesta (1997). They state the case management plan provides patient care data, length of stay information, and resource utilization data.

Data Issues

The quality of the data is also an issue for end-users. Without good data, it is hard to move along the continuum to decision making. Two concepts are used as a measure of data quality: validity and reliability. *Validity* refers to the meaningfulness of the data. It is the extent to which the data represent the phenomena. *Reliability* refers to accuracy of the data, that is, the repeated precision of the quantification process (Bauer, 1996). All three lenses use these concepts as indicators of quality data.

Health care is an information-intensive activity. One difficulty with health care data, in particular nursing data, is its dependence on textual information. It has long been a tradition to record narrative notes. These textual notes are extremely rich in nature but difficult to transform across the quantification continuum. According to Ozbolt and Graves (1993), "nurses have traditionally recorded narrative notes whose information content and form were as varied as the nurses authoring them (p. 409)." In many instances, the lack of consistent and atomic-level patient data has fostered the invisibility of nursing.

There have been many attempts to make visible the data elements related to nursing practice. Werley and Lang (1988) first addressed this issue in an invitational conference to identify approaches for delineating data elements essential for diagnosis, nursing intervention, and evaluation of care. The work eventually identified 16 data elements that would constitute the Nursing Minimum Data Set (NMDS). The NMDS identified patient demographic and other service data elements, but there was still work needed in the four nursing care elements: diagnosis, intervention, outcomes, and intensity of nursing care. To this end, several efforts were made to develop vocabularies and classification systems for these data elements. The seven vocabularies and classification schemes recognized by the American Nurses Association are as follows:

North American Nursing Diagnosis Association (NANDA) (Kim, McFarland, & McLane, 1984)
Iowa Intervention Project (NIC) (McCloskey & Bulechek, 1992)
Omaha Visiting Nurses Association (Martin & Scheet, 1992)
Home Health Care Classification System (HHCC) (Saba et al., 1991)
Nursing Outcome Classification (NOC) (Daly, Maas, & Johnson, 1997)
The Patient Care Data Set (Ozbolt, 1996)
Perioperative Nursing Data Set (AORN, 2000)

Although these efforts are making major strides in providing meaning to nursing data, there is still no one existing vocabulary or classification system that represents all that nurses do (Henry & Mead, 1997). The development of a unified nursing language system (UNLS) would identify the linkages and associations across the various vocabularies and classification schemes as well as retain their unique data elements.

Another issue related to data bases is the lack of information related to transactions that could describe the cost of nursing services as well as represent diagnoses, treatments, and outcomes from other disciplines. This is of particular importance for case managers who are using critical pathways designed to capture patient care using terminology across health care disciplines. Jones (1997) indicates that transaction data bases used by health care purchasers, policymakers, and health care organization administrators exclude information about the quality, type of, or cost of nursing services. The national health care transaction data bases consist of the International Classification of Diseases (ICD-9-CM0, Physician's Current Procedural Terminology (CPT) and the National Drug Code (NDC).

Data Management Issues

Data-based decision making in case management requires collecting the right information at the outset to manage outcomes appropriately. Outcomes management is "the enhancement of patient outcomes through development and implementation of exemplary health practices and services, driven by outcome assessment" (Luquire & Houston, 1997, p. 5). Even though the process is driven by outcomes assessment, it is imperative to collect the input and process data in order to determine the factors associated with outcomes achievement.

Outcomes management is rooted in the quality framework introduced by Donabedien (1966) who used systems theory to evaluate care. In his model, structures or inputs give rise to processes that influence outcomes. Holzemer and Reilly (1995) expanded this framework to add the dimensions of client, provider, and setting. The resulting matrix (Table 39-2) broadly illustrates the types of data required to facilitate outcomes management. For example, to evaluate the process of clinical pathways as a model of care delivery, you may monitor patient (length of stay), provider (cost of practitioner services), and/or institutional (patient satisfaction) outcomes.

One difficulty associated with outcomes assessment is that the data required are often dispersed throughout an organization, requiring "considerable time and energy to find, collect, and organize the data. Negotiation with the 'owners' of the data bases is required" (Schriefer, Urden, & Rogers, 1997, p. 18). To deal with this obstacle, Meistrell and Schlehuber (1996) propose the concept of a corporate data base. They further describe the corporate database as providing the following:

1. "Accessibility by a broad community of legitimate users, including clinicians, researchers, decision makers, and policy makers
2. Accountability for the accuracy of the data
3. Accessibility to definitions of the data elements, entities, and their relationships
4. Accessibility to definitions of the context in which the data are generated, including documentation of the operating assumptions of those responsible for data collection" (p. MS93).

It is important to distinguish between two data base types that are commonly referred to in the health care literature: data warehouse and clinical data repository (Waldo, 1998). A data warehouse contains clinical and financial data and is used by managers and analysts for population-based management. Data are comparative, trended, and aggregate. A clinical data repository, on the other hand, is designed to facilitate a clinician's decision making concerning individual patients. The focus of the repository is on operational and clinical data that are available in real time.

"The goal of clinical decision support is to present the 'right information' to the 'right person' at the 'right time,' in the 'right format'" (Broverman et al., 1996). Key choices regarding design of an effective clinical support system include the following:

- Passive versus active systems
- Aggregate versus individual patient-based
- Concurrent versus retrospective
- Systems integrated with patient data base versus stand-alone systems
- Proprietary versus standards-based encoding

Ideally, the decision support system should be active, patient-based, concurrent, integrated, and standards based. The decision support system should be active in that it processes information prospectively as opposed to waiting for input from the user. The system should be designed to facilitate decision making regarding specific individuals when they require care as opposed to decision making about a group of patients based on retrospective information. "Clinical decision support is intended as a front-line process that actively defines critical data required for real-time analysis and reporting.Specifically, the information is relevant to the provider within the context of the patient visit" (Orlando, 1998).

Table 39-2	THE OUTCOMES MODEL FOR HEALTH CARE RESEARCH (HOLZNER, REILLY, 1995)		
	INPUTS	**PROCESSES**	**OUTCOMES**
CLIENT (individual, family, school, community)	Personal characteristics, cultural values and beliefs, social support networks, personal strengths, concerns and needs, well-being, functional status, quality of life, and sociodemographic factors (level of education, ethnicity, income per capita, disability rates, and unemployment rates).	Self-care activities.	Mortality, complications, length of stay, readmission rates, physiological status, psychosocial status, functional status, behavior, knowledge, symptom control, quality of life, home functioning, family strain, goal attainment, safety, and resolution of nursing diagnosis.
PROVIDER (physicians, nurses, social workers, nontraditional healers)	Technical competence, interpersonal skills, level of experience, specialty certification, level of education, and personal characteristics.	Critical paths, care maps, standardized care plans, clinical practice guidelines.	Costs of health practitioner services, provider satisfaction, provider intent to stay or leave, and level of ongoing continuing education.
SETTING (formal and informal organizations for care delivery)	Values, attitudes, and beliefs of the organizations, as well as available resources, including financing, equipment, number and type of providers, size, ownership status, customers, average volume of service, facility type, and environmental and health conditions of communities. Staff mix, staffing levels, professional practice models, and patient acuity. Medical care resources, number of physicians per capita, percentage of physician specialists, number of beds per capita.	Implementation of total quality improvement principles, strategic planning, implementation and evaluation of policies and procedures, governing activities, communication among providers and different departments, evaluation of operational systems, decision making, and organizational interventions.	Patient satisfaction, provider turnover, morbidity, mortality, malpractice rates, costs of care, and readmission rates. Appropriateness, availability, continuity, effectiveness, efficacy, efficiency, respect and caring, safety, and timeliness.

It is also important that the information system be integrated across the care continuum. This means that the system should do the following:

- Facilitate data exchange among all system components
- Track patients from cradle to grave
- Provide real-time information to support clinical and administrative decision making
- Monitor quality of service, clinical outcomes, resource use, and financial performance measures (Kennedy, 1996)

Such a system must incorporate a data repository linked with a knowledge base and a user-friendly decision-support interface. The system must be enterprise-wide. Patient data must be linked from outpatient, acute, community-based, and home settings.

DATA ANALYSIS AND PRESENTATION

Where is the knowledge that we have lost in the information?
T.S. Eliot

This section presents three different approaches to analysis and presentation techniques. The first approach is a traditional statistical approach. The second approach introduces data mining from an information-processing perspective. The final approach presents data analysis through a continuous quality performance lens.

Statistical Approach

The first traditional method uses statistical techniques to analyze nursing data and standard graphing techniques to present data. Statistical techniques are tied to the research or evaluation questions generated by the end user. To ask appropriate questions the end user must understand the data set and recognize the data sources required to answer the questions. If these conditions are met, an end user can use statistical techniques. These techniques can employ either descriptive or inferential tools on either parametric or nonparametric data. Let's review the various tools available.

Descriptive statistical techniques are used when one wants to describe aggregated data. Depending on the level of data (nominal to ratio), difference measures are used to describe these aggregates. Two specific measures, central tendency and variability, describe aggregates. With interval-level data, the mean and the standard deviation are the specific measures. For nominal-level data, the mode and the range are considered the appropriate measures.

Let's take an example from case management: length of stay (LOS) as a standard outcome measure. In this case, length of stay is considered an interval-level measure, so the mean and standard deviation can be used to describe aggregated LOS data. For example, the mean LOS was 2.34 days with a standard deviation of 1.37 days. To best view these data, one could plot the frequency distribution of the data and examine the distribution (Figure 39-2).

In the second case the distribution is skewed with one or two cases exceeding the average LOS and thus inflating the mean and positively skewing the distribution. The mean of this distribution is 6.34 with a standard deviation of 5.75 and a median of 4. In this case the median is the appropriate measure of central tendency (Figure 39-3).

According to biostatistician Nina Kohn of North Shore University Hospital (Bean, 1995), the most effective method to display LOS is through the use of box plots. Kohn states that most people report

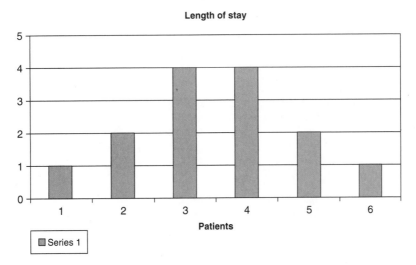

FIGURE **39-2** Length of stay with normal distribution.

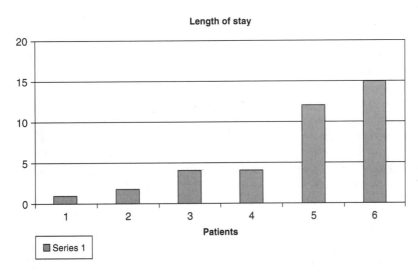

FIGURE **39-3** Length of stay with skewed distribution.

the average LOS when this does not give the most precise picture, since there is no zero point. Most LOS distributions are skewed, and it would be more appropriate to report the median value and the inter-quartile range as the measures of central tendency and variability. In a box plot, sometimes called a box and whisker plot, a box is drawn to represent the middle half of the scores with the lower hinge being the 25th percentile and the top hinge being the 75th percentile. The median is represented as a line across the box and the mean is the plus sign ($+$). The whiskers are drawn from the box to represent the lowest and highest values. In Figure 39-4, pre- and post-case management LOS is compared in two plots. Plot A represents the pre-implementation. Plot B represents post-implementation of the care management intervention. Pre-implementation, the distribution was positively skewed with the LOS

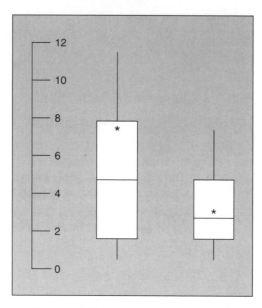

FIGURE **39-4**   Box and whiskers plot.

varying from 1 to 12 days with a mean of 7 and a median of 4. For the post-implementation phase the LOS decreased and varied less (1 to 7 days) with a mean of 3 and a median of 2.8.

Another set of statistical tools is used for inferential statistics in which the end-users ask questions about comparisons, relationships, or causality. Once again, various statistical techniques are related to levels of measurement. For example, if a case manager wanted to compare the outcomes of two different critical pathways for a specific chronic condition, one could use analysis of variance or t-test techniques to compare cost outcome data. If one wanted to compare the satisfaction of two different groups of clients using a nominal level satisfaction scale (1 = happy, 2 = not happy), one would use a chi-square analysis for the comparison. The results of these inferential statistics can be graphed to demonstrate comparison or relationships.

Grier and Foreman (1989) explicated guidelines for the presentation of scientific data in nursing research. The first guideline recommends that one clearly determine the intent of the presentation and select only the most relevant information to display. The second guideline recommends that one choose the most appropriate medium to clearly and precisely present the data. Within this guideline, there are specific recommendations for the use of graphic and tabular displays as well as the presentation of statistical descriptions.

Another resource for the presentation of data is Tufte (1983) who believes that "graphics reveal data (p. 13)." Data graphics, according to Tufte, visually display measured quantities through the use of various objects like points, lines, numbers, symbols, and color. He believes that graphics are tools for quantitative reasoning. In his book on the visual display of quantitative data, Tufte outlines his principles of graphic excellence. His principles are as follows:

Graphic excellence:

- Is the well-designed presentation of interesting data—a matter of substance, of statistics, and of design.
- Consists of complex ideas communicated with clarity, precision, and efficiency.
- Gives the viewer the greatest number of ideas in the shortest time with the least ink in the smallest space.
- Is nearly always multivariate.
- Requires telling the truth about the data.

Information Processing Approach

In the previous approach the end-user questions dictated the statistical analysis of the data to make decisions. The statistics served as a method to summarize data to make decisions. The end-user as an analyst was able to query the data and summarize the results of the question. This approach rapidly breaks down as the quantity of data grows and the number of dimensions increases (Fayyad & Uthurusamy, 1996). It is impossible as health care organizations collect voluminous data in large data warehouses for anyone to understand all the data sets and make reasonable sense of the data. To this end, there are a growing number of researchers and computer scientists who are interested in the problem of automating data analysis and have labeled these attempts as data mining and knowledge discovery in data bases (KDD). This growing field, whose core disciplines are from statistics and data base management, is joining forces to extract useful knowledge from the volumes of data in warehouses. According to Fayyad, Piatetsky-Shapiro & Smyth (1996), finding useful patterns in data is known by different names in different communities. Terms such as knowledge extraction, information discovery, information harvesting, data archeology and data pattern processing are but a few examples. To understand this concept, Fayyad, Piatetsky-Shapiro, & Smyth (1996) declare that KDD is the term used to describe the overall process of discovering useful knowledge from data. Here is a diagram of the KDD process:

DATA ⟶ Target ⟶ Pre-process ⟶ Transform ⟶ Patterns ⟶ Knowledge

The KDD process is both interactive and iterative. In the first step the end user learns about the data set and the goals. The creation of a targeted data set or subset on which the KDD is performed is the next step. Data cleaning and pre-processing, such as extraction of outliers, is the third step. Data reduction and other transformational methods are used in the next step to reduce the effective number of variables. Data mining, the application of specific algorithms for extracting patterns or models of the data, is the fifth step. In this step, one must choose the appropriate model to match the KDD process. Once the data are mined, the interpretation phase occurs in which patterns are examined for redundancy and irrelevance. The last phase is using the discovered knowledge and incorporating previous knowledge and proper interpretation. The one caution is data dredging, the blind application of data mining models to the data, which results in the discovery of meaningless patterns. To compare the statistical with the KDD approach, it is important to remember these following assumptions. The traditional statistical approach is predicated on hypothesis testing. In this approach, one is testing a conjecture against a body of data to confirm or reject that hypothesis. In many cases the data drive the discovery. In KDD, particularly in data mining, the end-user draws conclusions from the data, allowing the data to suggest the conclusion. Many propose that KDD is a combination of hypothesis testing and data-driven discovery.

Data visualization tools are used to facilitate KDD. Data visualization is the visual interpretation of complex relationships in multidimensional data using a host of graphic tools. These graphic tools include map (data displayed on a geographic map), scatter (data points shown in one to three dimensions), and tree visualizers (data are mapped to see hierarchical break downs). An example might be to use a map visualization to represent the incidence of a particular patient condition by age groupings in particular counties in Colorado. Data or information visualization (Walker, 1995) helps "to bridge the gap between the abstract, analytical world of the digital computer and the human world."

This relatively cursory view of KDD and data mining is merely an example of another approach to data-driven decisions. The intent was not to provide a detailed description of KDD and data mining but to raise awareness of other techniques that can be used to facilitate decision-making in organizations. An example of data mining relevant to case managers is from a health maintenance organization

(HMO) in Seattle, Washington. According to Moyer (1998), Group Health Cooperative is using "an innovative population management application that combines decision support tools with an online transaction system" to make better quality decisions. Using population management data (specific patient data with conditions) stored in a data warehouse, they use data mining tools to identify populations of patients, what resources these populations require, and how to adjust those resources to provide quality, cost-effective care.

CQI Approach

From a CQI perspective, data presentation techniques include those concerning idea generation (e.g., brainstorming, boarding, multivoting, decision matrices), portrayal of beliefs (flow diagrams, fishbone diagrams), display (check sheets, histograms, run charts), and analysis (Pareto charts, control charts, pie charts, scatter diagrams) (Wagner, 1995). For purposes of this chapter, display and analysis techniques will be discussed.

Display techniques for data presentation include check sheets, histograms, and run charts (Wagner, 1995). Check sheets are used to facilitate recording the frequency of an activity or event (McLaughlin & Kaluzny, 1994). For example, in case management this may be used to track prolonged LOS reasons for a population of patients. A sample check sheet for total hip arthroplasty patients is presented in Table 39-3.

Table 39-3	CHECK SHEET ILLUSTRATING REASONS FOR EXTENDED LOS			
REASON FOR INCREASED LOS	**WEEK 1**	**WEEK 2**	**WEEK 3**	**WEEK 4**
Pre-existing chronic condition	3	5	2	4
Surgical complication	1	3	2	1
Delay in ambulation	2	3	1	4
Lack of home support	1	2	2	1

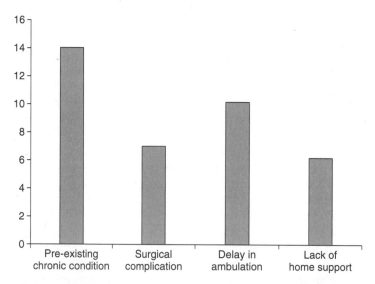

FIGURE **39-5** Histogram representing causes of delay in discharge.

The histogram is simply a bar chart that graphically presents the data from a check sheet. The categories are placed on the x-axis at equal intervals. The length of the bar on the y-axis represents the number of observations within that interval (Figure 39-5).

A run chart (Figure 39-6) allows for visualization of observations over time (Gaucher & Coffey, 1993). Assessing performance over time allows one to "(1) see what the temporal behavior of the process is and (2) establish the time of process performance changes so that they can be linked to the time of other possibly related events" (Gaucher & Coffey, 1993).

Of the analysis techniques for data presentation, Pareto charts and control charts will be discussed here. Pareto charts are named after a seventeenth-century Italian economist who noted that the greatest amount of wealth was distributed among a small group of people (McLaughlin & Kaluzny, 1994). "A Pareto chart (Figure 39-7) is used to display visually the significance of different factors, to separate the

FIGURE **39-6**   Run chart representing length of stay over time.

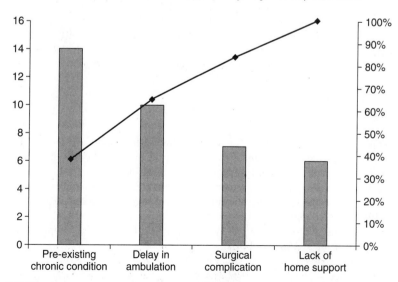

FIGURE **39-7**   Pareto chart representing the most frequently occurring reasons for discharge delay.

FIGURE **39-8**   Control chart with upper and lower control limits.

many from the vital few. This is similar to the '80-20 rule,' which ascribes 80 percent of the potential improvement to 20 percent of the issues" (Gaucher & Coffey, 1993).

A control chart is similar to a run chart, with the added feature of upper and lower control limits at 3 standard deviations above and below the mean. Control charts facilitate determining whether a variation is due to a special cause or a common cause (Gaucher & Coffey, 1993). For example, in the chart displayed (Figure 39-8), even though the average length of stay is 4.7 days, only a value of 10 falls outside the upper control limit and requires further analysis to the cause of the variation.

SUMMARY

We have provided three perspectives on which one may consider when building an infrastructure to support data-based decision making. The first method is use of traditional statistical theory, the second is use of an informatics perspective, and the third is through a CQI perspective. Regardless of approach, it is essential to carefully define the data to be collected before beginning.

References

AORN (2000). *Perioperative Nursing Data Set:* The perioperative nursing vocabulary. Denver: AORN.

Bauer, J. (1996). *Statistical analysis for decision makers in healthcare: understanding and evaluating critical information in a competitive market.* Chicago: Irwin Professional Publishing.

Bean, B. (1995). Issues in evaluating a clinical pathway program. *Issues and outcomes: The newsletter for mapping and managing care* (pp. 9-11). South Natick, Mass.: Center for Case Management.

Blum, B.L. (Ed.) (1986). *Clinical information systems.* New York: Springer-Verlag.

Broverman, C.A., Clyman, J.I., Schlesinger, J.M., & Want, E. (1996). Clinical decision support for physician order-entry: Design challenges. *AMIA,* 572-576.

Cleveland, H. (1985). *The knowledge executive: Leadership in an information society* (pp. 22-23). New York: Dutton.

Cohen, E.L., & Cesta, T.G. (1997). *Nursing case management: From concept to evaluation.* (2nd ed.). St. Louis: Mosby.

Daly, J.M., Maas, M.L., & Johnson, M. (1997). Nursing outcomes classification: An essential element in data sets for nursing and health care effectiveness. *Computers in Nursing, 15*(Suppl. 2), S82-S86.

Donabedien, A. (1966). Evaluating the quality of medical care. *Milbank Quarterly, 44,* 166-206.

Fayyad, U., Uthurusamy, R. (1996). Data mining and knowledge discovery in databases. *Communications of the ACM, 39*(11), 24-26.

Fayyad, U., Piatetsky-Shapiro, G., Smyth, P. (1996). The KDD process for extracting useful knowledge from volumes of data. *Communications of the ACM, 39*(11), 27-34.

Fields, W., Siroky, K. (1994). Converting data into information. *Journal of Nursing Care Quality, 8*(3), 1-11.

Gaucher, E.J., & Coffey, R.J. (1993). *Total quality in healthcare: From theory to practice.* San Francisco: Jossey-Bass.

Graves, J.R., & Corcoran, S. (1989). The study of nursing informatics. *IMAGE: Journal of Nursing Scholarship, 21,* 227-231.

Grier, M., & Foreman, M. (1989). In I. Abraham, D. Nadzan, & J. Fitzpatrick (Eds.), *Statistics and quantitative methods in nursing: Issues and strategies for research and education.* Philadelphia: Saunders.

Henry, S.B., & Mead, C.N. (1997). Nursing classification systems: Necessary but not sufficient for representing "what nurses do" for inclusion in computer-based patient record systems. *Journal of the American Medical Informatics Association, 4,* 222-232.

Holzemer, W.L. & Reilly, C.A. (1995). Variables, variability, and variations research: Implications for medical informatics. *Journal of the Medical Informatics Association, 2,* 183-190.

Jones, L.D. (1997). Building the information infrastructure required for managed care. *Image: Journal of Nursing Scholarship, 29,* 377-382.

Kennedy, M. (1996, March). Building information systems to manage care and improve clinical quality, *The Quality Letter,* 2-11.

Kim, M.J., McFarland, G.K., & McLane, A.M. (Eds.) (1984). *Classification of nursing diagnoses: Proceedings for the fifth national conference.* New York: McGraw-Hill.

Luquire, R., & Houston, S. (1997). Outcomes management: Getting started. *Outcomes Management for Nursing Practice, 1*(1), 5-7.

Martin, K.S., & Scheet, N.J. (1992). *The Omaha System: Applications for community health nursing.* Philadelphia: W.B. Saunders.

McCloskey, J.C., & Bulechek, G.M. (Eds). (1992). *Nursing interventions classification (NIC).* St. Louis: Mosby-Year Book.

McLaughlin, C.P., & Kaluzny, A.D. (1994). *Continuous quality improvement in health care: Theory, implementation, and applications.* Gaithersburg, Md.: Aspen.

Meistrell, M., & Schlehuber, C. (1996). Adopting a corporate perspective on databases: Improving support for research and decision making. *Medical Care, 34*(3), MS91-MS102.

Moyer, R. (1998). Making healthy decisions. http://www.sas.com/corporate/profiles/healthy.html

Orlando, M.L. (1998). Outcomes: Essential information for clinical decision support: An interview with Ellen B. White. *Journal of Health Care Finance, 24*(3), 71-81.

Ozbolt, J. (1996). From minimum data to maximum impact: Using clinical data to strengthen patient care. *Advanced Practice Nursing Quarterly, 1*(4), 62-69.

Ozbolt, J., & Graves, J. (1993). Clinical nursing informatics: Developing tools for knowledge workers. *Advances in Clinical Nursing Research, 28*(2), 407-425.

Rose, J.S. (1998). *Medicine and the information age* (p. 28). Tampa, Fla.: Hillsboro Printing.

Saba, V.K., O'Hare, P.A., Zuckerman, A.E., Boondas, J., Levine, E., Oatway, D.M. (1991). A nursing intervention taxonomy for home health care. *Nursing & Health Care, 12*(6), 296-299.

Schriefer, J., Urden, L.D., Rogers, S. (1997). Report cards: Tools for managing pathways and outcomes. *Outcomes Management for Nursing Practice, 1*(1), 14-19.

Stead, W.W. (1991). Systems for the year 2000: The case for an integrated database. *MD Computing, 8*(2), 103-110.

Tufte, E. (1983). *The visual display of quantitative information.* Cheshire, Conn.: Graphics Press.

Wagner, P.S. (1995). Guide to identifying, collecting, and managing data. In J.A. Schmele (Ed.), *Quality management in nursing and health care* (pp. 408-458). Albany: Delmar.

Waldo, B. (1998). Decision support and data warehousing tools boost competitive advantage. *Nursing Economics, 16*(2), 91-93.

Walker, G. (1995). Challenges of information visualization. *British Telecommunications Engineering, 14,* 17-25.

Werley, H.H., & Lang, N.M. (Eds.). (1988). *Identification of the nursing minimum data set.* New York: Springer.

Zielstorff, R.D., Hudgings, C.I., Grobe, S.J., & the National Commission on Nursing Implementation Project (NCNIP) Task Force on Nursing Information Systems. (1993). *Next-generation nursing information systems: Essential characteristics for professional practice.* Washington, D.C.: ANA.

Zubof, S. (1991, Summer). Informate the enterprise: An agenda for the Twenty-First Century. *Phi Kappa Phi Journal,* 3-7.

The Importance of Research in the Evaluation Process

CHAPTER OVERVIEW

Implementation of a case management model should include establishment of a nursing research methodology. Nursing research data provide the framework for evaluating and justifying the efficacy of the overall model.

This chapter explores methods for designing the research and provides samples for data analysis, including patients, staff, and length of stay for selected diagnosis-related groups (DRGs). Each organization must determine its own research design based on its goals for the model, but some sort of research base is recommended to provide a framework for evaluation.

DATA TALKS

Someone once said, "In God we trust. When all else fails, use data." Creating change in any organization is never an easy task. Obtaining the support and cooperation of hospital administration is necessary for complete integration of a nursing case management model. With such support the model can be viewed as both a nursing and a multidisciplinary model.

Perhaps the best way to obtain the support of the institution as a whole is through the use of data. This includes collecting, analyzing, and disseminating the results of a statistical data analysis as well as any anecdotal data collected. Some data will already exist and be available in the organization. Other data will need to be collected.

Obtaining the administration's support is only part of what is needed as the change to case management proceeds. A sound, valid evaluation process must be implemented to provide ongoing support as the model continues to develop and become part of the institution. It is imperative therefore that the elements to be monitored and evaluated be determined before any changes are implemented (Jennings & Rogers, 1986).

Case management provides an opportunity for nursing to conduct research, as well as to quantify the case management model. Research, broadly defined, is an attempt to find the solution to a problem so that it may be predicted or explained (Treece & Treece, 1973). Research has also been described as a formal method for carrying on the scientific method of analysis, which, in turn, involves the use of several problem-solving steps. These include problem identification, hypothesis formation, observation, analysis, and conclusion (Polit & Hungler, 1983).

These basic elements are no less important in the analysis of a case management model and all the changes that come about as a result of the integration of this system (Jennings & Rogers, 1986). Generally, research is divided into two categories. The first is basic research, the goal of which is to obtain knowledge for the sake of knowledge. The second category is applied research, which takes this process one step further as it seeks to apply the research to everyday situations (Nachmias & Nachmias, 1981). Case management research is applied research in its truest sense. Everyday questions concerning the efficacy of the model are asked, answered, and applied as the case management research data are collected and analyzed.

The methodology used for case management analysis can take several forms and can encompass several different elements. It need not be limited to one particular process but can include several steps and processes. Nursing research includes the clinical elements of the nursing profession, such as the steps of the nursing process: assessment, diagnosis, outcome identification, planning, implementation, and evaluation. Nursing research also involves the preparation and evaluation of practitioners and studies the systems in which nurses work and apply the steps of the nursing process (Corner, 1991).

EVALUATION VERSUS EXPERIMENTAL RESEARCH

Research involving case management can be approached as evaluation research. It can also be designed as an experiment or quasi-experiment. In evaluation research, data are collected and analyzed to evaluate or assess the effects of some project or change. This type of research helps to evaluate how well implementation of the program is going.

Experimental research tests the relationships between the variables being manipulated. A control group and an experimental group are used in classic experimental research. The control group symbolizes a normal representation of subjects, and the experimental group consists of those subjects for whom at least one variable has been altered.

In case management research it is difficult to devise a classic experimental design. If patients are compared, the researcher must be sure that the cases are similar enough to justify comparison. Some examples of factors to be controlled when choosing subjects are severity of illness, concurrent problems, gender, and age. In addition, random assignment to each group must be conducted. This process involves the admitting office, which ensures that certain previously evaluated patients are placed on particular units.

If nurses on nursing units are being studied for job satisfaction, for example, it would be impossible to separate those nurses who had been affected by the model from those who had not. Comparing nurses between nursing units can lead to some of the same methodology questions that arise when comparing some patients with others (Schaefer, 1989). The registered nurses could only be matched if differences were controlled in some way.

Even comparing one nursing unit with another is difficult. There are few institutions in which nursing-unit patient populations are so similar, and yet so randomized, that nurses' and patients' experiences could be said to be similar from one to the next. It is more likely that comparing one nursing unit with another is like comparing apples with oranges. Nursing units are often designated by specialty, and physicians will usually, whether formally or informally, prefer that patients be sent to a particular nursing unit because the physicians believe that unit is most suited to meeting their patient's nursing needs.

The Quasi-Experimental Approach

Because of the difficulties in matching subjects for control and experimental groups, it becomes practical to use each nursing unit as its own control. Once this takes place, the methodology becomes quasi-experimental. Unit data, including staff satisfaction, length of stay, and so on, are compared before and after implementation. Additional postimplementation data are collected and analyzed at predetermined intervals. A longitudinal approach of this kind cannot guarantee that the same staff members will be compared from one time frame to the next (Kenneth & Stiesmeyer, 1991). Whenever possible, the same nurses and staff members should be compared from one time period to the next. For those staff members who come and go during the study, global score comparisons can be made.

Certain intrinsic factors affecting internal validity are impossible to control (Lederman, 1991). One such intrinsic factor that always affects longitudinal studies is maturation. The nurses tested may have either an increase or a decrease in job satisfaction solely because of the passage of time. For some workers the passage of time provides a certain comfort that increases job satisfaction and sense of accomplishment. For others, longevity can lead to exhaustion, disillusionment, and decreased job satisfaction. In either case, these elements associated with maturation can probably not be controlled.

Another intrinsic factor is that of experimental mortality. One of the goals of case management is to decrease turnover rates among registered nurses, but there will always be a certain amount of turnover among any group of employees, no matter how happy they are with their work. Some may leave because they cannot deal with the changes accompanying the introduction of case management. In either case, it is clear that the researcher will not have the same sample at each stage of data collection. Dropouts from the study can prejudice the results. Unfortunately this factor cannot be controlled.

One way to account for the issue of experimental mortality or dropouts is to statistically analyze the entire sample size as a global unit, then match subjects from a previous data collection period with those in the current period and study this group separately.

Subjects serve as their own controls in a pretest-posttest design (Nachmias & Nachmias, 1981). The advantage to this design is that the variable is measured both before and after the intervention. In other words, the variable is compared to itself.

As the first step in either process, pre-implementation data and continuous data are obtained as the model goes forward. The provision of a solid nursing research base for evaluation lends credibility to the model for those evaluating it in 6 months, 1 year, 2 years, or longer (Rogers, 1992).

Typically when changes are made in nursing, very little data collection occurs during the implementation phase (Acton, Irvin, & Hopkins, 1991). This lack of data makes validation of results difficult, which in turn makes it difficult to maintain the momentum and support needed for change to progress.

To determine what to measure, the organization must first decide what it hopes to achieve by implementing the case management model. After identifying the goal of implementation it will be easier to formulate the questions that should be asked. Based on these questions the researcher can begin to form a hypothesis. The hypothesis indicates what the researcher believes to be the cause and effect of a given situation, and it states the relationship between the variables.

Basic research questions will not be affected by the type of methodology used, regardless of whether an evaluation or experimental methodology is chosen. These research questions are prospective and based on hoped-for outcomes. The outcomes will fall into several categories. Data collection will be longitudinal because it will probably be collected at predetermined intervals over a long period of time.

The changes attempted in case management will take years to take hold, so choosing an evaluation time period that is too short may make it appear as if implementation has failed to achieve the desired outcomes. On the other hand, some measure of changing trends will need to be shown within the first year of implementation to prove that things are moving in the desired direction.

The areas affected by the implementation of a case management model are diverse and complicated. They range from patients to staff to finance. Many of the changes are obtuse, intangible, and anecdotal, but others can be validated through stringent data collection and statistical analysis. Those changes to be measured must be determined in advance so that baseline data can be collected. These data will provide the foundation for comparison.

If a case management model is being implemented, the focus of evaluation must be on patients, finance, length of stay, and quality of care. Therefore some outcomes may be measured against changes occurring within the care delivery systems and processes. Some may have to do with changes in care management clinical interventions. Some outcomes are actually measuring programmatic changes associated with the implementation of case management, while others are measuring the clinical effects on patients when protocols and/or resource utilization is altered.

Consider the following factors when identifying organizationally specific outcomes:
Outcomes should be:

- Patient and family oriented
- Realistic and practical
- Clear and concise
- Measurable and observable
- Concrete and doable
- Time/interval specific

A non-unit-based case management model is broadly focused, and it may be difficult to prove a relationship between implementation of the model and level of staff satisfaction. Therefore this might not be a variable worth trying to measure.

In the unit-based case management model, certain changes affect particular nursing staff members in specific ways (Swanson et al., 1992). The response of these individuals can be measured and evaluated in terms of job satisfaction, turnover rates, absenteeism, and vacancy rates.

One of the most difficult but essential elements to measure in a case management model is quality of care. The basic tenet of case management is to move the patient through the hospital system as quickly and efficiently as possible. Because the hospital stay is being accelerated, some controls must be put in place to guarantee that quality care is not being compromised (Mitchell, Ferketich, & Jennings, 1998; Edelstein & Cesta, 1993).

Accrediting institutions, such as the Joint Committee on the Accreditation of Healthcare Organizations (JCAHO), are struggling with questions regarding the measurement of quality. These issues will undoubtedly continue into the next century (Williams, 1991).

Perhaps the most tangible measure, and possibly the most important in terms of hospital viability, is the length of stay. Decreases in length of stay have come to be associated directly with case management. It is difficult to address case management without also addressing the issues of hospital reimbursement and patient length of stay.

The prospective payment system provided the first and most potent incentive to hospitals to move toward reducing length of stay. Now with the rapid infiltration of managed care, other financial incentives are in the health care arena. These include capitation and negotiated per diem rates under managed care. These payment schemes provide for the same need to control cost and reduce length of stay as the prospective payment system did in the 1980s. These incentives are strictly financial.

Shorter hospital stays mean increased profits. It is only a matter of time before every institution in the United States will be looking at measures for reducing length of stay as well as controlling other costs.

Caution should be taken when studying and reporting length of stay statistics. The prospective payment system and diagnosis-related groups (DRGs) were designed to be used only as financial tools for determining reimbursement.

Because of a lack of other ways to tap into this information, the DRG has become the basis for studying length of stay and related clinical interventions. A serious analysis of many DRGs will reveal that the DRG is usually too broad and too heterogeneous to be used as a determinant of the effect of a particular clinical intervention.

To report this information with the utmost accuracy, it is more advantageous and appropriate to analyze the situation at a microlevel. For example, there is one DRG for chemotherapy, despite the fact that there are 1-day, 2-day, and 5-day chemotherapy protocols. The reimbursable length of stay is 2.6 days, no matter what the protocol. If a managed care plan is applied to a particular case for a specific chemotherapy protocol to determine the effectiveness of the plan, the researcher would have to identify more than just the DRG. If the plan is a 5-day plan, clearly the reimbursable rate is inadequate. But having this information would allow the investigator to determine, for example, whether the length of stay could have been shortened or whether quality care was provided.

Elements of Data Collection

One form of data collection is the questionnaire. Using questionnaires that have been previously determined to be valid and reliable can reduce or eliminate many of the problems associated with this technique. The content of the questions determines their ability to control bias, which could influence a respondent's answer in a particular way.

One way to test staff nurses is to compile packets of various questionnaires, including one on demographics, that the researcher can use to describe the sample itself. The questionnaires should take no longer than 15 to 20 minutes to complete (Kenneth & Stiesmeyer, 1991).

The consent form should clearly indicate that participation in the study will in no way affect the respondent's employment in the institution.

When questioning patients, nurses must ensure that patient care is not being disturbed. The researcher must also determine whether the patient is able to understand, read, and respond to the questionnaire appropriately. One way to do this is to provide questions on the demographic questionnaire that address the respondent's highest level of education, age, and ability to speak and understand English.

Box 40-1 presents some of the broad categories that an organization converting to a case management model might want to address when collecting data for determining success or failure of implementation. The list in the box is certainly not exhaustive. An organization on the brink of implementing case management may choose to study any or all of these questions. Questions may involve a multitude of benchmarks or only a few. There may be areas for study not listed in the box but still important to the organization in question. Each organization must decide for itself what is most important to measure and how it will be measured. The tools for measuring each of these expected outcomes are determined by the nurse researcher involved in the case management analysis. Valid and reliable tools exist to measure most variables, but others will have to be obtained from already-existing hospital information systems, DRG information, and managed care and hospital billing records. The areas from which to obtain the data vary from institution to institution. The finance department, the DRG office, and the managed care departments can be of great assistance to the nurse researcher evaluating a case

---

Box 40-1 ▸ **DATA COLLECTION MONITORS**

1. Improved staff satisfaction
   Outcome indicators:
   a. Registered nurse job satisfaction
   b. Physician job satisfaction
   c. Nursing assistant job satisfaction
   d. Decreased registered nurse burnout scores
   e. Decreased absenteeism
   f. Decreased turnover rate
   g. Increased recruitment
2. Improved patient satisfaction
   Outcome indicators:
   a. Patient satisfaction
   b. Family satisfaction
3. Improved quality care
   Outcome measures:
   a. Quality improvement data
   b. Patient satisfaction
   c. Readmission rate
   d. Uniform treatment of all cases
   e. Frequency and type of patient education
   f. Clinical outcome indicators
   g. Variance analysis data
4. Decreased length of stay
   Outcome measure: reduction in length of stay
5. Improved communication or collaboration among disciplines
   Outcome measures:
   a. Development of collaborative practice groups
   b. Opened lines of communication between all disciplines
   c. Development of case management plans
6. Decreased costs
   Outcome measures:
   a. Improved resource use (both product and personnel)
   b. Decreased absenteeism, turnover, and vacancy rates
   c. Decreased delays in waiting for tests and procedures
   d. Uniform treatment within physician groups
   e. Alteration of registered nurse and ancillary staff mix

---

management system. Each unit of analysis will require the use of the nurse researcher's expertise for selecting the most appropriate data with which to answer the research questions.

References

Acton, G.J., Irvin, B.L., & Hopkins, B.A. (1991). Theory-testing research: Building the science. *Advances in Nursing Science, 14*(1), 52-61.

Corner, J. (1991). In search of more complete answers to research questions. Quantitative versus qualitative research methods: Is there a way forward? *Journal of Advanced Nursing, 16,* 718-727.

Edelstein, E.L. & Cesta, T.G. (1993). Nursing case management: An innovative model of care for hospitalized patients with diabetes. *The Diabetes Educator, 19*(6), 517-521.

Jennings, B.M., & Rogers, S. (1986). Using research to change nursing practice. *Critical Care Nurse, 9*(5), 76-84.

Kenneth, H.K., & Stiesmeyer, J.K. (1991). Strategies for involving staff in nursing research. *Dimensions of Critical Care Nursing, 10*(2), 103-107.

Lederman, R.P. (1991). Quantitative and qualitative research methods: Advantages of complementary usage. *The American Journal of Maternal/Child Nursing, 16,* 43.

Mitchell, P.H., Ferketich, S., & Jennings, B.M. (1998). Quality health outcomes model. *Journal of Nursing Scholarship, 30*(1), 43-46.

Nachmias, D., & Nachmias, C. (1981). *Research methods in the social sciences.* New York: St. Martin's Press.

Polit, D., & Hungler, B. (1983). *Nursing research.* Philadelphia: J.B. Lippincott Company.

Rogers, B. (1992). Research utilization, *AAOHN, 40*(1), 41.

Schaefer, K.M. (1989). Clinical research: Gaining access to patients. *Dimensions of Critical Care Nursing, 8*(4), 236-242.

Swanson, J.M., Albright, J., Steirn, C., Schaffner, A., & Costa, L. (1992). Program efforts for creating a research environment in a clinical setting. *Western Journal of Nursing Research, 14*(2), 241-245.

Treece, E.W., & Treece, J.W. (1973). *Elements of research in nursing.* St. Louis: The C.V. Mosby Company.

Williams, A.D. (1991). Development and application of clinical indicators for nursing. *Journal of Nursing Care Quality, 6*(1), 1-5.

Documentation of Quality Care

CHAPTER OVERVIEW

For health care organizations to improve delivery of services, they must first determine their definition of quality. Recently, quality issues have moved from an organizational perspective to a consumer-oriented one, in which the needs and concerns of the customer count.

Among the elements measured in defining quality is patient satisfaction. Patients can be questioned directly through focus groups or indirectly through written questionnaires.

Each organization must determine its measures in relation to the incorporated case management documentation system. Patient, health care provider, and operational variances can be used to continuously improve quality. The case manager serves an important role in this process.

WHAT IS QUALITY?

The meaning of quality takes on a new twist when introduced as a concept relevant to health care. Quality may be seen in terms of its effect on the health care delivery system or on specific dimensions of the system (Institute of Medicine, 1976).

On the larger scale of the entire health care system, quality may include the availability and accessibility of health care services, credentialing requirements and standards of the providers, comprehensive assessment and documentation, collaborative and informed relationships with the patient and family, minimal injuries or complications in hospitalized patients, evaluation of new technology and resources, and effective management of health care resources (McCarthy, 1987).

The advent of the prospective payment system forced health care institutions to focus on health care as a business. Leaving good quality care to chance did not work and ultimately did not make good business sense. As organizations, regulatory agencies, and patient needs became more complicated, it became obvious that health care was no less a business than any other and that the product of the business was patient care. Increasingly, the value of that care depended on matching cost and quality. Before they could determine the value of the product, organizations had to know what the expected quality comprised.

Manufacturers, small-business owners, and large corporations have known for years that to provide quality, the organization or business must first determine its definition of quality (Davis, 1990). Discovering what attributes the organization wants to attain is one way to arrive at such a definition.

Health care organizations have already begun to realize that a change in the definition and measurement of quality is needed (Jones, 1991). The products of health care are often intangible items that are difficult to identify and measure. Quality assurance measures in the past have attempted to identify errors and then place blame on the individual who made the error. However, one could argue that counting the number of bedsores or medication errors only partially helps to define quality health care. It also did not provide a mechanism for monitoring and then *improving* quality.

Consumer Focus

As in business, it became obvious that one useful technique for defining quality health care was to ask the recipients of that care how they defined quality. This technique of asking consumers what they want often highlights issues to which the health care practitioner is blind. In the past, our definition of quality was to count the number of patient falls. If the organization came in below the desired threshold, it was providing quality care. However, the patient's definition of quality care was care given by a competent, pleasant employee who was familiar with the patient and the patient's needs, providing a clean and quiet healing environment, and good food!

Of course, the issue of falls is an important one in terms of assuring quality, and patients will surely consider this equally important if they have ever fallen. The point is, once the customer's needs have been queried and identified, an entirely new area can be addressed. Invariably the necessary dimensions of quality that the consumer identifies focus on the business end of health care. This area has been ignored in the past. Organizations believed they knew what patients needed and supplied it to them within the constraints and needs of the organization. The patient had to conform to the organization. There are occasions when this approach is truly necessary. But remaining forever in this mindset eliminates the possibility of ever going beyond providing basic services, and it does not allow for an atmosphere of continual improvement.

By determining what constitutes quality, it can be measured. Once measured, it can be managed. Managing care allows for a process of continual improvement toward excellence, and excellence is the definition of quality.

PATIENT SATISFACTION

With a renewed focus on patient needs, the issue of how to measure patient satisfaction has never been more important. Patient satisfaction is quickly becoming the benchmark for measuring quality health care (Roth & Schoolcraft, 1998). Customer needs not only are identified but also are the basis on which quality improvements are made. Within the mission statement of most health care organizations is a clause that cites patient satisfaction as a goal. Although the health care industry has always identified itself as a service industry, clearly this was a self-serving need. In most instances the attitude of health care providers was that the patient was lucky to be getting what he or she was getting.

How often have nurses used the following phrases in defense of a system that was obviously failing the patients and customers?

"You had to wait 5 days for a CAT scan? Well, Mrs. Jones had to wait 6 days. Aren't you lucky?"
"You haven't seen your surgeon since the operation? That is something you are going to have to accept if you want to have the best surgeon in this field."

The patients were certainly not lucky to be sick, to be in the hospital, or to be having surgery. When even minimal expectations are not being met, something is terribly wrong with the system.

Customer service will be what defines quality in the next century. Health care organizations that provide service to all customers, from physicians to patients to the community, will be the most successful. The focus must shift away from a purely organizational approach to one that blends consumer and organizational needs (Strasen, 1991).

Depending on the philosophy, resources, and goals of the organization, the approach for measuring patient satisfaction can be made in a number of ways. Generally a questionnaire is used to gauge the level of patient satisfaction. Such a survey can be administered while the patient is in the hospital or after discharge (Steiber & Krowinski, 1990). Generally an attempt is made to administer the questionnaire 24 to 48 hours before discharge. However, some patients may be intimidated by a questionnaire that is filled out while they are still in the hospital, fearing that if a bad report is given, one of the health care providers may retaliate with less than optimal care. On the other hand, patients' memories of their hospital stays will be most vivid if recorded while still in the hospital. Positive and negative impressions will be fresh in their minds, and these impressions can provide valuable information.

However, patients who are queried after discharge, in the safety and comfort of their homes, may be more likely to provide honest information because they have no fear of retribution. Unfortunately, positive and negative experiences can be quickly forgotten once the patient is home, which means valuable information can be lost if patients are questioned in this manner.

The pros and cons of each method must be evaluated by each organization. There is no perfect way, and it is possible that some form of patient satisfaction questioning is already in place. These data can be used both as pre-implementation data and for ongoing studies.

If the questionnaires are administered to patients while they are in the hospital, someone who is not directly involved in the patient's care should administer the survey. This method will help to diminish any potential for bias.

Because people who are ill or who have been ill recently are being questioned, care should be taken to select a questionnaire that has short, understandable questions. The focus of each question should be clear to the patient. Patients who are questioned while still in the hospital are more likely to be experiencing increased anxiety or other physical conditions that may affect their ability to participate.

It is best to select instruments that have been identified previously as valid and reliable. Most instruments use closed-ended questions in which a series of possible choices are given. This format is easiest to score and analyze statistically. Open-ended questions provide the investigator with less control of response content and are more difficult to analyze. Even so, the open-ended format may provide the most meaningful information. It may be beneficial to design an instrument that combines both closed-ended and open-ended questions. This allows for some control over responses and the opportunity to elicit useful anecdotal information.

The focus of the survey also may depend on the philosophy and goals of implementing the case management system. Many patient satisfaction surveys focus on hygiene needs, such as food, room comfort, noise, and so on. Although these factors are important, they may not be capturing the elements that a case management system is attempting to change. Therefore it may be necessary to find a questionnaire that focuses more on the professional care provided. In some cases the institution may have to develop its own instrument that clearly questions the patients with regard to this unique switch to case management.

Developing an instrument can be difficult. The decision to develop a unique questionnaire should not be taken lightly. If the organization is looking for immediately valid and reliable results, the use of a pilot instrument is not the best route to take. The use of more than one instrument is one way to address this dual requirement so that the needs of both the organization and the researcher can be met. Previously established questionnaires allow for a rapid compilation of information with which to measure implementation. In the long run, however, a new questionnaire, aimed at determining specific effects of the case management system on the patient, will contribute a great deal to the validation of the model's efficacy. In addition, the questionnaire can be used by other organizations that implement case management systems.

Another technique is the qualitative method. Qualitative assessment is used to compile data that can be used later in a self-report or paper-and-pencil questionnaire. Patient-focused groups and interviews provide data for the development of written questions. Qualitative approaches allow the researcher to see the situation through the experience of the patient. The patient's perceptions are used to compile information that is later categorized. These categories are then transformed into specific questions.

The qualitative method is time consuming. Personal interviews or focus groups last from 1 to 2 hours, but the researcher must devote even more time to use this form of data collection. However, the information gained can be invaluable.

Determining which patients to question is really a matter of good research technique. The sample should be as heterogeneous as possible to allow for the greatest deal of generalizability. Random sampling will provide this.

Every health care organization compiles statistics that are fed back to regulatory agencies. This information is generally used to determine accreditation and licensing and to analyze mistakes, untoward effects, and outcomes. Information categorizing the number and type of falls, infections, and medication administration errors has been tracked for years. Analysis of these data helps identify patterns or frequent offenders. Such a system has been referred to as the "bad apple" approach. If a health care practitioner makes a mistake, that person is counseled. If the practitioner makes the same kind of mistake repeatedly, more serious intervention on the part of the employer might take place. This system does not take into account possible system issues that may contribute to the problem. Instead, one person is seen as the cause of the problem as well as the means for fixing it.

This approach not only looks for the bad apple but also lies in wait for the accident or error. The approach does not provide a mechanism for addressing the larger elements of the problem, and it does nothing to control the recurrence of this problem. Nevertheless, most institutions evaluating case management systems have turned to the bad-apple approach in an attempt to improve quality patient care. A reduction in patient falls or patient infections might be reported as a result of the introduction of a case management model. In reality, the factors leading to a fall or an infection go beyond a managed care plan or a case manager.

If the goal of data analysis is to improve the quality of care, a method other than the bad-apple approach must be selected. Patient care is simply too multidimensional to be analyzed effectively by this method. Identifying more appropriate data to measure will come as a direct result of establishing a definition of quality. Case management data are positive outcome data because they focus on the expected outcomes of the interventions in which we participate as health care providers. The case management plan provides all the expected outcomes of care during hospitalization, from patient teaching expectations to expected resource use to expected length of stay. It also provides for the expected clinical outcomes of care.

These expected outcomes provide the foundation for determining quality care. By delineating these outcomes, each discipline is identifying the quality issues around a particular diagnosis or procedure (Baker, Miller, Sitterding, & Hajewski, 1998).

Additional indexes of patients' perceptions of quality can be identified. These indicators should be incorporated into any measure of quality. Until the organization has converted to a case management system or until the new case management plans are in place, it may be necessary to continue to report the quality assurance data to obtain baseline indexes of quality. Ultimately this format can be abandoned or combined with other quality indicators.

CRITERIA FOR MEASURING OUTCOMES

Some of the outcomes identified on the case management plan can be tracked during hospitalization. These outcomes are the day-to-day clinical, psychosocial, and teaching interventions. The case manager addresses these on a daily basis and ensures that the patient is moving along the continuum of health care in a timely fashion. If any outcome is not achieved, the case manager is responsible for determining why and correcting the problem or changing the plan.

The unit of analysis within the case management plan will vary depending on the increments in which the hospital stay is measured. For example, while most case management plans are developed on the basis of the 24-hour day, others may have longer or shorter units of analysis. In the neonatal intensive care unit, where the expected length of stay can run from 1 to 3 months, daily measures are not appropriate. In this case the managed care plans are "time-lined" in 1-week intervals, during which the expected outcomes should be achieved.

In some cases, such as an emergency room setting, the time frames may be short. Then the case management plan time frames are set at 15-minute or 30-minute intervals. During these shorter time periods, specific outcomes are expected. Whatever the time frame, it should realistically correlate to the clinical situation being planned. Once a unit of analysis or time period is chosen, analysis can begin.

In case management, anything that does not happen when it is supposed to happen is called a variance. Variances alert practitioners to changes in the patient's condition, or they highlight problems in the health care delivery system itself. Any variances that occur are identified daily as well as retrospectively. Every expected outcome on the plan is a potential variance, and, unless the outcome is achieved within a predetermined time period, it falls into the variance category. As outlined in Chapter 16, there are four causes for variances: the patient, the health care provider, operations, or unmet clinical indicators.

There are two types of patient variances. The first is a patient variance, comorbidity, or a condition identified on admission. These conditions may or may not require an alteration in the usual plan for that diagnosis or procedure. For example, a patient allergy identified on admission might mean that a drug usually considered standard for that diagnosis or procedure cannot be administered. As a result, the plan of care must be discussed with the physician, who decides either to refrain from using the drug or to replace it with a suitable alternative.

In some cases the variance is noted, but no change is made to the plan at that time. An example of this is a patient who has diabetes. The person admitting this patient reviews the plan and notes that no changes are needed. The patient's condition still must be noted in the Patient Exception on Admission section of the case management plan. This section may also be labeled as preexisting conditions or comorbidities. This alerts all health care providers that the patient has diabetes. It also indicates that the plan was individualized at the time of admission.

The other type of patient variance is one that the patient causes. In other words, this type involves situations in which an expected outcome cannot be achieved because of the patient's condition or noncompliance.

For example, a tuberculosis case management plan might call for collection of sputum specimens on the first, second, and third days of hospitalization. If the patient cannot produce sputum on the second day, that outcome cannot be achieved within the anticipated time frame. In such a case, specimen collection is moved to the third and fourth days.

An example of a patient variance caused by noncompliance might occur on the second postoperative day, when the plan calls for the patient to dangle the legs over the edge of the bed. Because of pain, the patient refuses. Despite pain medication, the patient continues to refuse. This refusal results in an inability to achieve the desired outcome, and the patient's plan must be adjusted accordingly.

By reviewing the patient's progress throughout the day and anticipating the course of recovery for the entire hospital stay, the case manager can adjust the plan so that the variance does not change the length of stay. If the patient refuses to ambulate, the "dangling" and "out-of-bed-to-the-bathroom" goals can be combined into expected outcomes for the following day, when the patient is feeling better. Another possibility might be to try the dangling step again on the next shift, when the pain medication is more effective.

Regardless of the reason for the variance, the case manager and the staff nurse should be aware of the recovery protocol and should attempt to get the patient back on track as soon as possible. This method helps avoid unnecessary delays and makes the patient's progress and expected plan well known and easily tracked. This in turn means that potential problems will be less likely to continue for several days without being noticed.

A health care provider variance is caused by an omission or error made by a health care practitioner. Institutions have unique regulations regarding documentation, and employees must acquaint themselves with these policies. However, mistakes are bound to occur.

An example of a health care provider variance might involve a transcription error. If a physician order for a medication is not transcribed by the nurse but the error is detected on the next shift, the patient might have missed a dose of the medication. Other health care provider variances involve changes in practice patterns that alter the patient's predetermined case management plan.

Operational variances are probably the most common variances. Operational variances include those that happen within the confines of the hospital as well as some caused by a condition outside the hospital.

A large-system variance, one that occurs because of something outside the hospital, might involve discharge placement. These types of variance would fall within the operational category. Sometimes a patient is assessed as appropriate for nursing home placement, so all the paper work is completed, and the patient is clinically ready for discharge, but no nursing home beds are available. As a result, the patient remains in the hospital until a bed becomes available, and the extended stay is classified as a large-system variance.

The most typical large-system variances are postdischarge problems in which a proper discharge location is not available. This type of variance is difficult to control. The best prevention is for the case manager to attempt to identify those patients who will need placement as early in the hospital stay as possible and begin to prepare the necessary paperwork so that delays can be avoided.

Other operational variances can occur because of the institution's infrastructure. Most health care institutions are large, complex places. Systems have developed over time, often without planning. Once these systems are in place, most workers are too busy to correct the operational problems. Instead, informal mechanisms are developed to work around the flaw in the system. Such operational problems can delay the patient's progress toward discharge. An inadequate patient-scheduling system may mean that the nursing unit is unaware of a scheduled procedure and the patient is not correctly prepped. Thus the procedure cannot be performed, which may increase the length of stay.

Other operational variances occur when equipment breaks. One such operational variance is an inability to complete a computed tomography (CT) scan because the machine is not functioning. Any equipment malfunction results in a delay, which in turn takes the patient off the case management schedule. Clinical quality indicators are those expected clinical indicators identified by the physician that may include intermediate and discharge outcomes. These indicators are used to assess clinical progress and quality of care. See Chapter 32 for more information on variances.

Any of these variances require the input of the case manager, whose responsibility it is to identify the variance and intervene to correct it. The goal is to minimize the effect the variance will have on the patient's length of stay.

The other responsibility of the case manager is to document the variance. Retrospective analysis of operational variances results in the identification of frequently occurring, but rectifiable, problems. It is important that variances also be documented for the purposes of utilization review and reimbursement.

References

Baker, C.M., Miller, I., Sitterding, M., & Hajewski, C.J. (1998). Acute stroke patients: Comparing outcomes with and without case management. *Nursing Case Management, 3*(5), 196-203.

Davis, W.W. (1990). Quality care and cost control? *The Case Manager, 1*(3), 24-29.

Institute of Medicine. (1976). Assessing quality in health care: An evaluation. (DHEW Publication No. 282-75-0437 PM). Washington, D.C.: National Academy of Sciences.

Jones, K.R. (1991). Maintaining quality in a changing environment. *Nursing Economics, 9*(3), 159-164.

McCarthy, C. (1987, Feb.). Quarterly health care inches closer to precise definition. *Hospital Peer Review,* 19-20.

Roth, T.A., & Schoolcraft, M. (1998). Patient satisfaction: The survey says. *Nursing Case Management, 3*(5), 184-189.

Steiber, S.R., & Krowinski, W.J. (1990). *Measuring and managing patient satisfaction.* Chicago: American Hospital Publishing.

Strasen, L. (1991). Redesigning hospitals around patients and technology. *Nursing Economics, 9*(4), 233-238.

The Link Between Continuous Quality Improvement and Case Management

CHAPTER OVERVIEW

The continuous quality improvement (CQI) process has gradually been adapted to the health care setting to improve quality without increasing costs. In traditional quality assurance models, quality is measured by the number of accidents or errors occurring. No provision is made for improving the conditions under which the errors occurred.

However, continuous quality improvement focuses on the processes used to achieve a goal. These processes may be clinical, financial, or operational issues. Each step in the process is analyzed; then a plan for improvement is tested and refined.

The three leaders in the CQI process are Deming, Juran, and Crosby. Each has made unique contributions toward improving the quality of work performed in the industrial setting. Now their concepts are being applied in the health care arena.

Case management and CQI are linked in philosophy and process. The steps of the CQI process can be applied to managed care plans from both clinical and financial perspectives.

INTRODUCTION TO CONTINUOUS QUALITY IMPROVEMENT (CQI)

The CQI process was officially introduced in 1991 as a more effective approach to improving the quality of health care. In that year the JCAHO announced that it would be introducing new standards requiring all chief executive officers of hospitals to be educated on CQI methods (*Hospitals*, 1991). This mandate went into effect for accreditation surveys as of January 1, 1992.

This seemingly abrupt switch from traditional quality assurance methods to an approach that had had tremendous success in the business arena was timely. Quality had become the promotional tool for many health care organizations as they adopted a more consumer-oriented approach (Naisbitt, 1982).

At the same time the prospective payment system had changed the speed and scope of health care delivery. Techniques that had been successful in the past were no longer financially feasible. Change, once considered something to be avoided, was hailed as the way to financial viability for the industry

(Kanter, 1983). The changes included new and more effective management styles that could provide quality under a cost-containment umbrella.

Another force driving the need for change was an emerging consumerism (Naisbitt, 1982). The average person had become an educated health care consumer who expected quality care. Consumers wanted to be involved in their care, which included participation in decisions involving treatment, cost, and self-care (O'Connor, 1984).

Continuous quality improvement falls in the realm of total quality management, a concept originated by W. Edward Deming (*Hospital Peer Review,* 1988). Quality improvement involves an analysis, understanding, and improvement of the processes of care. In the case of the health care industry, these processes include the hospital system, the personnel, the clinical management, and the financial structure surrounding each patient case.

In this format, quality is defined as the meeting or exceeding of customer requirements (Marszalek-Gaucher & Coffey, 1990). In other words, the customer defines quality. Suppliers and customers are involved in each of the above mentioned processes. The supplier is the one who passes on the patient, information, or equipment, and the customer is the one who receives the patient, information, or equipment.

One of the first steps in CQI is the identification and study of the individual steps that make up each of the processes of health care. This CQI extends beyond individual departments because the exchanges between departments are usually the areas that yield difficulties. Each process can be broken down into its working parts in various ways. One way involves use of a flow chart. The flow chart pictorially de-

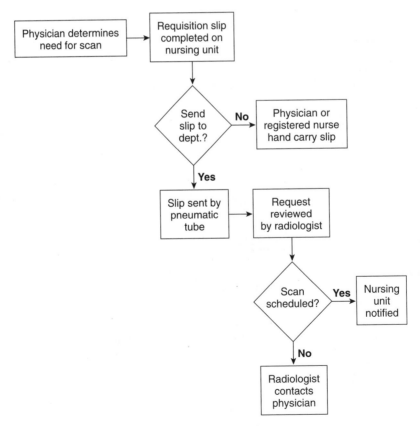

FIGURE **42-1**   Flow diagram of CT scan scheduling process.

scribes each step and helps identify where bottlenecks or overuse of resources is occurring. Fig. 42-1 is a simplified example of how a computed tomography (CT) scan scheduling process is broken down into its major steps.

Root causes of problems are identified through the flow chart. Once the root causes have been determined, more data can be gathered and the team can begin selecting solutions. It is necessary to pick the root cause that may result in the greatest initial improvement of the process. Additional causes can then be addressed after one solution has been tried. At this point, more data should be collected to evaluate whether the solution was given enough time to take hold and whether it was effective.

TRADITIONAL QUALITY ASSURANCE

The health care industry has been crippled by waste and misuse of resources (Marszalek-Gaucher & Coffey, 1990). Within this wasteful environment, quality care has always been difficult to measure (Goldfield & Nash, 1989). Compounding this difficulty is the unabated growth of industry inspection, which has resulted in an adversarial relationship between health care organizations and inspection agencies. Sanctions mandating quality as defined by agencies, such as the Peer Review Organizations (PRO), the Joint Commission on the Accreditation of Healthcare Organizations (JCAHO), the state licensing agencies, and others, have resulted in measures designed to ensure minimum expectations rather than continuous improvement (Laffel & Blumenthal, 1989).

Relatively arbitrary thresholds have been established within organizations. These thresholds define minimum expectations and identify bad apples but do not provide any mechanism for finding causes or suggestions for improvements. These techniques for assuring quality do not address health care's increasing need for improvement in all processes of the industry (Donabedian, 1980). It is clear that while quality must be maintained, systems have to be designed for improving business at all levels.

The traditional quality assurance process provides a system for identifying opportunities to improve care or solve problems. These opportunities are based on the collection of information regarding incidents or errors that have surpassed a predetermined threshold (Box 42-1). Factors affecting the occur-

---

Box 42-1 ▸ QUALITY ASSURANCE MONITORING AND EVALUATION

THE 10-STEP PROCESS
Assign responsibility for monitoring and evaluating activities.
Delineate the scope of care provided by the organization.
Identify the most important aspects of care provided by the organization.
Identify indicators (and appropriate clinical criteria) for monitoring the important aspects of care.
Establish thresholds (levels, patterns, trends) for the indicators that trigger evaluation of the care.
Monitor the important aspects of care by collecting and organizing the data for each indicator.
Evaluate care when thresholds are reached in order to identify either opportunities to improve care or problems.
Take actions to improve care or to correct identified problems.
Assess the effectiveness of the actions and document the improvement in care.
Communicate the results of the monitoring and evaluation process to relevant individuals, departments, or services and to the organization-wide quality assurance program.

Copyright 1990 by the Joint Commission on Accreditation of Healthcare Organizations, Oakbrook Terrace, Illinois. Reprinted with permission.

rence of the incidents, the systems affecting the errors, or processes for improvement are not identified.

In addition, errors or incidents are identified through individual finger-pointing based on the mistake of one person. Therefore each quality issue appears to be the fault of one particular person, acting independently. This focus removes all accountability from the organization or the systems within which the individual practitioner is working.

THE NEW HEALTH CARE AGENDA

Quality has become paramount on the health care agenda. Industrial models of quality improvement have been adopted and used successfully in the health care arena. Industry's goals, the reduction of costs and the improvement in the quality of the product, match those of health care. More than a decade ago, industrial leaders realized that to compete and survive in a world economy, quality improvement techniques were needed that would yield significant operational improvements (Drucker, 1991; Hickman & Silva, 1984; Naisbitt & Aburdene, 1985; Tichy & Devanna, 1986).

The three individuals most closely associated with these processes are Philip B. Crosby, W. Edwards Deming, and Joseph M. Juran. Crosby is probably the best known of the three quality experts. His approach is based on his *14 steps* for the quality improvement process (QIP) (Crosby, 1979):

1. Management commitment
2. Quality improvement team
3. Measurement
4. Cost of quality
5. Quality awareness
6. Corrective action
7. Zero defects planning
8. Employee education
9. Zero defects
10. Goal setting
11. Error cause removal
12. Recognition
13. Quality councils
14. Do it all over again

Crosby (1979) explains that his efforts differ from those of Juran or Deming in that these *14 steps* provide a complete process. This process, says Crosby, provides a methodology for improving quality, not just a series of quality improvement techniques.

W. Edward Deming is the leading figure in quality improvement. It was Deming who, working with Japanese manufacturers in the 1950s, was responsible for the tremendous improvements made in Japanese manufacturing. To make improvements, Deming relies on technical expertise as well as statistical analysis. His work helped place the Japanese in a completely different class of manufacturing.

Deming's (1986) approach places emphasis on 14 points, which have been used in the transformation of American industry:

1. Create constancy of purpose for improvement of product service.
2. Adopt a new philosophy.
3. Cease dependence on inspection to achieve quality.
4. End the practice of awarding business on the basis of price tag alone. Instead, minimize total cost by working with a single supplier.
5. Improve constantly every process for planning, production, and service.

6. Institute training on the job.
7. Adopt and institute leadership.
8. Drive out fear.
9. Break down barriers between staff areas.
10. Eliminate slogans, expectations, and targets for the work force.
11. Eliminate numerical quotas for the work force and numerical goals for management.
12. Remove barriers that rob people of pride of workmanship. Eliminate the annual rating or merit system.
13. Institute a vigorous program of education and self-improvement for everyone.
14. Put everybody in the company to work to accomplish the transformation.

Deming (1986) may be best known for his work in involving the employee in the quality improvement system. Concepts such as the "quality circle" or the "QC circle" grew out of the development of these processes, which involved groups of employees in problem identification and solving. Perhaps most relevant in adapting Deming's work to the health care industry is its focus on implementing intervention strategies to improve quality and reduce cost. Other aspects applicable to health care are the continuous improvement in quality and the use of employee teams trained in problem-solving techniques (Deming, 1986).

Juran was with Deming in the 1950s in Japan and had previously worked with Deming in the 1920s at the Hawthorne Western Electric Plant in Chicago. Juran, like Deming, is considered a pioneer and an expert in quality improvement technology. Best known for his *quality trilogy* (Juran, 1987, 1988), Juran broadened the quality approach to a wider operational or managerial perspective:

Quality planning: The process of developing the products and processes required to meet customer needs.
Quality control: The regulating process through which actual performance is measured and compared to standards and the difference is acted on.
Quality improvement: The organized creation of beneficial change.

The structure, process, and outcome approaches of these quality issues can be operationalized and evaluated for continuous improvement. With the patient as the focus, quality is identified as those factors most important to patient and family. If asked, the patient might identify many of the factors outlined in Fig. 42-2 as important to his or her care.

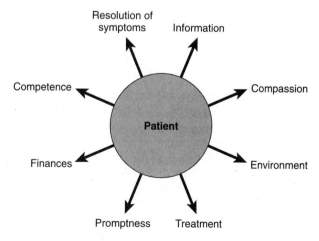

FIGURE **42-2** Patient care concerns.
(Courtesy A. Ron & M. Holtz.)

THE LINK TO CASE MANAGEMENT

Data for analysis in traditional quality assurance methods have focused on "unquality" or "disquality," such as infections, falls, medication errors, returns to the operating room, and deaths.

Some of these elements focus on the institution, such as global indicators of quality within the hospital. Examples of global indicators include morbidity and mortality and generic risk-management indicators. The focus of these elements has been on those identified as outliers.

Another traditional data base has been financial data and analysis, which tracks the cost of specific procedures or diagnosis-related groups (DRGs). The finance department uses this information to determine case mix index, which in turn helps determine the reimbursement rate.

Data related to individual practitioners have been more loosely followed. Utilization review evaluators and other quality management departments have focused on specific practice patterns.

Within case management, each of these elements can be followed more comprehensively. The data, once collected, are linked to CQI methods. The first step in a CQI process such as this is to identify problems that appear to be more than isolated events and to identify all of the issues that may be affecting the outcome. These issues might be linked to a DRG cost analysis as well as to individual practice patterns. In a case management framework, all practitioners are monitored for quality, use of resources, and length of stay. (Walrath, Owens, and Dziwulski, 1998.)

The case management plan is the foundation for this kind of data collection and analysis. The case management plan provides a guideline for administering care to a particular patient type. These plans take into consideration not only length of stay but also resource use. During the development of the case management plan the optimal treatment plan, one that streamlines care without compromising quality, is identified.

If planned correctly, these collaborative guidelines are agreed on by the group of practitioners for whom the guidelines are relevant. These plans, in essence, describe the one best treatment plan for a particular patient problem. By following these guidelines, quality issues are easily tracked. The case management plan provides the collection and evaluation of variances or complications or both. These data may or may not reveal the need to alter the plan to improve quality (Deming, 1986).

For example, a plan for the treatment of pneumonia may indicate that more than 50% of the patients managed by this plan develop some complication on the third or fourth day. This pattern is seen when retrospectively analyzing the variances documented on the case management plan. A review of this information may indicate the need for a change in the protocol. This may mean providing some element of the plan either earlier or later in the hospital stay.

The cost of the hospital stay can also be followed through the use of the case management plans. Performance within a particular DRG can be tracked financially or through a quality perspective. Comparing case-managed patients to similar patients who are not case managed is one way to do this tracking. Another method is to compare physicians' practice patterns and any deviations from the care plan. This information then can be evaluated for both quality and cost.

Monitoring length of stay or cost before and after implementation of the case management system allows particular nursing units to be their own controls.

If nursing documentation is a part of the managed care plan, the documentation is reviewed for completeness. The registered nurse documents against each expected outcome as it appears on the plan. Thus the documentation more accurately reflects the plan of care and the expected outcomes.

In any case, the processes surrounding the quality issue become the main focus when a CQI approach is taken. Theoretically this process makes continuous analysis and improvement possible because it pinpoints every imperfection in the process and opens the door for change (Berwick, 1989).

THE COST OF QUALITY

Poor quality is costly (Marszalek-Gaucher & Coffey, 1990) and can be assessed by the following:

Cost associated with giving wrong medications or treatments
Increased costs related to misuse of personnel or product resources
Cost of delays
Loss of sales because of dissatisfied patients or physicians

Crosby stresses a "cost of quality" determination as part of the quality improvement process (*Quest for quality,* 1989). His outline parallels actions used when developing a managed care plan. However, the development of the managed care plan takes Crosby's process one step further because it addresses issues and incorporates solutions into the plan of care:

Audit medical records to determine medically unnecessary tests, treatments, or procedures and other factors contributing to increased cost or length of stay.
Meet with a quality assurance or utilization review representative and review incident reports to determine opportunities for improvement.
Interview key members of the organization to identify barriers to the smooth operation and coordination of care.
Interview the medical staff to identify areas for improvement.
Review and analyze patient records to identify costs that can be eliminated.
Evaluate current reporting procedures, information related to operations, and data related to patient satisfaction.

The cost-of-quality analysis identifies a number of potential opportunities for quality improvement. From a case management perspective the information may lay the foundation for managed care plans by taking into account the best, most cost-effective method available.

THE CQI PROCESS

The CQI process consists of a number of specific steps. Although it is not necessary to follow the steps in a precise sequence, all steps should be evaluated and addressed (Marszalek-Gaucher & Coffey, 1990). The achievement of quality care and cost savings is the foundation of both case management and CQI. The process is a cycle that continuously repeats itself.

As with the case management implementation process, the first major step in the CQI process is that of planning and preparing to improve; the second step is to implement; and the third step is to innovate.

Preparing to improve involves seven essential steps (Marszalek-Gaucher & Coffey, 1990). Once again, it is not necessary to follow them in precise order, but each should be addressed in some manner:

1. Find a process. The first step is to find a process that needs quality improvement, cost control, or both. These processes may be within a clinical, operations, or financial setting from admitting, to medication distribution, to billing.
2. Assemble a team that knows the process. It has been said that those who know the process best are those working the front line or those who work within the process on a day-to-day basis. Therefore a large percentage of the team should be those directly involved in health care delivery. Management should also be included because this division can remove obstacles and facilitate change and improvement. The members of the team should know the process they are evaluating.

3. Identify the customers and the process outputs and measure the customer expectations of these outputs. Quality has been defined as meeting or exceeding customer expectations (*Hospital Peer Review,* 1988). Because of the complexity of health care, each process may be made up of several smaller processes. The first thing the team should do is identify its customers, the outputs of each process, and the customer expectations regarding these outputs. In some cases, such as clinical settings, the expectations may not be those of individuals but of the profession as a whole. These expectations may be based on profession-wide standards for the practice of nursing and medicine.

4. Document the process. The process consists of a series of steps or inputs, each of which is working toward a particular output. Each step can usually be broken down into subsets, which are hierarchical. A fundamental knowledge of the process is necessary to identify each of the steps accurately, and this is why the input of the front-line worker is so important. A process cannot be managed or improved without this fundamental knowledge.

5. Generate output and process specifications. Specifications are measurable, explicit attributes expected of the process and the output. Output specifications may involve the expectations of the customers, which are considered expectations external to the process. However, process specifications are the key internal process factors. Each of the specifications must be measurable. When these specifications are achieved, quality is achieved. Quality is maintained by conforming to these specifications, which is precisely what the managed care plan facilitates. The expected outcomes, if met, ensure quality care has been delivered for that particular problem. As these processes and outputs are evaluated, the process is adjusted to continuously improve it.

6. Eliminate inappropriate variation. The sixth step involves implementation. Each specification denotes a measurement point, which is evaluated. One major goal is to prevent quality failures or variations. Two types of variations will occur. The first is random variation. These variations result from factors inherent in the process, and they occur each time the process is played out. The other form of variation is the specific variation, which is a variation that occurs because of one specific component within the process. Once the processes for improvement are implemented, specific variation frequency should be reduced. The goal of the CQI process is to eliminate as many specific variations as possible (Deming, 1986). This results in consistently high-quality output. Within case management the managed care plans allow for the documentation of variations in clinical practice. By working as a team the health care professionals can differentiate between random variation and specific variation. The elimination of inappropriate variations results in an approach to health care delivery in which only random variations occur. Random variations are inherent within every process because every patient is different, and every response to treatment is slightly different. These "noises" in the system occur for every process and affect every output.

7. Document continuous improvement. This is the final process and the one that makes continuous improvement possible. Once the opportunities for specific or nonrandom variations have been reduced or eliminated, improvements or innovations are introduced. Team members can make changes that result in improved quality or increased productivity. Because the opportunity for variation has been reduced, it is easier to evaluate the impact of the innovation. After such evaluation the change either becomes permanent, or the team discontinues its use.

Walter A. Shewhart described this method of using a stable process to test innovations as the *plan-do-check-act cycle* (PDCA) (Deming, 1986). First developed in the 1930s, this process has become known as the Shewhart cycle (Fig. 42-3; Deming, 1986).

The PDCA cycle is applied to the process used in case management for addressing and improving health care delivery for particular patient types. Planning involves the identification of specific clinical areas for improvement. As discussed earlier, these areas are either patients in a specific DRG or nurses in a particular unit chosen to undertake the switch to case management.

The plan step involves determining the best case management plan. The do step involves implementation of the case management approach. The third step, check, involves the analysis of variances that hinder efficient use of the plan. The effects of such variances can be observed by changes in length of stay, patient satisfaction, staff satisfaction, or costs. In some cases the plan might need further revisions until these tangible results are noted.

Step 1   **Plan:** Outline a change.
Step 2   **Do:** Carry it out on a small scale.
Step 3   **Check:** Observe the effects of change.
Step 4   **Act:** Adopt or modify the plan.

FIGURE **42-3**   The Shewhart cycle.

The act step is for modifications if needed. Minimal case management variances indicate that the plan is usable and can be adopted at that point as the standard. If the variances are not minimal, the process begins again with the plan changed, tested, checked, and finally adopted.

The aim of the team is to continuously improve the process. In health care the process may never be brought to a conclusion because of the evolutionary nature of the treatment of disease. Changing technology, an aging patient population, and economic considerations, all have a prolonged effect on the delivery of health care. Therefore the process probably will remain open ended and continuous.

In any case, each process should be seen as one that unremittingly moves forward because today's goals may be tomorrow's standard.

THE NURSE CASE MANAGER IN THE CQI PROCESS

The case manager can play a vital role in the quality improvement efforts of any organization. CQI can occur through the use of formal teams or through case by case clinical process changes made at the patient level. The case manager plays a vital role in both.

Identification of CQI teams can be done through analysis of the variance data collected by the case manager and analyzed by the case management department. Generally the systems-related variances are most helpful in identifying opportunities for quality improvement efforts. By noting recurring, aggregated variances related to the system, the case manager identifies opportunities for process improvement teams or projects. On the other hand, patient- or family-related variances will generally not provide data for process improvement, but may provide data needed for revisions of an existing guideline or pathway.

A case manager should always be part of any process improvement team, particularly those that originate from the variance collection process. The leader of the team should be an individual who has the greatest familiarity with the process being studied. This may be the director of a department, or in the case of clinical processes, a physician. The case manager will play an important role as either the facilitator of the team or as a member. The facilitator is responsible for organizing the entire improvement process, including setting up meetings, taking minutes, and providing any data that the team may need during their assessment process. Team members should have a working knowledge of the process and be active participants on the team, bringing their clinical insights to the process.

An important mechanism for facilitating this process is through variance collection and analysis. The case manager identifies quality improvement opportunities through anecdotal discoveries as well as through aggregated data. The facilitation/coordination function of the case manager opens the door to the discovery of system patterns that may need analysis or improvement. In addition, the aggregate of these noted variances will support the discovery and provide the foundation for a quality improvement effort. CQI, therefore, has its basis in the variance collection and analysis process, a fundamental component of case management.

References

Berwick, D.M. (1989, Jan. 5). Sounding board. *The New England Journal of Medicine, 53-56.*

Bryce, G.R. (1991, Feb.). Quality management theories and their application. *Quality, 23-26.*

Crosby, P.B. (1979). *Quality is free: The art of making quality certain.* New York: McGraw-Hill.

Deming, W.E. (1986). *Out of the crisis.* Cambridge, Mass.: Center for Advanced Engineering Study, Massachusetts Institute of Technology.

Donabedian, A. (1980). *Explorations in quality assessment and monitoring. Vol. 1: The definition of quality and approaches to its assessment.* Ann Arbor, Mich.: Health Administration Press.

Drucker, P. (1991, Nov.-Dec.). The new productivity challenge. *Harvard Business Review, 67-79.*

Goldfield, N., & Nash, D.B. (Eds.). (1989). *Providing quality care.* Philadelphia: American College of Physicians.

Hickman, C.R., & Silva, M.A. (1984). *Creating excellence: Managing corporate culture, strategy, and change.* Ontario, NY: New American Library.

Hospital Peer Review. (1988). Deming's philosophy improves quality. *13*(10), 12-24.

Hospitals. (1991, Aug. 5). New JCAHO standards emphasize continuous quality improvement (pp. 41-44).

Joint Commission on Accreditation of Hospitals. (1990). *Quality assessment and improvement proposed revised standards.* Chicago: Author.

Juran, J.M. (1987). *Juran on quality leadership: How to go from here to there.* Wilson, Conn.: Juran Institute.

Juran, J.M. (1988). *Juran on planning for quality.* New York: Free Press.

Kanter, R.M. (1983). *The change masters: Innovations for productivity in the American corporation.* New York: Simon & Schuster.

Laffel, G., & Blumenthal, D. (1989). The case for using industrial quality management science in health care organizations. *Journal of the American Medical Association, 262*(20), 2869-2873.

Marszalek-Gaucher, E., & Coffey, R.J. (1990). *Transforming healthcare organizations.* San Francisco: Jossey-Bass.

Naisbitt, J. (1982). *Megatrends: Ten new directions transforming our lives.* New York; Warner Books.

Naisbitt, J., & Aburdene, P. (1985). *Reinventing the corporation.* New York: Warner Books.

O'Connor, P. (1984). Healthcare financing policy: Impact on nursing. *Nursing Administration Quarterly, 8*(4), 10-20.

Quest for quality and productivity in health services. (1989, Sept.). Excerpts from the 1989 Conference Proceedings. Washington, D.C.

Tichy, N.M., & Devanna, M.A. (1986, July). The transformational leader. *Training and Development Journal,* 27-32.

Walrath, J.M., Owen, S., Dziwulski, E. (1998). Case management: A vital link to performance improvement. *Nursing Economics, 14,* 117-122.

Job Satisfaction

CHAPTER OVERVIEW

Many variables affect job satisfaction in the workplace. Among these variables, autonomy, professional status, and socialization are consistently and positively related to increases in job satisfaction for registered nurses. Job satisfaction has also been positively related to retention of nurses.

Case management models integrate many of the elements associated with greater job satisfaction, including autonomy, a feeling of connectedness on the job, and professional status.

Two case studies show the relationship between a case management model and job satisfaction. The Nursing Initiatives Program at Long Island Jewish Medical Center in New York demonstrated that the introduction of the case manager role on three pilot units increased job satisfaction and reduced vacancy rates for registered nurses. This study was replicated at Beth Israel Medical Center in New York City. Data on three pilot units were collected before start-up and after 9 months. Outcomes demonstrated improved job satisfaction for staff registered nurses and case managers and reductions in vacancy and turnover rates.

JOB SATISFACTION AS A VARIABLE

Among the variables affected by the implementation of a case management model is staff job satisfaction. The introduction of a case manager to a nursing unit can improve the work environment and thus the level of job satisfaction of nurses working there.

The case manager plans and organizes the care of patients who have the most complex cases, assists with patient teaching, and follows through with discharge planning. In an era when many nurses complain that they spend more time documenting patient care, meeting regulatory documentation requirements, filling out requisitions, or making telephone calls than they do with patients, this model allows nurses to remain at the bedside while ensuring that all peripheral patient needs are met. Because the case manager relieves staff nurses of some of the indirect nursing functions related to their patients' care, many staff nurses report that they are able to spend more time in direct contact with their patients.

Clearly the case management model builds in a support system to help busy practitioners meet complex patient needs. The model promotes independent practice in those nurses providing the direct patient care. But it does not expect these same nurses to function in a vacuum without the proper support systems to meet all their patients' needs in a rapid-paced, complicated health care environment.

Job satisfaction has been related to nurses' job-turnover rates (Curry et al., 1985; Reich, 1984; Slavitt, Stamps, Piedmont, & Haase, 1978). Choi et al. (1989) demonstrated that nurses' overall dissatisfaction with their work was the strongest predictor of intent to leave the place of employment or current position. Job satisfaction has been directly related to nurse retention and turnover (Hinshaw & Atwood, 1982; Weisman, Alexander, & Chase, 1981). Therefore the importance of this variable should not be overlooked when a new nursing care delivery system is being designed or evaluated.

A case management model affects the staff nurses providing direct patient care as well as the case managers. The model takes a team approach to care. The team consists of the patient, the family, the physician, the case manager, the direct nursing care provider, the social worker, and others as needed. The model brings all members of the team together with a common focus. Whereas primary nursing led to feelings of isolation and separation for the direct care providers, the case management model does just the opposite. The model's structure works to bring everyone together. Each member supplies information relevant to the care of the patient, and value is placed on every member's input.

As a highly socialized model, case management allows for combined work units organized around a common goal: good patient care. Communication and conflict resolution become needed skills for each team member. If the members of the team cannot function as a group, the outcomes of care will not be achieved in a timely and efficient manner. Because these are among the primary goals of case management, group dynamics play a significant part in the success or failure of the model.

The case manager role, which fosters teamwork, also provides the nurse with an autonomous job that requires independent thought and action. The support provided by the case manager to the other nurse providers reinforces similar feelings of autonomy and independence in them (Alexander, Weisman, & Chase, 1982). It does this by positioning the direct-care provider in a strategic position. A team must rely on the information provided by each of its members, and it is the nurse responsible for direct patient care who provides the information that determines the clinical course of treatment, the teaching needs, and the discharge plan.

This enhanced role for nurses builds feelings of professionalism and self-esteem because nursing's input is valued and deemed important to the patient's progress. In the past, communication was of a hierarchical nature, with the physician dictating to the other members. In the case management model the nurse case manager serves as the thread that links all members of the team. Each member's input is needed so that appropriate and timely outcomes of care are achieved. In this system the staff nurse providing direct care at the bedside supplies the case manager and the rest of the team with valuable information.

As discussed in Chapter 35, clinical career ladders help organizations reward both experience and education. A case manager position allows clinically expert, educated, experienced nurses to take on increased responsibility while remaining close to the patient. The position provides for a new set of job responsibilities and a new wage scale that takes into account all these factors.

The case management model incorporates those elements that have been correlated to increased job satisfaction and decreased turnover. These elements include autonomy, a feeling of connectedness on the job, and salary (Johnston, 1991; McCloskey, 1990; Pooyan, Eberhardt, & Szigeti, 1990).

Some institutions have attempted to measure the satisfaction of their nurses when implementing a case management tool. Although it may be said that other factors can affect the nurses' feelings of satisfaction or dissatisfaction with their work—such as the physical work environment, the presence of a computerized clinical information system, the hours of work, or the fringe benefits—some of these other variables can be controlled by testing the same nurses before and after implementation.

CASE STUDIES

In 1988 as part of the United Hospital Fund's Nursing Initiatives Program, five hospitals—The Brooklyn Hospital Center, Long Island Jewish Medical Center, The Neurological Institute of the Presbyterian Hospital, The New York Hospital, and New York University Medical Center—were selected to orchestrate innovative methods for addressing the nursing shortage. Four of the sites proposed and tested new methods of structuring nursing care providers' work, with the goals of increasing nursing productivity, satisfaction, and retention. The fifth site, New York University Medical Center, introduced a stress reduction program with similar goals (Gould & Mezey, 1991).

Long Island Jewish Medical Center, New York

At Long Island Jewish Medical Center a new nursing position was created as part of the United Hospital Fund's program. The new position was titled patient care manager and became part of a case management delivery model. The position was designed specifically to match the nurse's expertise with the patient's needs and the severity of the illness. One of the reasons for the new position was to keep nurses at the bedside. The position provided the patient care manager with a challenging and rewarding role (Gould & Mezey, 1991).

Three data collection points were used to gauge nurses' job satisfaction. The first point was before implementation, the second at 1 year, and the third about 18 months into the project. Job satisfaction was measured by the Nursing Job Satisfaction Scale (Atwood & Hinshaw, 1981, 1984). The instrument, which has been tested for validity and reliability, was given to all nurses on all shifts at each collection point (Ake et al, 1991).

The medical center's implementation strategies were as follows:

Selecting expert registered nurses as patient care managers
Assigning patient care managers to coordinate care
Decentralizing unit decision making to registered nurses and physicians
Upgrading nursing attendant tasks
Establishing walking rounds

Registered nurse vacancy rates and registered nurse hours per patient were evaluated in addition to tracking nurse job satisfaction.

Nurses were chosen as patient care managers based on their clinical expertise and willingness to participate in what was, at that time, an experimental role.

The three units participating in the project were a 39-bed medical unit, a 32-bed surgical unit, and a 40-bed neonatal intensive care unit (NICU). At the end of the first 18 months of implementation, 20% of the registered nurses on each unit involved were patient care managers. They managed the care provided for one to three patients in addition to their regular direct care functions.

After about 1 year the patient care managers on the medical unit reported that this dual role was too difficult and stressful. At that time, one patient care manager was recruited to take on the role full-time and was removed from direct nursing role functions. This individual functioned in a truly autonomous and independent case management role.

Table 43-1	REGISTERED NURSE SATISFACTION BY SERVICE AND BY TITLE ON CASE-MANAGED PILOT UNITS AT LONG ISLAND JEWISH MEDICAL CENTER 1988-1990 (GOULD & MEZEY, 1991)					
	AT START-UP (1988)		**AT 12 MONTHS (1989)**		**AT 18 MONTHS (1990)**	
	N	**AVERAGE SCORE**	**N**	**AVERAGE SCORE**	**N**	**AVERAGE SCORE**
UNIT						
Medicine	20	87	26	90	19	94
Surgery	13	92	16	98	15	97
NICU	79	103	69	105	59	105
TOTAL	112		111		93	
Title						
Staff PCMs	26	99	17	104	15	110*
Other RNs	86	99	94	100	78	100
TOTAL	112		111		93	

*Patient care managers (PCMs) include all full-time and part-time PCMs.
NOTE: $p = .008$; lowest possible score: 23; highest possible score: 115.

Average nursing hours per patient remained relatively consistent throughout the project. However, the number of registered nurse hours per patient and the number of registered nurses on the unit decreased from 119.8 full-time equivalents (FTEs) at the start to 113.7 FTEs at 18 months, indicating an increase in productivity.

The registered nurse vacancy rate also improved during the 18-month period. On the medical unit the rate decreased from 8% to zero; on the surgical unit the vacancy rate decreased from 23% to zero; and in the NICU it remained constant at zero.

Among the most dramatic findings was the improvement in nursing job satisfaction, particularly comparing start-up scores to those at 18 months for nurses functioning as patient care managers and those working as staff nurses on the units (see Table 43-1).

Beth Israel Medical Center, New York, New York

The findings of the Nursing Initiatives Program at Long Island Jewish Medical Center pointed to a relationship between nurse roles and responsibilities and job satisfaction. The study was replicated at Beth Israel Medical Center in New York City to determine if the case manager role did indeed play an important part in the job satisfaction of registered nurses.

At the time of implementation of the three pilot units at the Beth Israel Medical Center in January 1991, all patient care managers were employed on a full-time basis, carrying a case load of 15 to 20 patients. Three pilot units were chosen for the study. These units included a 38-bed neurosurgical unit, a 12-bed acquired immunodeficiency syndrome (AIDS) unit, and a 45-bed medical/surgical unit for the chemically dependent. One case manager was employed on each unit on a full-time basis, meaning that all three were removed from direct care responsibilities.

Indirect care responsibilities included coordination and facilitation of services to the patient, multidisciplinary care planning, patient and family teaching, and discharge planning.

It was anticipated that the introduction of a case management model would increase employee job satisfaction. The case managers, working as staff nurses, remained close to the bedside. Relieved of any administrative responsibilities or direct nursing functions, the case managers were better able to provide not only indirect care to the patients but also assistance to other staff nurses.

The case manager was the only staff nurse working a 5-day-a-week schedule. The case manager was able to fill the information gaps caused by flextime schedules, which were fragmenting care. This built-in continuity factor allowed the staff nurse to spend more time in direct patient contact rather than in reviewing reports or trying to catch up on what happened to the patient in the nurse's absence.

It was also hypothesized that a case management documentation system would enhance registered nurse job satisfaction. With the new system, involving the use of multidisciplinary action plans (MAPs), the nurse could anticipate care needs on a daily basis. In addition, nursing documentation was collapsed onto the form itself, eliminating the need for long, narrative notes. Instead of paragraph notation, the nurse responded to a series of implementation strategies designed to achieve the goals outlined on the plan. Each 24-hour period was attended to separately, and enough room was provided so that all nurses caring for the patient within that period could document patient progress and outcomes.

The management of patient care provides a structure that addresses length of stay as well as quality of care. Because the case manager is not geographically bound within the nursing unit, this person is the primary caretaker for the patient and family from admission to discharge from the unit. The case manager's lack of geographic constraints and the 5-day-a-week schedule provide for continuity of care for the patient and family.

The case management system, which improves communication between staff members, leads to a greater feeling of teamwork and collegiality. In addition, the enhanced information base from which nurses function provides a greater level of autonomy in their practices.

All registered nurses working on the pilot units were tested for job satisfaction via the Nursing Job Satisfaction Scale (Atwood & Hinshaw, 1981, 1984). Testing took place before implementation and about 9 months after implementation of the case management model. Thirty registered nurses, or 70% of all nurses filling out questionnaires, completed the questionnaire at both data collection points. Of those 30, three were case managers and 27 were staff nurses. All three shifts were represented in the sample.

Job satisfaction scores before start-up and after 9 months indicate that there was a statistically significant increase in satisfaction for those nurses working on case-managed care units who were there for both data collection periods (Table 43-2). Comparisons of case managers to other staff nurses at both collection points indicated an increase for both groups (Table 43-2).

For all three units, both registered nurse vacancy rates and turnover rates decreased over the period of the pilot project (Table 43-3).

On neurosurgery the vacancy rate decreased from 17.33% at start-up to 6% at the end of 9 months. The turnover rate decreased from 21% to 12.5%. On the AIDS unit the vacancy rate went from 11% at start-up to 7% at the end of 9 months, and the turnover rate went from 9% to 7%. The medical/surgical unit for chemically dependent patients achieved a reduction in the vacancy rate from 9% to zero and a drop in turnover from 17% to 12% at the end of 9 months.

While largely anecdotal, there have been some recent studies measuring the work satisfaction of case managers in various settings. Lancero and Gerber (1995) studied the job satisfaction of nurse case managers as related to their control over nursing practice and their perceived job stress. These comparisons were made on two separate groups of nurse case manager, those working in a "within-the-walls" model, and those working in a "beyond-the-walls" model of case management. The within-the-walls model studied was the Acute Care Delivery (ACD) model practiced at Tucson Medical Center at Tucson, Arizona. The Carondelet Community based (CCB) Model was used to measure satisfaction within a beyond-the-walls model.

The ACD model, designed as a typical hospital-based model, had as its major goal to standardize the appropriate use of resources using standardized care planning methods. Case managers, with extensive

Table 43-2	REGISTERED NURSE SATISFACTION BY UNIT AND BY TITLE ON CASE-MANAGED PILOT UNITS AT BETH ISRAEL MEDICAL CENTER NEW YORK, NEW YORK			
	AT START-UP (12/90)		**AT 9 MONTHS (9/91)**	
	N	**AVERAGE SCORE**	**N**	**AVERAGE SCORE**
UNIT				
Neurosurgery	11	82	11	82
AIDS	9	88	9	91
Medical-surgical for chemical dependency	10	84	10	90
TOTAL	30		30	
TITLE*				
Patient care managers	3	78	3	86
Other RNs	27	84	27	89
TOTAL	30		30	

NOTE: T = 2.57, df = 29, p = 0.0157. Not significant at the .05 level. Lowest possible score: 23; highest possible score: 115.
*Data at both points.

Table 43-3	REGISTERED NURSE VACANCY AND TURNOVER RATES AT BETH ISRAEL MEDICAL CENTER BEFORE AND AFTER CASE MANAGEMENT INTRODUCED		
UNIT	**TIME**	**VACANY RATE**	**TURNOVER RATE**
Neurosurgery	Start-up	17.33%	21%
	9 Months	6%	12.5%
AIDS	Start-up	11%	9%
	9 Months	7%	7%
Medical/surgical for	Start-up	9%	17.6%
chemical dependency	9 Months	0	12%

clinical experience either functioned as unit-based case managers or across multiple in-patient units. The CCB model, a community-based model, links case managers to high risk patients with the goal of assisting them in achieving and maintaining their maximum level of wellness.

Both groups, the ACD and CCB, were tested on the 21-item Control Over Nursing Practice Scale (CONPS), the NCM Job Stress Index (NCMJSI), and the 29-item Work Satisfaction Index (WSI/NCM). Both groups were correlated positively with work satisfaction and negatively with job stress. A high degree of control over practice was highly correlated with positive work satisfaction. Both groups perceived the same amount of control over practice, whether they were working within the hospital or beyond the walls. One conclusion drawn by the investigators was that the role itself contributed to the sense of satisfaction rather than the setting in which the case manager was working. Interactions with physicians also contributed to higher job stress. The major conclusion of the study was that the high degree of autonomy in the role of case manager does contribute to less stress and greater job satisfaction.

Tonges (1998) studied the hypothesized differences between the characteristics of nurse case manager and staff nurse jobs, including intended positive effects and unintended negative effects. Nurse case managers reported significantly higher levels of autonomy, job identity, and collaboration with physicians. Conversely, they reported significantly more required interactions, which resulted in higher job stress, greater amounts of role conflict, ambiguity, and overload.

Goode's (1995) research demonstrated greater job satisfaction for staff engaged in multidisciplinary care map process and who provided care under a case management practice model. The effects indicated greater collaboration, autonomy, and satisfaction with quality of care. In addition, patients surveyed communicated increased satisfaction with their care and greater participation decision making.

References

Ake, J.M., Bowar-Ferris, S., Cesta, T., Gould, D., Greenfield, J., Hayes, P., Maislin, G., & Mezey M. (1991). The nursing initiatives program: Practice based models for care in hospitals. In *Differentiating nursing practice: Into the twenty-first century.* Kansas City, Mo.: American Academy of Nursing.

Alexander, C.S., Weisman, C.S., & Chase, G.A. (1982). Determinants of staff nurses' perceptions of autonomy within different clinical contexts. *Nursing Research, 31*(1), 48-52.

Atwood, J., & Hinshaw, A. (1981). Job stress: Instrument development program results. *Western Journal of Nursing Research, 3*(3), 48.

Atwood, J., & Hinshaw, A. (1984). Nursing job satisfaction: A program of development and testing. *Research in Nursing and Health.*

Choi, T., Jameson, H., Brekke, M.L., Anderson, J.G., & Podratz, R.O. (1989). Schedule-related effects on nurse retention. *Western Journal of Nursing Research, 11*(1), 92-107.

Curry, J., Wakefield, D., Price, J., Mueller, C., & McCloskey, J. (1985). Determinants of turnover among nursing department employees. *Research in Nursing and Health, 8,* 397-411.

Goode, C. (1995, Nov./Dec.). Impact of a CareMap and case management on patient satisfaction and staff satisfaction, collaboration, and autonomy. *Nursing Economics, 13*(6), 337-348.

Gould, D.A., & Mezey, M.D. (1991). *At the bedside: Innovations in hospital nursing.* New York: The United Hospital Fund of New York.

Hinshaw, A.S., & Atwood, J.R. (1982). Anticipated turnover: A preventive approach. *Western Journal of Nursing Research, 4,* 54-55.

Johnston, C.L. (1991). Sources of work satisfaction/dissatisfaction for hospital registered nurses. *Western Journal of Nursing Research, 13*(4), 503-513.

Lancero, A.W., & Gerber, R.M. (1995). Comparing work satisfaction in two case management models. *Nursing Management, 26* (11), 45-48.

McCloskey, J.C. (1990). Two requirements for job contentment: Autonomy and social integration. *Image, 22*(3), 140-143.

Pooyan, A., Eberhardt, B., & Szigeti, E. (1990). Work-related variables and turnover intention among registered nurses. *Nursing and Health Care, 11*(5), 255-258.

Reich, P.A. (1984). *The relationship between Jungian personality type and choice of functional specialty in nursing.* Unpublished master's thesis. Adelphi University, Garden City, N.Y.

Slavitt, D.B., Stamps, P.L., Piedmont, E.B., & Haase, A.M. (1978). Nurses satisfaction with their work situation. *Nursing Research, 27,* 114-120.

Tonges, M.C. (1998). Job design for nurse case managers. *Nursing Case Management, 3*(1), 11-23.

Weisman, C.S., Alexander, C.S., & Chase, G.A. (1981). Determinants of hospital staff nurse turnover. *Medical Care, 19,* 431-443.

Nurse Case Manager Job Characteristics and Effects on Well-Being*

Mary Crabtree Tonges

CHAPTER OVERVIEW

As managed care expands, nursing case management is becoming increasingly widespread. Yet little is known about the characteristics of the case manager job and its effects on nurses' workplace well-being. This study investigated hypothesized differences between the characteristics of the nurse case manager (NCM) and staff nurse (SN) jobs, including both intended positive and unintended negative effects associated with changes incorporated in the NCM job. NCMs reported significantly higher levels of autonomy, job identity, feedback from agents, and collaboration with physicians than SNs; however, they also reported higher levels of required interaction, role conflict, overload, and ambiguity. These findings have important implications for NCMs and the organizations that employ them, in relation to job design, career/candidate selection, and orientation and ongoing development.

Introduced in the mid-1980s (Ethridge, 1987; Zander, Ethridge, & Bower, 1987), hospital-based nursing case management is a relatively new innovation that has been widely implemented during the last decade (Sherer, 1993; Wake, 1990). Most hospitals currently have or are in the process of implementing some form of case management. With continued growth in managed care, particularly capitated contracts, this trend can be expected to continue.

Despite the growing popularity of nursing case management, however, little is known about the characteristics of this job and its effects on nurses' workplace well-being. Most of the studies that have been conducted focus on patient and organizational outcomes rather than effects on nurses (Lamb, 1992). While patient and organizational outcomes are clearly important, it is also recommended that hospital management monitor and evaluate the effects of changes in organizational design and nursing jobs on nursing personnel themselves (Institute of Medicine, 1996).

This research was partially funded by the American Organization of Nurse Executives Nursing Administration Research Award.
*Adapted with permission from Tonges, M.C. (1998). Job design for nurse case managers: Intended and unintended effects on satisfaction and well-being. *Nursing Case Management, 3*(1), 11-23.

This chapter presents summary findings from a study of the motivational characteristics of nursing jobs that examined links between these characteristics and nurses' job satisfaction, stress, and burnout. Building on these results, the study evaluated differences in the perceived characteristics of the nurse case manager (NCM) and staff nurse (SN) jobs, which is the primary focus of this discussion.

SIGNIFICANCE AND NEED FOR STUDY

As our nation's largest group of health professionals, nurses play an important role in the quality and cost of health care. Moreover, nurses can be part of the solution to key problems within the existing system by, for example, managing patients' care to achieve clinical outcomes more quickly and cost-effectively. Thus nurses' workplace well-being is a significant issue.

Job design theory directs "the design of the work itself—that is, changing the actual structure of the jobs that people perform" (Hackman & Oldham, 1980, p. 44) These changes are intended to increase the quality of employees' work experience as well as their performance. Many adults spend most of their waking hours at work, and workplace well-being has important personal consequences (Locke, 1983; Maslach, 1982; Motowidlo, Packard, & Manning, 1986).

From an organizational perspective, negative workplace well-being outcomes, including burnout (Maslach, 1982) and stress (Motowidlo, Packard, & Manning, 1986), are related to poor performance. Dissatisfaction (Price & Mueller, 1981, 1986) and burnout are also linked to turnover. In nursing specifically, job satisfaction is related to patient satisfaction, which is in turn associated with patients' compliance with care regimens (Weisman & Nathanson, 1985).

The Job Characteristics Model (JCM) developed by Hackman and his colleagues (Hackman & Lawler, 1971, Hackman & Oldham, 1976, 1980) is the most influential paradigm in contemporary job design theory and research. The JCM has provided the theoretical framework for hundreds of studies, and reviews of this evidence suggest that specified motivational characteristics of jobs are reliably related to personal and work outcomes (Berlinger, Glick, & Rodgers, 1988; Fried & Ferris, 1987). Yet it is important to note that the JCM grew out of research with industrial workers, which means that our current understanding of job design is rooted primarily in the study of manufacturing jobs. Given the transformation to a service economy, our knowledge of job design may no longer provide an adequate explanation of relationships between job characteristics and workers' responses.

In addition to the shift from manufacturing to service employment, other important changes are occurring in the world of work, including the redesign of existing jobs (Hammer & Champy, 1993). Based on a growing recognition of the need to focus on business processes rather than functional activities, many firms are reorganizing to enable one individual to ensure continuity in the performance of a series of tasks (e.g., fulfillment of a customer's order from beginning to end) (Hammer & Champy, 1993; Davenport & Nohria, 1994). This new approach, known as case management, redesigns business processes at the customer interface, (Tonges, 1989) and is characterized by the creation of a quintessential service role, in which case managers (CMs) buffer clients from the difficulties of dealing with complex organizational structures and processes (Hammer & Champy, 1993).

Davenport and Nohria pointed out that the CM job includes a number of elements, such as autonomy, that work motivation theorists identify as desirable (Davenport & Nohria, 1994). Yet they cautioned that the potential for satisfaction in these jobs may be paradoxically low. Potential sources of dissatisfaction include conflict with functional departments and existing procedures and a loss of face-to-face interactions in jobs mediated through a telephone or computer workstation. What these authors described is a common, yet under-researched phenomenon. Although real-life job design changes are often complex and may not create simple effects, our knowledge of how job dimensions combine to influence perceptions and reactions to work is limited.

Case management structures have been observed in various different industries, including banking (customer relationship management), insurance (underwriting and issuing new policies), and health care (patient care management) (Davenport & Nohria, 1994). Hospitals have been on the forefront of this trend. The change to prospective payment, coupled with nursing leaders' desire to enrich the SN job, led to the creation of the NCM job (Tonges 1989; Zander, 1988). Given its growing popularity and intended function as an enriched job, there is a pressing need to examine NCM job characteristics and links to nurses' well-being.

Purpose of Study

This study was designed to achieve the following: (1) test an extended model of job characteristics for human service professions and (2) investigate the characteristics of case management as a new job design expected to have mixed motivational consequences. Development and testing of the extended model have been reported in detail elsewhere (Tonges, 1997). This chapter focuses on the second component of the study—CM job characteristics—and provides an overview of the model testing component to create a context for presenting the CM findings.

Literature Review

As illustrated in Figure 44-1, the JCM identifies five core job dimensions (skill variety, task identity, task significance, autonomy, and feedback) that evoke three critical psychological states (CPS) (experienced

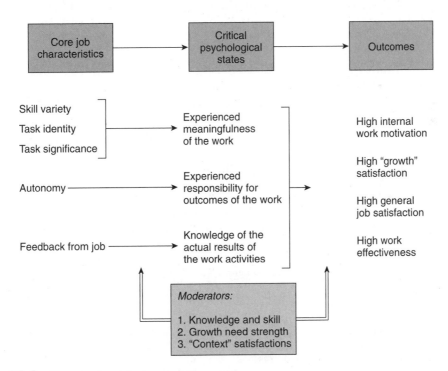

Figure 44-1   The complete job characteristics model.
(From Hackman, J.R., & Oldham, G.R. [1980]. Work redesign. Menlo Park, Calif. Addison-Wesley, p. 90. Reprinted with permission.)

meaningfulness of the work, experienced responsibility for outcomes of the work, and knowledge of the actual results of work activities). The CPS, in turn, lead to four desirable personal and work outcomes (high levels of internal work motivation, general job satisfaction, growth satisfaction, and work effectiveness) (Hackman & Oldham, 1976, 1980).

EXTENSION OF THE JCM

The JCM is generally a well-supported theory (Berlinger, Glick, & Rodgers, 1988; Fried & Ferris, 1987; Loher, Noe, Moeller, & Fitzgerald, 1985; Taber & Taylor, 1990); however, theory development is an evolutionary process, and a number of authors have recommended that job characteristics theory be modified or extended. Beginning with the characteristics and moving across the model, key recommendations concerning each set of constructs and responses to these potential limitations are summarized here.

Task Characteristics

Many researchers have suggested and/or found evidence that the five core dimensions of the JCM may not represent an exhaustive list of possible attributes (Sims, Szilagyi, & Keller, 1976; Stone & Gueutal, 1985; Taber & Taylor, 1990). Examples of additional job content characteristics that appear to have consequences for motivation and redesign efforts include speed, time, and physical danger (Jermier, Gaines, & McIntosh, 1989), as well as a service versus production orientation (Stone & Gueutal, 1985).

Other authors have called for an integration of job characteristics theory with role theory (Abdel-Halim, 1981; Loher, Noe, Moeller, & Fitzgerald, 1985; Tumulty, 1992). Such an integration would combine the narrower considerations of task design with more global aspects of role design, to gain a better understanding of individuals' reactions to their work, particularly in the service sector.

In addition to the five characteristics of the work itself specified by the JCM, this research evaluated the effects of an expanded set of interpersonal relationship and work role characteristics, thought to be especially relevant in service jobs (Mills, Hall, Leidecker, & Marguiles, 1983). These characteristics are defined as follows:

1. *Required interaction*—The degree to which the job requires an individual to work closely with other people (coworkers and/or clients) in carrying out the work activities (Hackman & Oldham, 1975).
2. *Collaboration with physicians*—The degree to which the interactions of nurses and physicians enable synergistic influence of patient care (Weiss & Davis, 1982).
3. *Influence with other disciplines*—The extent to which other professionals (e.g., social workers, discharge planners, and dietitians) consider the nurse's ideas in making decisions about patient care.
4. *Social integration*—The degree to which an individual has close friends among organizational members within the immediate work unit (Price & Mueller, 1986).
5. *Feedback from agents*—The degree to which the individual receives clear information about her performance from supervisors or coworkers (Hackman & Oldham, 1975).
6. *Role conflict*—The extent to which different members of a role set communicate disparate expectations that arouse motivational forces within the individual toward different behaviors (Kahn, Wolfe, Quinn, & Snoek, 1981).
7. *Role overload*—A specific type of role conflict in which members of a role set hold legitimate expectations that are compatible in the abstract, but impossible for the individual to completely fulfill because of time constraints (Kahn, Wolfe, Quinn, & Snoek, 1981).
8. *Role ambiguity*—The extent to which an individual lacks information required to perform the job (Kahn, Wolfe, Quinn, & Snoek, 1981).

Critical Psychological States

Investigators have also proposed and/or found evidence that other psychological states, not specified by the JCM, may mediate relationships between characteristics and outcomes (Fried & Ferris, 1987; Renn & Vandenberg, 1995). A new psychological state, experienced attachment to coworkers, has been incorporated in the model to link the effects of close, supportive relationships with coworkers to outcomes (Baumeister & Leary, 1995; Korman, 1992).

Outcomes

Researchers have found links between job characteristics and/or psychological states and outcomes that are not included in the JCM. Riordan and Griffeth, for example, found that friendship opportunities at work were strongly related to job involvement (Riordan & Griffeth, 1995). Mental health has also been evaluated as a dependent variable and was meaningfully related to the three CPS, especially experienced meaningfulness (r = 0.39) (Wall, Clegg, & Jackson, 1978).

In addition to general job and growth satisfaction from the JCM, this study included burnout and perceived job stress as dependent variables. Burnout refers to a "syndrome of emotional exhaustion and cynicism that occurs frequently among individual who do 'people-work' of some kind" (Maslach & Jackson, 1981, p. 99). Psychological stress occurs when a person has made an evaluation that external or internal demands tax or exceed her resources (Lazarus, 1991). These two workplace well-being constructs are particularly salient to the study of human service professionals (Maslach, 1982; Motowidlo, Packard, & Manning, 1986) and enhance our understanding of this type of job.

These characteristics, psychological state, and outcome constructs and their proposed interrelationships are depicted in Figure 44-2.

JOB CHARACTERISTICS RESEARCH WITH STAFF NURSES

Nursing has been the subject of a number of JCM studies (Holaday & Bullard, 1991; Joiner, Johnson, Chapman, & Corkrean, 1982; Roedel & Nystrom, 1988). A consistent pattern of findings has emerged (Joiner et al., 1982; Roedel & Nystrom, 1988) which shows that SNs perceive higher levels of significance and variety, about the same levels of autonomy and feedback from work, and lower task identity than those in other professional/technical jobs (Hackman & Oldham, 1980).

In their sample of 135 nurses, Roedel and Nystrom found statistically significant correlations between all five of the core dimensions and general satisfaction, ranging from a high of r = 0.30 ($p < 0.01$) with feedback from work to a low of r = 0.12 ($p < 0.10$) with significance (Roedel & Nystrom, 1988).

NURSING CASE MANAGEMENT JOB DESIGN RESEARCH

Review of the nursing case management literature suggests two general conclusions, which are supported by the findings of other reviewers: (1) this literature is largely anecdotal (Marschke & Nolan, 1993) and, as previously noted, (2) the research that does exist focuses primarily on patient and institutional, rather than nurses' outcomes (Erkel, 1993). A small body of relevant research was located, however, and descriptions and key findings from these studies are summarized in Table 44-1.

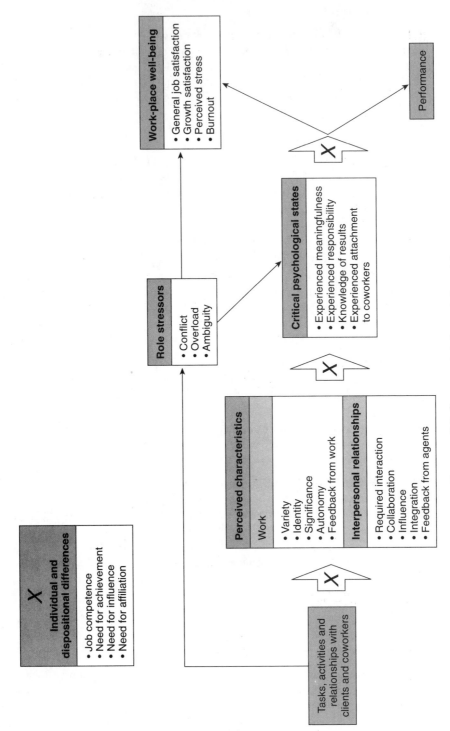

FIGURE **44-2**   Extended theoretical model.

| Table 44-1 | NURSING CASE MANAGEMENT STUDIES AND KEY FINDINGS | |

AUTHOR AND DATE	DESCRIPTION	KEY FINDINGS
Ethridge, 1987	Quantitative evaluation of Carondelet model	NCMs (n = 7) reported significantly higher levels of autonomy, enjoyment of work, and professional status than staff nurses (n = 72).
Newman, Lamb, & Michaels, 1991	Qualitative study of nursing case management practice at Carondelet	Nurses experience something different when practicing as NCMs. Specifically, NCMs (1) are not bound by time and space and establish ongoing partnerships with clients and (2) are organizationally empowered to carry out professional service. Relationships with hospital SNS were "sensitive" initially, but improved with time.
Van Dongen & Jambunathan, 1992	Qualitative pilot study examining role of psychiatric NCM in outpatient clinic	Both psychiatrists (n = 2) and NCMs (n = 5) described the NCM role as autonomous, yet collaborative with the psychiatrist.
Goode, 1993	Quantitative evaluation of Hospital Based Managed Care (HBMC) intervention combining CareMaps and case management	Nurses who applied and were selected for NCM positions had higher levels of collaboration than other nurses, reported higher levels of job satisfaction with quality of care, and their autonomy increased with time in the NCM job. Multidisciplinary team members had higher levels of collaboration than other multidisciplinary staff on the experimental unit.
Lancero, 1994	Quantitative examination of perceived control over nursing practice, job stress, and work satisfaction among 30 NCMs in two different models	Satisfaction was positively correlated with control ($r = 0.65$, $p = 0.01$) and negatively correlated with stress ($r = 0.43$, $p = 0.01$). Stress scale items NCMs reported as most unique to NCM practice included "focusing on continuum rather than episode," "having independence and autonomy," and "long-term relationships with clients and families."
McGill, 1994	Qualitative evaluation of the impact of the NCM role on leadership development within a hospital setting, based on data from two focus groups of NCMs (N = 16)	NCMs' relationships changed with physicians and other disciplines positively, but relationships with staff nurses changed negatively. Specifically, NCMs reported more collaboration and communication with MDs and other disciplines; however, they also described a sense of being in an ambiguous job separated from other nurses.

Continued

Table 44-1	NURSING CASE MANAGEMENT STUDIES AND KEY FINDINGS—cont'd	
AUTHOR AND DATE	**DESCRIPTION**	**KEY FINDINGS**
Rheaume et al., 1994	Qualitative study of the effects of case management on nursing practice, based on literature review and interviews with community-based NCMs (N = 17) in Canada	Case management has the potential to fundamentally alter usual lines of authority between nurses and MDs. Difficulties are encountered in relationships between NCMs and discharge planners and other nurses and health care workers, especially if the NCM role is not clearly understood. Despite the potential difficulties, however, case management appears to improve quality of working relationships in that it makes collaborative relationships feasible.

Motivational Characteristics of the NCM Job

The NCM job was developed in response to changes in hospital financing that presented an opportunity to enrich staff nursing and create a new job. Work redesign strategies focus on expanding the responsibilities of a job both horizontally, to increase characteristics such as variety and identity, and vertically, to increase autonomy.

These changes are intended to produce desired improvements in affective and behavioral outcomes, which have been reported in numerous studies (Fried & Ferris, 1987; Hackman & Oldham, 1980; Herzberg, 1966). Yet it has also been noted that the effects of work redesign initiatives are not always as intended (Joiner & van Servellen, 1984). I believe that the design of the NCM role has successfully introduced a number of theoretically important changes that should make it a more satisfying and motivating job. However, the design of this job is also expected to produce several unintended effects.

Unintended Effects From Job Redesign

Although not nearly as prevalent as reports of improved satisfaction and performance, there are occasional examples of unintended effects from job redesign scattered through the literature. Kopelman noted that job enrichment sometimes leads to decreased satisfaction with pay and supervision: employees may expect increased compensation for expanded responsibilities, and supervisors may interfere with the autonomy employees expect to receive (Kopelman, 1985). Moreover, because of the stimulating nature of highly motivating jobs, some employees may suffer stress and mental overload.

Two studies identify the potential for unintended effects from job enrichment in nursing, specifically the transition to nurse managed care (Shigemitsu & Tsushima, 1990; Wolf, 1993). Wolf's dissertation research described a number of negative outcomes associated with the shift to a professional nursing practice model in which nurses assumed responsibility for managing the care of a caseload of patients, such as increased intensity of work and decreased work group cohesion (Wolf, 1993).

As part of an evaluation of nurse managed patient care, Shigemitsu and Tsushima measured nurses' stress before and after implementation of a model that encouraged nurse-physician collaboration in managing patient care in accordance with predetermined protocols. Results suggested that a significant increase in nurse job stress occurred after the implementation of the care management program (Shigemitsu & Tsushima, 1990). In summary, although these models appear to be extensions of primary nursing more than the type of formal nursing case management system in this research, it appears that there is a need for balanced consideration of potential unanticipated consequences, as well as intended effects, in assessing the motivational characteristics of the NCM job.

THE NURSE CASE MANAGER JOB

From the job characteristics and role theory perspectives, what is the NCM job? Its design appears to create changes in the SN job that affect characteristics of the work itself, relationships with colleagues, and the work role.

CHARACTERISTICS OF THE WORK. Staff nurse jobs are known to be high in significance and skill variety (Joiner et al., 1982; Roedel & Nystrom, 1988). The NCM job is likely to be similar in these characteristics; however, it is expected that NCMs experience more job identity, autonomy, and feedback in their work than SNs.

As compared to the traditional SN job, the NCM has an expanded scope in terms of both a broader perspective on patient care and a view across a longer continuum. NCMs see the system of patient care more broadly in that they manage the entire hospitalization, as opposed to just the nursing care component on one unit. They also follow the same patients longitudinally across unit and institutional boundaries.

McGill's and Lancero's studies with NCMs provide support for increased task identity in this job (Lancero, 1994; McGill, 1994). Case managers in McGill's study described a change in their focus to the total picture of patient care, and Lancero's findings suggested that one of the most unique aspects of NCM practice is focusing on a continuum of care.

Previous research also suggests that NCMs experience greater autonomy in their jobs. Case managers in Lancero's study identified independence and autonomy as additional unique characteristics of their jobs. Ethridge explicitly demonstrated that NCMs report higher levels of autonomy than SNs (Ethridge, 1987), and Goode found that nurse autonomy increased over time in the NCM job (Goode, 1993). NCMs' jobs are less structured by schedules and routines than SNs' jobs, which allows NCMs greater latitude in organizing and managing their work. Because NCMs usually work with the most complex cases, they may also experience more independence in decision-making, as they are grappling with unique problems for which fewer standardized answers are available.

NCMs may also receive more feedback from their work, particularly if they are working with a clinical path/CareMap* system. These systems include concurrent and retrospective analysis of variances from the plan of care (Bower, 1993), which NCMs can use to assess effectiveness in facilitating a patient's progress through the hospitalization.

Bueno and Hwang (1993) described a sophisticated system developed at Robert Wood Johnson University Hospital that integrates variance analysis with the performance appraisal system for NCMs. Variance analysis data are entered into a data base and summary reports are prepared for each NCM that list the frequency for each case type and compare the average expected length of stay with the average actual length of stay. SNs generally do not receive this type of regular, quantitative performance feedback.

CHARACTERISTICS OF COWORKER RELATIONSHIPS. NCMs would be expected to have more influence with physicians and other disciplines because of their authority and responsibility for patients' movement through the hospital system. NCMs are in a better position to collaborate with physicians

---

*CareMap is a licensed trademark of The Center for Case Management, S. Natick, Mass.

than SNs because they can affect events that are important to physicians (e.g., arranging services patients need) and have access to comparative information about physicians' practice patterns and outcomes. Thus, while NCMs may not interact with physicians on a "level playing field," their relationships are more equitable. Descriptions of NCMs' interactions with physicians from McGill's research suggest a more balanced relationship in which nurses exert more control in relation to decisions about patient care (e.g., questioning a physician's assertion that a patient does not need a particular intervention) (McGill, 1994).

McGill's findings also indicate that NCMs have influence with other disciplines in the management of patient care. For example, in relation to a question about relationships with members of other professions, the focus group facilitator commented, "I see you all nodding your heads, so would you pretty well agree that, as you become the recognized experts, other departments also approach you, not just your own area?" (McGill, 1994, p. 40). This was confirmed by the participants. Similarly, Goode found that members of multidisciplinary care management teams, including physicians, NCMs, a dietitian, and a pharmacist, reported higher levels of collaboration than other multidisciplinary staff on the unit (Goode, 1993).

NCMs perform an integrator/expeditor function within hospitals (Zander, 1994) and occupy what can be described as an intraorganizational boundary spanning position (Adams, 1983). Because of their structural relationship to other roles, boundary positions have a number of unique properties. Boundary role individuals are more distant from other organizational members, may be viewed with suspicion, and must negotiate with multiple groups (Adams, 1983). Because NCMs move throughout the organization in the course of their work, they may have fewer opportunities to develop close relationships with coworkers in one geographic work area. In addition, the structure of their responsibilities may increase the potential for interpersonal conflict with other nurses and other professionals, such as social workers or discharge planners (McGill, 1994; Morse, 1991; Newman, Lamb, & Michaels, 1991; Rheaume, Frisch, Smith, & Kennedy, 1994).

In summary, nurses' jobs involve a great deal of interaction with others, and it is expected that both SN and NCM jobs are characterized by required interaction and feedback from agents; however, because of the design of their jobs, NCMs are expected to experience more collaboration and influence with other disciplines and less social integration than SNs.

WORK ROLE CHARACTERISTICS.   The boundary spanning nature of NCMs' roles may also contribute to role conflict. NCMs link patients, physicians, and other disciplines to each other and to the organization. Dealing with these multiple constituencies places the NCM at high risk for inter-sender role conflict. The shift from a clinical to a more administrative role noted by Rheaume and colleagues (Rheaume et al., 1994) may also create a form of intrapersonal role conflict in which the NCM feels torn because values as a clinician may suggest everything possible should be done for a patient regardless of cost, while role expectations require administrative attention to resource management. Thus it is predicted that NCMs will experience greater role conflict than their SN counterparts.

Work overload is an important factor in SNs' job dissatisfaction (Irvine & Evans, 1992). Similar to their colleagues in staff positions, NCMs report that they have difficulty completing their work within the time available (Lancero, 1994; McGill, 1994). It appears that role overload may characterize both jobs.

NCMs work in positions that are new and frequently incompletely defined. As previously noted, NCMs' jobs are also less structured by routines (e.g., medication administration schedules). Additionally, NCMs are frequently at risk for role blurring and diffusion between their new roles and SN responsibilities (Tonges, 1993). McGill's subjects explicitly described the experience of repeatedly explaining their jobs to others (McGill, 1994). Thus it is expected that NCMs experience more role ambiguity than SNs.

Table 44-2	HYPOTHESIZED DIFFERENCES IN CHARACTERISTICS OF NCM AND SN JOBS	
JOB CHARACTERISTICS	**NURSE CASE MANAGER**	**STAFF NURSE**
Autonomy	Higher	Lower
Job identity	Higher	Lower
Job feedback	Higher	Lower
Collaboration	Higher	Lower
Influence	Higher	Lower
Social integration	Lower	Higher
Role conflict	Higher	Lower
Role ambiguity	Higher	Lower

Hypothesized differences between the characteristics of SN and NCM jobs that were evaluated in this research are summarized in Table 44-2.

Method

A cross-sectional correlational design was used to collect data concerning relationships among perceived job characteristics and workplace well-being outcomes. More detailed descriptions of methodology are reported elsewhere (Tonges, 1997, 1998).

SUBJECTS, SAMPLE, AND SETTING
The sample comprised RNs employed as NCMs, unit-based care coordinators (CCs), and SNs; however, this report focuses on a comparison of NCMs and SNs. Nurses included in the sample (1) were female; (2) worked in acute care hospitals on inpatient units; (3) worked at least half-time; and (4) had a minimum of 2 years of RN experience. NCM subjects also had to be employed in that position for at least 1 year.

Data were collected from eligible NCMs and a random sample of SNs from eight not-for-profit, acute care hospitals ranging in size from 238 to 1000 beds. A total of 413 subjects provided usable responses, which represented a 29% response rate.

The mean age of respondents was 40 years (SD = 9.2). Thirteen percent had a diploma in nursing, 30% an associate's degree, 43% a baccalaureate, and 13% a master's degree or higher. Their mean years of experience was 14 (SD = 8.3). Distribution across clinical practice areas was as follows: 33% medical/surgical, 23% intensive care, 9% pediatrics, 6% obstetrics/nursery, and 28% other (does not total to 100% because of rounding and missing data).

INSTRUMENTS
Items from 11 instruments and a demographic data form were used to measure the variables in this study. Descriptions of their psychometric properties in previous research and this study are reported elsewhere (Tonges, 1997).

PROCEDURES
After receiving permission to access hospital staff, a list of eligible SNs and NCMs was obtained, and SN names were randomized. Surveys were coded and placed in envelopes labeled with subjects' names for internal distribution. Packets containing a cover letter, informed consent, demographic data form,

Table 44-3	DEMOGRAPHIC PROFILE OF RESPONDENTS FROM EACH JOB CATEGORY												
	AGE		**EDUCATION***				**YEARS OF RN EXPERIENCE**		**CLINICAL AREA**				
JOB TITLE	**M**	**SD**	**DIP**	**ADN**	**BSN**	**MSN OR HIGHER**	**M**	**SD**	**M/S**	**CC**	**PEDS**	**OB**	**OTHER†**
Staff nurse	40	9.8	17%	35%	46%	2%	14	8.4	29%	28%	10%	8%	25%
Case manager	40	9.2	—	7%	37%	56%	17	6.2	47%	10%	14%	4%	25%

*Does not add to 100% due to rounding/missing data.
†"Other" includes inpatient specialties such as telemetry, oncology, and psychology.

questionnaire, and prepaid return envelope were mailed to an on-site coordinator to be delivered to subjects.

Results

Hierarchical regression analysis was used to evaluate hypotheses concerning relationships predicted in an extended model. Findings suggest that characteristics of interpersonal relationships and work roles explain significant increases in variance, beyond that explained by the core dimensions of the JCM, in general and growth satisfaction, burnout, and job stress. Again, a detailed description of these findings is reported elsewhere (Tonges, 1997).

INTENDED AND UNINTENDED EFFECTS OF NCM JOB DESIGN

The demographic profile of the NCM and SN respondents who met criteria for inclusion in these comparisons is displayed in Table 44-3. One-way ANOVAs comparing the NCM and SN groups for age, education, and years of experience by job category indicated no significant difference in age at the 0.05 level. There were significant differences among the groups in education, with NCMs having more education than SNs. NCMs ($x = 16$) also had significantly more years of experience than SNs ($x = 14$). Effects of the demographic variables were controlled by entering the set of demographic covariates as step 1 in the regressions, and significant findings are reported here. The effect of site was evaluated in step 3 and reported elsewhere (Tonges, 1997).

Means and standard deviations for the job characteristic variables for NCMs and SNs are reported in Table 44-4. The number of subjects per category was further reduced because of missing data. A multivariate analysis of variance in job characteristics between job categories was significant at the $p < 0.01$ level. Based on this finding, analysis progressed to testing hypotheses concerning perceived differences in specific job characteristics between NCM and SN jobs.

Intended Positive Effects of NCM Job Design

Hypothesis 1 states that there is a significant relationship between working in the NCM job and perceived autonomy. For the sample of SNs and NCMs meeting the criteria for inclusion, the increment in

Table 44-4	MEANS AND STANDARD DEVIATIONS FOR JOB CHARACTERISTICS BY JOB CATEGORY			
	SN (N = 254)		CM (N = 53)	
VARIABLE	**M**	**SD**	**M**	**SD**
Autonomy	5.1	0.93	6.2	0.59
Job identity	4.2	1.10	4.8	1.10
Feedback from work	5.0	0.98	5.0	1.20
Collaboration	3.7	1.10	4.4	0.74
Influence	6.9	1.90	7.4	1.50
Social integration	3.7	0.69	3.7	0.79
Role conflict	3.4	0.99	3.7	0.92
Role ambiguity	3.4	0.77	3.9	0.94
Skill variety	5.7	0.90	6.0	0.75
Task significance	6.2	0.74	6.1	0.79
Feedback from agents	3.9	1.40	4.4	1.40
Required interaction	6.4	0.72	6.8	0.44
Role overload	3.7	1.60	4.6	1.30

R-squared for the variable representing the contrast coded vector for SN and NCM jobs was 0.144 ($p < 0.01$). This means that working as a NCM, rather than a SN, uniquely explains 14% of the variance in autonomy beyond that explained by demographic differences. Hypothesis 1 is therefore supported.

Hypothesis 2 states that there is a significant relationship between working in the NCM job and perceived job identity. The increment in R-squared for the contrast between SN and NCM jobs was 0.05 ($p < 0.01$), and hypothesis 2 is supported.

Hypothesis 3 states that there is a significant relationship between working in the NCM job and perceived job feedback. The increment in R-squared was 0.00001 ($p = 0.98$). This means that working as a NCM, rather than a SN, does not uniquely explain meaningful variance in feedback from work, and hypothesis 3 is not supported.

Hypothesis 4 states that there is a significant relationship between working in the NCM job and perceived collaboration with physicians. The R-squared for the set of covariates was 0.11 ($p < 0.01$). This means that demographic differences accounted for 11% of the variance in collaboration. Examining the betas for individual variables within the set revealed that the two strongest, significant explanatory variables were education (beta = 4.1, $p < 0.01$) and working in intensive care (beta = 3.36, $p < 0.01$).

The increment in R-squared for the contrast between SN and NCM jobs was 0.04 ($p < 0.01$). This means that working as a NCM, rather than a SN, uniquely explains 4% of the variance in collaboration, and hypothesis 4 is supported.

Hypothesis 5 states that there is a significant relationship between working in the NCM job and perceived influence with other disciplines. The increment in R-squared for the contrast was 0.002 ($p = 0.45$), and hypothesis 5 is not supported.

Unintended Negative Effects of NCM Job Design

Hypothesis 6 states that there is a significant relationship between working in the NCM job and perceived social integration. The increment in R-squared for the contrast between SN and NCM jobs was 0.002 ($p = 0.54$), and hypothesis 6 is not supported.

Hypothesis 7 states that there is a significant relationship between working in the NCM job and perceived role conflict. The increment in R-squared for the contrast was 0.03 ($p < 0.01$), and hypothesis 7 is supported. This means that working in the NCM, rather than the SN job, uniquely accounts for 3% of the variance in role conflict, beyond that explained by demographics.

Hypothesis 8 states that there is a significant relationship between working in the NCM job and perceived role ambiguity. The increment in R-squared for the contrast was 0.04 ($p < 0.01$), and hypothesis 8 is supported.

Although no differences were hypothesized between the NCM and SN jobs for the remaining five characteristics, contrasts were run to provide a comprehensive analysis. Findings from these regressions were as follows:

Variable	R^2 for Covariates	R^2 for Job
Skill variety	0.03 ($p = .23$)	0.01 ($p = .07$)
Significance	0.03 ($p = .25$)	0.003 ($p = .29$)
Required interaction	0.02 ($p = .49$)	0.035 ($p < .001$)
Feedback from agents	0.01 ($p = .83$)	0.016 ($p = .02$)
Role overload	0.07 ($p = .002$)	0.027 ($p = .002$)

These findings mean that for respondents in this study, working in the NCM job, as opposed to the SN job, uniquely explains significant increases in variance in required interaction, feedback from agents, and role overload, beyond that explained by differences in age, education, clinical area, and years of experience.

Regarding the other significant effects, all clinical areas except medical/surgical were significantly negatively related to role overload. This indicates that nurses working in the medical/surgical area reported significantly higher levels of role overload than nurses working in intensive care, pediatrics, obstetrics/nursery, and other inpatient areas.

Discussion, Conclusions, and Further Research

As compared to staff nursing, the NCM job appears to combine higher levels of both positive and negative characteristics. Specifically, NCMs report significantly higher levels of autonomy, job identity, collaboration with physicians, and feedback from agents; however, they also report considerably more required interaction, which was significantly related to job stress, as well as higher levels of role conflict, ambiguity, and overload. Because these characteristics have opposite effects on outcomes and are significantly negatively related to each other, increasing them simultaneously would be expected to have mixed effects.

Work redesign changes the structure of people's jobs in an attempt to increase their perception of positive job characteristics. Although the identification of links between specific tasks and perceived characteristics has not been a major research focus, some evidence suggests that activities can be related to more than one characteristic (Tonges, Rothstein, & Kikiras, 1998). Thus changes designed to increase a particular positive characteristic may also increase a negative one.

As an example, consider the possibility that cross-training an employee to perform additional functions may increase perceptions of skill variety, but may also increase feelings of role overload. In this case, each characteristic would be expected to exert opposite effects on job satisfaction and burnout (i.e., variety is related positively to satisfaction and negatively to burnout, and overload has the opposite pattern of relationships). Ultimately, effects associated with increases in the positive may be offset by increases in the negative characteristic.

Three of the hypothesized differences between characteristics of NCM and SN jobs were not supported: higher levels of job feedback, higher levels of influence with other disciplines, and lower social integration. A possible explanation for NCMs reporting higher levels than SNs of feedback from agents, but not feedback from work, is that information about issues such as length of stay and cost management may be received in reports from supervisors. Thus, although this information is about the results of NCMs' work, it comes through agents, rather than directly from the work itself.

Regarding the findings for influence, the wording of this scale asks about the frequency with which other disciplines ask and act on "nurses" opinions. Feedback was received from NCMs who completed the survey questioning which nurses' opinions the items referred to, SNs' or NCMs'. It is possible that the general nature of this wording contributed to a lack of differentiation between jobs. Revising the items to refer to "my opinion" should clarify this issue.

Three of the significant differences between NCM and SN job characteristics were not predicted: higher levels of required interaction, feedback from agents, and role overload. There was limited prior research to guide these hypotheses, and the findings of this study should prove helpful to other researchers in this regard.

In summary, results of this study suggest that the NCM job is associated with differences in a number of motivational characteristics found to have positive and negative consequences for workplace well-being. Further study of nursing and other types of case manager jobs is needed to continue to evaluate the characteristics and consequences associated with this job design.

IMPLICATIONS OF THIS RESEARCH

Given the growing popularity of the case management approach, results from this study have useful implications for individuals and organizations.

Implications for Individuals

Workplace well-being has important personal consequences. Work-related stress has been linked to depression (Motowidlo, Packard, & Manning, 1986), and burnout is characterized by a combination of negative feelings, including emotional exhaustion and low personal accomplishment (Maslach & Jackson, 1981). Clearly, it is in our best interests to know more about job characteristics and design and use this knowledge to enhance workplace well-being.

The conclusions concerning negative and positive characteristics in the same job and mixed consequences of work redesign imply that individuals must think about the possible cons, as well as the pros, associated with job changes. The implication for individuals is to learn as much as possible about a job in its entirety when contemplating a change or, more specifically, to evaluate all the ways the new job differs from one's current position, not just how it is different in some particular positive way. Nurses specifically must be aware of the potential for problems with role overload, conflict, and ambiguity in the NCM job.

Implications for Organization

The implication for practice of the conclusions concerning negative and positive characteristics and mixed consequences of work redesign is that we need to learn more about the combined effects of job design changes. This knowledge could help us to enrich a job without introducing unintended negative characteristics at the same time.

In view of the turmoil within health care (Lumsdon, 1995), this is especially valuable and timely information for nursing and other health care professions. Conclusions about NCM job characteristics imply a specific need for attention to role stressors in this job. To address these concerns, however, it is necessary to have more information about the specific aspects of the job that give rise to perceptions of role overload, conflict, and ambiguity.

Rizzo, House, and Lirtzman suggested that role stressors are intervening variables that mediate the effects of various organizational practices (Rizzo, House, & Lirtzman, 1970). Specifically, role conflict is associated with violations of the principles of unity of command and single accountability, and role ambiguity is related to conditions such as lack of a clear idea of job scope and responsibility, vague task definition, inconsistent direction from a supervisor, and lack of clarification regarding the function of each member in a group.

Findings from an organizational stress study with a sample of 158 RNs, licensed practical nurses, and aides suggest that administrative efforts to establish goals, to plan and coordinate, and to resolve interdepartmental conflict are linked to lower levels of role conflict among staff (Gray-Toft & Anderson, 1985). The same study found that representation, consultation, and involving staff in decision making (communication) directly and indirectly led to a significant reduction in role ambiguity among nursing staff.

Without more research concerning specific links between job activities and perceived characteristics, definitive recommendations for interventions to reduce perceived role stressors in the NCM job cannot be made. However, several suggestions are offered for evaluation.

There is a growing trend in hospitals to create NCM jobs by integrating utilization review/management, discharge planning, and, sometimes, quality improvement and social service functions into one position. Given the financial pressures hospitals are experiencing and the overlap among these jobs and case management, this approach is understandable; however, it appears to contribute to higher levels of role stressors.

For example, a NCM who is expected to inform patients that they need to go home because their insurance company is denying payment for further hospitalization (utilization review), while also trying to function as a patient advocate (clinical case management) may well experience feelings of role conflict. Similarly, adding the responsibility for responding to numerous calls from insurance companies for information (utilization review) to a day of seeing patients and families and working with other disciplines to expedite care (clinical case management) is likely to lead to feelings of role overload. The point is not that some additional functions cannot be integrated, but rather that tasks must be consistent with the purpose of the job and the resulting workload must be realistic.

While there may always be some ambiguity associated with a relatively new job, some possible interventions to clarify the NCM role include the following: (1) the development and distribution of a specific job description, (2) a thorough orientation, and (3) multiple opportunities for communication, including regular meetings with the manager and peer group.

The job description should include precise statements outlining the NCM's major responsibilities in the areas of clinical management, financial management, leadership, and self-development. Other essential functions may include performance improvement and consultation/education. This description should be augmented by a list of measurable cost/quality performance goals that are revised annually (e.g., "decrease length of stay for traditional DRG Medicare patients by 0.5 day" or "reduce readmission rates for COPD patients by 10%").

Orientation should focus on the desired behavioral outcomes of the job and include a combination of clinical, financial, and managerial content. If possible, introduction to the role should culminate in a precepted experience with a seasoned case manager mentor.

Communication opportunities should be provided through a combination of regular one-on-one and group meetings with the case management supervisor. Group meetings should include case presentations and peer consultation. Again, however, specific sources of role ambiguity and the effectiveness of such interventions must be evaluated.

The findings of this study also have implications for selection of candidates for NCM jobs. In addition to knowledge and skills in the clinical and financial arenas, results suggest that serious consideration should be given to applicants' tolerance for ambiguity, time management abilities, and interpersonal skills.

In conclusion, a revolution is occurring in the world of work, and a combination of factors—including the shift to service employment and the emergence of case management job design—have created the need for an expanded job characteristics model and a better understanding of the characteristics of case manager jobs. As work and assignments continue to evolve, the more we know about job characteristics and their links to workplace well-being, the better prepared we will be to design jobs that enhance personal and work outcomes. It is hoped that the results of this study will contribute to this goal.

References

Abdel-Halim, A.A. (1981). Effects of role stress–job design interaction on employee work satisfaction. *Academy of Management Journal, 24,* 269-273.

Adams, J.S. (1983). The structure and dynamics of behavior in organizational boundary roles. In M. Dunnette (Ed.), *Handbook of industrial and organizational psychology* (2nd ed.) (pp. 1175-1200). New York: Wiley.

Baumeister, R.F., & Leary, M.R. (1995). The need to belong: Desire for interpersonal attachments as a fundamental human motivation. *Psychological Bulletin, 117,* 497-529.

Berlinger, L., Glick, W., & Rodgers, R. (1988). Job enrichment and performance improvement. In J. Campbell & R. Campbell, and associates (Eds.), *Productivity in organizations* (pp. 219-254). San Francisco: Jossey-Bass.

Bower, K.A. (1993). Case management: Work redesign with patient outcomes in mind. In K.J. McDonagh (Ed.), *Patient-centered hospital care: Reform from within.* Ann Arbor, Mich.: Health Administration Press.

Bueno, M.M., & Hwang, R. (1993). Understanding variances in hospital stay. *Nursing Management, 24*(11), 51-57.

Davenport, T.H., & Nohria, N. (1994, Winter). Case management and the integration of labor. *Sloan Management Review,* 11-23.

Erkel, E.A. (1993). The impact of case management in preventive services. *Journal of Nursing Administration, 23*(1), 27-32.

Ethridge, P. (1987). Nurse accountability program improves satisfaction, turnover. *Health Progress, 5,* 44-49.

Fried, Y., & Ferris, G.R. (1987). The validity of the job characteristics model: A review and meta-analysis. *Personnel Psychology, 40,* 287-322.

Goode, C.J. (1993). *Evaluation of patient and staff outcomes with hospital-based managed care.* Unpublished doctoral dissertation, University of Iowa, Iowa City, Ia.

Gray-Toft, P.A., & Anderson, J.G. (1985). Organizational stress in the hospital: Development of a model for diagnosis and prediction, Part I. *Health Services Research, 19,* 753-774.

Hackman, J.R., & Lawler, E.E. (1971). Employee reactions to job characteristics. *Journal of Applied Psychology, 55,* 259-286.

Hackman, J.R., & Oldham, G.R. (1980). *Work redesign.* Menlo Park, Calif. Addison-Wesley.

Hackman, J.R., & Oldham, G.R. (1976). Motivation through the design of work: Test of a theory. *Organizational Behavior and Human Performance, 16,* 250-279.

Hackman, J.R., & Oldham, G.R. (1975). Development of the Job Diagnostic Survey. *Journal of Applied Psychology, 60,* 159-170.

Hammer, M., & Champy, J. (1993). *Reengineering the corporation: A manifesto for business revolution.* New York: HarperCollins.

Herzberg, F. (1966). *Work and the nature of man.* Cleveland: World Publishing.

Holaday, B., & Bullard, I.D. (1991). Pediatric staff nurses' reactions to job characteristics. *Journal of Pediatric Nursing, 6,* 407-416.

Institute of Medicine. (1996). *Nursing staff in hospitals and nursing homes: Is it adequate?* In G.S. Wunderlich, F.S. Sloan, & C.K. Davis (Eds.), Washington, DC: National Academy Press.

Irvine, D., & Evans, M. (1992). Job satisfaction and turnover among nurses: A review and meta-analysis. *Quality of Nursing Worklife Research Monograph Series,* Toronto, Canada.

Jermier, J.M., Gaines, J., & McIntosh, N.J. (1989). Reactions to physically dangerous work: A conceptual and empirical analysis. *Journal of Organizational Behavior, 10,* 15-33.

Joiner, C., Johnson, V., Chapman, J.B., & Corkrean, M. (1982). The motivating potential in nursing specialties. *Journal of Nursing Administration, 12*(2), 26-30.

Joiner, C., & van Servellen, G.W. (1984). *Job enrichment in nursing.* Rockville, Mo: Aspen.

Kahn, R.L., Wolfe, D.M., Quinn, R.P., & Snoek, J.D. (1981). *Organizational stress: Studies in role conflict and ambiguity* (Reprint ed.). Malabar, Fla.: Krieger.

Kopelman, R.E. (1985). Job redesign and productivity: A review of the evidence. *National Productivity Review, 4,* 237-255.

Korman, A.K. (1992). Seminar in organizational behavior: Work-place well-being. Baruch College of the City University of New York.

Lamb, G.S. (1992). Conceptual and methodological issues in nurse case management research. *Advances in Nursing Science, 15*(2), 16-24.

Lancero, A.W. (1994). *Work satisfaction among nurse case managers: A comparison of two practice models.* Unpublished master's thesis, University of Arizona, Tucson, Ariz.

Lazarus, R.S. (1991). Psychological stress in the workplace. *Journal of Social Behavior and Personality, 6*(7), 1-13.

Locke, E.A. (1983). The nature and causes of job satisfaction. In M. Dunnette (Ed.), *Handbook of industrial and organizational psychology* (2nd ed.) (pp. 1297-1350). New York: Wiley.

Loher, B.T., Noe, R.A., Moeller, N.L., & Fitzgerald, M.P. (1985). A meta-analysis of the relation of job characteristics to job satisfaction. *Journal of Applied Psychology, 70,* 280-289.

Lumsdon, K. (1995). Faded glory: Will nursing ever be the same? *Hospital and Health Networks, 69*(23), 30-35.

Marschke, P., & Nolan, M.T. (1993). Research related to case management. *Nursing Administration Quarterly, 17*(3):16-21.

Maslach, C. (1982). *Burnout: The cost of caring.* Englewood Cliffs, NJ: Prentice-Hall.

Maslach, C., & Jackson, S. (1981). The measurement of experienced burnout. *Journal of Organizational Behavior, 2*(2), 99-113.

McGill, R.L. (1994). *Nursing case management: Developing clinical leaders.* Unpublished master's thesis, College of St. Catherine, St. Paul, Minn.

Mills, P.K., Hall, J.L., Leidecker, J.K., & Marguiles, N. (1983). Flexiform: A model for professional service organizations. *Academy of Management Review, 8,* 118-131.

Morse, J.M. (1991). Negotiating commitment and involvement in the nurse-patient relationship. *Journal of Advanced Nursing, 16,* 455-468.

Motowidlo, S.J., Packard, J.S., & Manning, M.R. (1986). Occupational stress: Its causes and consequences for job performance. *Journal of Applied Psychology, 71,* 618-629.

Newman, M., Lamb, G.S., & Michaels, C. (1991). Nurse case management: The coming together of theory and practice. *Nursing & Health Care, 12*(8), 404-408.

Price, J.L., & Mueller, C.W. (1986). *Absenteeism and turnover of hospital employees.* Greenwich, Conn.: JAI Press.

Price, J.L., & Mueller, C.W. (1981). *Professional turnover: The case of nurses.* New York: SP Medical and Scientific Books.

Renn, R.W., & Vandenberg, R.J. (1995). The critical psychological states: An underrepresented component in Job Characteristics Model research. *Journal of Management, 21,* 279-303.

Rheaume, A., Frisch, S., Smith, A., & Kennedy, C. (1994). Case management and nursing practice. *Journal of Nursing Administration, 24*(3), 31-36.

Riordan, C.M., & Griffeth, R.W. (1995). The opportunity for friendship in the workplace: An underexplored construct. *Journal of Business and Psychology, 10*(2), 141-154.

Rizzo, J., House, R., & Lirtzman, S. (1970). Role conflict and ambiguity in complex organizations. *Administrative Science Quarterly, 13,* 150-163.

Roedel, R.R., & Nystrom, P.C. (1988). Nursing jobs and satisfaction. *Nursing Management, 19*(2), 34-38.

Sherer, J.L. (1993). Health care reform: Nursing's vision of change. *Hospitals, 67*(8), 20-26.

Shigemitsu, K., & Tsushima, G. (1990). Collaborative practice: Nurse managed care. *Straub Foundation Proceedings, 55*(3), 37-42.

Sims, H.P., Szilagyi, A.D., & Keller, R.T. (1976). The measurement of job characteristics. *Academy of Management Journal, 19,* 195-212.

Stone, E., & Gueutal, H.G. (1985). An empirical derivation of the dimensions along which characteristics of jobs are perceived. *Academy of Management Journal, 28,* 376-396.

Taber, T., & Taylor, E. (1990). A review and evaluation of the psychometric properties of the Job Diagnostic Survey. *Personnel Psychology, 43,* 467-500.

Tonges, M.C. (1998). Job design for nurse case managers: Intended and unintended effects on satisfaction and well-being. *Nursing Case Management, 3*(1), 11-23.

Tonges, M.C. (1997). *An extension of the job characteristics model for a service economy.* Unpublished doctoral dissertation. Baruch College of the City University of New York.

Tonges, M.C. (1993). Work designs: Sociotechnical systems for patient care delivery. *Nursing Management, 23*(1), 27-32.

Tonges, M.C. (1989). Redesigning hospital nursing practice: The Professionally Advanced Care Team (ProACT®) Model, Part 1. *Journal of Nursing Administration, 19*(7), 31-38.

Tonges, M.C., Rothstein, H.R., & Kikiras, H.C. (1998). Sources of satisfaction in hospital nursing practice: A guide to effective job design. *Journal of Nursing Administration, 28*(5), 47-61.

Tumulty, G. (1992). A model for nursing role redesign. In B. Henry (Ed.), *Practice and inquiry for nursing administration* (pp. 67-71). Washington, D.C.: American Academy of Nursing.

Tumulty, G. (1990). *The relationship of head nurse role characteristics, job satisfaction, and unit outcomes.* Unpublished doctoral dissertation, University of Texas at Austin.

Van Dongen, C.J. & Jambunathan, J. (1992). Pilot study results: The psychiatric RN case manager. *Journal of Psychosocial Nursing, 30*(11), 11-14.

Wake, M.M. (1990). Nursing care delivery systems: Status and vision. *Journal of Nursing Administration, 20*(5), 47-51.

Wall, T.D., Clegg, C.W., & Jackson, P.R. (1978). An evaluation of the Job Characteristics Model. *Journal of Occupational Psychology, 51,* 183-196.

Weisman, C.S., & Nathanson, C. (1985). Professional satisfaction and client outcomes: A comparative analysis. *Medical Care, 23,* 1179-1192.

Weiss, S.J., & Davis, H.P. (1982). Validity and reliability of the Collaborative Practice Scales. *Nursing Research, 34,* 299-305.

Wolf, K.A. (1993). *Professionalization at work: The case of nursing at Mill City Medical Center.* Unpublished doctoral dissertation, Brandeis University.

Zander, K. (1994). Case management series, Part I: Rationale for care-provider organizations. *The New Definition, 9*(3), 1-2.

Zander, K. (1988). Nursing case management: Strategic management of cost and quality outcomes. *Journal of Nursing Administration, 18*(5), 23-30.

Zander, K., Etheredge, M.L., & Bower, K.A. (1987). *Nursing case management: Blueprints for transformation.* Boston: New England Medical Center.

Measuring Cost-Effectiveness

CHAPTER OVERVIEW

Measuring cost-effectiveness is one of the most important tasks in the evaluation of nursing case management models. This chapter reviews various strategies for measuring cost savings in a case management system and provides examples of case studies using these approaches. In addition, suggestions for using these methods in further research are reviewed.

EFFECT OF CASE MANAGEMENT ON VARIANCES OF LENGTH OF STAY AND RESOURCE UTILIZATION

In a study done by the American Hospital Association titled *1990 Report of the Hospital Nursing Personnel Survey* (AHA, 1990), the case management model represented the largest increase of nursing care delivery systems most frequently used in the acute care setting. In light of this study and others, it is important to present some of the methods of evaluating the cost-effectiveness of nursing case management. The studies presented in this chapter represent some of the groundbreaking work done in measuring the cost-effectiveness of nursing case management and health care delivery approaches. In general, case management has been associated with reduced total costs per patient case, decreased patient length of hospital stay, increased patient turnover, and potential increase in hospital-generated revenues.

In a program instituted at Long Regional Hospital in Utah, cost savings were achieved through the use of a bedside-centered case management model (Bair, Griswold, & Head, 1989). With this approach the registered nurse controls the use of patient care resources, guides the outcomes of this care within acute care and community-based settings, and, as a member of a multidisciplinary care coordination team, monitors and evaluates the costs and quality components of hospitalization for patients within defined diagnosis-related group (DRG) categories.

The registered nurse was given the responsibility and accountability for assessing the inpatient and discharge care requirements and for developing and implementing the plan of care related to the prescribed length of stay and amount of patient care resources used. To determine actual costs, focus was placed on the clinical management of defined groups of patients within 10 DRGs or service lines. Each of these groups was analyzed with special emphasis placed on patient care services, length of hospitalization, treatment and educational outcomes, discharge and post-discharge care planning, and outpatient and community-based services. Some of the DRGs that were investigated included major joint procedures, angina, heart failure, chest pain, circulatory disorders, acute myocardial infarction, and pneumonia.

A cost-containment study that focused on reducing the average loss per DRG case type was implemented. A comparison was made of the actual cost per case and the average reimbursement for 10 DRGs. It was demonstrated that bedside case management resulted in cost savings associated with a decrease in length of stay of 0.4 day, an average hospital savings of $284 per case and overall cost savings of $94,572.

Additional savings were realized through strategic planning and better use of patient care resources as evidenced by a reduction in admissions to the intensive care unit by 0.7 day and through the accurate assessment and classification of Medicare reimbursement criteria related to inpatient and outpatient group status.

An investigation done by McKenzie, Torkelson, and Holt (1989) showed that interventions associated with nursing case management had a significant effect on patient resource consumption and expenditures.

Case management plans and critical paths were developed for specific high-volume DRGs associated with diseases and disorders of the circulatory system, coronary artery bypass, and catheterization. This study demonstrated an average cost saving per case that was equivalent to $350 for laboratory charges, $180 for radiology charges, and $766 for pharmaceutical charges for nursing case-managed patients. The average length of stay was also reduced by 1.1 days. Within a 1-year period, close to $1 million was saved by using the case management system of care.

Stillwaggon (1989) demonstrated the effect of a nurse model on the cost of nursing care and staff satisfaction. This study was conducted at Saint Francis Hospital and Medical Center in Hartford, Connecticut. An approach to the delivery of patient care called *managed nursing care* was developed and implemented. This model promoted collaborative practice arrangements, encouraged care based on individualized patient assessment and need, eliminated routine and non-nursing tasks, and established nursing practice guided by professional standards of care. In addition, the professional nurse was able to contract for services and care needed by the patient. This contracting eliminated the need for the traditional work schedule.

The study sample consisted of 100 cases of normal, spontaneous delivery without complication or comorbidity. Comparisons were made between the traditional nursing care delivery system and the new approach to patient care under the nurse managed care model. An assessment was made of the nursing care hours actually delivered and the staff's satisfaction with the nurse managed care model.

Results showed a reduction of 5 hours spent delivering nursing services and a $61.71 decrease in cost of care per case. Additional findings indicated a high level of nursing staff and patient satisfaction with the nurse managed care delivery system.

In another study, Cohen (1991) incorporated a cost-accounting methodology with a combined team nursing–case management model to investigate personnel factors and variable cost components such as pharmaceuticals and supplies under the nursing case management model. The purpose of this study was to substantiate the financial benefit of using the nursing case management model within the acute care setting.

It was predicted that cesarean section patients who received care under the nursing case management model would have a shorter length of stay than patients who received care under the existing practices. It was also predicted that the nursing case management system of care would result in an overall decrease in hospital costs and expenditures associated with the cesarean section patient (Cohen, 1991).

The study used a quasi-experimental design on the experimental and control units. The cesarean section case types, DRGs 370 and 371, were selected for study because of the high volume and long length of stay associated with these DRGs. The study sample consisted of 128 cesarean section patients who made up 768 total patient days in 1988. A nonrandom selection was used.

Because randomization was not used, homogeneity controlled for individual extraneous variables that may have affected patient length of stay. Restricting the patient sample to cesarean section helped to control for patient gender, type of diagnosis, and surgical operation.

The data needed for the study required the development and implementation of the nursing case management delivery system. Use of the case management model required thorough orientation for the nursing staff. This orientation period introduced nurses in the experimental group to care under a case management model and helped the case managers assume their roles. Those who were in the experimental group included registered nurses, licensed practical nurses, and nursing assistants. Critical paths and nursing case management care plans were also used.

Demographic data, length of stay, and comorbidity information were received and compiled from the patient subject group. An evaluation was made of professional staff mix as well as the amount of time spent by nurses in delivering patient care (Cohen, 1990, 1991).

Nursing staff members were expected to cooperate with the investigator of this hospital-based administrative research project. The implementation of the nursing case management model included the following guidelines:

1. The case manager (registered nurse) became responsible for the patient when she was admitted to the unit.
2. Case associates (co-case managers or primary registered nurses) and case assistants (licensed practical nurses and nursing assistants) were given responsibility for ensuring continuity of care and accountability throughout the patient's length of stay. Each of the co-case managers was assigned different schedules to avoid overlapping days on the unit. Each patient was designated one case manager whose caseload was covered by the co-case manager on the case manager's days off.
3. Each case manager was to collaborate with the attending physician in assessing and evaluating the outcomes of patient care and individualizing the case management plan and critical path.
4. Each case manager was trained to use the case management care plan and critical path to facilitate patient care.
5. The critical path was used for the change-of-shift report.
6. Variance from the case management care plan or the critical path required discussion with the attending physician and a nursing case management consultant.
7. The nursing case manager and physician were to communicate at least twice during the patient's length of stay.
8. The nurse case manager and the patient care coordinator (head nurse) were to collaborate daily to negotiate assignment planning that would optimize the use of nursing resources.
9. Daily documentation was to reflect the monitoring of patient progress and evaluation of outcomes specified in the case management care plan or variances on the critical path, or both (Cohen, 1990).

COST ACCOUNTING METHOD

One of the primary objectives of the nursing case management system is to develop a cost management information system that validates the patient's use of clinical resources and services and confirms the financial benefits of case management to the institution. In this investigative project a nursing case management concept was established with the cesarean section case type that incorporated the following fiscal priorities:

To maximize control over patient hospital stay by implementing definable and attainable patient goals within a short period of time.

To decrease service-related costs and enhance DRG reimbursement by reducing patient length of stay through anticipatory planning, early intervention, and the coordination and arrangement of services.

The cost accounting process used in this study involved the following four procedural steps.

Step I: Establishment of a Resource Use Profile on the Typical Cesarean Section Patient

A historical patient profile reflecting conventional practice patterns was developed from the hospital's management information system. This procedure involved a review of detailed charges based on the hospital's charge description and general ledger code reports. These charges were summarized and then compressed from 272 service codes into 14 major clinical use and expense categories. Those categories were then separated by sample group. The categories included routine care, delivery room, operating room, anesthesia, recovery room, laboratory or blood, radiology, respiratory physiology, general pharmacy, antibiotics, intravenous (IV) therapy, other pharmacy, routine treatment, and other.

A 2-month sample from 1988 medical records and bills was accessed so that clinical information, financial data, volume of tests and services, posted charge rates for room and board, and ancillary services could be analyzed. An average of the accumulated costs was obtained to arrive at the cost of a unit of service (i.e., patient day, tests, procedures, pharmaceuticals) for all clinically related resources used.

Step II: Establishment of a Resource Use Profile for the Cesarean Section Patient Based on the Nursing Case Management Concept

The historical data obtained from the patient profiles were used to develop a patient profile adjusted for nursing case management outcome standards. The major nursing, medical, and ancillary outcome indicators of care were derived from the cesarean section patients' critical paths and were used to assess the nursing case management model's efficacy and productivity. Cost standards were set by reducing patient length of stay by 2 days (from 6 to 4 days), streamlining tests and procedures, and initiating patient teaching early in the hospital stay.

Step III: Comparison of the Charge and Resource Use Associated With Comparable Cesarean Section Cases

A charge and clinical resource use comparison was made between the experimental (case management) and control (conventional practice) groups. The comparison involved correlating the average unit of service for both the experimental and control groups to establish the average clinical resource use for the cesarean section patient. For example, the following was identified: average number of tests incurred, average number of supplies used, average number of pharmaceuticals given, average number of nursing care hours provided, and average length of stay. This comparison established a mechanism for monitoring the change in resource use after switching from conventional practices to case management. Such monitoring helped ensure that efficient use of services was maintained. The results of this comparison substantiated the efficacy of the case management model.

Step IV: Determination of the Total Average Cost for the Nursing Case Management Model

The above analysis provided the total room and board charges. However, to more effectively determine the average cost of the nursing case management model as well as the required nursing care resources, the following methodology was used: (1) The total direct nursing care costs were computed for both sample groups; (2) nursing care was segregated from total room and board costs; and (3) the ratio of cost to charge (RCC) factor was applied. The comparisons in step III were then categorized by skill mix to determine the number of direct nursing care hours required under each system for the care of the cesarean section patient.

To determine the total direct nursing care costs associated with both the experimental and control groups, the following computation was completed:

Average base salary per skill mix by sample group ÷ 1,950 hours (the number of hours
worked in a year by an employee) = Average hourly wage rate

Average hourly wage rate × Sum total of direct nursing care hours provided by skill mix
(from the Nursing Case Management Activity form) × 1.25 (average fringe benefits) = Total average costs
of direct nursing care for the cesarean section patient.

The direct nursing care costs were then segregated from the total expenditures to arrive at the remaining room and board costs.

The method used for determining costs was the departmental RCC, which is the cost-accounting methodology most widely used by health care institutions. The RCC is delineated from the Institutional Cost Report, which is a cost statement used by the Medicare program for various reimbursement processes. This report contains revenue, cost, and clinical service use information by department.

The method involved taking the RCC for each major clinical use and expense category and applying it against the total charges to arrive at an approximate determination of the total cost per case. This provided the final pieces of data needed to establish the total average costs for the nursing case management model (Cohen, 1990, 1991).

Findings indicated that a significant reduction in patient length of stay was achieved. Length of stay declined by 1.16 days, or 19%, between the experimental and control groups ($p \le 0.0001$). Expenditure and cost analysis showed an increase in direct patient-centered nursing care hours and intensification in use of inpatient services and treatments. This intensification of nursing time and resource use led to the reduction in patient length of stay and a decrease in total overall costs.

The analysis further demonstrated a savings of $930.40 per patient case and a general decrease in hospital costs and expenditures associated with the cesarean section patient. This profit was made possible because of the increase in patient turnover and the availability of additional patient beds. Potential savings and revenues of more than $1 million were identified for the hospital (Cohen, 1991; Health Care Advisory Board, 1990).

Although an analysis of the demographic data showed comparability between the experimental and control groups, the rigor of this investigation can be strengthened by using matched sampling to decrease the likelihood of extraneous variance and by using randomized assignment of the sample groups.

At Beth Israel Medical Center in New York City the case management model is used as a vehicle for reducing patient length of stay. Coupled with other initiatives such as CQI, reductions in the length of stay for selected diagnoses were realized in the first year of implementing the case management model (Table 45-1).

Nursing, medicine, social work, administration, patient representatives, operations, and finance were among the departments that participated in the change to a case management delivery system. In some

| Table 45-1 | BETH ISRAEL MEDICAL CENTER CASE MANAGED INCREMENTAL REVENUE FOR SELECTED DIAGNOSES | | | | | |

DIAGNOSIS	DRGs	ALOs 1990*	NO. OF CASES 1990	ALOS 1991*	NO. CASES 1991	INCREMENTAL REVENUE†
Laminectomy	4/755/756/ 577/758/ 214/215	10.0	260	9.08	213	$238,000
Endocarditis	126	14.4	94	8.7	58	$900,000
Soft tissue infection	278	9.1	189	8.7	156	$28,000
Pneumonia	89	11.06 1/91- 6/91	298 1/91- 6/91	10.05 7/91- 2/92	257 7/91- 2/92	$196,000
Orthopedics	209/211/233/ 234/218/ 219/220/ 221/223/224	9.0	143	7/08	226	$489,000
				11/11/91-1/31/92		
Diabetes team						
Principal diagnosis	294/295/296/ 297/566	9.9	300	3.45	37	
				11/11/91-1/31/92		
Secondary diagnosis	—	11.8	—	10.5	29	
High-risk obstetrics	383	—	—	8.25	12	$438,000
					TOTAL	$2,289,000

*Average length of stay data compiled from an MIS download from the Charms systems.
†Incremental revenue calculated by Don Modzewleski, Assistant Vice President, Finance.

cases, specific medical or surgical departments or specialties were targeted for the development of multidisciplinary action plans (MAPs). These plans incorporated all professional disciplines in management of the patient's care and ensured outcome-related quality services. In other cases, specific diagnoses or DRGs were targeted for significant reductions in length of stay (Table 45-1).

The Pareto chart, a statistical tool to determine which diagnoses or procedures to target, was used for the development of managed care plans and financial analysis (Fig. 45-1). If an annual review is being conducted, the number of cases for the top volume DRGs can be tallied. These are then placed on the chart in the form of a bar graph in descending order. On the right side of the chart the percentage of the total cases that each number of cases represents is placed on a cumulative line graph. For example, DRG 707 represented 63 cases, or 31% of the total number of cases. The next highest volume, DRG 277, represented a total of 50 cases, or 24% of the total number of cases. These two percentages are represented cumulatively as 55% of all cases. This means that these two DRGs represented 55% of all cases admitted to the unit. In most instances, one would study the top 80%, in this case DRGs 707, 277, 708, and 89, which represent approximately 80% of all cases. In this way it is clear that a fair representation of all cases has been included.

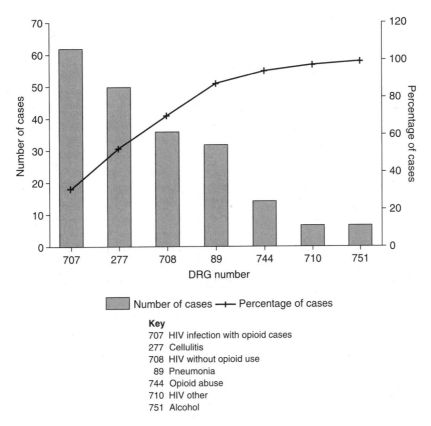

FIGURE **45-1**   DRG Pareto chart showing patient cases for 1991.

Non-unit-based case management teams are committed to following all patients of a specific case type who are admitted to the medical center. They are also responsible for monitoring length of stay, resource use, and quality. The teams also provide in-service training sessions to house staff and nursing personnel to maintain appropriate treatment of these patients.

Two teams, one for diabetes and one for asthma, consisted of several physicians, a nurse case manager, a nurse clinician, and other clinically relevant disciplines. In the case of the diabetes team a nutritionist was included and functioned as a full-time member who saw all patients assigned to the team.

The managed care plan is used to guide care and to provide a framework for keeping the length of stay in check. The length of stay on the plan is determined by studying the region, state, and federal lengths of stay for those DRGs relevant to the diagnosis or procedure. The physician practice patterns are then reviewed, and length of stay for the institution is established for that diagnosis.

Two groups for case management, unit-based case managers and non-unit-based case managers, were developed. The unit-based case managers assumed the same role as the non-unit-based case manager. However, the unit-based manager's primary responsibility was on an individual unit level and involved more than one diagnosis and many different physicians. The unit-based case manager can be equally effective because that person sees the patient several times during the day, intervening whenever necessary. The non-unit-based case managers, on the other hand, may spend a portion of the day traveling from one unit to another. Therefore their time with each patient is more limited.

Both groups, the non-unit-based case managers and the unit-based case managers, were able to demonstrate significant cost reductions within the first few weeks and months of implementation. Once the targeted diagnoses had been identified, the institution's prior length of stay history was obtained. These data allowed the team to determine what the expected length of stay would have been if the conventional model of patient care had been used.

After implementation of case management the length of stay was tracked on a monthly basis for those patients followed by the case management approach. Patients with certain diagnoses or surgical procedures were targeted and followed by the case manager.

Stringent data collection was necessary for accurate cost accounting. Preimplementation length-of-stay data provided the framework for determining whether the length-of-stay goals were achieved.

RELATIVE WEIGHTS AND FINANCIAL ANALYSIS

Some diagnoses fall within a single DRG. For example, pneumonia will almost always be coded within DRG 89. Conversely, many surgical procedures can be classified within a number of DRG categories. For example, laminectomy can be coded within as many as seven DRGs. Each of these DRGs may have a different financial weight.

The weights applied to each DRG are called *relative weights*. The relative weight is a value applied to the DRG based on the average complexity and resource consumption for patients within that DRG. The relative weight for carpal tunnel release will be much lower than the relative weight for major chest procedures, which is one of the most highly weighted DRGs. The relative weight will apply differently for Medicare versus other third party payers.

Institutions performing a larger number of procedures with higher relative weight values will see a higher overall reimbursement, reflected in the case mix index (CMI) for each department and ultimately the institution. The CMI provides an indication of the relative cost of providing care and is determined by taking an average of all the service intensity weights over all discharges for the institution. The service intensity weights are the average of all the weights of all DRGs seen on a particular service.

For example, transplants carry an extremely high relative weight. Therefore a large number of transplants will inflate the overall CMI, resulting in a better financial appearance. Complexity and intensity form the basis of the CMI system. Although there is no clear definition of complexity, it generally refers to the types of services rendered, while intensity refers to the number of services per patient day or hospital stay (Luke, 1979).

There is some incentive in this system for health care organizations to bring in larger numbers of patients whose DRG will be of a higher relative weight. Often hospitals emphasize these types of services to the detriment of lower paying groups.

Beth Israel Medical Center used the relative weight values as a basis for determining the financial gain or loss of each of the diagnoses or procedures tracked under the case management system. If the diagnosis being evaluated falls within one DRG, the process is much easier. In the case of endocarditis the length of stay for case managed patients decreased from 14.4 days in 1990 to 8.7 days in 1991. This length-of-stay reduction was analyzed against the number of cases at the shorter length of stay and the relative weight for the DRG.

A relative cost weight is obtained by dividing the adjusted national cost per DRG by the adjusted national cost per case for all DRGs. The larger the relative cost weight, the greater the relative costliness of a DRG (Grimaldi & Micheletti, 1983).

An assumption was made that for each day's reduction in length of stay, the bed was "back-filled" with a patient falling into a DRG with the same or greater relative weight. In this way, although the length of stay was decreased, available beds were used.

In other cases the surgical procedure being analyzed fell under more than one DRG, as in the case of laminectomies. In this circumstance the relative weight for all possible DRGs must be averaged.

With case management teams that potentially could be managing several DRGs, the same process would be followed. The average relative weight would be averaged for all possible DRGs, again assuming the beds would be back-filled with similar patients.

Although this type of cost-accounting system is not precise, it does give a good indication of the approximate incremental revenue savings for the diagnosis or surgical procedure under analysis.

More recent studies have shown similar results of decreased length of stay and costs (Blegen, Reiter, Goode, & Murphy, 1995).

IMPLICATIONS FOR FURTHER RESEARCH

All the studies reviewed share common implications for clinical and professional practice. One implication is in the area of assessing the quality of the critical path analysis and MAPs. Both the critical path and MAP were used to set clinical resource and cost standards and were responsible for most of the planning, coordination, and integration activities of the nursing case management model. Future research would be helpful for evaluating the critical path's and MAP's reliability and validity. Additional research should also focus on the treatment and practice protocols developed by the critical path and MAP analysis as they relate to patient care and clinical practice outcomes.

One other major implication is in objectively measuring the contributions of the nursing case management model to the quality of patient care, in particular, its effects on patient care resources, and in assessing patient and provider satisfaction. Additional research is needed to look at the effects of nursing case management on professional autonomy and decision-making opportunities for nurses, collaborative practice arrangements between nurses and physicians, nursing case management staffing and assignment allocations, payment and reimbursement mechanisms for nursing case management services, and the types of nursing case management interventions used and the effects of these interventions on patient outcomes. Other general implications for nursing follow:

- The changes in practice patterns associated with nursing case management can help to reduce overall expenditures related to hospitalization.
- Nursing case management can provide substantial improvements in the cost-effectiveness of patient care.
- Nursing case management focuses on collaborative practice arrangements between nurses and physicians to help shorten length of hospital stay and maintain effective use of money and materials, thereby having a significant effect on the hospital's fiscal bottom line and viability.
- Nursing case management has the potential to equate the effects of clinical nursing services and outcomes with resource allocation, costs, and reimbursement systems.
- Nursing case management has the potential to positively affect the present nursing care shortage by reorganizing delivery systems to maximize professional decision-making opportunities for nurses and allowing for continuity of patient care.
- Nursing case management can relate the cost savings of nursing interventions to specific patient populations in the acute care setting.
- Nursing case management can enhance the management of nursing services and substantiate the economic accountability and contribution of nurses to consumers of health care services.

Nursing case management provides the baseline for further research and evaluation of the functional competencies and uses of different skill levels in delivering nursing care services to patients and their families. This approach allows for more efficient integration of various levels of support staff by defining role expectations. Cohen's (1990) study successfully used the registered nurse as the case manager and case associate with the nursing assistants as support staff. The nurse case manager coordinated, assessed, evaluated, and participated with the case associates in the delivery of patient care. The nursing assistants carried out tasks associated with the patients' activities of daily living as delegated by the nurse case manager.

References

American Hospital Association. (1990). *1990 report of the hospital nursing personnel survey.* Chicago: Author.

Bair, N., Griswold, J., & Head, J. (1989). Clinical RN involvement in bedside-centered case management. *Nursing Economics, 7*(3), 150-154.

Blegen, M.A., Reiter, R., Goode, C.J., & Murphy, R. (1995). Hospital based managed care: Cost and quality. *Obstetrics & Gynecology, 86*(5), 809-814.

Cohen, E. (1990). *The effects of a nursing case management model on patient length of stay and variables related to cost of care delivery within an acute care setting.* Dissertation Abstracts International, 51-07B, 3325 (University Microfilm No. 90-33878), Ann Arbor, Mich.: University Micro Films International.

Cohen, E. (1991). Nursing case management: Does it pay? *Journal of Nursing Administration, 21*(4), 20-25.

Grimaldi, P.L., & Micheletti, J.A. (1983). *Diagnosis related groups.* Chicago: Pluribus Press.

Health Care Advisory Board. (1990). Tactic #1 potential savings of more than $1 million from change in delivery system, use of critical paths for two DRGs. Superlative clinical quality: Special review of pathbreaking ideas, clinical quality (1) (pp. 23). Washington, D.C.: Advisory Board Co.

Luke, R.D. (1979, Spring). Dimensions in hospital case mix measurement. *Inquiry, 16,* 38-49.

McKenzie, C., Torkelson, N., & Holt, M. (1989). Care and cost: Nursing case management improves both. *Nursing Management, 20*(10), 30-34.

Stillwaggon, C. (1989). The impact of nurse managed care on the cost of nurse practice and nurse satisfaction. *Journal of Nursing Administration, 19*(11), 21-27.

Case Management Evaluation

The Use of the Cost-Effectiveness Analysis Method

Hussein A. Tahan

CHAPTER OVERVIEW

The widespread restructuring of health care has created an urgent need for strategies that optimize the health condition of the people, their access to a wide variety of care services, and the quality and cost-effectiveness of these services. One strategy that has gained considerable attention and recognition is case management. There is growing consensus that case management enhances the value of health services (i.e., cost and quality), accessibility to care services, and client (patient, family, and significant other/care giver) and professional (health care providers and staff) satisfaction. Yet the research data to support this conclusion are still limited. Increasingly, administrators of case management programs of care delivery are called on to provide evidence that their decisions are, in fact, contributing to strategic quality and cost goals. This chapter explores how case management evaluation studies should be conducted so that better decisions regarding effective patient care delivery systems, health services, and health policy can be made and the utility of the case management systems can be widely supported. A review of select case management research studies (Appendix 46-1) is also presented to support the discussion and recommendations made.

Case management is defined according to the American Nurses Association as follows:

> Dynamic and systematic collaborative approach to providing and coordinating health care services to a defined population. It is a participative process to identify and facilitate options and services for meeting individuals' health needs, while decreasing fragmentation and duplication of care and enhancing quality, cost-effective clinical outcomes. The framework for nursing case management includes five components: assessment, planning, implementation, evaluation, and interaction (1999, p. 3).

However, since the practice of case management is not limited to nursing, it is essential to include the definition of case management advocated for by the Case Management Society of America, an international, multidisciplinary, not-for-profit organization with members from various disciplines, including nursing, medicine, managed care organizations, workers compensation, social work, physical therapy and durable medical equipment company representatives. The Case Management Society of America defines case management as follows:

Collaborative process which assesses, plans, implements, coordinates, monitors, and evaluates options and services to meet an individual's health needs through communication and available resources to promote cost-effective outcomes (1995, p. 8).

Examining these definitions one may note that they are very similar and basically contain the same elements of the case management process, specifically, assessment, planning, implementation, facilitation, coordination and collaboration, monitoring, and evaluation. These elements are important when considering a research process for evaluating the effectiveness of case management programs. The variables studied should reflect these essential elements.

The case management research literature reviewed and critiqued in Appendix 46-1 shows that case management programs are rarely appropriately evaluated and, in some instances, variables are loosely defined or used. The research design methods, data collection, and sampling methodologies seem to be an "afterthought." These research studies are for the most part retrospective attempts at validating the value of case management programs and neglect the use of cost-effectiveness analysis methods despite the fact that they claim to evaluate cost. None of these studies discuss any confounding variables that may have influenced the results obtained. Therefore these studies are of minimal significance for health policy and health services decision-making practices. In addition, they are weak studies and can be deemed minimally effective if used by health care administrators to promote the practice of case management as a patient care delivery model. Issues of cost, quality, access to care, and scope of services should be examined when evaluating case management delivery systems so that their implications for health policy decisions can be heightened. Very rarely more than one of these variables are examined in the studies shared herein. The following section discusses the extent to which different variables are examined in the reviewed studies.

THE PROCESS, STRUCTURE, AND OUTCOME VARIABLES

One of the most complex tasks is to design a study that evaluates the interconnectedness and relationships of the process, structure, and outcome variables of any care delivery system, not just case management. However, researchers should attempt to maximize the significance of their studies by including a mix of variables that address important process, structure, and outcomes variables of their care delivery systems. The reviewed case management studies were found to be lacking in this area. A select list of the most commonly examined variables in the case management studies reviewed and summarized in Appendix 46-1 is presented in Box 46-1. Most of the case management process variables were addressed in a descriptive and conceptual way (Edelstein & Cesta, 1993; Erkel et al, 1993; Ethridge & Lamb, 1989; Goode, 1995; Polinsky, Fred, & Ganz, 1991; Rubin, 1992; Trella, 1993), and the information shared was not based on research outcomes, but rather on the case management model design at the specific institution where the study was conducted. Descriptive statistics (mean, median, standard deviation, frequency, and percentage) were primarily used in the analyses of these studies; regression analysis or other inferential techniques were seldom applied.

A few qualitative studies described the nurse case manager's activities and attempted to identify the case management process(es) of care delivery (Goodwin, 1994; Newcomer, Arnsberger, & Zhang, 1997; Sohl-Kreiger, Lagaard, & Schorrer, 1996; Van Dongen & Jambunathan, 1992; Williams et al, 1993). Researchers should rely on the results of these studies when they design quantitative studies for the evaluation of case management programs. A few other studies examined the structure of case management by evaluating the uncertainty and ambiguity of the work environment, extent of staff autonomy, col-

> Box 46-1

VARIABLES EXAMINED IN THE CASE MANAGEMENT STUDIES REVIEWED

STRUCTURE
Case management team
Nurse case manager qualities
Collaboration
Autonomy
Need for transportation
Available housing
Availability of providers/service
Participation in decision making
Work environment (uncertainty, ambiguity, predictability)
Telephone-based case management
Hospital-based care
Clinic-based care
Community-based care
Client outreach programs
Use of advanced practice nurses/clinical nurse specialists
Role conflict, identity,
Role overload
Interactions with other providers

PROCESS
Case management activities/process (assessment, planning, interventions, evaluation, monitoring, etc.)
Transfer to skilled nursing facility
Access to case managers/health care provider
Access to prenatal care
Access to immunization services
Discharge process
Telephone-based case management
Patient/family teaching
Client outreach process
Care coordination process
Referral process
Client advocacy
Information sharing

OUTCOMES
Length of stay
Blood glucose control
Patient satisfaction
Staff satisfaction
Social stability
Number of clinic visits
Length of time spent with the patient
Physical and functional abilities
Level of dependence/independence
Emotional status
Physiological outcomes (blood pressure, respiration rate, ejection fraction, oxygen saturation, etc.)
Direct cost

Continued

> **Box 46-1**   VARIABLES EXAMINED IN THE CASE MANAGEMENT
> STUDIES REVIEWED—cont'd

OUTCOMES—CONT'D
Indirect cost
Cost per case
Cost per patient day
Hospital charges per case
Average daily charges
Discharge destination
Nosocomial infections
Adverse events (urinary tract infection, pressure ulcer, bacteremia)
Patient/family health knowledge
Number of telephone calls
Emergency department visits
Readmissions
Infant mortality and morbidity
Resource utilization
Estimated reimbursement
Nurse case management hours per patient day
Cost of nurse case management hours per patient day
Medications
Nutritional status
Weight loss
Pain

laboration with other providers, and role conflict and overload (Allred et al, 1995; Arford & Allred, 1995; Tonges, 1998).

As to the outcomes of case management services, many studies identified the effect of case management on patient satisfaction, staff satisfaction, length of stay, number of clinic visits, cost of care, complications, readmissions, and other variables (refer to Appendix 46-1, and Box 46-1). Some studies evaluated the relationships between two types of variables: either process or structure with outcome variables.

THE SCOPE, ACCESS, COST, AND QUALITY VARIABLES

Regardless of the setting where case management is practiced (e.g., ambulatory, acute, community, long-term), the type of health care professional (discipline or specialty) responsible for the case manager's role, or the type of health care organization (e.g., private, academic, research, non-for-profit, etc.) and geographical location, the goals of case management remain the same. Case management care delivery models are basically implemented to:

1. Expand the scope of services provided to the population
2. Increase access to health care services
3. Reduce cost of health care services
4. Improve outcomes of the care delivered
5. Improve quality of care.

The scope of services is considered a structure variable, while cost and quality are outcome variables. Access to health care services, on the other hand, may be a process or a structure variable. As a process, it entails the way a person accesses health care services, for example, via telephone or home care visit. As a structure, it is concerned with availability of services that enhance patient accessibility to care. None of the case management studies reviewed examined the relationships of these four types of variables at the same time. The combination of variables most commonly used was scope, cost and quality, or access, cost, and quality. This may have resulted from the difficulty of conducting a study that combines the four variables. Such studies are known to be complex, costly, and time consuming and require the coordination of a professional with a specialized knowledge base.

In the studies reviewed in Appendix 46-1, cost and quality are the most commonly examined outcome variables in case management. However, this does not mean that the quality outcomes of case management delivery systems are well supported by research and well documented in the literature. The most frequently examined variables are cost per case, length of stay, readmission rate, and complication rate. These variables are defined by some researchers as quality of care indicators and by some others as cost indicators. The confusion as to whether these indicators are quality or cost variables may have contributed to the present lack in the use of cost-effectiveness analysis (CEA) method in case management evaluation studies.

Studies that incorporate the CEA method in their evaluation enhance better decision making regarding health policy and health services practices. Thus conducting such research is a priority if case management is to be endorsed as a desired care delivery system. Health policy makers cannot and will not support such endorsement unless the cost-effectiveness of these systems is validated using health services research designs; that is, examining the relationship between cost and quality of case management delivery systems and demonstrating that these systems are more cost-effective than the standard/traditional care delivery approaches. Cost and quality variables are integral to CEA research. Eliminating the confusion surrounding which variables constitute quality and which ones constitute cost is important before conducting case management evaluation studies that have implications for health policy and health services research.

COST-EFFECTIVENESS ANALYSIS IN NURSING CASE MANAGEMENT

Lately, interest in applying economic methods to the evaluation of health care interventions, options, and delivery systems has increased. CEA is one economic method commonly used to evaluate outcomes and costs of interventions and treatments or delivery systems designed to improve the person's state of health (Allred et al, 1998).

CEA is defined as a method for evaluating the health outcomes and resource costs of patient care treatments and interventions (Russell et al., 1996; Stone, 1998). Its central function is to show the relative value of alternative interventions implemented for improving the health condition of an individual patient or the health status of a population. Such analysis leads to information that can assist the decision maker weigh the alternatives and select the best one(s). Cost of the alternative interventions is measured in monetary values. However, outcomes effectiveness is measured using nonmonetary terms (e.g., health-related quality of life, life years gained) (Chan & Henry, 1999). Arford and Allred (1995) developed a quality index measure and used it to evaluate the effectiveness of nursing outcomes. It is feasible to employ this quality index measure when applying the CEA method for the evaluation of case management systems.

Although the influence of CEA in the development of health care policy is not well documented (Allred et al, 1998; Chan & Henry, 1999), this method allows the making of more influential health policy decisions. The CEA framework is also an effective mechanism for making decisions regarding health care resource allocation, scope of services, accessibility of the public to health care, and especially those decisions that involve the delivery of nursing care and improvement of clinical care quality outcomes. Thus CEA as a case management evaluation method is perfectly appropriate because it facilitates and promotes a better decision-making process regarding the essential strategies that improve the scope of and access to health care services while maintaining or enhancing quality outcomes and reducing cost.

The CEA method is a preferred approach to evaluating the effectiveness of case management systems of patient care delivery because it does not necessitate the conversion of outcomes/benefits into dollar values, unlike the cost-benefit analysis method, which cannot be applied unless benefits are quantified using dollar amounts (Chan & Henry, 1999; Udvarhelyi et al., 1992). Outcomes of case management systems are not limited to cost. Quantifying some of the outcomes such as patient and family satisfaction, continuity of care, and quality of life in dollar amounts is a challenge.

The CEA method has been advocated widely since the early 1990s by federal agencies, including the Agency of Health Care Policy and Research (known today as the Agency for Healthcare Research & Quality (AHRQ), the National Institute of Health, the Health Care Financing Administration, and the Centers for Disease Control and Prevention (Chan & Henry, 1999). The use of this method in evaluating nursing case management has been lacking. Although the financial and quality-related variables and outcomes of nursing case management systems for patient care delivery have been widely studied, this method has been applied in few cases only (Allred et al, 1995; Arford & Allred, 1995; Erkel, et al, 1993). In a review of medical, nursing, and health services literature for the years 1990 through 1996, Chan and Henry (1999) identified 88 articles that applied cost analysis methods, of which four were attributed to nursing. Of these articles, 36 used the CEA method, including only two studies conducted by nurses. The lack of CEA studies in the field of nursing may be attributed to nursing's lack of knowledge and training in financial-cost analyses, and the difficulty and complexity of such evaluations. It was not until 1997 that cost analysis research was recommended as an area of study in nursing administration education (American Association of Colleges of Nursing, 1997).

In the evaluation studies reviewed in this chapter, the CEA method was applied on three occasions only, but it could have been appropriately used in 16 studies. To bring case management systems to the forefront of health care delivery and public/health policy decisions, health services research applying the CEA method is highly needed.

Often the goal of CEA is to compare the cost-effectiveness of a new alternate intervention (Allred et al, 1995; Russell et al, 1996; Stone, 1998) or care delivery system (in this case the use of case management care delivery system) to current/traditional standards. Cost-effectiveness studies of case management are influential in health policy making, since the goals of case management are similar to those of health policy, which are to increase accessibility to care services, improve quality of care, and reduce the incurred cost. Other goals that are integral to case management are services coordination, integration, and brokerage, as well as the use of preventive services such as wellness and health promotion programs. Studies addressing these goals are of interest to the payers, providers, and consumers of health care alike, but especially to health policy makers, lobbyists, and public advocates.

OVERVIEW OF THE COST-EFFECTIVENESS ANALYSIS METHOD

Conducting case management evaluation studies using the CEA method must comply with the six principles of cost analysis identified and defined by Udvarhelyi et al (1992) and Stone (1998), and applied by Chan and Henry (1999) in their review of the literature on cost analyses in the disciplines of nursing, medicine, and health services. These principles define the minimum acceptable standard (minimum requirement) for conducting and reporting a CEA study. Udvarhelyi and his colleagues designed these principles based on a review of the theoretical literature regarding the methods of cost analysis and the economic evaluation of health care practices. The six principles recommended are the ones found to be most commonly advocated for in the literature reviewed (Udvarhelyi et al, 1992). These principles help clarify any misunderstandings of the methodology applied, prevent faulty techniques, and avoid inconclusive or incorrect procedures. These principles are summarized here.

PRINCIPLE 1.   **Explicit statement of the analytic perspective** which usually addresses who pays specific costs (e.g., payers such as managed care organizations and the federal government) and who benefits from an intervention (e.g., patients and society).

PRINCIPLE 2.   **A description of the anticipated benefits** of the intervention (in this case the case management care delivery system). If the benefits are unproven, one can make explicit the assumed benefits. Examples of the anticipated benefits of case management systems may include reduced readmission/rehospitalization rates, patient and family satisfaction with care, increased patient and family knowledge of illness, health condition, and health needs.

PRINCIPLE 3.   **A specification of the types of costs** used or considered that are carefully derived from the statement of the analytical perspective. Examples of costs as they relate to the practice of case management are cost of case managers (i.e., salaries), costs of services such as utilization reviews/managed care reviews, including the cost of the method used for communication and costs of equipment (e.g., computers, fax machines) and supplies (e.g., paperwork). Cost can also be defined as the cost per case, that is, the cost incurred while caring for a particular patient.

PRINCIPLE 4.   **Adjusting for differential timing,** which is called discounting. This process is important when the costs and benefits studied accrue during significantly different time periods, usually greater than 1 year. Frequently the timing of costs and the noted benefits are different. It is essential to account for this difference in the analysis, so future costs and benefits are adjusted back to their present values. As for case management, discounting is necessary if the CEA evaluation is performed in a time period greater than 1 year.

PRINCIPLE 5.   **Conducting a sensitivity analysis** to test the robustness of conclusions to variations in the underlying assumptions and estimates. The sensitivity analysis usually explores whether alternative assumptions explain the costs and benefits noted. It reinforces the validity of the conclusions made.

PRINCIPLE 6.   **Including a summary measurement of efficiency** such as a cost-effectiveness ratio (C/E ratio). The use of a C/E ratio is essential to facilitate the comparison of the alternative interventions. The ratio is usually expressed using incremental cost-effectiveness terms to compare and prioritize one intervention with the next least expensive or the next least effective/beneficial. In case management, for example, the interventions compared can be the use of disease-based case managers versus patient care unit-based case managers (i.e., general case managers), or a fragmented case management role versus an integrated role (i.e., combined clinical management, utilization management, and transitional planning).

The question CEA is designed to address must be clearly stated. Often the goal is to compare the cost-effectiveness of one intervention or model to either the current standard or to one or more other variations on the model. The question asked delineates what outcomes should be included and evaluated in the analysis. Therefore the question must be stated explicitly. In case management the practice of case management may be compared to the traditional way of delivering patient care or different variations of the case management system can be compared among each other. Either way, the purpose of the CEA evaluation and the question should be clearly asked before the data are collected and the analysis is performed. Different questions demand different types of cost and benefit data collection and analyses.

The benefits evaluated in case management CEA are the outcomes of the case management system as defined by the individual institution implementing this system of patient care delivery. The appropriate outcomes depend on the purpose of the analysis. Since outcomes of case management systems may not be considered society-based, quality-adjusted life years as an outcome is considered inappropriate. Developing a specific case management quality index measure based on the quality index developed by Arford and Allred (1995) can result in a better determined outcome measure for case management systems. The outcomes considered in the development of the Arford and Allred's quality index are occurrence of urinary tract infection, occurrence of bacteremia, skin breakdown, patient satisfaction, and length of stay. Two of these outcomes are appropriate for case management, specifically, patient and family satisfaction and length of stay. Other case management–based outcomes can be determined by the individual institution in relation to the specific goals of the case management system. Among these outcomes are staff satisfaction, readmission/rehospitalization rates, emergency department visits, unplanned primary care provider's visits, rate of reimbursement denials, rate of denied appeals, patient/family knowledge of illness and treatment regimen, carve-out days (these are hospitalization days the payer denies payment for), patient/family perception of health and quality of life, continuity of care, and others as desired.

To estimate the cost of resources incurred by the case management system, different types of costs must be considered. Traditionally, costs have been classified as "direct" or "variable" and "indirect" or "fixed." Direct/variable costs are those incurred in providing direct care for patients. Indirect/fixed costs, however, are those of overhead (e.g., salaries, utilities, etc.). Health care organizations determine these costs differently depending on specific factors such as payer mix, patient mix, staffing patterns, or the cost accounting system they employ. In acute care case management, for example, determining the cost per patient is important when performing a CEA.

Arford and Allred (1995) identified a method for CEA incorporating a quality index. The quality index is multidimensional, hence, it captures the multidimensionality of the outcomes of case management systems. The steps involved in this method are outlined here.

Step 1.   **Identifying the outcomes/benefits or indicators** used to measure the effectiveness of case management systems.

Examples of these outcomes are presented in Table 46-1. It is important to determine the threshold of the indicators (desired level/criterion) that cannot be reported in a percentage figure. For example, patient and family satisfaction is reported as an average score based on a rating scale of 1 to 5, with 1 being poor and 5 being outstanding. A threshold for such indicator could be patient and family satisfaction with care ratings of 4 and above. Similar indicators can then be incorporated in the case management quality index score as the percentage of patients meeting or exceeding the predetermined threshold; for example, percentage of patients reporting their rating of satisfaction with care as 4 or above. Other similar indicators that require building a threshold for are staff satisfaction, patient and family knowledge of illness and treatment regimen, and patient's perception of health and quality of life.

Step 2.   **Weighing the outcomes** in terms of importance to quality care and to measuring the effectiveness of case management systems.

Weights can be established using an expert panel of case management providers applying appropriate research methods. The expert panel can use a 10-point rating scale to rate their perception of the importance of each indicator in the benefits/outcomes of case management systems. The weights assigned to each of the outcome indicators correspond to the indicator's mean importance rating. The mean weights are then standardized by dividing each weight by the total value of all the assigned weights. For example, based on the hypothetical examples presented in Table 46-1, the mean rating (i.e., assigned weight) for length of stay is 8.6 and the total weight is 90.0, so the standardized weight for length of stay becomes 0.0956. The standardized weight is important for calculating the quality index.

Step 3. **Measuring the outcomes** using appropriate methodologies as indicated by the type of outcome indicator.

For example, questionnaires are used to measure patient and family satisfaction, and length of stay can be determined based on data extracted from the Admit-Discharge-Transfer (ADT) automated system. It is important to be clear up-front on the best method(s) to be followed in outcomes data collection.

Step 4. **Calculating the case management quality index (CMQI) score.**

The quality index is calculated based on the unit of analysis identified in the purpose and question of the CEA study. In CEA the unit of analysis is related to the alternative ways of accomplishing the outcome indicators. The CMQI score (Box 46-2), for example, may include the environment of delivering patient care (i.e., case management versus no case management). The formula shared here is derived based on the formula developed by Arford and Allred (1995). The outcomes incorporated in the current formula compared to the ones found in the original formula are considered more reflective of the practice of case management.

The case management quality index score is calculated as described in Box 46-2. As illustrated, the numerator is derived by determining the proportion of patients in the case management practice environment that demonstrated each of the 10 quality indicator/attributes, then multiplying the proportion of accomplishing each indicator by its associated standardized weight, shown in Table 46-1, and finally totaling the 10 products (i.e., resulting values). The denominator is calculated in the same way, however, the proportion of the total patients accomplishing the quality indicator/attribute is calculated based on both practice environments (i.e., case management and no case management). Table 46-2 presents a practical example on the application of the quality index. Data presented in this example are hypothetical and shared for clarification purpose only.

Table 46-1	**OUTCOME INDICATORS/ATTRIBUTES FOR THE CASE MANAGEMENT QUALITY INDEX**	
INDICATORS/ATTRIBUTES	**AVERAGE ASSIGNED WEIGHT**	**STANDARDIZED WEIGHT**
a. Length of stay reduction (%)	8.6	0.0956
b. Patient and family satisfaction (% meeting the threshold)	9.3	0.1033
c. Staff satisfaction (% meeting the threshold)	8.5	0.0944
d. Rate of readmissions/rehospitalizations (%)	9.4	0.1044
e. Rate of reimbursement denials (%)	9.6	0.1067
f. Rate of emergency department visits (%)	8.9	0.0989
g. Rate of unplanned primary care provider visits (%)	8.6	0.0956
h. Patient and family knowledge of illness and treatment regimen (% meeting the threshold)	9.0	0.1000
i. Patient's perception of health and quality of life (% meeting the threshold)	9.1	0.1011
j. Carve-out days (%)	9.0	0.1000
TOTAL	**90.0**	**1.0**

NOTE: The weights shared are hypothetical and presented for clarification purposes only.

| Box 46-2 | **FORMULA FOR CALCULATING THE CASE MANAGEMENT QUALITY INDEX (CMQI) SCORE** |

$$CMQI = \frac{\sum_{i=1}^{10} W_i \cdot n_{ti}/N_t}{\sum_{i=1}^{10} W_i \cdot n_{oi}/N_o}$$

Where: $CMQI$ = the case management quality index for each of the practice environments (case management versus no case management)

n_{ti}/N_t = the proportion of patients, in the case management practice environment, who demonstrated the accomplishment of the quality attribute/indicator

n_{oi}/N_o = the proportion of the total patients in both practice environments that demonstrated the accomplishment of the quality attributes/indicators

W_i = the standardized weight for each of the quality attributes/indicators

Σ = summation across all 10 quality attributes/indicators (the number of attributes/indicators is adjusted based on the actual number of indicators measured)

NOTE: Modified from Arford, P. & Allred, C. (1995). Value = quality + cost. *Journal of Nursing Administration, 25*(9), 64-69.

Step 5. **Calculating patient care costs (direct and indirect).**

Patient care costs are calculated differently in different health care organizations. The more sophisticated an organization is in its cost accounting system, the more accurate the resulting cost estimate is. However, since the environment of health care reimbursement is no longer based on fee for service, the calculated cost reflects a relative estimate rather than 100% accurate dollar amounts. In any case, it is important to determine the average cost per patient for both the case management and no case management practice environments. The average cost per patient is determined by dividing the total costs per environment accrued in a specific time period (usually the time period of the CEA study) by the total number of patients cared for in that environment during the same time period. These figures are needed for calculating the associated cost-effectiveness ratios.

Step 6. **Calculating the cost-effectiveness ratio.**

The C/E ratio (Box 46-3) is a measure of value of case management. It is constructed with the cost as the numerator and the net benefits as the denominator (Arford & Allred, 1995; Stone, 1998). Therefore the average cost per patient makes the numerator and the CMQI makes the denominator. A lower C/E ratio is desired because such ratio indicates better outcomes and lesser costs. The greater the C/E ratio, the lower its associated value is. The higher the CMQI is, the lower the C/E ratio becomes. The C/E ratio aids in determining which practice environment is relatively better, the case management or no case management environment. Box 46-3 presents an example of how to calculate a C/E ratio.

The CMQI and the C/E ratio can be used to evaluate the outcomes of case management systems over time. The application of these methods is not limited to comparing case management and no case management environments of care. Health care organizations who have implemented case management systems several years ago as their patient care delivery models can still apply these methods. However, a different type of comparison is employed. The objective of using the CMQI and the C/E ratio in such organizations is shifted to studying the environment of care in terms of comparing the financial and quality outcomes of the different services (e.g., cardiac, geriatric, obstetrics, oncology, pediatrics, pulmonary, etc.) or different case managers (e.g., cardiac case manager, geriatric case manager, obstetric

Table 46-2	EXAMPLE OF CALCULATING THE CASE MANAGEMENT QUALITY INDEX SCORE

Sample A consists of 100 patients who received case management services and Sample B consists of 100 patients who did not receive case management services. All patients were cared for in an acute care setting. Assuming that the patients in both samples have similar case mix index and the following data on the 10 quality indicators prospectively determined as the attributes/benefits of case management services, calculate the CMQI. Note that the average length of stay before case management was 7.0 days.

INDICATOR	SAMPLE A	SAMPLE B	ALL PATIENTS
a. Length of stay reduction	2.8 (40%)	1.4 (20%)	2.1 (30%)
b. Patient and family satisfaction	89%	78%	83.5%
c. Staff satisfaction	95%	89%	92%
d. Rate of readmissions/ rehospitalizations	3%	7%	5%
e. Rate of reimbursement denials	2%	5%	3.5%
f. Rate of emergency department visits	2%	3.5%	2.75%
g. Rate of unplanned primary care provider visits	4%	6%	5%
h. Patient and family knowledge of illness and treatment regimen	88%	79%	83.5%
i. Patient's perception of health and quality of life	85%	78%	81.5%
j. Carve-out days	1%	2.5%	1.75%

QUALITY INDEX FOR THE CASE MANAGED POPULATION (SAMPLE A) =

$$QI = \frac{\begin{array}{c}(0.0956)(0.4) + (0.1033)(0.89) + (0.0944)(0.95) + (0.1044)(0.03) + \\ (0.1067)(0.02) + (0.0989)(0.02) + (0.0956)(0.04) + (0.1)(0.88) + (0.1011)(0.85) + (0.1)(0.01)\end{array}}{\begin{array}{c}(0.0956)(0.3) + (0.1033)(0.835) + (0.0944)(0.92) + (0.1044)(0.05) + (0.1067)(0.035) + \\ (0.0989)(0.0275) + (0.0956)(0.05) + (0.1)(0.835) + (0.1011)(0.815) + (0.1)(0.075)\end{array}}$$

QI = 1.0363

QUALITY INDEX FOR THE NON-CASE-MANAGED POPULATION (SAMPLE B) =

$$QI = \frac{\begin{array}{c}(0.0956)(0.2) + (0.1033)(0.78) + (0.0944)(0.89) + (0.1044)(0.07) + (0.1067)(0.05) + \\ (0.0989)(0.035) + (0.0956)(0.06) + (0.1)(0.79) + (0.1011)(0.78) + (0.1)(0.025)\end{array}}{\begin{array}{c}(0.0956)(0.3) + (0.1033)(0.835) + (0.0944)(0.92) + (0.1044)(0.05) + (0.1067)(0.035) + \\ (0.0989)(0.0275) + (0.0956)(0.05) + (0.1)(0.835) + (0.1011)(0.815) + (0.1)(0.075)\end{array}}$$

QI = 0.9676

case manager, oncology case manager, pediatric case manager, pulmonary case manager, etc.). In this case the C/E ratio is used to evaluate whether cost and quality outcomes are maintained or improved over time and how these ratios are compared across services and/or case managers. The same methods and formulas discussed in Table 46-2 and Box 46-3 are applied. However, the population of patients used to compute the values of the numerators and denominators of these formulas are defined differently and based on the patient populations of the particular services or who are cared for by the individual case managers.

| Box 46-3 | CALCULATING THE COST-EFFECTIVENESS RATIO (C/E RATIO) |

Assume that in the same example presented in Table 46-2, the average cost per patient is $15,000.00 in Sample A and $18,600.00 in Sample B. Calculate the C/E ratios

C/E Ratio = Average cost per patient/Quality index

C/E Ratio for the case-managed population (Sample A) = $15,000/1.0363 = $14,474.57

C/E Ratio for the non-case-managed population (Sample B) = $18,600/0.9676 = $19,222.82

If the cost-effectiveness comparative analysis is completed in relation to the different services, the numerator is computed for each of the services separately (i.e., cardiac), and the denominator is then computed, considering all the services combined, including cardiac. However, if the comparison is made in terms of the different case managers, then the numerator is computed for each of the case managers (i.e., cardiac patient population served by the cardiac case manager), and the denominator is computed for all the populations cared for by the case managers combined, including cardiac. After these values are computed, the results of the CMQI are used to compute the C/E ratios. The C/E ratios are compared and the service or the case manager who is most cost-effective is determined.

To use this comparison over time, it is important to determine the frequency of completing such CEA and the time period for which data are collected. Because the method is time consuming, a time interval of 4 to 6 months is recommended (i.e., two to three times per year). A threshold for the C/E ratio should also be predetermined. The value of the threshold communicates the minimum acceptable cost-effectiveness standard. This value is not arbitrary; it is determined based on the baseline data and the expectations of the health care organization. Usually it is desirable to have an observed C/E ratio that is lower than the threshold. This means that the performance of the case management system or case managers are more cost-effective. It is also desired to have a downward trend in the C/E ratios observed over time. Such a trend indicates improvement in cost-effectiveness.

Cost-effectiveness analysis allows health care organizations, decision makers, and health policy advocates to convey the value of case management services delivered based on cost information for an anticipated level of quality outcomes and health care benefits. CEA, especially, the use of the C/E ratio, facilitates a process of decision making regarding what services to advocate for based on the relationship between their attached cost and quantifiable outcomes. Standardizing the CEA procedures can improve the quality and facilitate comparability of studies (Stone, 1998). The method described herein allows for such standardization and enhances a better way of analyzing the effectiveness of case management systems; thus providing a state of better health policy decisions considering the cost and value of case management services are better understood and measured.

Change today is very different. It is continuous and happening faster than ever before; it is more complex; its implications are more serious; and it is taking place on all levels: personal, professional, organizational, and societal. Applying the CEA method in case management evaluation practices presents a great challenge for all involved. It is an example of professional and organizational change that requires patience and perseverence. The results of such change affect the health of the society/population in that the outcomes of the CEA studies assist in making more appropriate decisions regarding access, scope, cost, and quality of health care services. The discussion and argument presented in this chapter make it clear that a revolutionary change in the way case management evaluations are done is necessary. It also provides a process for applying such analyses that can be used for expanding one's knowledge, alleviating fears and uncertainties, and reinforcing a positive attitude toward the necessity of such leap in nursing practice. The use of the CEA method in evaluating case management programs is essential for moving the practice of case management into a higher level of sophistication. The practical examples shared in this chapter can be used by health care administrators, executives, educators, and researchers as a step-by-step guide for applying the CEA method in case management program evaluations.

References

Allred, C., Arford, P., Mauldin, P., & Goodwin, L. (1998). Cost-effectiveness analysis in the nursing literature, 1992-1996. *IMAGE: Journal of Nursing Scholarship, 30*(3), 235-242.

Allred, C., Arford, P., Michel, Y., Dring, R., Carter, V., & Veitch, J. (1995). A cost-effectiveness analysis of acute care case management outcomes. *Nursing Economics, 13*(3), 129-136.

American Association of Colleges of Nursing. (1997). *Joint position statement on education for nurses in administrative roles.* Washington, D.C.: Author.

American Nurses Association. (1999). *Modular certification examination catalog.* Washington, D.C.: American Nurses Credentialing Center.

Arford, P., & Allred, C. (1995). Value = quality + cost. *Journal of Nursing Administration, 25*(9), 64-69.

Baker, C., Miller, I., Sitterding, M., & Hajewski, C. (1998). Acute stroke patients: Comparing outcomes with and without case management. *Nursing Case Management, 3*(5), 196-203.

Case Management Society of America. (1995). *Standards of practice for case management.* Little Rock, Ark.: Author.

Chan, W., & Henry, B. (1999). Methodologic principles of cost analyses in the nursing, medical, and health services literature, 1990-1996. *Nursing Research, 48*(2), 94-104.

Cohen, E. (1991). Nursing case management: Does it pay? *Journal of Nursing Administration, 21*(4), 20-25.

Crawley, W., & Till, A. (1995). Case management: More population-based data. *Clinical Nurse Specialist, 9*(2), 116-120.

Edelstein, E., & Cesta, T. (1993). Nursing case management: An innovative model of care for hospitalized patients with diabetes. *Nursing Care Management, 19*(6), 517-521.

Eggert, G., Zimmer, W., Hall, J., & Friedman, B. (1991). Case management: A randomized controlled study comparing a neighborhood team and a centralized individual model, *Health Services Research, 26*(4), 471-507.

Erkel, E., Morgan, E., Staples, M., Assey, V., & Michel, Y. (1993). Case management and preventive services among infants from low-income families. *Public Health Nursing, 11*(5), 352-360.

Ethridge, P., & Lamb, G. (1989). Professional nursing case management improves quality, access and costs. *Nursing Management, 20*(3), 30-35.

Fitzgerald, J., Smith, D., Martin, D., Freedman, J., & Katz, B. (1994). A case management intervention to reduce admissions. *Archives of Internal Medicine, 154,* 1721-1729.

Fleishman, J., Mor, V., & Piette, J. (1991). AIDS case management: The client's perspective. *Health Services Research, 26*(4), 448-470.

Goode, C. (1995). Impact of a CareMap and case management on patient satisfaction and staff satisfaction, collaboration, and autonomy. *Nursing Economics, 13*(6), 337-348.

Goodwin, D. (1994). Nursing case management activities: How they differ between employment settings. *Journal of Nursing Administration, 24*(2), 29-34.

Helvie, C., & Alexy, B. (1992). Using after-shelter case management to improve outcomes for families with children. *Public Health Reports, 107*(5), 585-588.

Johnson, K., & Proffitt, N. (1995). A decentralized model for case management. *Nursing Economics, 13*(3), 142-165.

Lamb, G., & Stemple, J. (1994). Nurse case management from the client's view: Growing as insider expert. *Nursing Outlook, 42*(1), 7-13.

Lynn, M., & Kelly, B. (1997). Effects of case management on the nursing context: Perceived quality of care, work satisfaction, and control over practice. *IMAGE: Journal of Nursing Scholarship, 29*(3), 237-241.

Mahn, V. (1993). Clinical case management: A service line approach. *Nursing Management, 24*(11), 48-50.

Mawn, B., & Bradley, J. (1993). Standards of care for high-risk prenatal clients: The community nurse case management approach. *Public Health Nursing, 10*(2), 78-88.

McKenzie, C., Trokelson, N., & Holt, M. (1989). Care and cost: Nursing case management improves both. *Nursing Management, 20*(10), 30-34.

Micheels, T., Wheeler, L., & Hays, B. (1995). Linking quality and cost effectiveness: Case management by an advanced practice nurse. *Clinical Nurse Specialist, 9*(2), 107-111.

Morrison, R., & Beckworth, V. (1998). Outcomes for patients with congestive heart failure in a nursing case management model. *Nursing Case Management, 3*(3), 108-114.

Newcomer, R., Arnsberger, P., & Zhang, X. (1997). Case management, client risk factors, and service use. *Health Care Financing Review, 19*(1), 105-120.

Polinsky, M., Fred, C., & Ganz, P. (1991). Quantitative and qualitative assessment of a case management program for cancer patients. *National Association of Social Work, 16*(3), 176-183.

Rogers, M., Riordan, J., & Swindle, D. (1990). Community-based nursing case management pays off. *Nursing Management, 22*(3), 30-34.

Rubin, A. (1992). Is case management effective for people with serious mental illness? A research review. *National Association of Social Workers, 17*(2), 138-150.

Russell, L., Gold, M., Siegel, J., Daniels, N., & Weinstein, M. (1996). The role of cost-effectiveness analysis in health and medicine. *Journal of the American Medical Association, 276*(14), 1172-1177.

Sands, R., & Canaan, R. (1994). Two methods of case management: Assessing their impact. *Community Mental Health Journal, 30*(5), 441-456.

Sizemore, M., Bennett, B., & Anderson, R. (1989). Public hospital-based geriatric case management. *Journal of Gerontological Social Work, 13*(3), 167-179.

Sohl-Kreiger, R., Lagaard, M., & Schorrer, J. (1996). Nursing case management: Relationships as a strategy to improve care. *Clinical Nurse Specialist, 10*(2), 107-113.

Stone, P. (1998). Methods for conducting and reporting cost-effectiveness analysis in nursing. *IMAGE: Journal of Nursing Scholarship, 30*(3), 229-234.

Thompson, M., Curry, M., & Burton, D. (1998). The effects of nursing case management on the utilization of prenatal care by Mexican-Americans in rural Oregon. *Public Health Nursing, 15*(2), 82-90.

Tonges, M. (1998). Job design for nurse case managers: Intended and unintended effects on satisfaction and well-being. *Nursing Case Management, 3*(1), 11-23.

Topp, R., Tucker, D., & Weber, C. (1998). Effect of a clinical case manager/clinical nurse specialist on patients hospitalized with congestive heart failure. *Nursing Case Management, 3*(4), 140-145.

Trella, R. (1993). A multidisciplinary approach to case management of frail hospitalized older adults. *Journal of Nursing Administration, 23*(2), 20-26.

Twyman, D., & Libbus, K. (1994). Case management of AIDS clients as a predictor of total inpatient hospital days. *Public Health Nursing, 11*(6), 406-411.

Udvarhelyi, S., Colditz, G., Rai, A., & Epstein, A. (1992). Cost-effectiveness and cost-benefit analysis in the medical literature. *American College of Physicians, 116*(3), 238-244.

Van Dongen, C., & Jambunathan, J. (1992). The psychiatric RN case manager: Pilot study results. *Journal of Psychosocial Nursing, 30*(11), 11-14.

Williams, F., Warrick, L., Christianson, J., & Netting, F. (1993). Critical factors for successful hospital-based case management. *Health Care Management Review, 18*(1), 63-70.

APPENDIX 46-1

Summary of Selected Case Management Evaluation Studies

Author, Year	Aim(s)	Indicators			Services				Design	CEA	Findings	Limitations/ Comments
		P	St	O	Sc	A	C	Q				
Ethridge & Lamb, 1989	Evaluate the impact of continuum-based nursing case management model			✓	✓	✓	✓		Retrospective review Varied patient population	N	Reduced cost and length of stay	Nonspecific procedure for data collection and instruments
McKenzie, Trokelson, & Holt, 1989	Evaluate the effectiveness of case management and its impact on cost and patient and staff satisfaction		✓	✓			✓	✓	Unclear design Retrospective MR review Comparative analysis of intervention and nonintervention groups	N	Reduced cost and length of stay Improved satisfaction	Actual satisfaction data are not shared
Sizemore, Bennett, & Anderson, 1989	Examine the evidence of success of a geriatric case management program implemented in a large public teaching hospital	✓	✓	✓	✓	✓			Retrospective descriptive program evaluation	N/A	Elderly patients had serious multiple health and social problems Successful program implementation	Good program model Results are tentative No report of readmissions or the need for institutionalization after hospital discharge Convenient sample
Rogers, Riordan, & Swindle, 1990	Examine the effectiveness of a community-based case management model	✓		✓			✓		Pre-/post-comparison	N	Reduced length of stay, admission rate, and cost of services	Only one process discussed: patient referral to community services Unclear data collection and sampling methods

P, Process; St, structure; O, outcome; Sc, scope; A, access; C, cost; Q, quality; ✓: yes/related-indicators applied in the study; CEA, cost-effectiveness analysis.

Continued

Author, Year	Indicators			Services				Design	CEA	Findings	Limitations/ Comments
	P	St	O	Sc	A	C	Q				
Cohen, 1991 Study the effects of a nursing case management model on the care of patients hospitalized for cesarean section delivery	✓	✓	✓			✓	✓	Quasi-experimental	N	Significant reduction in length of stay and cost. Increased direct care hours in the experimental group	Nonexplicit content of case management intervention. Nonrandom sample. Excellent cost accounting method described
Eggert, Zimmer, Hall, & Friedman, 1991 Compare two types of community-based case management models: individual vs team approach	✓	✓	✓	✓		✓	✓	Randomized controlled trial	N	Team approach less costly, higher hospital admission rate, much lower length of stay	No report of reliability and validity of instruments. Excellent study design
Fleishman, Mor, & Piette, 1991 Compare a community-based and clinic-based case management model for AIDS patients	✓	✓	✓		✓		✓	Qualitative comparative	N/A	Clinic-based patients are more likely to be disadvantaged, some patients had no contact with case managers at all	Weak design. Data reported quantitatively, although authors claim to use a qualitative approach
Polinsky, Fred, & Ganz, 1991 Evaluate a social work, telephone case management model	✓	✓	✓		✓		✓	Unclear/ unidentified Qualitative	N/A	Identified the needs, problems, and concerns of newly diagnosed cancer patients	Results reported in a quantitative format even though interviews were conducted for data collection
Helvie & Alexy, 1992 Examine the benefits of offering families after-shelter case management services	✓	✓	✓		✓			Descriptive	N/A	Case management services reduce length of stay in a shelter, increase housing stability after discharge	Unclear what made the difference; no description of the intervention. Unspecified sampling method

Study	Purpose	P	St	O	Sc	A	C	Q	Design	CEA (Y/N/A)	Findings	Comments
Rubin, 1992	Review of eight studies conducted between 1987 and 1991 on case management to identify common, significant case management elements	✔		✔	✔			✔	Descriptive	N/A	Controversial and conflicting outcomes from the studies regarding quality of life, functional abilities, and social functioning	Research literature review found no common elements in case management models
Van Dongen & Jambunathan, 1992	Examine client satisfaction with RN case management			✔	✔				Pilot study Exploratory	N/A	Description of the qualities of nurse case managers and their most frequent interventions and services	Convenient sample No report of validity or reliability of instruments No quantitative data are reported
Edelstein & Cesta, 1993	Evaluate the effect of an acute care case management model on the outcomes of care for patients with diabetes	✔	✔	✔	✔			✔	Pre- and post-comparison Retrospective chart review	N/A	Team case management approach was found to have better outcomes: length of stay, readmission rate, and blood glucose control on discharge	Convenient samples No discussion of the comparability of the samples
Erkel, Morgan, Staples, Assey, & Michel, 1993	Determine the impact of case management services on use of child health clinic and immunizations in low-income families	✔		✔	✔		✔	✔	Quasi-experimental Retrospective record review	Y	Continuous case management was found to be better than fragmented approach and with better cost-effectiveness ratio	Nonrandom convenient sample Excellent application of the cost-effectiveness analysis method

P, Process; St, structure; O, outcome; Sc, scope; A, access; C, cost; Q, quality; ✔: yes/related-indicators applied in the study; CEA, cost-effectiveness analysis.

Continued

Author, Year	Aim(s)	Indicators			Services				Design	CEA	Findings	Limitations/ Comments
		P	St	O	Sc	A	C	Q				
Mahn, 1993	Examine the effectiveness of an acute care case management model for patients with coronary artery bypass surgery		✓	✓			✓	✓	Comparative Intervention and nonintervention groups	N	Case management approach revealed better outcomes: length of stay, cost, readmission rate, and adverse events	Nonrandom convenient samples; Patients matched based on preoperative risk using risk stratification guidelines
Mawn & Bradley, 1993	Describe the process of developing a risk stratification tool for use in case management programs			✓	✓	✓		✓	Unclear	N/A	Work in progress Tool not shared	Excellent review of the literature; No validity or reliability reporting
Trella, 1993	Evaluate the cost and quality outcomes of a geriatric acute care case management model	✓	✓	✓			✓	✓	Unclear, intervention and nonintervention and pre- and post-groups comparison	N	Case management group had better length of stay, cost per patient day, reimbursement index, and patient and staff satisfaction	No procedure for data collection shared; No discussion whether the groups are comparable
Williams, Warrick, Christianson, & Netting, 1993	Identify the basic elements of case management models	✓	✓	✓	✓	✓	✓	✓	Unidentified phenomenology	N/A	Successful and unsuccessful characteristics of case management models are identified	Provide insights for successful program development; Convenient sample; Unclear the cost implications of each program

Study	Purpose	P	St	O	Sc	A	C	Q	Design	CEA	Findings	Critique
Goodwin, 1994	Examine the activities of case managers functioning in home health settings compared to other case management groups: insurance, independent, and HMOs	✓	✓	✓		✓			Descriptive, exploratory	N/A	The use of case management activities was identified by case manager type and setting	Nonrandom convenient sample, small size. Unclear whether same patients were followed by more than one case manager (duplication)
Fitzgerald, Smith, Martin, Freedman, & Katz, 1994	Examine the effects of telephone case management program for patient after acute hospitalization	✓	✓	✓	✓	✓			Randomized controlled trial	N	Frequent contacts by case managers for patient/family education and care accessibility were not effective in reducing nonelective readmissions	Good study design. Examining cost-effectiveness of the program could have been beneficial
Lamb & Stemple, 1994	Obtain patients' perspective regarding working with nurse case managers	✓	✓	✓	✓	✓			Grounded theory	N/A	Understanding the impact of case management on patient care. Design of a model of how patients perceive case management	Solid design and data analysis method. Results provide a perfect structure for future research in case management effectiveness
Sands & Canaan, 1994	Compare case management community treatment teams and intensive case management teams			✓		✓			Comparative groups retrospective review	N/A	Similar outcomes in the two groups except for length of hospitalization, which was longer for community team	Random selection of subjects

Continued

P, Process; St, structure; O, outcome; Sc, scope; A, access; C, cost; Q, quality; ✓ yes/related-indicators applied in the study; CEA, cost-effectiveness analysis.

Author, Year	Aim(s)	Indicators			Services				Design	CEA	Findings	Limitations/ Comments
		P	St	O	Sc	A	C	Q				
Twyman & Libbus, 1994	Examine whether deceased AIDS patients who received case management services had shorter hospitalizations						✓		Retrospective chart review Intervention and nonintervention Comparative groups	N	No significant differences were noted Only length of stay was examined	Random selection of the case management group only Convenient control group Quality and cost were not evaluated
Allred et al., 1995	Cost-effectiveness analysis of acute care nursing case management system		✓	✓			✓	✓	Descriptive Exploratory	Y	Moderate environmental uncertainty is best factor for cost-effectiveness	Stratified random sampling technique Excellent application of the CEA method
Arford & Allred, 1995	Development of the quality index measure		✓	✓			✓	✓	Descriptive Exploratory	Y	Case management is most cost-effective in an environment of moderate uncertainty	Random sampling Combines nurses and case managers in same group
Crawley & Till, 1995	Evaluate the cost and quality outcomes of case management		✓	✓			✓	✓	Unidentified	N	Case management approach improved outcomes of care	Unclear sampling methodology No cost-effectiveness analysis
Goode, 1995	Examine the impact of a CareMap and case management systems on patient and staff satisfaction, collaboration, and autonomy	✓	✓	✓				✓	Patients: cohort pre- and post-intervention Staff: pre- and post-test	N/A	Results supportive of case management services in both groups; patients and staff—no difference in collaboration scores	No discussion of patient care outcomes (clinical) Confusing sampling methodology

Author/Year	Purpose	P	St	O	Sc	A	C	Q	Design	N	Findings	Comments
Johnson & Proffitt, 1995	Examine the impact of an acute care case management model on cost and satisfaction (patient and staff)	✓	✓	✓			✓	✓	Unidentified (?) Comparative	N	Reduction in length of stay and cost after case management. No data on satisfaction	Unclear sampling method
Micheels, Wheeler, & Hays, 1995	Examine the relationships between advanced practice nurse case management, patient acuity, and length of stay	✓		✓				✓	Retrospective chart review. Comparative groups	N	No significant differences between the two groups. Those case managed by advanced practice nurse were of higher acuity and shorter length of stay	Small size, convenient samples
Sohl-Kreiger, Lagaard, & Schorrer, 1996	Examine the case management activities of clinical nurse specialists functioning as case managers	✓		✓					Unidentified	N/A	Description of the process of case management and its related activities	Unclear method and sample size. Cost data provided, but unclear implications. Very weak study
Newcomer, Amsberger, & Zhang, 1997	To develop a typology of nurse case manager activities	✓		✓					Retrospective/qualitative chart review	N/A	Typology of six major case management activity categories was developed	Probability sampling technique, large size. Excellent study design
Baker, Miller, Sitterding, & Hajiewski, 1998	Examine the effectiveness of unit-based nursing case management model vs. standard nursing care	✓		✓			✓	✓	Retrospective chart review. Intervention and nonintervention comparison groups	N/A	Case-managed patient groups showed significantly better care outcomes and quality	Random sampling. Small groups. Pilot study. Unclear whether groups are comparable

P, Process; St, structure; O, outcome; Sc, scope; A, access; C, cost; Q, quality; ✓: yes/related-indicators applied in the study; CEA, cost-effectiveness analysis.

Continued

Author, Year	Aim(s)	Indicators			Services				Design	CEA	Findings	Limitations/ Comments
		P	St	O	Sc	A	C	Q				
Morrison & Beckworth, 1998	Describe the outcomes of care of patients with heart failure in a hospital-based nursing case management model	✓	✓				✓	✓	Descriptive Retrospective chart review	N	Descriptive results of several cost and quality variables are reported	Weak design No report of nursing-sensitive outcomes, although one of the study goals was to do so
Thompson, Curry, & Burton, 1998	Evaluate the effectiveness of prenatal nursing case management services for rural, low-income, Mexican-American families	✓	✓		✓	✓		✓	Quasi-experimental Retrospective chart review	N/A	Intervention group had more prenatal visits No statistical differences in initiation and number of visits	Secondary data analysis–type study Small sample size
Tonges, 1998	Test an extended model of nurse case manager's job characteristics. Compare nurse case managers, care coordinators, and staff nurses	✓	✓	✓				✓	Cross-sectional correlational	N/A	Nurse case manager's job appeared to combine higher levels of positive (autonomy, identity, collaboration) and negative (role conflict, ambiguity, overload) characteristics	Random sample from eight large national hospitals
Topp, Tucker, & Weber, 1998	Evaluate the effect of case management on hospital length of stay and cost for patients with heart failure	✓	✓	✓			✓		Retrospective chart review Comparison groups	N	Case-managed patients had lower length of stay and lower hospital charges	Convenient sample No discussion of groups comparability

P, Process; St, structure; O, outcome; Sc, scope; A, access; C, cost; Q, quality; ✓: yes/related-indicators applied in the study; CEA, cost-effectiveness analysis.

Quality and Outcomes

An Overview

Michelle M.O. Boylan

CHAPTER OVERVIEW

The health care market of the 1990s is consumed with mergers, partnerships, acquisitions, and consolidations, as well as with becoming large community-wide organizations that are accountable to the health care consumer, third party payers, consumer groups, and taxpayers. The demand for quality cost-effective health care services is a trend that will take the case manager well into the next century. The literature describes United States health care as the world's largest service industry. Quality service is benchmarked characteristics that shape the experience of care beyond technical competence and influence the quality of life and the consumer's perception of quality.

CASE MANAGER PARADIGM

A paradigm is a theoretical framework for performing a typical task that easily becomes habit; it's the way things are usually done. Case managers have many paradigms to deal with to be successful in today's health care marketplace. The new paradigm values teamwork and collaboration over individualism. Health care is focused on the consumer and the consumer's family rather than short-term profits in maintaining an operating margin. The paradigm recognizes the value of innovation, prevention, and creativity while appreciating the value of a multicultural, diverse patient population and consumer base. Organizations are based on networks of alliances, partnerships, and collaboration with other organizations (Paradigms for Postmodern Manager, 1992). Case managers interact with baby boomers, baby busters, generation Xers, and consumers of various class and ethnic backgrounds, all with different needs. The new health care team is made up of partners, suppliers, third party payers, health care professionals, allied health providers, administrators, and, most importantly, the consumer. How does the case manager break through the old paradigm to the new paradigm? How does the case manager bring together the various levels of the health care system, known as the strategic, tactical, and operational levels of an organization, to meet the needs of the consumer? How does the case manager create a successful mix of providers on the health care team to provide quality services?

Organizational Awareness for Success

The strategic level of an organization or health care system is expressed in the mission, vision, and goals. It represents the direction the organization is taking to maintain its market share. Strategically, the key is to create a work environment that brings the organization's goals, consumers' needs, and employer's goals together to meet the financial bottom line. The tactical level of the organization is expressed in written policy and procedure. Tactically, the case manager brings together policies, procedures, and regulations that support placing the right mix of people on the health care team to support the patient's needs. The operational level of the organization is where everything comes together and outcomes are generated. Operationally, the case manager, with the health care team, provides the right services in the right setting at the right time to the right patient with the right funding to promote quality patient outcomes.

Challenges for the Case Manager

Linking consumers, third party payers, suppliers, and health care team members to the strategic needs of the health care system is one of the two greatest challenges for case managers. This coordination simply means getting everybody from the top of the organization to the bottom doing things to implement the strategy of the health care system effectively. A basic assumption of the case manager must be that the system is dynamic and will constantly change. The change will be created by events that impact both internal and external characteristics of the organization. External characteristics are economy, local community beliefs, influences, and geographic location. Organizational structure, culture, environment, technology, and politics represent internal characteristics.

Philosophy of case management is expressed in statements defining business values and culture in the health care system. Philosophy can be expressed through professional standards but routinely is specialized to define how to treat and value people and patients in a particular health care system. An example of this is an organization's code of ethics. Policies are shared values that establish guidelines for action on people-related business issues and case management programs. An example of this is a policy that expresses the relationships between discharge planning, case management, and care coordination. Programs are articulated as case management strategies and can be population specific. Frequently these strategies are represented as clinical pathways and outcome measures. It coordinates efforts to facilitate change and address major people-related business and health care issues. Practices guide leadership and management in operational roles in motivating and reinforcing needed behaviors of the health care team. At a minimum, use of written mission, vision, and goals provide the case manager, health care team, and case management program with the infrastructure necessary to promote quality outcomes and success.

Quality Defined

The Institute of Medicine has defined quality as "the degree to which health services for individuals and populations increase the likelihood of desired health outcomes and are consistent with current professional knowledge" (Lohr 1990). Quality simply defined is the five rights (5 Rs). The five Rs represent the right patient, at the right time, in the right setting, receiving the right care at the right cost. Truly this means appropriate services are offered to the patient and family in a technically competent manner with participative decision making and clear communication. Clear communication, understanding of the patient's desires, and sensitivity to culture, age, and religious belief contribute to positive outcomes of care. Communication with third party payers, suppliers, and insurers heavily influences the potential outcomes for the patient, family, and health care system.

Quality can further be defined by perception (understanding through the senses). Perception poses the second greatest challenge for the case manager and the health care team. In today's world of educated consumers and medical necessity, the right care at the right time in the right setting at the right cost may be perceived by the health care team as quality care and may not be enough to satisfy the patient, although everything medically has been done. This can lead to less than desirable outcomes for the patient and family, health care team, and health care system. The health care team can become dissatisfied when the patient refuses to receive the recommended care, thus interfering with the medically indicated treatment and traditional definition of quality care.

Perception of care further defines poor quality. Poor quality can be defined as too much care (providing unnecessary/redundant tests, medications, extended treatment), wrong care (providing uncomplete information about a procedure, or a unnecessary procedure), or too little care (not providing the necessary procedure, medication, or test). Inadequate technical competence, questionable service quality, and unclear communication lead to questionable outcomes.

OUTCOMES DEFINED

"Outcomes are the changes, either favorable or adverse in the actual or potential health status of persons, groups, on communities that can be attributed to prior or concurrent care" (Donabedian, 1985). Outcome measurement is the assessment, at a specific point in time, of one or more of the variables defined as "outcomes," or results of interaction between a patient and the health care delivery system. Outcomes monitoring refers to the repeated assessment, over time, of variables defined as outcomes in a manner that allows causal inferences about what (care, services, resources) produced the observed results. Outcomes management is the use of information and knowledge gained from outcomes-monitoring activities and related sources to continually improve the process of decision making, patient care management, and service delivery to achieve optimal outcomes for the patient and the health care system (Davies & Halpern, 1993). Successful outcomes management uses information from all levels of the organization, outcomes monitoring activity, and awareness of the health care marketplace. Outcome measures are being linked to payment incentives even though there is no formal consensus about which outcomes should be measured. Scrutiny of outcomes is most intense in high-cost, high-volume patient populations that are easily defined and have significant morbidity and mortality (Higgins, 1998).

QUALITY SYSTEMS APPROACH

Quality should be evaluated as a system; structure, process, and outcomes (Donabedian, 1980). Structural quality evaluates organizational characteristics as defined at the organization's strategic level. Process quality assesses interactions between the internal and external characteristics of an organization and interactions between the health care team and consumer as defined at the organization's tactical and operational levels. Outcome quality shows evidence about changes in the patient's health status, whether actual (remission of cancer, lowering of blood pressure) or perceived (feeling of hopefulness, decrease in pain). It also demonstrates levels of performance in the health care system.

Quality health care does not happen by accident. It takes time, energy, personal mastery of technical skills, a shared vision, and team learning (Senge, 1990). Systems thinking requires an awareness of the entire health care system, realizing sometimes fixing one part of the system only brings difficulties to other parts of the system (i.e., providing supplies at discharge that the insurance company will not reimburse). Some decisions actually look good in the short term, but produce marginal results and crisis in the end. The really effective decisions often produce difficulties in the short term, but create better quality outcomes in the long term.

Health care organizations can learn only when individuals on the health care team learn. Personal mastery, which is the discipline of personal learning and growth, where people are continually expanding their ability to create a quality outcome, is key for success. It is consistently finding better ways to improve individual and system performance.

A shared vision is a force the drives people, creating a sense of purpose that provides energy and focus for learning. Shared vision is important because it may be the beginning step to get people with different views to work together. Working together promotes effective communication and quality outcomes.

Team learning can be challenging in an organization of specialists whose performance depends on one another's individual excellence and how well they work together. Team alignment, where a group functions as a whole unit rather than as individuals working to cross-purposes, is the basis for quality outcomes. When a health care team is aligned, its energies are focused and harmonized. Members of the health care team need not sacrifice their own interests. Alignment occurs when the shared vision becomes an extension of personal vision. Alignment is a necessary condition to empower others and ultimately empower the health care team.

Mastering team learning, having a shared vision, and personal mastery enhance dialogue and discussion between members of the health care team, the health care consumer, and the third party payer. The performance of the system as a whole depends on the members of the team, as do service quality and outcomes.

Quality and Outcome Measurement

Measurement of quality and outcomes depends on the culture and values of the health care system, the internal and external characteristics, and the specific consumer population. Data must reflect the performance of the system and be significantly tied to the health care system's strategic, tactical, and operational goals. Appropriately selected criteria or metrics for measurement can successfully demonstrate an organization's performance and improvement activities. The criteria must reflect critical points in the process, be easy to measure, and be quantifiable. Criteria must be selected during the beginning phases of a process so a clear measure of success and evaluation can be established.

Quality indicators describe a process that should occur for a particular type of patient. Indicators are based on standards of care determined by research literature, professional organizations, or subject matter experts. Indicators are clinically focused and measure the patient's progress toward a state of health as defined by the patient and traditional medicine. Indicators can be nationally benchmarked and are used to compare disease-specific populations across the United States. Indicators are widely accepted as a measure of quality outcomes and organizational performance.

High-Performance Health Care Organizations

Health care organizations in today's marketplace do not want to merely survive; they want to be effective, efficient, provide for customer demands, and maintain the bottom line. People are the foundation on which to build.

High-performance organizations have many things in common, including a vision, systems thinking, and the ability to learn and maximize organizational effectiveness through the health care professional's ability to respond directly to changing conditions. This does not happen by accident. The quality functions are well developed throughout the organization and implemented with a purpose. The purpose is to implement corporate strategy through people. It is key to place the right people in the right job at the right time with the right skill set to provide the right care to the consumer.

Steps in an outcomes-based quality program include determining the purpose of the process, identifying the process to be analyzed, explaining the process to members of the health care team, determining their level of involvement, collecting the information, and organizing the information so it is easily understood. Success is only achieved when the information is applied to everyday practice. Outcomes are affected only when the information creates new opportunities for choice. Performance is affected when information and choice become an improvement in the process. Quality is affected when information, choice, and outcomes are perceived by the patient and health care team as the right thing to do. Successful case managers and organizations will use the quality process to have a clear understanding of the strategic, tactical, and operational levels of the health care system and its importance in developing quality outcomes.

Quality is a system of elements and functions that represent the organization. Health care team members who successfully adapt to change and the new paradigms will become the leaders of the future and managers for the millennium.

KNOWLEDGE, NOTICE, AND BUILDING PARADIGM BREAKTHROUGHS

How does the case manager break through the old paradigm to the new paradigm? How does the case manager bring together the various levels of the health care system to meet the needs of the consumer? How does the case manager create a successful mix of providers? The key is simple and links people to business through knowledge, noticing the environment, and building communication and cultural awareness through the quality improvement processes. Active listening and an acute awareness of the environment are necessary for success. To break into the new paradigm through business, the knowledge needed is as follows:

- Know the organization's mission, vision, and goals
- Know the organizational strategy and business needs
- Know the local health care marketplace, business alliances, and partnerships
- Know the organization's financial status and where to find funding
- Know the regulatory environment
- Know the specific needs of the consumer population

To break into the new paradigm, it is necessary to notice the environment through cultural awareness. National and ethnic culture can be addressed through 10 key observations:

- Notice the consumer's sense of self and personal space
- Notice the communication style and language (verbal and body) patterns
- Notice dress and appearance
- Notice food and dietary/eating habits
- Notice use of time and time consciousness
- Notice interpersonal relationships
- Notice values and norms
- Notice beliefs and attitudes
- Notice mental process, ability, and willingness to learn
- Notice work and leisure habits and practices

Box 47-1	PARADIGM BREAKTHROUGH SELF-ASSESSMENT		
1. I understand my organization's mission, vision, and goals.		**Yes**	**No**
2. I understand my organization's business strategy and direction.		**Yes**	**No**
3. I know where my organization's case management program fits into the organization's business strategy.		**Yes**	**No**
4. I am aware of the regulations, policies, and procedures and third party requirements that affect the case management process.		**Yes**	**No**
5. I am consistently aware of the specific ethnic and cultural needs of the consumer population.		**Yes**	**No**
6. I routinely consider ethnic and cultural differences in making decisions and putting together the health care team.		**Yes**	**No**
7. I consistently and intentionally treat others with respect.		**Yes**	**No**
8. I actively listen without interrupting.		**Yes**	**No**
9. I build activities that promote prompt, honest, and direct questions and answers.		**Yes**	**No**
10. I routinely create a sense of urgency to meet consumer needs.		**Yes**	**No**
11. I have built efficiencies into my work practices to improve organizational performance.		**Yes**	**No**

To break into the new paradigm requires collaboration, alliance building and teamwork, as follows:

- Build collaborative and collegial relationships with health care team members
- Build respect into the work environment, including respect for diversity, open communication, and functional trust
- Build in time to listen without interruption
- Build activities that promote prompt, honest, and direct questions and answers
- Build efficiencies into the system
- Build a well-thought-out plan of care and communicate it
- Build a sense of importance and urgency to meet consumer needs

Breaking the paradigms requires the development of innovative strategies for health care excellence. Take a few minutes to complete the self-assessment tool (Box 47-1) to find out where your opportunities to make a difference exist. "The one thing you don't want to be accused of is not noticing . . . noticing that you can make a difference" (Don Shula).

If any of the answers to the questions are "no," you have some work to do. Take time to increase your knowledge base.

References

Davies, A.R., & Halpern, R. (1993, Sept.). Health care outcomes: An introduction. Irving, Tex.: *Voluntary Hospitals of America.*

Donabedian, A. (1985). *Explorations in quality assessment and monitoring* (vol. 1). *The Definition of Quality and Approaches to Its Assessment.* Ann Arbor, Mich.: Health Administration Press.

Higgins, T.L. (1998). Quantifying risk and assessing outcome in cardiac surgery. *Journal of Cardiothoracic and Vascular Anesthesia 12,* 330-340.

Lohr, K.N. (Ed.) (1990). *Medicare: A strategy for quality assurance.* Washington D.C.: National Academy Press.

Paradigms for Postmodern Manager. (1992, Nov.). Reinventing America. *Business Week,* Bonus Issue.

Senge, P.M. (1990). *The fifth discipline. The art and practice of the learning organization.* New York: Doubleday.

Linking the Restructuring of Nursing Care With Outcomes

Conceptualizing the Effects of Nursing Case Management

Arthur E. Blank

CHAPTER OVERVIEW

Government, employers, and insurers are trying to restructure the delivery of health care. This restructuring of care has created opportunities for innovation as well as questions about the consequences of altering the delivery of health care. Nursing case management is one such innovation and as such needs to be studied. The Medical Outcomes Study (MOS) approach offers a conceptual guide to assessing the impact of nursing case management, but the MOS is not specific enough to document adequately the consequences of nursing case management. To make the MOS approach more germane, nursing case managers need to accomplish three tasks: (1) identify how case managers change the structure and process of care, (2) identify what clinical, administrative, physiological, and patient outcomes are influenced by these changes, and (3) develop reliable and valid measures. Accomplishing these three tasks will enable hospitals, nurses, and policy makers to assess whether nursing case management has "worked." Some ideas about how to proceed with each of these tasks are presented.

The delivery of health care is changing. National, state, and local governments are redefining the financing and delivery of health services to slow growing public expenditures. Employers are restructuring employee benefits and premiums to control their escalating health benefit costs per employee. And under pressure from employers, insurance companies, and government, health care providers are working to become more cost-effective without sacrificing quality.

These efforts to redefine how health care is provided and paid for have also engendered counter pressures. Employers, government, health care providers, and patients or consumers have started to question whether health care choices are being arbitrarily restricted, whether the quality of care is being sacrificed, and, in everyone's worst nightmare, whether lives are being unnecessarily jeopardized. These apprehensions remind us that change is taking place within another, more abstract context, one of uncertainty. We are not trading one well-defined system of care for another. We are trading for a system of care whose basic parameters are still undefined.

As providers or consumers of care, we are in the midst of a societal, institutional, and personal struggle to balance opportunity and fear, or, more modestly, concern: opportunity, because the structural pressures to reconfigure the delivery of care supports leaders who are willing to innovate; concern, because the consequences of these changes, whether they be at a societal, institutional, or personal level, will not be known for some time.

How can we as health care professionals, as researchers, as policy makers, and as citizens assess the consequences, or outcomes, of these various and varied attempts to reconfigure the delivery of health care? One way is to undertake outcome studies. These studies describe how the structure and process of medical care have been refashioned and identify a set of measures—outcomes—that can be used to determine the consequences of those changes. When done well, these studies tell us how well opportunity and concern have been balanced, and the results become part of a broader social metric. But these studies can be part of the metric only if we identify and measure how components of the structure and process of care are conceptually linked with outcomes of care—health as well as financial—and at a societal as well as an institutional or personal level.

What has all of this to do with nursing case management? It suggests that the Medical Outcomes Study (MOS) approach be used as a *conceptual guide* for studying the consequences of nursing case management. After all, nursing case management is fundamentally an alteration in the structure and process of care.* As such it is an intervention, an opportunity to reshape the delivery of in-patient care.† But it is also an intervention whose consequences are unknown (Lamb, 1995). The task then is not only to define and identify the organizational changes in the structure and process of care that nursing case management has brought about but also to articulate our concerns so we can link the restructuring of care with its consequences, with its outcomes.

Traditionally, clarifying the conceptual relationships between shifts in the organization of care and the outcome(s) of care is a critical step in designing a research study. But there is a complementary step not often well attended to in health care: ensuring that our design appropriately measures the relationships and constructs we are interested in. At a technical level the challenge is about the *validity* of our measures: are they conceptually nuanced and robust enough to reflect the relevant dimensions of change introduced by nursing case management?‡ Unfortunately, designing valid measures is no less daunting a task than is designing a rigorous study.

This chapter then has four objectives: (1) to briefly review how valid measures are constructed, (2) to review how the MOS both conceptualized the structure, process, and outcomes of care and developed valid health status measures, (3) to raise questions about whether the definitions and measures used in the MOS research can be directly applied to the study of nursing case management, and (4) to suggest some directions and issues for nursing case management research.

A PARTIAL§ MEASUREMENT REFRESHER: DEVELOPING VALID MEASURES

For many years, health care's consequences were assessed by measures of morbidity and mortality. Identifying the time of death, diagnosing whether the individual has an infection, or interpreting a par-

---

*Because *nursing case management* is not a term that means the same thing in every institution where it is practiced, these local variations are important to identify and document if we are to understand how the structure, process, and outcomes of care are linked.

†This chapter presumes nursing case management is being used in a hospital setting.

‡The concern in this chapter is with developing measures for, not the design of, outcome studies. Clearly both the study design and the measures will determine the scientific credibility of the results.

§This discussion is partial because it deals only with validity. There is no discussion of reliability, about how to write scale items, or about how to statistically assess the information collected.

ticular laboratory result, for example, was—and is—relatively straightforward. When our measures were this concrete, little attention needed to be devoted to thinking about whether we were capturing what we intended to measure. But as health professionals' interest in the consequences of care became nuanced and abstract, more attention had to be devoted to guaranteeing that we measured what we wanted to (Stewart, Hays, & Ware, 1992; Streiner & Norman, 1989) and ensuring that we knew how to interpret the results (Kane, 1992; Messick, 1995; Streiner & Norman, 1989). For example, measuring blood pressure is straightforward, as for the most part is the interpretation of the result. When we measure depression or patient or job satisfaction, we may be both less certain that we have accurately assessed the construct and less certain about how to interpret the resulting score. Some measures of inpatient satisfaction, for example, focus on hotel services such as the food, cleanliness of the room, and efficiency of the admitting or discharge process. Yet other measures focus on the nurses' responsiveness to pain, the clarity of information provided by physicians or nurses, and the compassion of the staff. Is one measure a more valid measure of satisfaction than the other? How do we measure and feel intellectually confident that we are correctly measuring and interpreting these more abstract consequences of health interventions?

As we approach our consideration of validity, it is essential to remember that there is a critical, interrelated step: to define, or more pointedly limit, what we are referring to when we talk about "outcomes." The concept of outcomes is broad and nonspecific and takes on a precise meaning only in the context of a particular intervention. In that context, outcomes must be defined in a way that is responsive to the intervention. This simple setting of boundaries, these definitional decisions, must not be made lightly. In the psychometric or scale development literature, defining the boundaries of the concept is usually treated as the purview of the expert. The expert's knowledge is based on his or her experience in the field as well as on a knowledge of the literature. This expertise will help determine which conceptual domains should be included or excluded. For example, are measures of pain, patient satisfaction, functional status, well-being, cost of care, hospital readmission, and length of stay conceptually relevant when we want to document the effects of nursing case management?

If a peer-reviewed literature exists, experts are clearly beneficial. But they may be less helpful if the topic is new or if the literature is out of date. In this context, convening a panel of experts and "users" to discuss the concept's boundaries may help. This need to harness the experience of a diverse group of individuals can be important even in well-established areas of study. For example, the outcome measures discussed in the MOS have been criticized by some as capturing outcomes more sensitive to the work of physicians than of nurses (Kelly et al., 1994), which raises a caution and a simple reminder: definitions set limits. They decide what to include and exclude. These decisions should be explicit and public, not tacit and hidden.

Once we know the domains we want to assess, the issue of whether our scales and surveys measure what we intend them to measure falls under the rubric of validity (Crocker & Algina, 1986; Nunnally, 1978; Portney & Watkins, 1993; Streiner & Norman, 1989; Thorndike, 1982). For abstract constructs, developing valid instruments is time consuming and difficult. In the field of psychometrics validity is usually discussed in terms of four different types: (1) face, (2) criterion, (3) content, and (4) construct validity.*

Face validity, the weakest form of validity, is perhaps the easiest to use and develop. With face validity, items on a survey or questionnaire *appear* to address the question we are interested in. There is, however, no empirical test of this assumption. Content validity tries to ensure that the various *items* that comprise the measure, or which tap the conceptual domain, adequately *sample* the content of the concept or domain being measured. Some of the questions raised earlier about patient satisfaction surface

---

*Health care researchers have turned to the social sciences and in particular to psychometricians to help develop indices and measures of abstract constructs. For one critique of this approach as it relates to assessing clinical change see Feinstein (1987).

here. Should patient satisfaction include hotel services as well as the thoroughness and clarity of the information provided? Part of the answer would be to review existing instruments, but it would also be useful to convene a panel of experts* to ensure that important items or concerns are not excluded inadvertently. But however the items are put together, content validity, like face validity, is still primarily subjective. The advantages of content validity is that it ensures that the item pool has been thoroughly documented and that the items reflect the concept being assessed *before* the measure is administered.

More rigorous—that is, more empirically based—tests of validity are possible with both criterion and construct validity. Criterion-related validity indicates that the test developed can be used in place of an already established test—a "gold standard." We may be interested, for example, in constructing a shorter version of a longer, more time-consuming scale. To determine whether the shorter test is valid, the long and the short tests are administered to the same set of subjects. If the two sets of scores are highly correlated, the shorter test is valid. Although this is an objective way to proceed, for many abstract constructs such as satisfaction a gold standard is not available. In these cases another approach, construct validation, is called for. Part of construct validity relies on content validity: that is, we have to have an item pool that adequately assesses the complexity of the concept. But the thrust of construct validity is to confirm that the measure accurately captures the construct by empirically ascertaining whether the new measure correlates with hypothetically related constructs.

Construct validity can be approached from a number of directions, but one common approach is that of convergent and discriminant validity (Cronbach & Meehl, 1955). Simply put, like measures should correlate highly with other measures of the same or similar theoretical constructs—convergent validity—but should not correlate, or show low correlations, with measures of dissimilar constructs—discriminant validity. If researchers are constructing a new measure to assess the impact of an illness on a person's life, the new measure should correlate highly with comparable illness burden measures but only minimally with measures of quite different constructs. The pattern of correlations documents whether the new measure is succeeding. But in the absence of a gold standard it is hard to absolutely know how well we have done. Consequently, for some researchers construct validity is an ongoing process, needing always to refine and test the measures (Messick, 1995; Stewart et al., 1992; Streiner & Norman, 1989). Within this framework, construct validity cannot be decided with the results of a single study.

THE MOS APPROACH: AN EXAMPLE OF HOW TO LINK THE STRUCTURE, PROCESS, AND OUTCOMES OF CARE

If we are to use the MOS approach as a guide for conceptualizing how to gauge the consequences of nursing case management, it is beneficial to review that study with two aims in mind: (1) to see how the components of structure, process, and outcomes were defined and (2) to see how a new generic measure of a patient's health status was validated.

The MOS was a "2 year observational study designed to help understand how specific components of the health care system affect the outcomes of care" (Tarlov et al., 1989). The study was conducted at multiple sites across the United States and sampled 502 physicians in group and solo practice, in health maintenance organizations (HMO), and in fee-for-service (FFS) systems of care. Information was collected from physicians using self-administered forms and telephone interviews. Patient data were collected using surveys, clinical examinations, and telephone interviews.

---

*Experts need to be thought of broadly. For example, the Picker Commonwealth Survey of Patient Satisfaction used patient focus groups to identify the dimensions of care that were important to them (Gerteis, Edgman-Levitan, Daley, & Delbanco, 1993).

The MOS study was unique, in part, because of its explicit emphasis on developing measures that could capture the consequences of medical care from the patients' perspective (Stewart & Ware, 1992; Tarlov et al., 1989). In arguing for the need to supplement traditional clinical outcomes such as mortality, laboratory values, and symptoms and signs, the MOS study faced issues comparable to those case management research now faces: MOS researchers had to define outcomes, in this case from the patients' perspective, which should be conceptually responsive to changes in the structure and process of care. Of course, MOS researchers also had to clarify how the components of structure and process would be measured.

For the concept *structure of care,* three broad domains were identified: (1) system characteristics, (2) provider characteristics, and (3) patient characteristics (Tarlov et al., 1989). System characteristics identified five components, including financial incentives, access or convenience, and specialty mix. Provider characteristics included seven components: age, gender, specialty training, economic incentives, job satisfaction, preferences, and beliefs and attitudes; and the eight patient characteristics included age, gender, diagnosis, severity, comorbidity, health habits, beliefs and attitudes, and preferences. The *process of care* had two broad categories: technical and interpersonal style. Technical style included among its eight items medications, referrals, test ordering, expenditures, continuity, and coordination of care; and interpersonal style's four items were communication level, counseling, patient participation, and interpersonal manner. The *outcomes of care* had four components: clinical endpoints, functional status, general well-being, and satisfaction with care. As with the structure and process of care, each of these components was specified in more detail. For example, a patient's functional status was described by measuring a patient's physical, mental, social, and role functioning.

To develop and test the generic patient-centered health outcome measures being sought by the MOS, researchers built on scales that had been developed as part of RAND's Health Insurance Experiment (HIE) or by other researchers (Stewart & Ware, 1992). Over time the MOS staff examined the existing literature on measures of physical functioning, psychological distress or well-being, health perceptions, social and role functioning, pain, and physical and psychophysiological symptoms (Stewart & Ware, 1992). By incorporating new items and including a multitude of already developed measures into their study design, MOS researchers could test the validity of their measures.* Face validity was not discussed, and content validity was checked by assessing the literature to determine whether the relevant concepts were captured in the set of measures being used. Criterion validity was used, when available, to see how new measures compared to established old measures. For example, would a new shorter measure of depression correlate with a gold standard measure of depression (e.g., the Diagnostic Interview Schedule in the third edition of the *Diagnostic and Statistical Manual of Mental Disorders* [DSM-III] published by the American Psychiatric Association) or would a shorter measure of physical functioning correlate highly with a longer measure of physical functioning (Hays & Stewart, 1992; Stewart et al., 1992)? Both convergent and discriminant validity were used to examine the construct validity of the measure. In principle, if we are developing new measures of well-being or pain, these measures should correlate highly with scales that measure similar constructs. But we would not expect these measures to correlate with those unrelated to either well-being or pain. More specifically, as the MOS authors indicate, "measures of physical functioning, mobility, and satisfaction with physical abilities were expected to correlate at least moderately with one another because they all assess physical functioning. [and] physical functioning would not be expected to be highly related to a measure of depression or of loneliness" (Stewart et al., 1992, p. 315).

---

*The MOS covers more than the four types of validity identified in this chapter. Furthermore, it breaks down content, criterion, and construct validity in more detail than is offered here (Stewart & Ware, 1992). Even though there are important refinements that can be made, the general points and theme do not change.

Under construct validity, Stewart et al. (1992) also discuss known-groups validity. Identified by Kerlinger (1973), known-groups validity involves comparing groups of individuals who should differ on the concept being measured. So, for example, on a measure of pain, mean scores should be higher for those patients known to be in pain than for those who are not.

This approach to developing an outcomes scale resulted in the MOS Short Form (SF-36). The MOS SF-36 is a generic 36-item measure of the patients' perception of their health status. This measure can be used across populations and across illness to measure the consequences of changes in the structure and process of care. The scale, demonstrated to be reliable and valid, captures eight health care concepts: (1) limitations in physical activities because of health problems, (2) limitations in social activities because of physical or emotional problems, (3) limitations in usual role activities because of physical health problems, (4) bodily pain, (5) general mental health (psychological distress and well-being), (6) limitations in usual role activities because of emotional problems, (7) vitality (energy and fatigue), and (8) general health problems (McHorney, Ware, & Raczek, 1993; McHorney, Ware, Rachael Lu, & Sherbourne, 1994; Ware & Sherbourne, 1992).

NURSING-BASED CHALLENGES TO THE MOS

The MOS's tripartite *conceptualization* of the delivery of health care has become an important framework for assessing the restructuring of health care. But we should not uncritically accept the specific details of the MOS approach without reassuring ourselves that the definitions of the structure, process, and outcomes of care are germane to studying the effects of nursing case management. Does the MOS approach define and capture what is unique to case management?

Nursing-Based Criticisms of the MOS Outcomes

With the successful development and validation of the SF-36, changes in the structure and process of care can now, in principle, be captured from the patients' perspective. For those interested in the patients' perspective, the SF-36 is a valuable addition to a researcher's measurement tools. The question remains, however, as to whether the SF-36 is sufficiently sensitive to reflect the *specific* structural and process changes introduced by nursing case management. If we assume that nursing case management has some similarities to nursing care in general, the articles by Brooten & Naylor (1995), by Kelly et al. (1994), and by Naylor, Munro, and Brooten (1991) suggest the answer is no.

Two different concerns are raised in these articles: First, the SF-36 is dominated by outcome measures sensitive to physician practices. Consequently, there is a need to construct measures that can capture "nurse sensitive patient outcomes" (Brooten & Naylor, 1995). And second, since the research was begun before all the current changes in the health care environment took place, the MOS—as an approach to effectiveness research—neglects a number of important domains, especially the effects of provider mix, that is, that many different professionals care for the patient (Kelly et al., 1994). This latter point is critical. For we not only must identify what these nurse-sensitive measures are but also must assure ourselves that these measures reflect only what nurses offer and not what other providers of care offer. This chore becomes harder to accomplish, and perhaps is not even achievable, as patient care becomes more interdisciplinary.

Some Suggested Nursing Case Management–Sensitive Outcomes

In their discussion of how to measure the consequences of nursing care, Brooten and Naylor (1995) identify a number of potential indexes: functional and mental status (these two domains are captured on the SF-36), stress level, satisfaction with care, caregiver burden, and the cost of care. Brooten and Naylor expand their suggested list of nurse-sensitive outcomes by incorporating a number of outcome categories identified in Lang and Marek's review of outcomes: physiologic status, psychological status, behavior, knowledge, symptom control, quality of life, home functions, family strain, goal attainment, utilization of service, safety, resolution of nursing problems, patient satisfaction, and caring (cited in Brooten & Naylor, 1995).

These suggested outcome measures continue in the tradition of developing patient-focused outcomes, but there are other outcomes introduced by nurses or nursing case management that also must be documented. Perhaps most basically, reconfigurations in health care have meant a redefinition of nursing responsibilities. What does this imply for nurses? Will they be more or less integrated in the delivery of care? Will they feel less autonomous or more autonomous in their roles, more or less fragmented with their varied responsibilities? Will nurses leave their jobs more often? Will sick leave increase or decrease? These too are outcomes of changes in nursing case management and should not be slighted when we identify the range of outcomes to be studied.*

Of course, comparable questions could be asked of physicians, especially as their relationships with nurses change. It must be stressed that identifying outcome categories does not end the process; it starts it. The task is to move from the outcome categories to valid outcome measures.

Nursing Case Management and the Structure and Process of Care

Clearly, outcomes studies are critical, as they correct many past oversights. But particular outcomes should not be identified, or agreed to, without first specifying how they are conceptually linked to the structure and process of care. Functional status, mental status, and relief from pain are important outcome measures because we expect them, under certain conditions, to be responsive to medical treatment, to the process of medical care. Similar efforts are needed for nursing case management: We must construct outcomes that are responsive to the specific changes introduced by nursing case management. So just as the MOS description of outcomes may not be fully germane for studying the effects of nursing case management, its description of the structure and process of care may also be deficient for studying case management. But Lamb (1995) has reminded us that there is a good deal of ambiguity regarding what nursing case managers do. Without knowing what case managers do, it is unclear whether the nursing-sensitive outcomes listed above are sensitive to alterations in the structure and process of care introduced by nursing case management. And it is unclear whether these outcomes are, in the words of Brooten and Naylor (1995), "sensitive to nursing alone." How does nursing case management change the structure and process of care?

We can, in a sense, work backward to answer this question. The outcomes suggested by Brooten and Naylor and others imply certain changes, or perhaps clarification, in some MOS definitions of the structure and process of care. For example, consider the process of care. If an outcome of case management is enhanced patient knowledge regarding his or her illness, we have presumed that nurses are educating their patients. Is this different from what is specified in the MOS component of interpersonal style, which "includes many aspects of the way clinicians relate to patients[?]. It encompasses friendliness, courtesy, respect, and sensitivity; the extent to which patients participate in making decisions and share responsibility for their treatment; whether the clinicians counsel patients about their health habits, the need to comply with treatment recommendations, and personal and emotional problems, and the overall level of communication" (Tarlov et al., 1989). Is nursing education distinctive enough to be

---

*The MOS approach characterizes provider satisfaction as a structural component, but in a dynamic environment it could also be considered as an outcome.

considered a unique component of the process of care? Do nurses engage in this process differently from other clinicians? Furthermore, do nursing case management programs change how the process of care is organized, a topic that would fall under the MOS idea of technical style? Related questions could be asked about relief from stress, reductions in caregiver burden, or the cost of care? What is it about the process of care that would reduce a patient's stress level, alter a caregiver's burden, or reduce the costs of care?

These questions can also be used to inquire about needed modifications in how the MOS study defined the structure of care. The MOS study, under system characteristics, talks about specialty mix. But Brooten and Naylor's (1995) argument that nurses are working in environments where the skill mix of nursing staff has changed suggests that the idea of specialty mix must be expanded. In addition, the interdisciplinary nature of case management suggests that how care is organized may need to be amplified. Questions about team structure and about how well teams function may need to be incorporated into the MOS's definition of the structure and outcomes of case management.

PUTTING IT ALL TOGETHER: SOME FUNDAMENTAL QUESTIONS

Brooten and Naylor's (1995), Kelly et al.'s (1994), and Naylor et al.'s (1991) critiques are forceful, not because they question the conceptual framework of the MOS approach or the validity of the SF-36 but because they pose fundamental questions about definitional and conceptual boundaries regarding the structure, process, and outcomes of care as it relates to, in our case, nursing case management. These critiques suggest the need not only to augment the MOS categories but also to construct measures that capture the unique aspects of nursing case management, the unique role of nurses, and the unique nurse-sensitive outcomes that are conceptually distinct from those identified in the MOS approach.

In essence, just as the generic SF-36 should be used in conjunction with specific illness measures so that researchers can capture nuances not measured by the SF-36, the MOS conceptualization of structure, process, and outcomes must be modified according to the specific intervention being studied. To use the MOS approach to its full advantage, we need to formally conceptualize the linkages among the structure, process, and outcomes of care that are specific to nursing case management.

The need to articulate how nursing case management reshapes the delivery of patient care and the need to document the impact of those changes is underscored in Lamb's (1995) recent review of the case management literature. Lamb raises a series of questions that should be undertaken as a challenge:

> The task of researchers is complicated by the popularity and visibility of case management. As the number of professions and individuals with a stake in the future of case management expands, it is increasingly difficult to cut through the debate and rhetoric to get to some basic questions, such as: What is case management? Who needs it? Who provides it? For how long? What are its outcomes? What are its costs? Does it save money by keeping people from higher levels of care?

Lamb's questions bring us full circle: if we are to study the consequences of nursing case management, we must know what nurse case managers do. What are the linkages among the structure, process, and outcomes of care?

· · ·

For the past few years there have been research studies at our institution to try to determine the consequences of various nursing innovations. Part of our charge, as usual, was to determine if the innovation "worked." This charge is difficult in the best of circumstances but is especially difficult in dynamic environments. With the need to develop cost-effective institutions, hospital administrators are introducing multiple innovations, are introducing them system wide, and are concerned with knowing what worked. Administrators were quite willing to listen to researchers' caveats and hesitancies about proceeding, and in some cases we mutually decided that it did not pay to do an analysis, since the results would be uninterpretable. Reaching this decision was part of the job and was not particularly the hard part of the job. The hard part was trying to get staff to detail what they did and what they thought were the specific consequences of their efforts.

Rather than presume we knew what the "right" consequences were or that the literature had the "right" concepts, we would ask staff to describe their jobs and to tell us whether they thought they were having the impact they had expected to have. This was our way of trying to ensure that we were capturing the correct domains and also a way to start thinking about our item pools. For most staff this effort, conducted in lay terms, was not at all straightforward. Of course, some staff were adept at helping us. At times we used the MOS study descriptions as a foil, as a way of probing whether the specifics of what staff were doing differed from how the MOS defined the structure, process, and outcomes of care.

Although we did not systematically interview or sample staff, when answers regarding nursing interventions were provided, they seemed to fall into three categories: (1) helping the patient relax and making him or her less anxious, (2) being more attentive to a patient's and the family's emotional well-being, and (3) educating patients about their illness. Of course, all staff felt they were helping patients with their physical well-being. Clearly the nurses we spoke to may be atypical, but note that two of these items—helping a patient relax and being attentive to a patient's emotional needs—may be different from the list of nurse-sensitive outcomes mentioned earlier in the chapter.

These conversations all worked to frame the questions raised earlier. We struggled with nurses to have them specify what they did, to have them detail the consequences of what they did, and to have them suggest how we could measure these activities and outcomes. It took us some time to resolve these issues, and in many ways they remain unresolved. But it was this specific need to identify how particular nursing innovations could be analyzed within the framework of the MOS approach that generated in a pragmatic way all the more abstract questions raised earlier. We struggled with every measure, concerned with whether it reflected the effect of nurses alone and with whether we were measuring what we thought we were measuring.

It was also clear that telling our story about what "worked" would be enhanced to the extent that we could document that we had the "right" measures and the "correct" outcomes. As we grappled with these issues, other institutions facing similar innovations approached us asking for assistance. So we quickly learned we were not alone.

This chapter, then, puts our struggle in reverse order. It raises general issues about studying the effects of nursing case management as if it preceded our efforts. Rather these concerns followed our efforts. Our efforts drove home the point that the MOS approach provides a general framework for assessing the consequences of care. The real effort is to develop valid measures that capture the interrelations among the structure, process, and outcomes of care that are germane to the particular intervention being put in place. If we can accomplish this, we can truly gauge the unique consequences of nursing case management.

References

Brooten, D., & Naylor, M.D. (1995). Nurses' effect on changing patient outcomes. *IMAGE: Journal of Nursing Scholarship, 27*(2), 95-99.

Crocker, L., & Algina, J. (1986). *Introduction to classical and modern test theory.* New York: Harcourt, Brace, Jovanovich.

Cronbach, L.J., & Meehl, P.E. (1955). Construct validity in psychological tests. *Psychological Bulletin, 52,* 281-302.

Feinstein, A.R. (1987). *Clinimetrics.* New Haven: Yale University Press.

Gerteis, M., Edgman-Levitan, S., Daley, J., & Delbanco. (1993). *Through the patient's eyes.* San Francisco: Jossey-Bass.

Hays, R.D., & Stewart, A.L. (1992). Construct validity of MOS health measures. In A.L. Stewart & J.E. Ware (Eds.), *Measuring functioning and well-being: The Medical Outcomes Study approach* (pp. 325-342). Durham, N.C.: Duke University Press.

Kane, M.T. (1992). An argument-based approach to validity. *Psychological Bulletin, 112*(3), 527-535.

Kelly, K.C., Huber, D.G., Johnson, M., McCloskey, J.C., & Maas, M. (1994). The Medical Outcomes Study: A nursing perspective. *Journal of Professional Nursing, 10*(4), 209-216.

Kerlinger, F.N. (1973). *Foundations of behavioral research* (2nd ed.). New York: Holt, Rinehart & Winston.

Lamb, G.S. (1995). Case management. In J.J. Fitzpatrick & J.S. Stevenson (Eds.), *Annual Review of Nursing Research, 13,* 117-136.

McHorney, C.A., Ware, J.E., Rachael Lu, J.F., & Sherbourne, C.D. (1994). The MOS 36-Item Short-Form Health Survey (SF-36): III. Tests of data quality, scaling assumptions, and reliability across diverse patient groups. *Medical Care, 32*(1), 40-66.

McHorney, C.A., Ware, J.E., & Raczek, A.E. (1993). The MOS 36-Item Short-Form Health Survey (SF-36): II. Psychometric and clinical tests of validity in measuring physical and mental health constructs. *Medical Care, 31*(3), 247-263.

Messick, S. (1995). Validity of psychological assessment. *American Psychologist, 50*(9), 741-749.

Naylor, M.D., Munro, B.H., & Brooten, D.A., (1991). Measuring the effectiveness of nursing practice. *Clinical Nurse Specialist, 5*(4), 210-214.

Nunnally, J. (1978). *Psychometric theory.* New York: McGraw-Hill.

Portney, L.G., & Watkins, M.P. (1993). *Foundations of clinical research: Applications to practice.* Norwalk, Conn: Appleton & Lange.

Stewart, A.L., Hays, R.D., & Ware, J.E. (1992). Methods of validating MOS health measures. In A.L. Stewart & J.E. Ware (Eds.), *Measuring functioning and well-being: The Medical Outcomes Study approach* (pp. 309-324). Durham, N.C.: Duke University Press.

Stewart, A.L., & Ware, J.E. (1992). *Measuring functioning and well-being: The Medical Outcomes Study approach.* Durham, N.C.: Duke University Press.

Streiner, D.L., & Norman, G.R. (1989). *Health measurement scales: A practical guide to their development and use.* New York: Oxford University Press.

Tarlov, A., Ware, J.E., Greenfield, S., Nelson, E.C., Perrin, E., & Zubkoff, M. (1989). The Medical Outcomes Study: An application of methods for monitoring the results of medical care. *Journal of the American Medical Association, 263*(7), 925-930.

Thorndike, R.L. (1982). *Applied psychometrics.* Boston: Houghton Mifflin.

Ware, J.E., & Sherbourne, C.D. (1992). The MOS 36-Item Short-Form Health Survey (SF-36): I. Conceptual framework and item selection. *Medical Care, 30*(6), 473-483.

An Overview of Assessing Health Through Quality of Life Indicators

Kathryn Nold

CHAPTER OVERVIEW

Various outcome indicators have been established as measurements of successful case management programs. Some of these indicators are resource utilization outcomes, institutions' economic outcomes, patient-centered outcomes, and process outcomes. As an additional outcome measure, quality of life indicators, or health status surveys, should be considered as essential tools for a case management program.

A population's health status, as defined by quality of life results, can be used externally by customers to purchase services or internally to improve outcomes. Customers, in this context, are payers, patients, and other health care providers and institutions. This chapter describes the basics of quality of life measurements, outlines the selection of an instrument, and concludes with a case study using liver transplantation recipients.

WHY MEASURE QUALITY OF LIFE?

"Quality of life" (QOL) is an outcome measure that can document the effectiveness of medical interventions such as treatment of a disease, surgery, or use of drug therapy. It assesses patients' perceptions of their health, satisfaction with life, and/or general sense of personal well-being that can provide insights about the strengths and weaknesses of diagnostic and treatment therapies (Spilker, 1996). QOL can also be defined as "the gap between the patient's expectations and achievements" (Calman, 1984).

Acknowledgments: Members of the Liver Transplant Program at the University of Colorado Health Sciences Center and Hospital who contributed to the Case Study are:

Tracy Steinberg, RN, MS (Transplant Coordinator and Case Manager)
Michael Talamantes, LCSW (Transplant Team Social Worker)
Igal Kam, MD (Professor/Chief of Transplant Surgery)
Gregory Everson, MD (Professor/Director Hepatology)
Steve Hartwell, BS, MSEM (Database Administrator)

The greater the gap, the lower is the quality of life. If the goal setting by the patient and the provider is realistic, the expectations of the patient may more closely align with the achievements.

One of the basic questions asked at institutions is "Why measure quality of life (health status)"? Some health care providers have viewed QOL analysis as subjective psychosocial assessments that lack scientific methods (Spilker, 1996). Confusion comes in the assumption that something subjective cannot be as valid as physical measures. This narrow view of health does not account for today's complex environments. Both subjective and objective findings can be measured and meet reliability and validity standards. Some of the non-biomedical model components that can be assessed in QOL data are values, beliefs, coping abilities, spiritual status, social networks, vocational status, cultural and religious opportunities, government and insurance policies, transportation and communication systems, and available medical facilities and services. Some researchers say that there are no perfect QOL instruments or surveys to measure the benefits of medical care, so it may not be possible to completely formulate definitive conclusions. Even with some controversy, the use of QOL measures is spreading and receiving increasing acceptance as an indicator for measuring effectiveness and efficacy and, therefore, accountability.

CATEGORIES OF QOL

The following categories are important to include in a QOL survey:

- Physical functioning (limitations attributed to physical problems)
- Social functioning (limitations attributed to social interactions/participation)
- Psychological functioning (limitations attributed to emotional problems)
- General well-being (general health perceptions)
- Economic resources (costs and access to care)

Various studies have been published using only one or two of these categories, sometimes referred to as domains (Granger et al., 1990; Lloyd et al., 1992). Without knowledge of the instrument's validation process, the novice should be cautioned about making an assessment of QOL by aggregating results across all domains. One single overall score for QOL may not reflect the differences in the domains. The physical functioning category may reflect improved outcomes while the psychological category exhibits decreased outcomes. It is essential to understand the properties and limitations of the measurement tool being used.

SPECIFIC INSTRUMENTS

A broad range of health status data is being collected and reported in clinical trials. Clinicians and researchers use disease-specific, general non-disease-specific, population-specific (age), function-specific, problem-specific, or psychologically specific tools. Generic instruments address various domains and can identify aspects that are affected by the disease or therapy. Generic measures, however, may fail to examine detailed aspects such as symptoms or functions. Disease-specific instruments have the advantage of addressing areas that are unique to a population. The disadvantages of disease-specific surveys are not providing a comparison of QOL between populations with or without other diseases and the potential for eliminating a domain. For example, if physical functioning is decreasing, what effect does this have on emotional functioning? Or did the decreasing emotional functioning lead to the decreasing physical functioning?

Examples of QOL instruments are as follows:

1. Non-disease-specific (generic): Short Form-36-Health Survey (Ware, 1996)
2. Disease-specific: Arthritis Impact Measurement Scales (Meenan, 1996)
3. Population-specific: The OARS Multidimensional Functional Assessment Questionnaire (OARS Duke University, 1996)
4. Function-specific: The Rapid Disability Scale (Linn, 1996)
5. Problem-specific: The McGill Pain Questionnaire (Melzack, 1996)
6. Psychologically specific: The Psychological General Well-being Scale (Dupuy, 1996), Rand Mental Health Inventory (Ware, 1996)
7. Psychosocially specific: Sickness Impact Profile (Bergner, 1996)

There are varying opinions as to the use of disease-specific surveys versus general surveys. Some clinical studies have used general and disease-specific scales for comparison. Choosing the instrument(s) where the expected differences are greatest in the domains measured by that instrument may lead to biases or overestimate the benefits of a therapy.

SELECTING AN INSTRUMENT

The number of surveys available is vast, and they differ in acceptability by experts in this field. The choice of a measure must be determined by the purpose and needs of the population and provider. Variables to consider are as follows:

What population(s) are you surveying? What are their characteristics?
How many subjects will participate in the assessment? Does this represent an adequate number for the outcome question you are asking?
How are you going to access this population?
Will your population(s) have special needs in completing a survey? (task perseverance, comprehension)
What outcomes are you measuring?
What is your purpose? (describe, predict, evaluate)
How many domains will you measure?
What "unit" are you interested in profiling? Patient? Family? Community?
What is in the current literature? (surveys and results for comparison data)
Will you use normative QOL measures where floor/ceiling effects could be encountered?
Will you use one or more surveys?
How are data reliability and validity tested? Has the survey been shown to be valid for your application? (measuring mortality, measuring functional ability)
What time treatment phases are you interested in surveying? (pre- and post-treatment, intervals of months or years)
How will the data be collected? (technical issues of collection)
Who will be the data collectors?
How are you going to handle missing data?
Is a scoring method defined? How will you analyze and report the data?
What are the costs?
How will feedback be given to the patients and providers?

McDowell and Newell (1996) have published a guide that can assist in selecting a credible instrument. These authors offer a review of over 80 surveys or instruments and address the measurement purpose and the reliability and validity results of each instrument. *Reliability* or *consistency* measures the reproducibility in obtaining the same results when the test is repeated, and *validity* measures the accuracy in measuring what it is supposed to measure. When available, an example of the instrument and the scoring method is included to aid clinicians in selecting the appropriate survey for their population. McDowell and Newell (1996) suggest that validated and reliable surveys should be used in clinical studies and that the creation of a new survey may not be necessary when an existing instrument is obtainable.

CASE STUDY: QOL AFTER LIVER TRANSPLANTATION

In measuring the success of surgical treatment, it is important to judge the results both in the traditional terms of operative mortality and operative morbidity, and in terms of the side effects that may impair function and health. Clinical decisions are often based on the patient's subjective feelings or physical abilities. This descriptive study summarizes the investigation of the biopsychosocial status of patients who have undergone orthotopic hepatic transplantation at a single institution. The results have not been published, so the findings reported are limited to preliminary observations. The purpose of this QOL review is to compare and describe, not to predict or evaluate.

The population reviewed is patients admitted for liver transplantation at the University of Colorado—University Hospital. Numerous factors contribute to their experiences and can impact results, including life-threatening illness, major surgery, financial issues, medications, and hepatic encephalopathy. These areas are additional opportunities for future research.

The National Institute of Diabetes and Digestive and Kidney Diseases (NIDDK) Liver Transplant Database (LTD) QOL questionnaire published by a multicenter study was selected as the instrument for measurement at the University of Colorado. Its selection was based on the published study and potential comparability to this population (Belle et al., 1997). A few demographic questions were added for

Table 49-1	**MEASURES OF DISEASE** **Average Presence or Absence of 21 Physical Symptoms***		
		PRE-TRANSPLANT	**POST-TRANSPLANT**
University of Colorado		14 symptoms	9.51 symptoms
Multicenter study		13.8 symptoms	10 symptoms

Multicenter study reported by Belle et al., 1997.
*Results were significant at <0.001.

Table 49-2	**MEASURES OF DISEASE** **Average Severity of Physical Symptoms*†**		
		PRE-TRANSPLANT	**POST-TRANSPLANT**
University of Colorado		29.62 severity	15.66 severity
Multicenter study		32.1 severity	17.8 severity

Multicenter study reported by Belle et al., 1997.
*Results were significant at <0.001.
†Scale: 0, Not at all, sequentially to 4, extreme; maximum score of 84.

this institution's analyses. The following domains were represented in the questionnaire: measures of disease, psychological status, personal function, social and role function, and general health perception.

The initial observations evaluated the outcome of 43 patients who completed a pre-transplant baseline questionnaire and a 1-year post-transplant questionnaire. Data were obtained at the time of transplantation listing and 6 and 12 months after liver transplant. An additional follow-up survey is planned after 2 years. The greatest improvements were shown in the post-transplant 1-year scales measuring physical symptoms (measures of disease) and psychological complaints. The University of Colorado results were equivalent to those of the multicenter study (Belle et al., 1997), which had over 300 patients were enrolled. The changes in number and severity of physical symptoms (Tables 49-1 and 49-2) and psychological complaints (Tables 49-3 and 49-4) were statistically significant. Moreover, a generalized improvement in all domains was found when compared to the same individual's pre-transplant status, a finding to be viewed as preliminary. Overall, most liver transplant recipients were satisfied with their QOL even with considerable economic strains and occasional personal distress.

FUTURE DIRECTIONS

Marketing QOL

The University of Colorado Hospital has been asked to quantify and qualify our services for prospective buyers. As our clinical data bases grow, we believe we will be able to include QOL data in contract negotiations. Because we believe QOL is an important evaluative element and effective categorizing element, combining these outcomes with severity of illness adjustments might result in a marketing advantage. A template should be established for pricing based on the predicted value to patients (efficacy)

Table 49-3	PSYCHOLOGICAL STATUS Average Presence or Absence of 5 Psychological Symptoms*	
	PRE-TRANSPLANT	**POST-TRANSPLANT**
University of Colorado	3.87 symptoms	2.38 symptoms
Multicenter study	3.7 symptoms	3 symptoms

Multicenter study reported by Belle et al., 1997.
*Results were significant at <0.001.

Table 49-4	PSYCHOLOGICAL STATUS Average Severity of Physical Symptoms*†	
	PRE-TRANSPLANT	**POST-TRANSPLANT**
University of Colorado	7.91 severity	3.53 severity
Multicenter study	8.1 severity	5 severity

Multicenter study reported by Belle et al., 1997.
*Results were significant at <0.001.
†Scale: 0, Not at all, sequentially to 4, extreme; maximum score of 84.

or on cost-effectiveness. This value is the increase in or maintenance of the patients' QOL. The payer may ask at what cost is this increased QOL? A standard that assists in weighing the economic advantages and disadvantages of treatment is the quality-adjusted life-years (QALY) (Glasziou et al., 1998). This standard can be calculated by using symptom reports or QOL surveys to show correlations of cost, effectiveness, and QOL gains. An example is the Veterans Administration Cooperative Study (Takaro et al., 1976), which estimated that net cost per QALY gained from coronary artery bypass graft surgery (CABG) ranged from $3,500 in left main artery disease to $30,000 in one-vessel disease. Subsequent studies have revealed that the medical management costs and medication usage of not having CABG surgery can result in higher costs than those associated with surgery (Rogers, 1985).

Case Management

If your case management program has not assisted in the development, measurement, and assessment of QOL at your institution, you may be forgetting a valuable professional resource. It is important to reiterate that QOL can be defined as "the gap between the patient's expectations and achievements" (Calman, 1984). The case manager is in an ideal position to assist in narrowing that gap through realistic goal setting. QOL results can be used by case managers to predict outcomes for patients, identify patient needs and services and meet those needs, and advise providers of systems improvements. For example, if joint replacement patients' psychosocial domains (ability to adequately perform social, occupational, and domestic roles) are lower immediately postoperatively than preoperatively, the case manager can provide patients with information and/or services to improve this outcome and advocate for systems development.

References

Belle, S.H., Porayko, M.K., Hoofnagle, J.H., Lake, J.R., Zetterman, R.K. (1997). Changes in quality of life after liver transplantation among adults. *Liver Transplantation and Surgery, 3*(2), 93-104.

Bergner, M. (1996). Sickness impact profile. In I MacDowell & C. Newell (Eds), *Measuring health, a guide to rating scales and questionnaires* (pp. 431-437). New York: Oxford University Press.

Calman, KC. (1984). Quality of life in cancer patients:an hypothesis, *Journal of Medical Ethics, 10,* 124-127.

Dupuy, J. (1996). The psychological general well-being schedule. In I MacDowell & C. Newell (Eds), *Measuring health, a guide to rating scales and questionnaires* (pp. 206-213). New York: Oxford University Press.

Glasziou, P.P., Cole, B.F., Gelber, R.D., Hilden, J., & Simes, R.J. (1998). Quality adjusted survival analysis with repeated quality of life measures. *Statistics in Medicine, 17,* 1215-1229.

Granger, C.V., Cotter, A.C., Hamilton, B.B., et al. (1990). Functional assessment scales: a study of persons with multiple sclerosis. *Archives in Physical Medicine and Rehabilitation, 71,* 870-875.

Linn, M.W. (1996). The Rapid Disability Rating Scale. In I. MacDowell & C. Newell (Eds), *Measuring health, a guide to rating scales and questionnaires* (pp. 82-88). New York: Oxford University Press.

Lloyd, C.E., Matthews, K.A., Wing, R.R., Orchard, T.J. (1992). Psychosocial factors and complications of IDDM. The Pittsburgh Epidemiology of Diabetes Complications Study, VIII. *Diabetes Care, 15,* 166-172.

McDowell, I., & Newell, C. (Eds.). (1996). *Measuring health, a guide to rating scales and questionnaires.* New York: Oxford University Press.

Meenan, R.F. (1996). The Arthritis Impact Measurement Scales. In I. MacDowell & C. Newell (Eds), *Measuring health, a guide to rating scales and questionnaires* (pp. 383-391). New York: Oxford University Press.

Melzack, R. (1996). McGill Pain Questionnaire. In I. MacDowell & C. Newell (Eds), *Measuring health, a guide to rating scales and questionnaires* (pp. 346-351). New York: Oxford University Press.

OARS Duke University. (1996). The OARS Multidimensional Functional Assessment Questionnaire. In I. MacDowell & C. Newell (Eds), *Measuring health, a guide to rating scales and questionnaires* (pp. 464-472). New York: Oxford University Press.

Rogers, W.J. (1985). Medical vs. surgical management of ischemic heart disease: Implications of the coronary artery surgery study. *Ala Journal of Medical Science, 22,* 416-422.

Spilker, B. (Ed). (1996). *Quality of life and pharmacoeconomics in clinical trials,* Philadelphia & New York: Lippincott-Raven.

Stewart, A., & Ware, J., (1992). *Measuring functioning and well-being, The medical outcomes study approach.* Durham & London: Duke University Press.

Takaro, R., Hultgren, H.N., Lipton, M.J., et al. (1976). The VA Cooperative Randomized Study of Surgery for Coronary Occlusive Disease. II. Subgroup with significant left main lesions. *Circulation, 54*(Suppl. III), 107-117.

Ware, J.E., (1996). Short Form 36 Health Status. In I. MacDowell & C. Newell (Eds), *Measuring health, a guide to rating scales and questionnaires* (pp. 446-456). New York: Oxford University Press.

Ware, J.E. (1996). The Rand Mental Health Inventory. In I. MacDowell & C. Newell (Eds), *Measuring health, a guide to rating scales and questionnaires* (pp. 213-219). New York: Oxford University Press.

Ware, J.E., Kosinski, M., & Keller, S.D. (1994). *SF-36 Physical and Mental Health Summary Scales: A user's manual.* Boston: The Health Institute.

Expanding Our Horizons

Managing a Continuum of Care

Jean A. Newsome

CHAPTER OVERVIEW

Patient education, a case management model of care, and continued outpatient contact and support have a positive effect on outcomes in caring for the diabetic patient. This chapter explores the driving forces behind the assessment of care outcomes at Brookwood Medical Center, Birmingham, Alabama: improving the quality of life for the diabetic patient, assessing and meeting consumer needs, providing holistic care, and expanding the focus on health and wellness. Among the topics considered herein are organizational factors such as evaluating and improving resource utilization, decreasing the cost of care, increasing the value of services provided, positioning the institution for increased competition, and positively influencing the morbidity, mortality, and hospital length of stay of the diabetic population.

As with most chronic illness, diabetes presents multiple challenges to the patient and the health care providers. Those challenges are manifested in all areas of the patient's life, in the lives of his or her family, and within the health care environment. Maintenance of quality of life, preservation of wellness, inhibition of deterioration, and management of financial impacts of the disease act singularly and in combination to create the need for holistic plans of care with which the patient willingly participates and contributes. Several authors writing on care for the diabetic population have recognized the need

Acknowledgment: The Diabetes Outcomes Project at Brookwood Medical Center was a progressive and successful attempt to positively affect quality of the overall care for a patient with diabetes. That project was successful only because of the committment and excellence of the members of the Diabetes Outcomes Project:

Patsy Kanter, RN (Certified Diabetes Educator)
Judy Baker, RN (Diabetes Educator)
Nancy Martin, RN (Diabetes Educator)
Debbie Miller, RN (Case Manager)
Joye Taylor, M.S. (Registered Dietitian, Certified Diabetes Educator)
Anita Floyd (Registered Dietitian)

for long-term patient follow-ups after educational and therapeutic interventions, yet those projects have yet to be well represented in current literature (Ary, Toobert, Wilson, & Glasgow, 1986; Glasgow, McCaul, & Schafer, 1987; Glasgow, Wilson, & McCaul, 1985; Johnson, 1992; Kurtz, 1990; Rosenstock, 1985). It has been well documented in the literature addressing other chronic illnesses, however, that continued education and outpatient support increase compliance rates and decrease rates of complications from the given illness.

The long-term effects of diabetes on the individual body systems vary from person to person with little consensus regarding factors that provide predictability of those effects. Past research in the area of complication avoidance has failed to demonstrate health-related behaviors or patterns that conclusively correlate with minimizing diabetic complications. Consistently low glycosylated hemoglobin levels, however, appear to offer a measure of avoidance of diabetic complications (American Diabetes Association, 1994; Haas, 1993; Jacobson et al., 1991; Orchard et al., 1990; Walsh & Roberts, 1993). The Diabetes Outcomes Project recognized this variable as a critical indicator of the quality of the education and monitoring of the diabetic patient.

An appropriate summation of the goals of this project team was found in Johnson's 1992 study: "Adherence behaviors have not been examined in relationship to health-related daily functioning. More adherent patients may be hospitalized less, miss school or work less, and experience fewer debilitating or distressing symptoms" (p. 1664).

Based on desires to improve patient compliance, decrease rates of diabetic complications, and realize financial improvements for the diabetic population at Brookwood Medical Center in Birmingham, Alabama, a longitudinal project was initiated, targeting improvement in all of the areas identified. That ap-

FIGURE **50-1**   The Diabetes Outcomes Project conceptual model.

proach to evaluating patient outcomes has been recommended by a number of authors (Ary et al., 1986; Jacobson et al., 1991; Johnson, 1992; Mazzuca et al., 1986; Rosenstock, 1985).

The Diabetes Outcomes Project at Brookwood Medical Center was based on the conceptual model presented in Fig. 50-1.

Determining the Clinical Process Variables

The Diabetes Outcomes Project team identified several variables as the most accessible and measurable within the time frame of their project. The variables were chosen both for their impacts on patient morbidity and for their impacts on the cost of patient care. The design of the project called for evaluation of the process variables at the time of the patient's initial hospitalization (with diagnosis-related group [DRG] 294), and again at 3 months, 6 months, and 12 months after that hospitalization. The project team recognized that the variables were not all inclusive in the complication, morbidity, and mortality of diabetes mellitus. Compliance with physician follow-up visits and patient education were considered inherent in the successful outcome of each area. Certain variables were targeted as reflecting long-term outcomes that could be positively influenced by patient education along with regular professional intervention and support (Box 50-1).

IDENTIFYING CLINICAL OUTCOMES

The clinical outcomes to be evaluated at the end of the 12-month tracking period were based on known potential complications of diabetes as well as on assumed consequences of that disease. Following are the clinical outcomes selected by the project team:

Patient morbidity
Patient mortality
Cost of care
Length of stay

Box 50-1 ► **CLINICAL PROCESS VARIABLES**

Compliance with recommended physician office visits
Self–blood glucose monitoring (SBCM) practices
Blood pressure monitoring
Weight control adherence
Adherence to caloric restrictions
Compliance with recommended ophthalmologic appointments
General well-being scores
Hospital days since initial hospitalization
Emergency room visits since initial hospitalization
Work or school days missed since initial hospitalization
Incidence of lower extremity cellulitis
Incidence of urinary tract infections
Incidence of lower extremity amputation

Caring for the Diabetic Patient

Compliance by the typical diabetic patient is similar to that of patients with other chronic illnesses. Unique to the diabetic population, though, are the complexity of the treatment programs and their direct impact on all body systems. Although past research on diabetic compliance is inconclusive, several themes may be identified. In general, rates of compliance and noncompliance reveal no patterns or predictability among individuals or subgroups within the diabetic population; compliance within one or two areas of diabetes self-care does not reflect or guarantee compliance within others; trends in patient-identified barriers to compliance have been tentatively identified and are currently being tested for validity; and the greater the complexity of diabetes and self-care, the less is the rate of consistent adherence to those self-care practices.

Psychosocial Factors

The psychosocial variables associated with positive outcomes in diabetic care have not yet been clearly identified or researched. The fact that diabetic care is long term does not appear to present the same set of psychosocial patterns that often emerge in persons with other chronic illnesses. Social support, education, and overall outlooks and adaptive responses have been only tentatively identified as indicators of positive outcomes in the diabetic population. The questions of psychosocial influences on long-term behaviors and outcomes of diabetic patients remains one that deserves exploration and elaboration.

Patient Education

Educating the diabetic patient is without question an essential element of care, yet current research in that area is lacking evidence of long-term results. Studies reported vary in the amount of importance placed on education as it affects metabolic control, and most studies are prompt to point out that education and metabolic control must not be viewed synonymously. There is, however, agreement within the literature that increased efforts must be made by health care professionals to evaluate the effects of education on overall patient outcomes and over longer periods of time than have been reported previously. At least one study has demonstrated positive outcomes by a diabetes educator on hospital length of stay (LOS) (Feddersen & Lockwood, 1994).

Morbidity and Mortality

Macroangiopathy is responsible for 60% of the deaths in diabetes (Vinicor, cited in Haas, 1993, p. 72). Strokes are at least twice as common in diabetic persons as in the general population and also are accompanied by a higher rate of recurrence and mortality. Coronary artery disease is also more severe in diabetic patients. Morbidity and mortality for both strokes and coronary artery disease are highest in patients with poor glucose control (American Diabetes Association, 1994; Haas, 1993). The Centers for Disease Control (1991) estimates that over 945 diabetics will have lower extremity amputations each year in Alabama alone; Haas (1993) writes that more than 50% of nontraumatic lower limb amputations result from diabetes mellitus. More than 250 cases of blindness will occur each year in Alabama (Centers for Disease Control, 1991), and there will be approximately 12,000 new cases of legal blindness throughout the United States as a result of diabetes (American Diabetes Association, 1994). Nephropathy will progress to end-stage renal disease (ESRD) in up to 40% of patients who have type I diabetes; up to 60% of diabetic patients will develop symptomatic neuropathy (Haas, 1993). Waclawski (1990) conducted a study that demonstrated a striking difference between diabetic and nondiabetic employees in working days lost because of illness.

The Centers for Disease Control (1991) estimated the following:

Over 2000 Alabamans will die each year from diabetes.
Alabama's death rate per 100,000 persons ranks forty-sixth highest among all states and the District of Columbia
Approximately 47,000 annual hospitalizations in Alabama are directly related to diabetes
Diabetes will cost the state of Alabama at least $375 million per year in medical care and lost productivity

Financial Implications

On a national level the cost of diabetes is staggering. The American Diabetes Association (1994) reports that over $37 billion was spent on diabetes inpatient care, with a total cost of $90 billion for the United States in 1992. Chronic complications of diabetes cost $410 billion for inpatient care. Almost 48,000 persons were permanently disabled because of diabetes in 1992, resulting in lost productivity and premature mortality.

The consequences of diabetes mellitus, and certainly of diabetes mellitus that is not well controlled, are far reaching and dramatic for both patients and health care providers. Early and consistent education, support, and intervention have proved effective in altering negative outcomes from both anecdotal and professional reports.

SAMPLE AND SETTING

Adult patients admitted to Brookwood Medical Center with the diagnosis "diabetes out of control" (DRG 294) were asked to participate in the project during that hospitalization. Only adults age 18 years or older who were not mentally impaired were included.

The project was designed to begin during hospitalization and to include the incidence of the variables under study for 1 year after that hospitalization. All subjects had read and signed a standardized informed consent document before their involvement in this project. Our practice patterns of initiating diabetic education while the patient was hospitalized and of providing consistent outpatient support and education were hypothesized to positively influence many outcomes of the diabetic population we serve.

The final sample consisted of 28 adults, ranging in age from 39 to 80 years. Seven of those adults were newly diagnosed with diabetes at the time of the hospitalization. The length of known diabetes among the remaining 21 participants ranged from 2 to 23 years, with an average of 9.5 years.

INSTRUMENTATION

Three instruments were used in this project to collect and evaluate information pertinent to the patient population. The standardized Diabetes Teaching Outline, the General Well-Being Instrument, and the Diabetes Outcome Data Collection Tool were employed with each patient who participated.

The Diabetes Teaching Outline, a two-page outline used for diabetic teaching at Brookwood Medical Center, had been used for several years before this project began. The outline consisted of categories of information, with each category itemizing specific areas of instruction to be addressed. The categories were self-monitoring, medications, hypoglycemia, hyperglycemia, exercise, diet, personal care, complications, sick days, and psychosocial factors. Subjects were graded as "competent," "requires assistance," or "no knowledge." "Competent family" was another grading option.

The General Well-Being Instrument, a two-page standardized multiple-choice questionnaire, was designed to evaluate general attitudes and outlook. Validity of the instrument was determined by its concurrent comparison with several other self-report scales. The General Well-Being survey demonstrated statistical significance in its ability to differentiate emotional status of subjects within an overall sample. The General Well-Being Instrument was either self-administered by the patient or verbally administered by the diabetes educator.

The Diabetes Outcome Data Collection Tool was developed in 1993 by an interdisciplinary health care team at Brookwood Medical Center in anticipation of this project. Both inpatient and outpatient information that it was deemed essential to monitor by that team was formatted into a one-page data collection form. That form allowed information to be recorded at the time of hospitalization and at 3 months, 6 months, and 1 year after hospitalization.

Information on the data collection form was recorded at each of the proposed time intervals. Patient information was recorded in the outpatient diabetes center to allow follow-up phone contacts at the proposed intervals after hospitalization. The outpatient diabetes center director and the internal medicine case manager regularly reviewed charts and data collection forms for consistency and accuracy within the process. Regular team meetings of the case management specialty nurses and outpatient diabetes center staff were conducted to discuss patient criteria, to solve problems, and to maintain consistency in process. Several limitations were recognized by the data collection team involved in this project.

OBJECTIVE OUTCOMES

Following is a brief discussion of the findings of the Diabetes Outcomes Project, along with graphs that depict results for some of the variables. Table 50-1 summarizes the findings for variables that are not accompanied by a graph.

Physician Office Visits

There was a definite decline in physician office visits related to problems with diabetes after the ongoing educational intervention. The average number of physician office visits concerning problems with diabetes before the educational intervention was 3.24 per quarter; after the ongoing education the average number of visits reported was 1.76.

Hospital Days Associated With Diabetes

Patients with new-onset diabetes were not rehospitalized during this project. Only one patient with preexisting diabetes was rehospitalized during the project time period.

Emergency Room Visits

There was no appreciable change in the average number of emergency room visits per quarter.

Missed Days of Work or School

Sixteen of the 28 project participants were retired or disabled. Of the 12 participants who were employed or were students, none reported missed work or school days after the project began.

Table 50-1	SUMMARY OF PROJECT OUTCOMES*
VARIABLE	**OUTCOME**
Average number of physician office visits per quarter	3.24 before educational intervention
	1.76 after educational intervention
Hospital days associated with diabetes	No newly diagnosed patients rehospitalized during project
	1 patient with preexisting diabetes rehospitalized
Average number of emergency room visits per quarter	No appreciable change
Missed days of school or work	23 days during 3 months before project began
	None after project began
Cost of care per case during hospitalization	No appreciable change, remained stable throughout project
Education outcomes: test scores before and after teaching session	Average test score at initial hospitalization: Before teaching session: 27% After teaching session: 98% Average test score 12 months after hospitalization: Before teaching session: 82% After teaching session: 97%
Average length of hospital stay (ALOS)	ALOS throughout project remained less than critical path projection of 5 days
Mortality	2 patients died before 3-month follow-up (deaths not directly attributable to diabetes)
Medical benefits	3 patients experienced significant weight loss; 2 of them were able to discontinue insulin therapy; the third patient could discontinue hypertensive medication
Cellulitis	No occurrences in year preceding or during project
Urinary tract infections (UTIs)	1 patient had a UTI during year of project
	1 patient had a UTI during 3 months after project began and 2 UTIs between 6- and 12-month follow-up
Lower extremity amputations	None in year preceding or during project

*Number of patients in study, 28.

Education Scores

Tests were given before and after each teaching session at the time of hospitalization, and at 3 months, 6 months, and 12 months after that initial hospitalization. The pre-teaching session test scores of those patients with newly diagnosed diabetes were not averaged into the first set of pre-teaching session tests. During the initial hospitalization, pre-teaching session test scores of those persons with preexisting diabetes ranged from 15% to 74%, with an average score of 38%.

Cost Per Case

There was no appreciable change in cost of hospital care per case.

Length of Stay

The critical path for DRG 294 at our hospital projects a length of stay of 5 days. The average length of stay (ALOS) during the project time period was fractionally less than that critical path projection.

Mortality

Two participants died before the 3-month follow-up session; neither of those deaths was directly attributable to diabetes.

Medical Benefits

Three patients experienced dramatic medical benefits because of their lifestyle changes. Two of these three lost a significant amount of weight and were able to discontinue insulin therapy. The third participant lost weight and no longer required antihypertensive agents.

Cellulitis

No participants in the project experienced cellulitis during the year preceding the project or during the actual project.

Urinary Tract Infection

One participant reported a urinary tract infection within 1 year of the hospitalization; another participant reported a urinary tract infection within 3 months after the hospitalization; that same subject reported two urinary tract infections between the 6-month and 12-month follow-up assessments.

Lower Extremity Amputation

No participant in this project underwent amputation before or during the project.

PSYCHOLOGICAL OUTLOOK

Psychological outlook was measured by the General Well Being Instrument during the hospitalization and at 3, 6, and 12 months after that stay. The instrument consisted of 14 questions, eight of which referred to negative outlooks or emotions. (Example: Have you been anxious, worried, or upset?) Five of those questions assessed positive outlooks or emotions. (Example: Have you been feeling emotionally stable and sure of yourself?) The questionnaire assessed reports of nervousness, self-control, sadness, stress, personal satisfaction, anxiety, alertness, discomfort, health fears, and fatigue.

The final analysis of the General Well Being Instrument provided surprising results. All participants had essentially no change in their self-perception of the measured variables over the year of data collection. Those who began with high negative responses remained so, as did those with high positive responses. Approximately half of the population scored high negative consistently, and the other half scored low negative consistently. Only two questions demonstrated a significant decline in negative responses: Have you been bothered by nerves? and Have you felt sad, discouraged, or hopeless?

Those persons scoring high negative consistently were not found to be only the persons who were noncompliant or with low pre-teaching session test scores. Although neither statistically sound nor scientifically controlled, these outcomes present an interesting premise: a person's self-perceived negative well-being does not negatively impact (certain) health care behaviors or knowledge levels.

COMPLIANCE BEHAVIORS

Participants diagnosed with new-onset diabetes (seven participants) at the time of hospitalization were not included in the initial compliance assessment. It is interesting to note that those subjects' compliance behaviors were those consistently adhered to by all the project participants for the year after the diagnosis.

Self-Blood Glucose Monitoring (SBGM)

Before hospitalization, SBGM was markedly poorly maintained, with half of the project participants reporting regular noncompliance. A significant increase in SBGM compliance was reported during the actual project. The greatest decline in compliance was between the 6-month and 12-month follow-up contacts. The cost of glucometer strips was reported as a reason for noncompliance by three subjects as the year progressed (Fig. 50-2).

Caloric Adherence

Poor adherence to prescribed caloric intake was reported by two thirds of the participants before hospitalization. There was a dramatic increase in the reports of compliance 3 months after hospitalization, but that behavior slowly declined as the time period progressed. The greatest decline was noted between the 6- and 12-month follow-up contacts (Fig. 50-3).

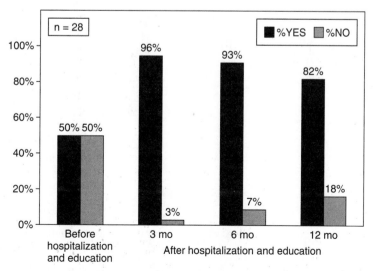

FIGURE **50-2**   Maintenance of self-blood glucose monitoring over a 1-year period.

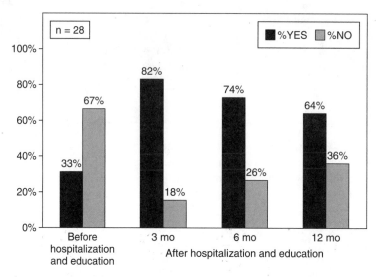

FIGURE **50-3**   Caloric adherence over a 1-year period.

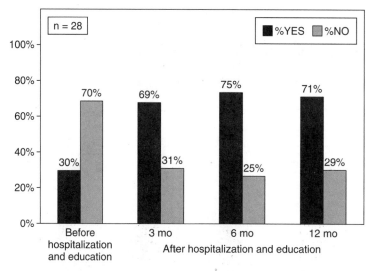

FIGURE **50-4**   Weight control goals met over a 1-year period.

Weight Control

As would be expected, weight control was also consistently an area of poor compliance before the hospitalization (noncompliance in 70% of subjects). Compliance in that behavior was markedly improved by self-reports, with approximately 70% of the participants compliant during the project (Fig. 50-4).

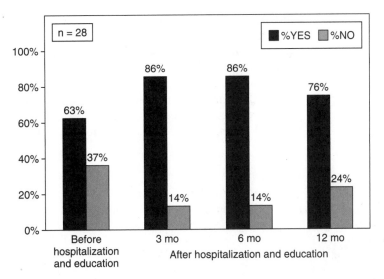

FIGURE **50-5**   Compliance with ophthalmology examinations over a 1-year period.

Ophthalmology Examinations

Recommended eye examinations were poorly complied with before hospitalization according to patient reports. Reported compliance rose by 20% during the project, with a notable drop between the 6- and 12-month follow-up contacts (Fig. 50-5).

Blood Pressure Monitoring

An overwhelming majority of patients in this project sample reported consistent compliance with blood pressure monitoring as prescribed by their physician.

Physician Office Visits

Almost universal compliance with physician visits also was reported for this study sample. Two of the three noncompliant subjects stated that finances were the reason for not visiting their physician as recommended.

SUMMARY OF THE PROJECT'S RESULTS

The project was designed to evaluate the impact of educational efforts and regular follow-up contacts by a team of diabetes educators at Brookwood Medical Center. It was theorized that greater educational efforts would decrease the overall incidence of complications, rehospitalization rates, and cost per case and length of stay for hospitalizations. Increases in knowledge scores, compliance behaviors, productivity, and psychosocial well-being perceptions were anticipated.

The final outcomes demonstrated no complications, with the exception of urinary tract infections, which plagued two of the participants. No patient in the project was rehospitalized during the year of the study.

Knowledge scores and self-reported compliance behaviors did indeed improve dramatically and were well maintained. It is notable that the greatest decreases in those two areas occurred between the 6- and 12-month follow-up contacts consistently, leading to the assumption that a 6-month delay in caregiver contact is detrimental to patient outcomes. The number of missed days of work or school decreased, and psychological well-being perceptions did not change.

The project was an aggressive attempt to improve the quality of care, quality of life, and efficiency in resource utilization for the patient with diabetes. The outcomes of that project, while not scientifically sound, deserve consideration in the planning of optimum care for the diabetic patient.

References

American Diabetes Association. (1994). *Diabetes 1993 vital statistics.* (ISBN #0-94544823-6).

Ary, T., Toobert, D., Wilson, W., & Glasgow, R. (1986). Patient perspectives on factors contributing to nonadherence to diabetes regimens. *Diabetes Care, 9*(2), 168-172.

Brown, S. (1988). Effects of educational interventions in diabetes care: A meta-analysis of findings. *Nursing Research, 37*(4), 223-230.

Cassileth, B., Lusk, E., Strouse, T., Miller, D., Brown, L., Cross, P. & Tenaglia, A. (1984). Psychosocial status in chronic illness: A comparative analysis of six diagnostic groups. *The New England Journal of Medicine, 311*(8), 506-511.

Centers for Disease Control (1991, May). *Diabetes in the United States: A strategy for prevention.* U.S. Department of Health & Human Services.

Cerkoney, K., & Hart, L. (1980). The relationship between the health belief model and compliance of persons with diabetes mellitus. *Diabetes Care, 3,* 594-598.

Chandalia, H., & Bagrodia, J. (1979). Effects of nutritional counseling on the blood glucose and nutritional knowledge of diabetic subjects. *Diabetes Care, 2*(4), 353-356.

Davis, M. (1966). Variations in patients' compliance with doctors' orders: Analysis of congruence between survey response and results of empirical investigations. *Journal of Medical Education, 41*(11), 1037-1048.

Diabetes Education Record. Birmingham, Alabama: Brookwood Medical Center, Outpatient Diabetes Center.

Diabetes Outcome Data Collection Tool. (1993). Birmingham, Alabama: Brookwood Medical Center, Outpatient Diabetes Center.

Feddersen, E., & Lockwood, D. (1994). An inpatient diabetes educator's impact on length of hospital stay. *The Diabetes Educator, 20*(2), 125-128.

Garrard, J., Mullen, L., Joynes, J., McNeil, L, & Etzwiler, D. (1990). Clinical evaluation of the impact of a patient education program. *The Diabetes Educator, 16*(5), 394-400.

General Well-Being Schedule. (1977). (DHEW Publication No. HRA 78-1347) U.S. Department of Health, Education and Welfare. National Center for Health Statistics, Hyattsville, Md.

Glasgow, R., McCaul, K., & Schafer, L. (1986). Barriers to regimen adherence among persons with insulin-dependent diabetes. *Journal of Behavioral Medicine, 9*(1), 65-77.

Glasgow, R., McCaul, K., & Schafer, L. (1987). Self-care behaviors and glycemic control in Type I diabetes. *Journal of Chronic Disease, 40*(5), 399-412.

Glasgow, R., Wilson, W., & McCaul, K. (1985). Regimen adherence: A problematic construct in diabetes research. *Diabetes Care, 8*(3), 300-301.

Haas, L. (1993, March). Chronic complications of diabetes mellitus. *The Nursing Clinics of North America, 28*(1), 71-85.

Holmes, D. (1986). The person and diabetes in a psychosocial context. *Diabetes Care, 9*(2), 194-206.

Jacobson, A., Adler, A., Derby, L., Anderson, B., & Wolfsdorf, J. (1991). Clinic attendance and glycemic control: A study of contrasting groups of patients with IDDM. *Diabetes Care, 14*(7), 599-601.

Johnson, S. (1992). Methodological issues in diabetes research. *Diabetes Care, 15*(11), 1658-1667.

Korhonen, T., Huttunen, J., Aro, A., Hentinen, M., Ihalainen, O., Majander, H., Siitonen, O., Uusitupa, M., & Pyorala, K. (1983). A controlled trial on the effects of patient education in the treatment of insulin-dependent diabetes. *Diabetes Care, 6*(3), 256-260.

Kurtz, S. (1990). Adherence to diabetes regimens: Empirical status and clinical applications. *The Diabetes Educator, 16*(1), 50-56.

Legge, J., Massey, V., Vena, C., & Reilly, B. (1980). Evaluating patient education: A case study of a diabetes program. *Health and Education Quarterly, 7*(2), 148-158.

Mazzuca, S., Moorman, N., Wheeler, M., Norton, J., Fineberg, N., Vinicor, F., Cohen, S., & Clark, C. (1986). The diabetes education study: A controlled trial of the effects of diabetes patient education. *Diabetes Care, 9*(1), 1-10.

Orchard, T., Dorman, J., Maser, R., Becker, D., Ellis, D., LaPorte, R., Kuller, L., Wolfson, S., & Drash, A. (1990). Factors associated with avoidance of severe complications after 25 years of IDDM. (1990). *Diabetes Care, 13*(7), 741-747.

Rosenstock, I. (1985). Understanding and enhancing patient compliance with diabetic regimens. *Diabetes Care, 8*(6), 610-616.

Rubin, R., Peyrot, M., & Saudek, C. (1989). Effects of diabetes education on self-care, metabolic control, and emotional well-being. *Diabetes Care, 12*(1), 673-679.

Rubin, R., Peyrot, M., & Saudek, C. (1991). Differential effect of diabetes education on self-regulation and life-style behaviors. *Diabetes Care, 14*(4), 335-338.

Stevens, J., Burgess, M., Kaiser, D., & Sheppa, M. (1985). Outpatient management of diabetes mellitus with patient education to increase dietary carbohydrate and fiber. *Diabetes Care, 8*(4), 359-366.

Waclawski, E. (1990). Sickness absence among insulin-treated diabetic employees. *Diabetic Medicine, 7*, 41-44.

Walsh, J., & Roberts, R. (1993, Nov.). Uncomplicating diabetes. *Diabetes Interview, 14*, 8.

Watkins, J., Williams, F., Martin, D., Hogan, M., & Anderson, E. (1967). A study of diabetic patients at home. *American Journal of Public Health, 57*(3), 452-457.

Wilson, W., Ary, D., Biglan, A., Glasgow, R., Toobert, M., & Campbell, D. (1986). Psychosocial predictors of self-care behaviors (compliance) and glycemic control in non-insulin-dependent diabetes mellitus. *Diabetes Care, 9*(6), 614-622.

Developing Outcome Management Strategies

An Intensive DRG-Focused Study

Bill Brodie

CHAPTER OVERVIEW

In July, 1994 the Department of Psychiatry at Brookwood Medical Center, Birmingham, Alabama, initiated an intense diagnosis related group (DRG)—focused outcome study that would involve patients who met the American Psychiatric Association's *Diagnostic and Statistical Manual of Mental Disorders* third edition revised (DSM IIIR) criteria for DRG 426, depressive neurosis. The goal was a 6-month study of 70 patients to identify and prioritize opportunities for measurable improvement in the delivery of patient services. This study was the first attempt undertaken at this medical center to identify areas on which to focus to improve quality in medication compliance and discharge planning.

The DRG 426 outcome team, which included psychiatric case managers, identified several measurable variables that would best represent barriers to achieving the desired outcomes: decreased readmission rates, increased functional capacity, increased medication compliance, decreased cost of care, decreased length of stay, and increased understanding of symptom management. Tracking these variables and re-

Acknowledgments: Voyaging into psychiatric case management was not without risk, and I would like to recognize those brave individuals who took the voyage and, together with the patients who volunteered for the study, are charting its future course. The hope of the Depressive Neurosis Outcome Study Team's collaborative effort is to create a map that will decrease the symptoms endured and prejudices experienced by those who suffer from mental illness:

To Glenda Brogden and Derek Spellman, who "mastered the risk" and provided the vision and support needed to implement nursing case management successfully within psychiatry.

To the DRG 426 Depressive Neurosis Outcome Study Team: Dr. Ed Logue, Albertha Lyas, Jean Newsome, Linda Lind, Gloria Sandlin, Sara Romano, Sue Trant, Sharon Beal Fowler, Gary Tate, Joan Witt, Karen Litwiniec, and Ellen Hitchcock, who provided the expertise, guidance, and professional assistance that allowed us to meet the goals and initiatives identified for this study.

A personal thank you to Elaine L. Cohen for being my long-distance friend and for recognizing the efforts and contributions that nursing case management is bringing into the 21st century.

viewing the final data revealed two key areas that needed to be addressed to help achieve major improvements in care delivery: (1) the patient's ability to pay for medications and (2) educational deficits related to symptom management during and after hospitalization. In the future the outcome team will undertake a more detailed study of the outcomes identified and will further evaluate some new interventions that the team introduced.

Patients diagnosed with DRG-426 depressive neurosis typically consume considerable inpatient resources as well as a large proportion of limited public mental health care resources. Concern over these areas led a DRG-focused team at Brookwood Medical Center to perform an intense clinical and financial review of patients frequently hospitalized and rehospitalized within the Department of Psychiatry. A retrospective chart review revealed that patients diagnosed with depressive neurosis have high readmission rates, high rates of self-harm, poor compliance with outpatient medication regimens, poor attendance at inpatient therapeutic activities, an unstable home environment, a lack of understanding of the disease process, longer lengths of stay, and higher costs.

The following resources were used to further substantiate these initial chart findings:

A cost analysis report for DRG 426 provided by the medical center's cost accounting department
Resource consumption trending reports for DRG 426 provided by the data processing and adjunctive
    therapy departments

THE STUDY

In June, 1994 this DRG 426–focused team from the Department of Psychiatry at Brookwood Medical Center in Birmingham, Alabama began to develop a 6-month study of 70 patients diagnosed with depressive neurosis. The goal of this team was to identify and prioritize opportunities for measurable improvement in the delivery of patient care services within the Department of Psychiatric Services. The DRG 426 outcome team consisted of health professionals with various clinical backgrounds, including psychiatrist, psychologist, psychiatric case managers, pharmacist, occupational therapist, and psychiatric registered nurses. The qualifications for team members included leadership ability, clinical expertise, knowledge of case management principles, continuous quality improvement experience, and point of care contact with patients.

Input was elicited from the cost accounting department, the psychiatric quality assurance committee, and the psychiatric strategic business unit committee to assist in profiling potential participants. These committees confirmed DRG 426 depressive neurosis as a population of psychiatric patients who were high volume, high cost, and problem prone. In addition, the quality assurance committee and a medical focus group had identified these patients as having high rates of recidivism and poor outpatient follow-up compliance. Further input from the cost accounting department demonstrated that DRG 426 accounts for 28% of all inpatient psychiatric admissions and lengths of stay of 9.02 days. Based on recommendations of the quality assurance committee and the medical focus group, patients diagnosed with DRG 426 depressive neurosis would be the identified population for the intense DRG outcome study.

CLINICAL OUTCOMES

The outcome team identified eight measurable outcomes to be evaluated during the time frame of their study:

1. Decreased readmission rates
2. Decreased acts of self-harm

3. Increased compliance with inpatient therapeutic treatment activities
4. Improved functional capacity
5. Increased medication compliance
6. Increased understanding of symptom management at discharge
7. Decreased cost of care
8. Decreased length of stay

METHODS USED

The outcome study began July 1, 1994, and initial data collection lasted through August 31, 1995. During this time 70 patients who met the DSM IIIR criteria for DRG 426 depressive neurosis were asked to participate in a 6-month outcome study. Only patients age 18 years and older who exhibited no associated axis 1 diagnosis and no associated medical complications were included in the outcome study. The outcome study began during hospitalization and concluded 6 months after that initial hospitalization.

Each participant read and signed a consent form for participation in the DRG 426 Depressive Neurosis Outcome Study. All records reviewed and collected by the outcome team were kept in secured areas of the hospital. Only persons directly involved with the outcome study were permitted access to patient materials. Patients also agreed to be interviewed and to take the Beck Depression Inventory (BDI) on admission, at discharge, and at 3- and 6-month intervals after discharge. Additionally, each participant was informed that this intense study would require that they divulge information relating to their family or social structure, social and economic levels, medication compliance or noncompliance, treatment plan compliance, and discharge teaching comprehension. Post-discharge compliance and any identified acts of self-harm would be assessed by the outcome team during scheduled follow-up telephone interviews. This information would assist the outcome team in determining whether these variables positively or negatively influenced the outcomes of the psychiatric patients studied.

Two data collection instruments were used during this outcome study to collect and evaluate information relevant to the study population: the BDI and the Depressive Neurosis Data Collection Measurement Tool. The BDI measures the affective variables of anxiety and depression. The inventory can be completed by the subject in as short a time as 5 minutes. The BDI, therefore, is an excellent quick and easy aid in detecting the individual suffering from depression when an evaluation might not otherwise be made (Beck & Beamesderfer, 1974).

The Depressive Neurosis Data Collection Measurement Tool (Fig. 51-1) was developed by the outcome study team. The final tool was implemented after revisions were made during a 10-patient pilot period. The final two-page tool addressed 15 key areas. Each key area captured information relevant to the expected patient outcomes. The tool itself was used to record both inpatient and outpatient information over the 6-month study period. Confidentiality was of utmost importance to this study population and outcome team.

STUDY RESULTS

In November, 1995 the 6-month data collection period ended for all 70 participants. Final data analysis is presented in Boxes 51-1 and 51-2.

The outcome team reviewed the final data analysis and divided the data into three categories:

1. Patient economics
2. Educational deficits
3. Medication compliance

DRG/IC-9:

Patient Name: _____   Insurance Company: _____
Medical Record #: _____   Unit: _____
Patient Date of Birth: _____   Admitting Physician: _____
Planned Admit: _____ Emergency Admit: _____   Admitting Physician: _____

I. Criteria For Admission
A. Symptoms met DSM III R Criteria   Yes _____ No _____

II. Previous Admission   *Please check*
A. Within last month _____
B. Within last 3 months _____
C. Within last 6 months _____
D. More than 6 months ago _____
E. More than 1 year ago _____

III. Family Social Structure
A. Care provider _____
B. Relationship to patient _____
C. Current living arrangements _____
   Alone _____   Domiciliary _____
   With family _____   Nursing home _____
   Foster homes _____   Boarding home _____
D. Service assistance
   _____ Dept. human resources   _____ Case worker
   _____ Home health care   _____ Other

IV. Social Economics Level
Vocation _____
Social Security _____   Social Sec. disability _____
Retirement/Pension _____   Other _____
Est. monthly income _____

Please check
<$12,000/year _____ $15,000-$25,000/year _____ $25,000-$35,000/year _____
$35,000-$50,000/year _____   >$50,000/year _____

DATA COLLECTION

Case Manager: _____
Specialty Nurse: _____
Open Adult: _____
Geriatrics: _____

V. Level of Cognition
Mini Mental Score _____

IV. Medication Compliance/Noncompliance
(Prehospitalization)
A. Taken as prescribed   Yes _____ No _____
B. Multiple medications prescribed (list) _____

C. List most bothersome side effects _____

VII. On admission was
A. Previous medical record available   Yes _____ No _____
B. Social history obtained   Yes _____ No _____
C. Previous therapies reviewed   Yes _____ No _____
   • Previous activities (list) _____

   • Assigned activities (list) _____

VIII. Functional Capacity
Beck Depression Inventory Scale   *Please indicate score*
   • Admit day _____
   • Day of Discharge _____
   • 3 months after discharge _____
   • 6 months after discharge _____

FIGURE **51-1** Depressive Neurosis Data Collection Measurement Tool developed by the DRG 426 outcome team.

IX. Inpatient Therapeutic Treatment Plan Compliance

A. Standard process (prevention) % activities attended

100%_____ 75%-100%_____ 50%-75%_____ <50%_____

B. Inpatient therapeutic treatment plan compliance

Reasons for nonattendance

Refused _____
Disruptive _____
Unavailable _____

C. Interrupted process (after intervention) % activities attended

100%_____ 75%-100%_____ 50%-75%_____ <50%_____

Interventions/strategies to increase attendance:

1.1 intervention_____   MD order_____
Other_____

X. Discharge Understanding Teaching/Screening

(able to verbalize)

A. Has a mangement of symptoms plan   Yes_____ No_____
B. Understands disease process   Yes_____ No_____
C. Has clear discharge goals   Yes_____ No_____

List:_____

D. Interventions and strategies planned to meet education deficit

List:_____

E. Were discharge criteria met?   Yes_____ No_____

XI. After Discharge—Did Patient Comply with

A. Prescribed office visits   Yes_____ No_____
B. Support group attendance   Yes_____ No_____

If no, indicate why:_____

XII. Prescribed Medication

A. Inpatient. List:_____

B. At discharge. List:_____

XIII. Acts of Self-harm

Use scale

1 0-3 months **3** >6 months
2 3-6 months **4** During hospital stay

A. Overdose _____
B. Self-inflicted wound _____
C. Ideation _____
D. Suicide/death _____

XIV. Inpatient Tracking

A. Estimated length of stay
B. Actual length of stay
C. Total cost per case
D. Variable cost per case
E. Variance from critical path
Please indicate all diagnostic testing/consultations

_____

XV. Other Treatment Used

A. Electroconvulsive therapy   Yes_____ No_____
#
B. Individual psychotherapy   Yes_____ No_____

FIGURE **51-1, cont'd**   Depressive Neurosis Data Collection Measurement Tool developed by the DRG 426 outcome team.

Box 51-1 ▶ SUMMARY OF DATA ANALYSIS

18.6% of study patients previously had been hospitalized with the same diagnosis twice within a
   6-month window.
27.3% of study patients had annual combined household incomes of $25,000 or less.
5.6% of study patients had annual combined household incomes of $12,000 or less.
9.4% of study patients were unable to convey an understanding of their disease process on discharge.
15.8% of study patients were unable to identify a management-of-symptoms plan on discharge.
22.4% of study patients were unable to identify clear discharge goals.
17% of study patients admitted to a self-harm act within the 6 months following hospitalization.
22.5% of study patients had not complied with their inpatient treatment plan.
37.9% of study patients self-reported noncompliance with medication administration.

Box 51-2 ▶ BECK DEPRESSION SCORES

COMBINED STUDY PATIENT SCORES (N = 70)
Admission score = 36
Discharge score = 23
3-month postdischarge score = 28
6-month postdischarge score = 22

DEPRESSION SEVERITY LEVELS
0-9 Minimal
10-14 Borderline
15-20 Mild to moderate
21-30 Moderate
31-40 Severe
41-63 Very severe

These three categories allowed the outcome team to capture the clinical picture and patient management needs of this defined patient population. Each category was then further analyzed, and the data indicated the following:

1. *Patient economics:* 32.2% of the study patients had combined household incomes of less than $25,000.
2. *Educational deficits:* 47.6% of the study patients had no clear discharge plans
3. *Medication compliance:* 37.9% of the study patients reported noncompliance with medication administration.

OUTCOMES EVALUATION

In November, 1995 the outcome team presented the final data analysis and outcome questions to the psychiatric quality assurance team and the Department of Psychiatric Services chairperson. All persons present at the meeting agreed that the data findings and literature review would support associations between medication compliance and patient education as predictors of patient outcomes. The outcome team also hypothesized that improving medication compliance and patient education among this population of patients would reduce readmission rates and increase treatment plan compliance.

To substantiate these hypotheses the outcome team was challenged to develop tools to address these two areas of patient outcome improvement. The tools developed were a Psychotropic Medication Cost Card (Fig. 51-2) and a Patient Education/Orientation Manual.

The Psychotropic Medication Cost Card indicates costs for 30-day outpatient prescriptions. Cost codes are provided for high and low dosing. The card includes generic availability for the listed medications and common adverse side effects, and it identifies outpatient mental health care centers' formulary codes to ensure medication availability as the patient moves from the inpatient setting to the outpatient setting. The card does not include every medication available for each category, but most of the medications prescribed within the Department of Psychiatric Services.

During inpatient management, study patients revealed that noncompliance with outpatient medication has a variety of causes, including inability to tolerate adverse side effects of certain medications and insufficient funds to buy some prescriptions. The Psychotropic Medication Cost Card could serve as a reference card for the psychiatrist prescribing medications. The admitting psychiatrist can discover the patient's financial status on admission by reviewing the financial statement provided by the financial planning liaison. The psychiatrist could take this financial information into consideration when prescribing medication as well as the availability of the medication at the patient's outpatient mental health care center and his or her tolerance for side effects.

Development of the Patient Education/Orientation Manual was based on the identified need to improve inpatient treatment plan compliance and to address deficits identified in discharge planning. The Patient Education/Orientation Manual would serve as a patient guide throughout the patient's hospitalization and after discharge. The patient would record his or her experiences within the therapeutic milieu daily. The staff, along with the patient, would use this tool as a teaching and learning guide.

The Patient Education/Orientation Manual is divided into several clinical sections. Each section focuses on the patient's individual treatment plan. Therapeutic activities and program group descriptions are defined, and short- and long-term patient goals are identified. Each section clearly defines the patient's treatment plan, diagnosis, and medication management and treatment objectives. On discharge the manual is reviewed with the patient, with emphasis placed on discharge goals, inpatient therapeutic educational deficits, outpatient management, support mechanisms, and follow-up medical appointments. The Patient Education/Orientation Manual helps the care provider ensure that after discharge the patient has a management of symptom plan, a follow-up appointment, a clear understanding of the need to take the medication as prescribed, and the means to purchase the medication.

Implementing the first step of the DRG 426 study and reviewing the final data analysis made it clear that a major contribution to the delivery of care can be made by addressing the economic ability of patients to pay for medications at the beginning of hospitalization and by identifying educational deficits related to symptom management during and after hospitalization. Nurse case management played an important role in achieving the project's desired outcome of identifying areas on which to focus to improve medication compliance and quality in discharge planning.

FUTURE STUDY

The next step for the outcome team is to undertake a more detailed study of the clinical outcome benefits of the Psychotropic Medication Cost Card and the Patient Education/Orientation Manual. The information gained will enable the outcome team to develop optimal outcome management strategies to predict which patients are most at risk for noncompliance with medication administration and poor

ANTIDEPRESSANTS

Drug	Cost
Wellbutrin (bupropion HCl)	$$-$$$
Prozac (fluoxetine)	$$$-$$$$
Paxil (paroxetine)*	$$$-$$$$
Zoloft (sertraline)*	$$$-$$$$
Luvox (fluvoxamine)	$$$-$$$$
Serzone (nefazodone HCl)	$$-$$$
Elavil (amitriptyline HCl)*	$
Anafranil (clomipramine)*	$-$$$$
Sinequan, Adapin (doxepin HCl)*	$
Tofranil (imipramine)*	$
Surmontil (trimipramine)	$$-$$$
Asendin (amoxapine)	$$
Norpramin (desipramine)*	$$-$$$$
Aventyl HCl, Pamelor (nortriptyline)*	$
Vivactil (protriptyline)	$$-$$$$
Effexor (venlafaxine)	$$-$$$
Ludiomil (maprotiline HCl)	$$$-$$$$
Desyrel (trazodone)	$$$
Nardil (phenelzine)	$$-$$$
Parnate (tranylcypromine)	

ANTICONVULSANTS

Drug	Cost
Tegretol (carbamazepine)	$$
Depakene (valproic acid)	$

ANTIANXIETY AGENTS

Equanil (meprobamate)	$
Xanax (alprazolam)*	$$-$$$$
Librium (chlordiazepoxide)*	$-$$$$
Tranxene (clorazepate)*	$$$$
Valium (diazepam)*	$$$$
Paxipam (halazepam)	$-$$$
Ativan (lorazepam)*	$$-$$$$
Serax (oxazepam)*	$
Klonopin (clonazepam)	$$-$$$$
BuSpar (buspirone HCl)	$$-$$$
Atarax (hydroxyzine HCl)	$$-$$
Vistaril (hydroxyzine pamoate)*	$-$$
Sinequan, Adapin (doxepin HCl)	$
Trancopal (chlormezanone)	$-$$

SEDATIVES/HYPNOTICS

Drug	Cost
Ambien (zolpidem tartrate)	
Noctec (chloral hydrate)	
Placidyl (ethchlorvynol)	
Dalmane (flurazepam HCl)	
Restoril (temazepam)*	
Halcion (triazolam)*	
Doral (quazepam)	
Phenobarbital	
Nembutal sodium (pentobarbital sodium)	

ANTIPSYCHOTICS

Haldol (haloperidol)*	$
Moban (molindone HCl)	$$-$$$$
Loxitane (loxapine)	$$-$$$$
Clozaril (clozapine)	$$$$
Risperdal (risperidone)	$$$$
Orap (pimozide)	$-$$$
Thorazine (chlorpromazine HCl)*	$$-$$$$
Sparine (promazine HCl)	$
Mellaril (thioridazine HCl)*	$$-$$$$
Serentil (mesoridazine)	$$-$$$
Trilafon (perphenazine)	$$-$$
Prolixin (fluphenazine HCl)	$-$$
Stelazine (trifluoperazine HCl)	$
Navane (thiothixene)*	$
Eskalith (lithium carbonate)*	$-$$
Lithobid (lithium carbonate)	

PSYCHOTHERAPEUTIC AGENTS

Etrafon, Triavil (perphenazine and amitriptyline HCl)	$
Hydergine (ergoloid mesylates)	$-$$
Ritalin (methylphenidate HCl)	$$-$$$
Cognex (tacrine HCl)	$$$
Deprol (meprobamate and benactyzine HCl)	
Limbitrol DS 10-25 (chlordiazepoxide and amitriptyline)	$$$-$$$$

*A good, effective medication recommended for treatment of specific disorders.
Bold Print: Generic drug availability

FIGURE **51-2**   Psychotropic Medication Cost Card developed by the DRG 426 outcome team.

COST CODE   The Cost Code provides approximate cost information for a 30-day prescription. Pharmacy prices will vary.

$ <$ 25.00 $$ <$ 50.00
$$$ <$ 100.00 $$$$ >$ 100.00
$-$$$$ The drug is inexpensive at low doses but becomes expensive with higher doses.

MEDICATION INFORMATION

1. Selective serotonin reuptake inhibitors (SSRIs) are emerging as the preferred first-line option for panic disorder. Of these agents, when a patient requires 50 mg/d, sertraline 100 mg tab (½ tab/d) will be less expensive. Otherwise, Paxil may be less expensive.

2. Imipramine and clomipramine are useful in panic disorders. Imipramine is inexpensive, and clomipramine becomes costly at higher doses.

3. The recommended steady-state serum lithium levels are 0.8-1.0 mmol/L during acute mania, and 0.5-0.8 mmol/L for prophylaxis. Lithium is excreted renally. Risk factors, e.g., reduced sodium intake, dehydration; signs of lithium toxicity, e.g., slurred speech, unsteady gait, coarse tremor.

4. Antipsychotics control manic symptoms; side effects (e.g., extrapyramidal, anticholinergic, antiadrenergic, neuroleptic malignant syndrome) may not be well tolerated.

5. Recommend triazolam (Halcion) for short-term insomnia. Zolpidem (Ambien) costs 4 to 5 times more than triazolam and should be reserved until patient has failed treatment with a benzodiazepine for 10 to 14 nights in a 14-day period.

6. Clomipramine (Anafranil), fluvoxamine (Luvox), paroxetine (Paxil), and fluoxetine (Prozac) are FDA approved for treatment of obsessive-compulsive disorder. Presently, clomipramine (Anafranil) is the least expensive, then paroxetine (Paxil).

7. **Common side effects:** Benzodiazepines, sedation; tricyclic antidepressants, anticholinergic effects, orthostatic hypotension, sedation, sexual dysfunction, weight gain; SSRIs, nausea, headache, nervousness, insomnia, sexual dysfunction; MAO inhibitors, food and drug interactions; lithium, nausea, fatigue, tremor, thirst, edema, weight gain; chlorpromazine, sedation, postural hypotension, weight gain, anticholinergic and occasional extrapyramidal effects; antipsychotic drugs, extrapyramidal effects.

8. Antidepressants require several weeks to achieve maximum therapeutic benefit.

9. Clozaril may be effective in schizophrenic patients resistant to other antipsychotics. Check with manufacturer for assistance with expense for this drug.

FIGURE **51-2, cont'd**   Psychotropic Medication Cost Card developed by the DRG 426 outcome team.

outpatient symptom management leading to readmissions. It is anticipated that the DRG 426 Depressive Neurosis Study will continue collecting further data for the next 6 months. Further study is necessary to investigate the refinements made in the delivery of care to these patient types.

The DRG 426 Depressive Neurosis Study was the first attempt at improving quality in the areas of medication compliance and discharge planning ever undertaken at the Department of Psychiatry, Brookwood Medical Center. This outcome study was the first progressive initiative to combat the traditional questions and answers with user responses that would produce true patient outcomes. Through this experience the outcome team learned the value of a focused study and how that can uncover areas of intervention never before realized. Finally, by understanding the continuum of care involved in a chronic illness, steps were taken to positively affect that entire continuum.

Reference

Beck, A.T., & Beamesderfer, A. (1974). Assessment of depression: The depression inventory. *Psychological Measurements in Psychopharmacology, 7,* 151-169.

Outcomes Effectiveness and Evidence-Based Practice

Colleen J. Goode

CHAPTER OVERVIEW

Evidence-based practice is conceptually defined as the use of current best evidence when making patient care decisions. When patient care interventions are based on the best evidence available, optimal outcomes are more likely to occur. Effectiveness is the degree to which the desired outcomes are achieved. Heater, Becker, and Olson's (1988) meta-analysis demonstrated that evidence-based practice produced more effective outcomes. The purpose of this chapter is to help case managers understand evidence-based practice, its influence on outcomes, and their role in practicing from an evidence-based practice framework.

EVIDENCE-BASED DECISION MAKING

Gray (1997) believes decisions about groups of patients or patient populations are made by combining evidence, values, and resources. These three factors also influence individual patient care decisions made by case managers. Evidence related to a specific intervention's effectiveness or management of a disease should drive the clinician's decision-making process, but sometimes the values of either the health care provider or the patient drive it, sometimes the availability of resources (i.e., money, staff, and equipment) is the motivating factor, and often a combination of all three factors influences decision making.

Case managers provide evidence-based care because quality is enhanced and outcomes are improved. Payers and policymakers have become interested in evidence-based clinical practice because of a desire to identify health care costs that do not result in benefit to the patient, thereby freeing resources for other uses. Case managers provide care from a quality perspective, linking practice to outcome. Evidence-based practice reduces variation in practice patterns. Tanner (1998) defines the aim of evidence-based practice as reducing wide variations in individual clinician practices, eliminating worst practices, and enhancing best practices, thereby improving quality and reducing costs. Case managers, payers, and policymakers must ensure that the best value is obtained from the resources available. A number of surveys have demonstrated that clinical decisions are often not based on the best evidence

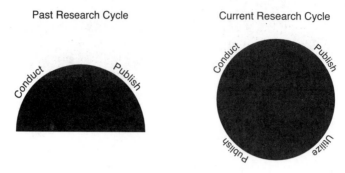

FIGURE **52-1**   Research cycle.

(Brett, 1987; Coyle & Sokop, 1990; Gibbs, Mead, Hager, & Sweet, 1994; Institute of Medicine, 1992). The current managed care climate emphasizes cost reduction but also demands positive patient outcomes. Evidence-based practice is an important vehicle for achieving these goals.

THE RESEARCH CYCLE

The evolution to a scientific basis for nursing practice has been slow. Figure 52-1 demonstrates the research cycle that was part of this evolution. In the early years the focus was on conducting and publishing research. Most of the research was done by those in academia, and it was often focused on studies related to nursing students, administration, or education, with few clinically focused studies. Today nursing research is very clinically focused and the cycle has expanded to include utilization of findings and publishing of outcomes when findings are used in practice.

The body of knowledge needed to conduct research differs from that needed for utilization of research. For example, utilization of a new research-based intervention on a busy medical surgical unit requires knowledge related to how to educate the providers about the change and convince them that there is value in changing their practice. Gathering support for the practice change, sustaining the change, and evaluating the effect of the change on patient outcomes are also parts of the utilization process. Changing behavior is complex, involves many systems, and usually cannot be achieved solely by education (Thomson, 1998). This process requires skills and knowledge that are not traditionally included in research courses that focus on conducting research.

EVIDENCE-BASED PRACTICE MODEL

Health care providers have evolved beyond research utilization to include other forms of evidence as a basis for practice. Figure 52-2 depicts a Multidisciplinary Evidence-Based Practice Model. Evidence is obtained through the synthesis of knowledge obtained from research; retrospective or concurrent chart review; quality improvement and risk data; international, national and local standards; infection control data; pathophysiology; cost-effectiveness analysis; benchmarking data; patient preferences; and clinical expertise. The process of evidence-based practice involves critically analyzing the evidence, selecting appropriate evidence-based interventions, implementing them, and evaluating outcomes.

Exploration of the evidence begins in the center or core of the model. Case managers should use **current and valid research** as the basis for clinical decision making whenever there is an adequate re-

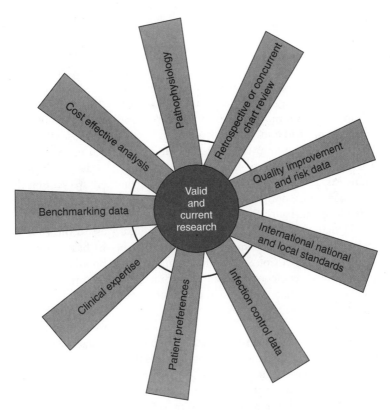

FIGURE **52-2**   Evidence-Based Multidisciplinary Practice Model.
(Courtesy University of Colorado Hospital, Denver, Colorado.)

search base available to guide practice. Evaluating clinical studies to determine if they are valid involves critically appraising both the merits and the limitations of the studies. All types of research should be evaluated for their contributions to the evidence. Results from experimental, nonexperimental, and qualitative studies may be synthesized to form the research base. No one would want to begin a drug regimen that had not been determined to be safe and effective in a randomized controlled trial. However, if we only use randomized controlled trials as the basis for our practice we are missing important evidence. For example, descriptive research that focuses on the stresses and problems of caregivers of patients with Alzheimer's disease provides evidence that can be used to improve care to this vulnerable patient population. In addition, analysis of the cost-effectiveness of care models designed to meet the needs of the Alzheimer's patient and their family can guide public policy related to this problem.

Research skills and knowledge of statistics are required to evaluate and interpret a study. In general, there are four major sections of a research report: introduction, methods, results, and discussion. A set of questions can be used in the critique of each section to help the reader determine the value and significance of the study. The reviewer must look for the most current research so the latest evidence is included in the review. Haller, Reynolds, and Horsley's (1979) criteria for selecting studies to be used in the research base include using studies that are scientifically sound, replicated, and cause no harm to patients. Changes in practice should not be based solely on one study with one small sample.

THE NINE EVIDENCE SOURCES

The nine sources of evidence attached to the research core can supplement evidence obtained from research. When research is not available, these provide the best available evidence.

Pathophysiology is a frequent source of evidence used by the case manager. The science of the function of cells, tissues, and organs and how these functions are altered by disease is evidence that helps the case manager plan for the appropriate level of care for the patient. For example, understanding the type of stroke the patient has had and what portion of the brain is affected will help the case manager understand the type of services and level of care the patient will need to aid in recovery.

Cost-effectiveness analysis aids the case manager in determining whether the benefit is sufficient relative to the risks and costs. Effectiveness alone does not imply that an intervention should be adopted. The neonatal case manager may decide it is more cost effective to send a newborn home on an apnea monitor and have the hospital absorb the cost of monitor rental than it is to keep the baby in the hospital for an extended length of stay. The case manager must clearly assess the skills and abilities of the parents and the risk to the infant in making this decision. Having the baby in the home environment rather than the sterile environment of the hospital might enhance bonding and improve outcomes.

Benchmarking data provide evidence related to best practices. Some institutions have better quality and cost outcomes than others for certain patient populations. For example, hospitals that belong to the University Health System Consortium, an organization located in Chicago, share clinical data and costs. The case manager learns that hospital X's pulmonary unit has a shorter length of stay, lower costs, and fewer complications for patients with chronic obstructive pulmonary disease (COPD) than similar facilities caring for patients with the same diagnosis. These data are adjusted for severity and regional variation in costs. By studying the evidence from the "best practice" hospital, the case manager can determine what must be changed to improve outcomes in his or her practice setting.

Clinical expertise involves clinical judgment based on reflection and knowledge of the patient and is an important source of evidence. Whether an intervention can be applied to a specific patient cannot always be deduced from the evidence. There may be biological, social, or other differences that influence the effect of an intervention. Clinicians move from a status of novice to expert as they acquire proficiency and judgment through clinical experience. Clinical expertise must be integrated with other sources of evidence.

Infection control data provide evidence related to the incidence of infections, the organisms involved, and methods to prevent transmission. As case managers work with patients in their homes, they need this evidence to prevent spread of the infection to other family members. Case managers who work with patients who are human immunodeficiency virus (HIV) positive rely heavily on evidence provided by infection control to plan appropriate care and provide needed education to prevent transmission.

International, national, and local standards of care often provide evidence that guides practice. The oncology case manager will draw on the standards from the Oncology Nursing Society when working with a patient who is receiving chemotherapy. Another example is using the Centers for Disease Control and Prevention (CDC) standards when planning for intravenous (IV) therapy in the home. Standards from the American Association of Critical Care Nurses will provide evidence related to appropriate care of arterial lines. The trauma case manager is guided by local community standards that determine where trauma patients will be cared for and the level of care that patients can expect to receive.

Quality improvement and risk data provide evidence to the case manager that can be used to support implementation of protocols to address problems. For example, if risk data indicate an increase in fall injuries in the neurosurgery population, the case manager can act on this evidence by providing instruction to caregivers and family members related to interventions to prevent falls. If quality data show an increased incidence of skin breakdown in the Intensive Care Unit (ICU), the ICU case manager can use this evidence to support implementation of a new protocol to reduce skin breakdown.

Retrospective or concurrent chart review provides a wealth of evidence such as patient allergies or changes in vital signs. The record provides the case manager with a rich history telling how the patient responded to a specific medication, procedure, or treatment in the past. Evidence related to response to current interventions and diagnostic testing influences decision making. The patient record also provides the payer source, and this information can drive decision making. In today's market, it is essential that the case manager seek this piece of evidence when doing discharge planning. Often the patient's health plan will dictate where the patient may receive skilled care, the home care agency that may provide care, and the approved pharmacy where the patient must obtain prescriptions. If the patient is sent to an agency not covered in the health plan, he or she may pay large out-of-pocket expenses.

Patient preferences, such as religious or cultural preferences or treatment preferences, and other patient information such as living wills and advance directives are an essential source of evidence. Case managers must respect the preferences of the patient and family and provide ample opportunity for the patient to have input into the decision making process. The patient is no longer a passive participant allowing the clinical provider to make all of the decisions. In contrast, many patients are quite vocal about their desire to participate in decisions affecting their health. This is a positive change, but one that some providers may have trouble accepting. Patient preferences contribute significantly to evidence-based practice.

These are just some examples of how the nine sources of evidence can contribute to decision making. Finding the best evidence, critically appraising it, integrating it with the case manager's clinical expertise and the patient's unique preferences, and applying the results to practice is what evidence-based case management is all about.

PROVIDING EVIDENCE FOR PATIENTS AND FAMILIES

Nurse case managers must communicate evidence-based information to patients and their families so they can make informed decisions about their plan of care. Whenever there is a research base for an intervention, it is helpful to share that information with the patient and family. For example, the case manager must share research evidence related to the effectiveness of combined medications in the treatment of HIV. The neonatal case manager should encourage parents of a low birth weight infant to participate in kangaroo care and should share with the parents the research related to this intervention. Obviously, clinicians must present information in a form that can be understood by the patient. Recipients of care are becoming very informed about health and illness and are asking thoughtful questions. It is possible that those who use the Internet to seek health information may be well informed about the current best evidence.

Case managers should provide information to support patients' participation in choosing treatments and strategies to manage their health. The information must be in concert with available evidence and be presented in a form that is understandable and useful if patients are to be active participants in decisions about their care. Educational pamphlets should be used to supplement and reinforce information provided by the case manager, but the information must conform to the highest standards of scientific accuracy. In most handouts, benefits of interventions are emphasized and risks and side effects often glossed over. The growth and wider availability of the Internet will greatly increase access to health information. It is quite possible that the patient will bring to the attention of the case manager the most current evidence related to a health problem. Accurate evidence-based information has the potential to enhance the quality and appropriateness of health care.

Evidence-Based Clinical Pathways

Case managers have a significant role to play in the development of clinical pathways. They often co-chair the multidisciplinary team with the physician in the development, implementation, and evaluation of the clinical pathway. Pathways that are evidence based are highly valued because their efficacy is greater. A caesarian section pathway contained an intervention to remove the Foley catheter within the first 24 hours postoperatively (Goode, 1995a; Goode & Blegen, 1993). This decision was based on research indicating that leaving the catheter in longer than 24 hours increased the chance of urinary tract infections. In addition, the pathway contained the appropriate antibiotic and dosage for prophylactic treatment of women who had premature rupture of the membranes. This decision was again based on current research. The evidence-based multidisciplinary model described earlier should be used when developing the pathway. The team should seek evidence from research and from all nine evidence sources as they construct the clinical pathway.

Evidence Related to Organizational Features

Organizational contextual variables (nonclinical variables) interact with specific treatments to influence patient care outcomes. We know more about the effectiveness of specific treatments than we do about the effectiveness of the health care system. Aiken, Sochalski, and Lake (1997) have demonstrated that nurse autonomy, nurse accountability, and registered nurse (RN)/physician relations affect patient care outcomes. Blegen, Goode, and Reed (1998) demonstrated that RN skill mix affects outcomes related to adverse occurrences. Attention must be paid to the context in which patients receive their care because this knowledge will help to improve quality and patient outcomes (Aiken et al., 1997). Drawing on this research, it would seem that better outcomes might be achieved by case managers who work collaboratively with physicians, are autonomous, and are accountable for their actions.

When case managers work in an organization where evidence-based practice is valued, they are more likely to base their practice on the current best evidence. The literature indicates that organizational factors explain 80% to 90% of the variance in research utilization, environmental factors account for 5% to 10% of the variance, and individual characteristics contribute only 1 to 3% (Thomson, 1998). It appears that unless nurses work where evidence-based practice is an expectation, the likelihood of nurses using research is minimal. The organizational characteristics associated with evidence-based practice include administrative support; education related to evidence-based practice, including expectations for evidence-based practice in job descriptions and performance evaluations; rewarding and recognizing staff who use research in their practice; linking these activities to quality improvement; and providing time and resources for staff to participate in evidence-based projects. Case managers, when functioning at an advanced practice level, must be leaders in the evidence-based practice movement (Stetler et al., 1998).

Measuring Outcomes From Evidence-Based Practice

The outcomes from evidence-based practice are determined by the strength of the evidence and by the management and delivery of the interventions. If the interventions are not carried out as intended, the expected outcomes may not occur. The research and other supporting evidence may indicate the intervention is extremely effective, but if the intervention is not carried out appropriately, the positive outcomes may not occur. We see this sometimes in interventions related to pain management. An evidence-based pain management protocol may not be effective because providers are not assessing pain appropriately and intervening in a timely manner, or there may be resistance from providers, or system issues, that make it difficult to implement the evidence-based pain management intervention.

Gray (1997) indicates that an intervention designed to prevent mortality was initially expressed only in terms of the number of extra years of life. Evidence later indicated that quality of life was also important, which lead to a formula for "quality-adjusted life-years." Case managers should support the collection of patient satisfaction data, quality of life data, and specific clinical outcome data for the patients they manage. Case managers can evaluate outcomes related to the appropriateness of moving the patient to the next level of care by measuring the rate of returns to a higher level of care. A tracking system should be in place to record the case manager interventions implemented to allow a patient to return home in a timely manner.

When an evidence-based practice change is made, it is essential that a plan is in place to evaluate the expected outcomes (Goode, 1995b). It is important to gather baseline data related to current practice. Sometimes these data come from quality improvement monitoring. The outcome variables to be measured are determined from the original research base. Horsley and Crane (1983) recommend that at least two dependent variables from the original research base be included as a measure of effectiveness. For example, when implementing an evidence-based guideline for the treatment of asthma, it would be important to gather data about current practice such as what drugs and treatments are currently being ordered. After the guideline is implemented, it would be important to measure whether the new guideline was used by the providers and whether it was effective in treating the asthma.

SUMMARY

Case managers must learn about evidence-based practice, embrace it, and help to create a culture where there is an expectation that care will be based on the best available evidence. Patient care should be based on evidence and not on tradition, opinion, or custom. Evidence-based care encourages a questioning and reflective approach to clinical practice and emphasizes the importance of life-long learning. Incorporating the current best evidence into the case manager's decision making will increase the proportion of patients to whom current best care is offered.

References

Aiken, L.H., Sochalski, J., & Lake, T.L. (1997). Studying outcomes of organizational change in health services, *Medical Care, 35*(11), NS6-NS18 Supplement.

Blegen, M.A., Goode, C.J., & Reed, L. (1998). Nurse staffing and patient outcomes, *Nursing Research, 47*(1), 43-50.

Brett, J.L. (1987). Use of nursing practice research findings. *Nursing Research, 36*(6), 344-349.

Coyle, L.A., & Sokop, A.G. (1990). Innovation adoption behavior among nurses. *Nursing Research, 39*(3), 176-180.

Gibbs, R.S., Mead, P.B., Hager, W.D., & Sweet, R.L. (1994). A survey of practices in infectious diseases by obstetrician-gynecologists. *Obstetrics & Gynecology, 83*(4), 631-636.

Goode, C.J. (1995a). Impact of a CareMap™ and case management on patient satisfaction and staff satisfaction, collaboration, and autonomy. *Nursing Economics, 13*(6), 337-348, 361.

Goode, C.J. (1995b). Evaluation of research-based nursing practice. In M.G. Titler & C.J. Goode (Eds), *Nursing clinics of North America.* Philadelphia: W.B. Saunders.

Goode, C.J., & Blegen, M.A. (1993). Developing a CareMap(for patients with a cesarean birth: A multidisciplinary process. *The Journal of Perinatal Neonatal Nursing, 7*(2), 40-49.

Gray, J.A.M. (1997). *Evidence-based healthcare.* New York: Churchill Livingstone.

Haller, K.B., Reynolds, M.A., & Horsley, J.A. (1979). Developing research based innovation protocols: Process, criteria and issues. *Research in Nursing and Health, 2,* 45-51.

Heater, B.S., Becker, A., & Olson, M. (1988). Nursing interventions and patient outcomes: A meta-analysis of studies. *Nursing Research, 37*(5), 303-307.

Horsley, J.A., & Crane, J. (1983). *Using research to improve nursing practice: A guide.* New York: Grune & Stratton.

Institute of Medicine (1992). *Guidelines for clinical practice: from development to use.* Washington, DC: National Academy Press.

Stetler, C.B., Brunell, M., Giuliano, K.K., Morsi, D., Prince, L., & Newell-Stokes, V. (1998). Evidence-based practice and the role of nursing leadership. *JONA, 28*(7/8), 45-53.

Tanner, C.A. (1998, May). *Clinical judgement and evidence-based practice.* Paper presented at the Western Institute of Nursing, Communicating Nursing Research Conference and WIN Assembly, Phoenix, Ariz.

Thomson, M.A. (1998, Jan.). Closing the gap between nursing research and practice. *Evidence-Based Nursing 1*(1), 7-8.

The Carondelet Community-Based Nurse Case Management Program

*Yesterday, Today, and Tomorrow**

Gerri S. Lamb, Donna Zazworsky

CHAPTER OVERVIEW

For more than a decade, the Carondelet Nurse Case Management program has been a model for leadership and innovation in nursing practice. This nationally recognized program anticipated and evolved with major trends in managed care, disease management, and outcome-based performance evaluation. In this final chapter, two of Carondelet's well-known leaders chronicle and celebrate the history of case management at Carondelet and highlight its lessons for the future.

Carondelet's nurse case management program has a well-deserved reputation for innovation and commitment to excellence in professional nursing and patient care. Many of the case management programs that have been recognized recently as best practices contain features that have characterized Carondelet's model for over a decade (Boult, Kane, Pacala, & Wagner, 1999). Carondelet's model is best known for patient-centered care across the continuum. Within this model, at-risk patients and their families have direct access to highly skilled professional nurses who provide education and support and assist them to manage their health needs across multiple settings.

Over the course of approximately 15 years, Carondelet's case management program took shape and became a leading example of "the beyond-the-walls" model of care coordination for numerous at-risk populations. It evolved through and took advantage of significant changes in the Tucson marketplace. The rapid growth of managed care in the late 1980s set the stage for the first nursing health maintenance organization (HMO) and the development of one of four national Community Nursing Organizations. Carondelet's case managers were among the first nurses to experiment with capitated financing for high-risk case management services. Ten years later, dramatic shifts in financing

*Acknowledgement: This chapter was written and the story updated with respect, humility, and love. The case managers of Carondelet are an extraordinary group of nurses. We believe that the story of Carondelet's nurse case managers belongs to each one of the nurses who contributed to the creation of a dynamic and ever-evolving professional practice model. This is our version of the story, what we have learned, and our vision and hope for the future.

arrangements between health plans and providers established new priorities and directions for case managers.

The evolution of case management at Carondelet illuminates a fascinating interplay between vision and financial reality. It offers an extraordinary case study in the stages of development of new practice models from innovation to consolidation to a struggle for survival. The story is rich with numerous nurses who were and continue to be passionate about the potential for nurses to improve health care for vulnerable populations.

The purpose of this chapter is to trace the history of case management at Carondelet and to share our interpretation of the implications of its evolution for the future of nurse case management practice.

THE STORY UNFOLDS

The story of Carondelet's case management program is best understood in the context of the history of professional nursing at Carondelet and the growth of what ultimately became a turbulent and unpredictable managed care environment. In the early years, prospective payment and managed care were the backdrop for the emergence of a new community-based case management model. In the later years, managed care moved to center stage and played a pivotal role in shaping case management practice and payment for it. The interplay between Carondelet's case management model and health care reimbursement and reform is shown in Figure 53-1.

The foundation of the Carondelet model has been and remains professional nursing practice and the nurse-patient relationship (Hey, 1993). The model is firmly grounded in an understanding and respect for the patient's and family's right to identify their own health care needs and priorities. The nurse case manager's role is that of facilitator, advocate and coach. One of Carondelet's most significant contributions to the evolution of nurse case management has been the exploration and description of the process of how a nurse case manager assists at-risk individuals to build self-care skills and negotiate the health care system. Carondelet nurse case managers have been in the forefront of developing systems of care that foreshadowed and ultimately transitioned into current models of population-based care and health and disease management.

The changing health care scene in Tucson, Arizona offered an incredible opportunity to experiment with practice elements that subsequently became core to successful care coordination systems. In the course of 15 years, the case management program expanded to include automated risk assessment and chronic illness management. It was linked to health promotion and risk reduction services for less at-risk populations. Practice guidelines were integrated and outcomes measured. What began as a pilot program to empower hospital-based nurses to work with vulnerable patients across the care continuum evolved into a cutting-edge delivery system for healthy and at-risk populations.

THE EARLY YEARS

The story begins with the introduction of the new prospective payment system for Medicare and the vision of one nurse. Not long after diagnostic related groups (DRGs) and prospective payment were initiated, policy people and health care administrators noted the decline in hospital length of stay accompanied by higher readmission rates, particularly for debilitating chronic illnesses like heart failure and obstructive pulmonary disease.

Phyllis Ethridge, who was Vice President for Patient Care Services at Carondelet, saw this scenario as an opportunity for innovation and change. Her initial plan was to prepare hospital-based nurses to

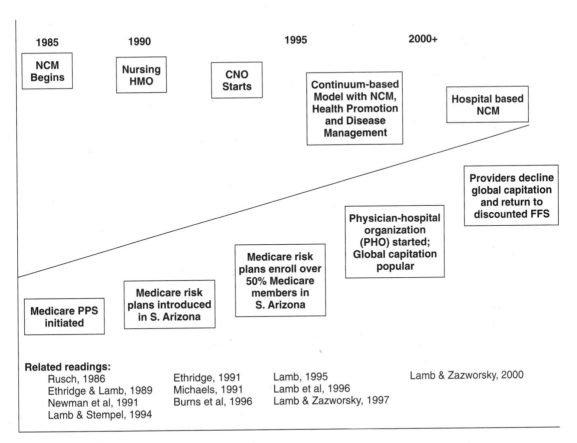

FIGURE **53-1**   Landmarks in Carondelet Nurse Case Management (NCM) and Health Care Reimbursement and Reform.

transition home with patients requiring skilled nursing care. Selected nurses from each hospital unit were educated about home care practices and documentation. With the support and mentoring of home health nurses led by Susan Rusch, Carondelet's Home Health Director, these nurses began to work with patients from hospital to home (Rusch, 1986).

The patients and families loved having the same nurse during their hospital stay and their transition to home. The nurses who participated in this experiment reported vast new insights into the challenges patients and their families face in managing their health care needs after hospitalization. Unfortunately, the nurses did not grasp the nuances of home health documentation quickly enough to avoid significant numbers of Medicare denials for home health services. After several months of learning and refining, Ethridge and colleagues decided to build on the strengths of a professional nursing care delivery model for transitional care that they had discovered and, at the same time, distinguish this model from traditional home health care. Thus from the lessons of a brief experiment in hospital-based home health emerged the seeds of Carondelet's nurse case management program.

Armed with the knowledge that patients and nurses valued transitional care from hospital to home, Ethridge decided to try an experiment. Two unit-based nurses were asked to observe admission and re-admission patterns on their units, to identify patients they felt would benefit from better continuity of care, and to work with them across settings. Salaries for these nurses came from the unit budget, and expenses were attributed to a pilot project to improve quality of care and reduce length of stay. The nurses were given little structure or guidelines—only the encouragement to use the nursing process and exercise their professional judgment. The two nurses became the core of a new nurse case management practice. In retrospect, it is interesting to note that the model emerged from a population-based practice focused on two high-risk patient groups.

By the beginning of 1989, the nurse case manager group had grown from two to 10 nurses, some of whom were unit-based specializing in selected populations, including patients with orthopedic, pulmonary, oncology, cardiac, and behavioral health conditions. Other case managers were generalists, including one nurse who focused on high-risk Native American patients. During these early years, there were few regulatory demands or payment constraints on case management practice. The nurses were free to explore how their relationships evolved with patients, the effectiveness of various nursing interventions, and the impact of their work within a broader health care delivery perspective.

At the same time that the nurse case management practice was evolving, core elements of professional nursing systems were being developed and debated locally and nationally. The nurse case managers of Carondelet designed new systems of care coordination in a broader nursing environment that had previously been recognized as a magnet hospital and embraced shared governance and exempt salary status for all nurses. While the relationship between these has not been formally studied, it was clearly a fertile time for innovation and Carondelet nurses worked in an environment that resonated with professional development and pride.

As the first nurse case managers were encouraged to explore their practices with at-risk populations, efforts began to translate their experiences into outcome data and information. Two doctorally prepared nurses, Cathy Michaels and Gerri Lamb, were brought into the practice to assist with the evaluation. Initial discussions with the nurse case managers highlighted their passion for understanding their relationships with patients, the process of case management, as well as their insights into their impact on patient outcomes. Observations about the process of case management practice led to collaboration with Margaret Newman, a prominent nurse theorist, who discovered that Carondelet's nurse case management model embodied key concepts within her theory of health as expanding consciousness (Newman, Lamb, & Michaels, 1991). The nurse case managers' belief that "something different was going on" in their nursing care led to qualitative research from which the theory of nurse case manager as "insider-expert" emerged (Lamb & Stempel, 1994). This study stands as one of the few systematic qualitative explorations of the nurse case manager–patient relationship.

At the same time that the process of case management was being explored, members of the group practice made beginning attempts to demonstrate the link between case management interventions and patient outcomes. Initially, extensive descriptive data were compiled to look at common diagnoses of nurse case manager patients, visit frequencies, and visit patterns over time. Interviews with patients and nurses conducted as part of qualitative studies suggested several key outcomes for further evaluation, including quality of life, self-care abilities, symptom management, functional status, and service use outcomes of reduced hospitalization and emergency room visits.

Initial exploration of descriptive data led to important insights about potential differences in impact with acute and chronic conditions (Ethridge & Lamb, 1989). Many of the case managers pursued their hypotheses about their practice in their graduate work and subsequent theses (Chapman, 1990; Doerge, 1992; Huggins, 1996). An experimental study of the impact of case management on well-being, symptom management, personal power, satisfaction, and health service use for individuals with progressive multiple sclerosis reinforced the importance of the nurse-patient relationship in understanding the process-outcome connection (Lamb et al., 1993).

THE MANAGED CARE YEARS

Toward the end of the 1980s and into the beginning of the 1990s, managed care plans entered the local market and grew rapidly. The first Medicare risk plan in southern Arizona attracted thousands of members, and soon several other plans followed. Within a short time, payment shifted from discounted fee-for-service to capitation as plans and providers experimented with various risk-sharing arrangements. Capitated payment seemed to be an ideal way to drive the development of more integrated delivery systems and generate financial profit.

For nursing, participation in managed care and new capitated arrangements was an exciting invitation to shaping new delivery systems, particularly for at-risk populations. As the local market moved rapidly through the stage of managed care from low to high penetration and from limited to global capitation, interest grew in effective strategies for managing high-cost populations as well as in health promotion, disease prevention, and more integration across settings.

Seeing the opportunities and the fit for nurse case management in this new environment, Phyllis Ethridge went to the first Medicare risk plan on the scene and offered them case management services. She proposed that Carondelet would provide case management and home health care within the same capitated package for approximately the same monthly capitation the plan paid for home health care alone. This venture would accomplish several goals. Most importantly, the agreement would launch case management as a reimbursed service within managed care (Ethridge, 1991). Within this pilot, Carondelet would identify the costs of nurse case management for subsequent contracting efforts and gain experience delivering services in a new venue. It also provided an opportunity for the nurse case managers to better differentiate and integrate their care with home health services.

Entry into capitated contracting was an eye-opening, invigorating, and occasionally overwhelming experience for the nurse case managers. Virtually overnight, the nurse case managers became responsible for identifying and coordinating services for at-risk members of a large and growing Medicare risk plan (Michaels, 1991). Risk assessment systems had to be put in place. New referral systems to communicate with primary care physicians and home health and community providers were needed. Meanwhile, the clock was ticking and every admission and readmission began to be examined as a potentially preventable event.

Carondelet's plunge into managed care capitalized on and consolidated many of the strengths of the case management program. Insights about how to identify at-risk individuals were translated into screening tools used by the case managers and nursing staff. In the world of managed care, it was essential to find at-risk people early and offer case management assistance in monitoring, symptom management, and coordination.

Initially, the nurse case managers found that they were more effective and efficient in identifying risk than other members of the health care team. Waiting for others to find vulnerable patients often resulted in missed opportunities and readmissions. The nurse case managers began to explore differences between patient and professional perceptions of risk (Nichols, 1996). The demands for patient and data tracking systems became evident. Hand-tallied readmission rates were common and a source of significant frustration. Smooth hand-offs to home health nurses required extensive dialogue about referral criteria and scope of practice and service. Carondelet's Nursing HMO was off and running! The stories behind the scenes told as much about hard work, perseverance, and commitment to a vision as they did to the exhilaration of playing at the contract table.

Evaluation of the Nursing HMO experience took many forms. There were the monthly data runs to evaluate admission and readmission rates. Managed care terms and indicators, such as bed days/1000 members, became very familiar. Judi Papenhausen worked extensively with the nurse case managers to measure and track their interventions (Papenhausen, 1996). In the most extensive quantitative analysis conducted to that point, Burns, Lamb, and Wholey (1996) compared hospitalization and service use in the Nursing HMO patients and a control group. Amassing and cleaning the required demographic, clinical, and financial data for this study required months of tedious work getting separate and distinct information systems to talk to each other. After rigorous methodological review, these findings were published in the journal *Inquiry* and represent one of the first efforts to evaluate the impact of integrated nursing care delivery systems.

THE COMMUNITY NURSING ORGANIZATION AND BEYOND

After years of waiting for the Community Nursing Organization legislation passed in 1987 to be implemented, Carondelet applied for and was selected to participated in the national Community Nursing Organization Medicare demonstration (CNO) in 1992. The goal of the CNO was to design, implement, and evaluate a nurse-managed model of community-based services for Medicare beneficiaries. Services included in the CNO were specified in the original legislation and included home health, outpatient therapies, durable medical equipment, and ambulance service. Case management was mentioned in the legislation as an optional service. Implemented as a randomized controlled experiment, the CNOs would be evaluated on the health status of their members as well as their functional status, satisfaction with health care services, service use, and Medicare costs.

At Carondelet the CNO was viewed as a wonderful vehicle to showcase and advance everything that had been learned about nurse case management within a fully capitated program. In addition, the CNO offered the opportunity to extend and link a primarily high-risk model with nursing delivery systems for low- and moderate-risk individuals. The CNO was required to enroll all eligible individuals, which included anyone who applied who had Medicare Part A and Part B and lived in the specified geographic areas. Members in the CNO range from older adults who are active and have few health problems to those who are extremely high risk with complex sets of acute and chronic conditions.

Carondelet's experience with case management formed the core of the CNO design. Carondelet and the other three CNO sites convinced the Health Care Financing Administration (HCFA), the sponsoring organization for the demonstration, that case management should be a mandatory rather than an optional feature of the CNO. HCFA used the experience of the CNO sites to establish initial rates for case management services.

The Carondelet CNO model incorporated and advanced case manager tools for risk assessment, documentation, and evaluation (Lamb, 1995). While Carondelet was the only site that differentiated case management practices for at-risk and low- or moderate-risk populations in the beginning of the demonstration, all four sites moved to some form of risk-adjusted practice model during the first few years.

The CNO currently is in its sixth year of operation after several extensions by HCFA and Congress. Nurse case managers in the CNO continue to provide their care and services to targeted high-risk populations. They work closely with the "nurse partners" for low- and moderate-risk members assisting them to identify cues for changes in risk status and transition patients when their health care needs intensify. The impact of the nurse case managers is of particular importance in the CNO, since their care is targeted to the highest risk and potentially most expensive members of the CNO population.

CASE MANAGEMENT, DISEASE MANAGEMENT, AND INTEGRATED CARE DELIVERY

As the CNO was growing, the health care scene in southern Arizona rapidly progressed from a Stage II to a Stage IV highly penetrated managed care market with hospitals and physicians taking on greater financial risk under capitation. In the mid to late 1990s, attention turned, along with significant financial incentives, to integrated delivery systems and managing care. Innovations from case management and the CNO were exported for use in managed care contracts. More systematic processes for risk assessment and disease management were developed and implemented.

Soon after the shift to global capitation, Carondelet called on the case management and community programs to design and implement a network-wide program to manage high-volume and high-cost populations across the continuum. The initial pilot study focused on congestive heart failure, the diagnosis associated with the greatest number of hospital admissions in the Carondelet system. Designed by an interdisciplinary team consisting of nurse case managers, home health nurses, social workers, and physicians, the heart failure project incorporated evidence-based guidelines for risk assessment and nurse case management interventions for symptom management, exercise, and nutrition (Lamb, Mahn, & Dahl, 1996). Results of the pilot showed significant improvement in health status, patient functional performance, and self-care performance, as well as a significant reduction in 30-day readmission rates.

The heart failure project led the way to a network-wide, continuum-based model for disease management. Rather than waiting for high-risk patients to be admitted or readmitted to the hospital, standardized risk assessment tools used in the CNO were used with all managed care members with high-risk diagnoses. A systematic approach for finding, triaging, and intervening with at-risk patients was developed and implemented (Lamb & Zazworsky, 2000). Once identified, these patients were tracked over time to assure timely access to services that would enable them to manage their health care needs in the least acute and costly setting.

The shift to global capitation provided the long-awaited incentive to integrate services across the continuum, particularly for the high-risk members of managed care plans. Finally, the time was ripe for one systematic approach to risk assessment and the implementation of interdisciplinary, continuum-based practice guidelines, reaching from the primary care offices into the hospitals, the skilled facilities, home health services, and the home. Case management figured prominently in all of the disease management guidelines, in new efforts at integrating information system support, and in referral tools used throughout the network. Along with the rest of the network, the nurse case managers experimented with new strategies to improve care for their patients and increase the efficiency and effectiveness of the evolving systems of care.

THE WIND CHANGES

Unlike the smooth-staged progression of managed care outlined in the literature, the market in southern Arizona progressed through Stage IV penetration and global capitation and went into meltdown. Plans continued to reduce provider rates beyond what was considered sustainable. In a matter of months, hospitals and physicians began refusing capitated contracts and demanded to return to discounted fee-for-service payment. Financial incentives for prevention, risk assessment, disease management, and service integration declined on the provider side and shifted almost immediately back to the plans. Once again, the plans assumed the majority of risk for managing the health needs of their enrolled populations.

The combination of capitation and the effects of the new Balanced Budget Act regulations took a severe toll on many of the health care organizations in southern Arizona. Profit margins, which had been diminishing, now plummeted. Carondelet, along with other hospitals, home health agencies, and skilled facilities, took stock, prioritized its core business, and went into a cost-cutting strategy designed to align priorities and resource use with current incentives. Case management, a centerpiece of disease management and integrated delivery systems under global capitation, now was needed to shift attention back into managing hospital stays under reduced fee-for-service and prospective payment.

In anticipation of the dramatic and rapid shift in incentives, administrators of Carondelet's community and hospital-based case management programs moved quickly to redesign the case management system. The new model incorporated risk assessment and population-based approach with emphasis on management of the hospital stay. The model built in the opportunity for case managers to transition from hospital to the community for particularly vulnerable and expensive populations, including high-risk mothers and infants. The intent in designing this new model was to shift case management skill sets to the emergent need as well as to maintain a strong "memory trace" of community-based management when sanity and money were restored.

The community case managers who applied for the newly redesigned hospital-based case manager positions were viewed as extraordinary models for professional practice and systems expertise. Not surprisingly, the community nurse case managers also were seen as highly desirable by the health plans that now held most of the risk for effective population-based care. Several of the case managers chose to continue their community practice on the plan side rather than to return to hospital-based practice.

Today, community nurse case managers continue to practice in the CNO at Carondelet and as members of a predominantly hospital-oriented model of case management. Several have left Carondelet and are spreading their knowledge and experience in new nursing roles.

THE LEGACY OF CARONDELET: YESTERDAY, TODAY, AND TOMORROW

For the past 15 years, Carondelet's nurse case management program has epitomized what we now consider the hallmarks of successful health care programs: leadership, professionalism, vision, flexibility, and innovation. In many cases the nurses of Carondelet anticipated and led the changes and, in some, worked furiously to keep vision and dream alive as health care plunged into the vast unknown.

It is important to highlight the features of Carondelet's nurse case management model that have stood fast for more than a decade, and still characterize the practice of Carondelet nurses who have remained at Carondelet and have now spread into the surrounding communities. These features are central to the vision of nurse case management as professional nursing practice.

Carondelet's model of nurse case management is first and foremost a model that demands, acknowledges, and celebrates nursing. While the nurse-patient relationship has evolved through face-to-face, group, and telephonic versions over the last 15 years, this relationship remains central to the work of case managers and is the core context in which quality and cost outcomes are achieved. Concepts of health as expanding consciousness and insider-expert are just as important today as when they were first explored at Carondelet. Interviews with patients and families today reveal the same themes that were heard 15 years ago. Patients of nurse case managers value their caring presence, their accessibility, their expert knowledge, and their commitment to making systems work better for highly vulnerable people.

While the essence of the nurse-patient relationship has not changed significantly, competencies and skills required for nurse case manager practice have evolved substantially. Group and telephonic case management require a new model of interpersonal negotiation and collaboration. Maintaining a strong relationship over time and settings via the whole new range of communication technologies is challenging. Demands for more systematic risk assessment have required transitioning from experiential and paper-based tools to automated standardized instruments. Practical experience and expertise in case management have been critical in assuring that these tools and other instruments used by case managers are relevant to their practice and will achieve the desired goals.

The Carondelet case managers anticipated the demand for outcome data. Over the course of 15 years, hundreds of reports, presentations, and publications attempted to capture the impact of community-based nursing practice on quality of care and cost outcomes. Even today, however, there has still not been sufficient advances in information technology support to bring together the requisite clinical and cost data in a timely way. While there are exciting and effective software available to support continuum-based case management, the majority of case managers practice in settings without them. Demonstrating the value of case management remains one of the most daunting and frustrating challenges. At Carondelet and for nurse case managers nationwide, the lack of "real-time" outcome data is the greatest threat to survival.

Carondelet's nurse case management program was among the first of the nursing programs to enter into risk contracts with managed care plans. Today, this is not as uncommon as it was 10 years ago. In several states, nursing programs hold Medicare, Medicaid, and commercial contracts. However, many of the same barriers to contracting continue to reduce opportunities to influence health care delivery, including financial payment systems that encourage fragmentation over integration, unaligned incentives across providers and settings, and contractors who understand finance much better than clinical practice.

Carondelet's story certainly would not be complete without a final emphasis on the close ties between nursing innovation and our national health care scene. What evolved at Carondelet was not coincidental. It was, in fact, a cataclysmic coming together of vision, opportunity, and a willingness to take risk. From Phyllis Ethridge's leap into managed care to the Community Nursing Organization to the crisis-precipitated redesign of Carondelet's care coordination system, at the center of it all is a fervent belief that nursing is integral to making our health care system better. Carondelet's story is a tribute to the drive to keep trying and the belief that our American health care system will be infinitely improved if nurses can get to the table and stay there.

References

Boult, C., Kane, R.L. Pacala, J.T., & Wagner, E. (1999). Innovative healthcare for chronically ill older persons: Results of a national survey. *The American Journal of Managed Care 5*(8), 1-11.

Burns, L.R., Lamb, G.S., & Wholey, D.R. (1996). Impact of integrated community nursing on hospital utilization and costs in a Medicare risk plan. *Inquiry 33*(1), 30-41.

Chapman, E. (1990). *Nurse case management and hospital length of stay.* Unpublished master's thesis, University of Arizona, Tucson, Ariz.

Doerge, J. (1992). *Cost effectiveness of nurse case management compared to an existing system of care.* Unpublished master's thesis, University of Arizona, Tucson, Ariz.

Ethridge, P. (1991). A nursing HMO: Carondelet St. Mary's experience. *Nursing Management 22*(7), 22-27.

Ethridge, P., & Lamb, G.S. (1989). Professional nursing case management improves quality, access and costs. *Nursing Management 20*(3), 30-35.

Hey, M. (1993). Nursing's Renaissance: An innovative continuum of care takes nurses back to their roots. *Health Progress, 74*(8), 26-32.

Huggins, D.B. (1996). *Nurse case management: Impact on costs and outcomes.* Unpublished master's thesis. University of Arizona, Tucson, Ariz.

Lamb, G.S. (1995). Early lessons from a capitated community-based nursing model. *Nursing Administration Quarterly 19,* 18-26.

Lamb, G.S., Donaldson, N., & Kellogg, J. (1998). *Case management: A guide to strategic evaluation.* St. Louis: Mosby.

Lamb, G.S., Mahn, V., & Dahl, R. (1996). Using data to design systems of care for adults with chronic illness. *Managed Care Quarterly 4*(3), 46-53.

Lamb, G.S., & Stempel, J. (1994). Nurse case management from the client's view: Growing as insider-expert. *Nursing Outlook 42*(1), 7-14.

Lamb, G.S. & Zazworsky, D. (1997). The Carondelet experience. *Nursing Management 28*(3), 27-28.

Lamb, G.S., & Zazworsky, D. (2000). Improving outcomes fast. *Advances for Providers for Post-Acute Care 3*(1), 28-29.

Lamb, G.S., Zazworsky, D., Stempel, J., Martin, D., Gibson, B., Carlson, A., & Rapacz, K. (1993). Comprehensive case management for individuals with progressive multiple sclerosis: An experimental study. Report to the National Multiple Sclerosis Society.

Lancero, A. (1994). *Work satisfaction among nurse case managers.* Unpublished master's thesis. University of Arizona, Tucson, Ariz.

Michaels, C. (1991). A nursing HMO: 10 months with Carondelet St. Mary's hospital-based nurse case management. *Aspen's Advisor for Nurse Executives 6*(11), 1, 3-4.

Newman, M., Lamb, G.S., & Michaels, C. (1991). Nurse case management: The coming together of theory and practice. *Nursing & Health Care 12*(8), 404-408.

Nichols, C. (1996). Older adults who remain at risk: uncertainty in decision-making. Unpublished master's thesis. University of Arizona, Tucson, Ariz.

Papenhausen, J.L. (1996). Discovering and achieving client outcomes. In E. Cohen (Ed.), *Nurse case management in the 21st century* (pp. 257-268). St. Louis: Mosby.

Rusch, S. (1986). Continuity of care: From hospital unit into home. *Nursing Management 17*(12), 38-41.

Index

Italics following page number indicates: *t*=table; *b*=box; and
capital letter following page number indicates: A=Appendix

591